MANUAL OF
ASTHMA
MANAGEMENT

MANUAL OF

ASTHMA

MANAGEMENT

EDITED BY

PAUL M. O'BYRNE & NEIL C. THOMSON

W.B. Saunders Company Ltd
London   Philadelphia   Toronto   Sydney   Tokyo

W.B. Saunders Company Ltd 24–28 Oval Road
London NW1 7DX

The Curtis Center
Independence Square West
Philadelphia, PA 19106-3399, USA

Harcourt Brace & Company
55 Horner Avenue
Toronto, Ontario M8Z 4X6, Canada

Harcourt Brace & Company, Australia
30–52 Smidmore Street
Marrickville, NSW 2204, Australia

Harcourt Brace & Company, Japan
Ichibancho Central Building,
22–1 Ichibancho
Chiyoda-ku, Tokyo 102, Japan

A catalogue record for this book is available from the British Library

ISBN 0-7020-1781-7

Typeset by Photo·graphics, Honiton, Devon, UK
Printed in Great Britain by the University Press, Cambridge

CONTENTS

Assessment and Treatment of Asthma

Management of Asthma

LIST OF CONTRIBUTORS

C J Allen MA BM BCh MRCP (UK) FRCPC
Respiratory Medicine
Firestone Regional Chest and Allergy Unit
St Joseph's Hospital
Hamilton, Ontario
Canada, L8N 4A6

S D Anderson PhD DSc
Department of Respiratory Medicine
PCP9, Royal Prince Alfred Hospital
Missenden Road
Camperdown, NSW 2050
Australia

N C Barnes
Consultant Physician
The London Chest Hospital
Bonner Road
London E2 9JX, UK

P J Barnes MA DM DSc FRCP
Department of Thoracic Medicine
National Heart and Lung Institute
Dovehouse Street
London SW3 6LY, UK

F M Baroody MD
Associate Professor of Otolaryngology – Head and Neck Surgery
The University of Chicago
5841 South Maryland Avenue – MC 1035
Chicago, Illinois 60637
USA

R Beasley MBChB FRACP MD
Professor of Medicine
Department of Medicine
Wellington School of Medicine
PO Box 7343, Wellington South
Wellington, New Zealand

A B Becker MD FRCPC
Associate Professor
Section of Allergy and Clinical Immunology
Department of Pediatrics and Child Health
University of Manitoba
AE 101, 840 Sherbrook Street
Winnipeg, Manitoba
Canada, R3A 1S1

R Bhagat MBBS MD
Division of Respiratory Medicine
Department of Medicine
Royal University Hospital
Saskatoon, Saskatchewan
Canada, S7N 0W8

J Bousquet
Professor
Service des Maladies Respiratoires
Hôpital Arnaud de Villeneuve
Avenue du doyen G Giraud
34295 Montpellier-Cedex 5
France

W W Busse MD
Professor of Medicine
Department of Medicine
Section of Allergy and Clinical Immunology
University of Wisconsin
H6/367 Clinical Science Center
600 Highland Avenue
Madison, Wisconsin 53792
USA

A Cartier MD FRCP(C)
Respirologist
Associate Professor of Medicine
University of Montreal; and
Head, Division of Respiratory
Medicine
Hôpital du Sacré-Cœur de Montréal
5400 boulevard Gouin Ouest
Montréal, Québec
Canada, H4J 1C5

N Chanarin MB ChB MRCP
University Medicine (centre block)
Level D, Centre Block
Southampton General Hospital
Tremona Road
Southampton SO16 6YD, UK

P Chanez
Service des Maladies Respiratoires
Hôpital Arnaud de Villeneuve
Avenue du doyen G Giraud
34295 Montpellier-Cedex 5
France

M Chan-Yeung
Respiratory Division
Department of Medicine
University of British Columbia
Vancouver General Hospital
Vancouver, British Columbia, Canada

A. Ciaccia
Professor
Institute of Infectious and Respiratory
Diseases
University of Ferrara
44100 Ferrara, Italy

T J H Clark MD BSc FRCP
Dean and Professor of Pulmonary
Medicine
National Heart and Lung Institute
Dovehouse Street
London SW3 6LY, UK

G M Cochrane FRCP
Consultant Physician and Senior
Clinical Adviser
Department of Thoracic Medicine
Guy's Hospital
London SE1 9RT, UK

D W Cockcroft MD FRCP(C)
Professor, Department of Medicine
Division of Respiratory Medicine
Royal University Hospital
Saskatoon, Saskatchewan
Canada, S7N 0W8

A L Cogo
Assistant Professor
Institute of Infectious and Respiratory
Diseases
University of Ferrara
Via Borsari 46
44100 Ferrara
Italy

J M Corne MA MRCP
University Medicine
Level D, Centre Block
Southampton General Hospital
Tremona Road
Southampton SO16 6YD, UK

P Cosma
Resident
Institute of Infectious and Respiratory
Diseases
University of Ferrara
Via Borsari 46
44100 Ferrara
Italy

J Crane MBBS FRACP
Department of Medicine
Wellington School of Medicine
PO Box 7343, Wellington South
Wellington, New Zealand

**G K Crompton MBChB FRCPE
FCCP**
Respiratory Unit
Western General Hospital
Crewe Road South
Edinburgh EH4 2XU, UK

B Dahlén
Asthma and Allergy Research at
Division of Pulmonary Medicine
Department of Internal Medicine
Karolinska Hospital
Stockholm
Sweden

S E Dahlén MD PhD
Department of Physiology and
Pharmacology
Division of Asthma Research
Karolinska Institutet
S-171 77 Stockholm
Sweden

J M Drazen MD
Parker B. Francis Professor of
Medicine
Harvard Medical School
Chief, Pulmonary Division
Brigham and Women's Hospital
75 Francis Street
Boston, Massachusetts 02115
USA

W D'Souza MBChB
Department of Medicine
Wellington School of Medicine
PO Box 7343, Wellington South
Wellington, New Zealand

S R Durham MA MD MRCP
Senior Lecturer and Honorary
Consultant Physician
Department of Allergy and Clinical
Immunology
Royal Brompton/NHLI
Dovehouse Street
London SW3 6LY, UK

L M Fabbri MD
Associate Professor
Institute of Infectious and Respiratory
Diseases
University of Ferrara
Via Borsari 46
44100 Ferrara
Italy

J Garrett MB ChB FRACP
Clinical Director, Respiratory Services
Green Lane Hospital
Private Bag
Auckland
New Zealand

DM Geddes MD FRCP
Consultant Physician
Department of Respiratory Medicine
Royal Brompton Hospital
Fulham Road
London SW3 6HP, UK

PG Gibson MBBS (Hons) FRACP
Airway Research Unit
Respiratory Medicine Unit
John Hunter Hospital
Newcastle
2305 NSW
Australia

A Guidoboni MD
Research Fellow
First Medical Clinic
University of Milan
20100 Milan, Italy

F E Hargreave MD FRCPC
McMaster University and St Joseph's
Hospital
Firestone Regional Chest and Allergy
Unit
50, Charlton Avenue East
Hamilton
Ontario
Canada, L8N 4A6

**B D W Harrison MA MB BChir
FRCP FCCP**
Consultant Physician
West Norwich and Norfolk Hospitals
Bowthorpe Road
Norwich
Norfolk NR2 3TU, UK

B Hickey MBBS FRACP
Department of Respiratory Medicine
Alfred Hospital and Monash
University Medical School
Commercial Road
Prahran, Victoria 3181
Australia

S T Holgate MD DSc FRCP
University Medicine
Level D, Centre Block
Southampton General Hospital
Tremona Road
Southampton SO16 6YD, UK

P H Howarth BSc (Hons) DM FRCP
University Medicine (centre block)
Level D, Centre Block
Southampton General Hospital
Tremona Road
Southampton SO16 6YD, UK

E Israel MD
Assistant Professor of Medicine
Howard Medical School
Director, Clinical Research,
Pulmonary Division
Brigham and Women's Hospital
75 Francis Street
Boston, Massachusetts 02115
USA

J W Jenne MD
Professor, Department of Medicine
Division of Pulmonary and Critical
Care Medicine
Loyola University of Chicago Stricth
School of Medicine; and The Edward
Hines, Jr Veterans Administration
Hospital
Hines, Illinois 60141
USA

E F Juniper MCSP MSc
Associate Professor
Department of Clinical Epidemiology
and Biostatistics
McMaster University Faculty of Health
Sciences
1200 Main Street West
Hamilton, Ontario
Canada, L8N 3Z5

H A M Kerstjens
Department of Pulmonology
University Hospital
Oostersingel 59
9713 EZ Groningen
The Netherlands

K J Killian
Professor of Medicine
Ambrose Cardio-Respiratory
Department
McMaster University Medical Center
1200 Main Street West
Hamilton, Ontario
Canada, L8N 3Z5

S J Lane PhD
Department of Allergy and
Respiratory Medicine
4th Floor, Hunt's House
Guy's Hospital
London SE1 9RT, UK

T H Lee MD
Professor
Department of Allergy and
Respiratory Medicine
4th Floor, Hunt's House
Guy's Hospital
London SE1 9RT, UK

M L Levy MBChB FRCGP
The Prestwood Avenue Surgery
32a Prestwood Avenue
Kenton
Middlesex HA3 8JZ, UK

J-L Malo
Department of Chest Medicine
Université de Montréal
Hôpital du Sacré-Cœur
5400, boulevard Gouin Ouest
Montréal, Québec
Canada, H4J 1C5

R J Martin MD
Head, Pulmonary Division
National Jewish Center for
Immunology and Respiratory
Medicine and Professor of Medicine,
University of Colorado
1400 Jackson Street, Room J116
Denver, Colorado 80206
USA

F-B Michel
Service des Maladies Respiratoires
Hôpital Arnaud de Villeneuve
Avenue du doyen G Giraud
34295 Montpellier-Cedex 5
France

R Naclerio MD
Professor and Chief of
Otolaryngology – Head and Neck
Surgery
The University of Chicago
5841 South Maryland Avenue –
MC 1035
Chicago, Illinois 60637
USA

**M T Newhouse MD MSc FRCPC
FACP**
Firestone Regional Chest and Allergy
Unit
St Joseph's Hospital
Hamilton, Ontario
Canada, L8N 4A6

**P M O'Byrne MB FRCPI
FRCP(C)**
Professor, Department of Medicine
Head, Division and Respiratory
Medicine
McMaster University, 1200 Main Street
West, Hamilton, Ontario, Canada L8N
3Z5

D Ortega-Carr MD
Midwest Allergy and Asthma
Associates
85 E. Wilson Bridge Rd
Worthington, OH 43085; and
Medical Teaching Staff
Riverside Methodist Hospital
3535 Olentangy River Rd
Columbus, OH 43214, USA

C I M Panhuysen
Department of Pulmonology
University Hospital
Oostersingel 59
9713 EZ Groningen
The Netherlands

M R Partridge MD FRCP
Chest Clinic
Whipps Cross Hospital
Whipps Cross Road
Leytonstone
London E11 1NR, UK

J Y Paton MD MRCP
Department of Child Health
Royal Hospital for Sick Children
Yorkhill
Glasgow G3 8SJ, UK

R Pauwels MD PhD
Professor of Medicine
Head of Department of Respiratory
Diseases
University Hospital
De Pintelaan 185
Ghent B9000, Belgium

J K Peat PhD
Senior Research Officer
Department of Medicine
University of Sydney
Sydney, Australia

S. Pedersen
Department of Pediatrics
Kolding Hospital
DK-6000 Kolding
Denmark

T A E Platts-Mills MD
University of Virginia Health Sciences
Center
Department of Internal Medicine
Division of Asthma and Allergic
Diseases
Charlottesville
Virginia 22908
USA

D S Postma
Department of Pulmonary Diseases
University Hospital
Oostersingel 59
9713 EZ Groningen
The Netherlands

C E Reed MD
Professor of Medicine, Emeritus
Mayo Medical School
200 First Street SW
Rochester, Minnesota 55905
USA

N Saltos MBBS FRACP FRCP FRCPI FCCP
Respiratory Medicine Unit
John Hunter Hospital
Newcastle
NSW 2305
Australia

P S Thomas MD MRCP
Senior Registrar
Department of Respiratory Medicine
Royal Brompton Hospital
Fulham Road
London SW3 6HP, UK

P. Venge, MD PhD
Director of Asthma Research Centre
Professor and Head of the
Department of Clinical Chemistry
University of Uppsala
University Hospital
S-751 85 Uppsala
Sweden

E H Walters MA DM FRCP FRACP
Professor
Direstor, Department of Respiratory
Medicine
Alfred Hospital and Monash
University Medical School
Commercial Road
Prahran, Victoria 3181
Australia

A J Woolcock AO MD FAA FRACP
Professor of Resiratory Medicine
University of Sydney
Sydney; and
Director, Institute of Respiratory
Medicine
Page Chest Pavilion
Royal Prince Alfred Hospital
Sydney NSW 2050
Australia

J G Wyman MD
University of Virginia Health Sciences
Center
Department of Internal Medicine
Division of Asthma and Allergic
Diseases
Charlottesville
Virginia 22908
USA

O Zetterstrom
Asthma and Allergy Research at
Division of Pulmonary Medicine
Department of Internal Medicine
Karolinska Hospital
Stockholm
Sweden

B Zimmerman MD FRCP(C)
Allergy and Immunology
Asthma Centre
The Toronto Hospital Western
Division
Toronto
Ontario
Canada, M4T 2A7

PREFACE

Asthma is the commonest chronic disease of children and adults and there is compelling evidence that the prevalence is rising in many western countries. The morbidity and mortality from asthma is considerable. The purpose of developing this book was to provide comprehensive, yet practical and easily accessed advice on the key issues of asthma management. It is intended that the manual will aid all those involved with the care of asthmatic patients to apply the recently published national and international guidelines on the diagnosis and treatment of asthma. We hope that the manual will be used to answer day-to-day clinical problems in asthma management and that in this way it will allow an individualised approach to treatment. We have selected internationally recognised experts on asthma as contributors and have asked them to write for a readership of physicians and other health care professionals who are involved in the day-to-day management of patients with asthma. We are grateful for the enthusiastic way they have helped us to undertake this project. We hope that the book will be of value to general internalists, general practitioners and specialists in respiratory medicine, pulmonology, allergy and paediatrics. Finally we wish to thank Margaret Macdonald and Maria Khan of W.B. Saunders for all their help and encouragement.

Paul O'Byrne
Neil Thomson

Epidemiology and Pathogenesis of Asthma

1

DEFINITION, CLASSIFICATION, EPIDEMIOLOGY AND RISK FACTORS FOR ASTHMA

Ann J. Woolcock and Jennifer K. Peat

INTRODUCTION

In 1983, Gregg summarized the epidemiological studies that had been conducted to that time and concluded that "... in spite of all the studies, the science of epidemiology has contributed little to the knowledge of asthma".[1] It is clear that this is no longer the case. In the last 10 years, carefully conducted epidemiological studies have revealed a great deal about the nature, the likely causes and the natural history of asthma. This information is relevant both to present-day management and to the prevention of asthma in future generations.

Epidemiological studies are the only way in which the risk factors associated with this disease can be measured in populations. Knowledge of prevalence and risk factors is important for resource allocation, for designing interventions to reduce severity and for preventing the development of disease at an early stage. In order to use epidemiological information precisely to prevent or manage the disease in specific individuals or populations, it is essential to define the disease, to classify it according to severity and to have accurate information about both prevalence and risk factors. These aspects of epidemiology are discussed in this chapter with the aim of increasing awareness of the concept of preventing asthma.

DEFINITIONS

ASTHMA

In this chapter "asthma" refers to an underlying abnormality of the airway walls that is associated with episodes of airway narrowing. Such episodes are referred to as "acute attacks" if they are short-lived and easily reversible, or "exacerbations" if they last longer than a day. No consensus has yet been reached on the exact definition of asthma but there are three definitions that are commonly used.

- Asthma is a disease of the airways that makes them prone to narrow excessively in response to a variety of provoking stimuli.[2] This is a clinical definition that can be used for epidemiological studies.

- Asthma is a disease of the airways characterized by chronic inflammation with infiltration of lymphocytes, eosinophils and mast cells together with epithelial desquamation, thickening and disorganization of the tissues of the airway wall. This is a pathological definition.

- Asthma is a clinical syndrome characterized by increased responsiveness of the tracheo-bronchial tree to a variety of stimuli. The major symptoms of asthma are paroxysms of dyspnoea, wheezing and cough, which may vary from mild and almost undetectable to severe and unremitting (status asthmaticus). The primary physiological manifestation of this hyperresponsiveness is variable airways obstruction. This can take the form of spontaneous fluctuations in the severity of obstruction following bronchodilators or corticosteroids, or increased obstruction caused by drugs or other stimuli.[3] This is the American Thoracic Society definition.

ALLERGY
In this chapter "allergy" refers to increased levels of circulating IgE, specific to environmental allergens. The terms "atopy", "atopic state", "allergy" and "sensitized" are often used interchangeably. Allergy is usually measured by skin-prick tests.

AIRWAY HYPERRESPONSIVENESS
This is an abnormal response of the airways to a provoking stimulus.

CLASSIFICATION OF ASTHMA

CLASSIFYING BY SEVERITY
In the clinic the severity of asthma is usually assessed by a combination of measurements, including severity and frequency of symptoms, peak flow variability, airway hyperresponsiveness (AHR) and lung function tests. In epidemiological studies the clinical criteria of severity, such as peak flow values, are not always available and the symptom history comes only from a questionnaire. Although AHR can be measured, it is not possible to class-ify the severity of the disease solely according to the degree of AHR because many subjects with AHR do not report symptoms, and vice versa. There-fore, a classification of asthma that incorporates both measurements of recent symptoms and the presence of AHR is more informative for describ-ing the range of severity of asthma that occurs in populations. This type

of classification has proved useful for comparing different populations, for describing prognosis and for determining treatment requirements.[4] Table 1.1 shows a classification based on spirometric function, AHR, symptoms and treatment requirements that can be used to rank severity from the most severe to the most trivial.

A detailed description of each severity category follows.

Obstructed Asthma

This is characterized by asthmatic symptoms and reversibility of the forced expiratory volume in 1 s (FEV_1) but airflow limitation persists after maximal treatment with bronchodilators and oral corticosteroids. AHR can be demonstrated by both direct and indirect stimuli (but is usually not measured because of poor lung function). The pathological changes that are responsible for the irreversible airflow limitation have not been described.

Persistent Asthma

This is characterized by frequent symptoms (unless these are under control with treatment) and airway abnormality as demonstrated by AHR to both direct and indirect stimuli and increased variability of daily peak flow readings at a time when the subject is symptom free. The histological changes in biopsies from subjects with mild persistent asthma has been well described.[5,6] This form of asthma is persistent throughout life but may go into remission during adolescence, with symptoms returning in later life.[7]

Current Asthma

In our epidemiological studies this term describes subjects studied at a single point in time who have both AHR and a history of wheeze in the previous 12 months. Most current asthmatics prove to have persistent disease but some lose their AHR and are then classified as "episodic". Longitudinal studies show that most children with "current asthma" have a more severe condition than children with AHR only or symptoms only.[4,8] It is probably the best definition with which to compare the disease in different populations.

Episodic Asthma

This is characterized by episodes of symptoms of sufficient severity to require medication but during the symptom-free interval there is no detectable AHR. Episodic asthma is the most common form of asthma in young children and in pollen-sensitive asthmatics. It also occurs early in the course of occupational asthma.[9] Children who have asthmatic episodes induced by viral infections usually have this form of asthma and it has also been described in non-allergic individuals.[11] The histological changes in the airways have not been described.

Asthma in Remission

The presence of AHR and a history of asthma needing treatment but no symptoms or treatment in the previous year are signs of asthma in remission.

TABLE 1.1: *Classification of asthma*

Description of airway disease	Baseline FEV$_1$	AHR (direct stimuli)	AHR (indirect stimuli)	Symptoms of asthma at any time	Symptoms of asthma previous year	Medications used previous year
Obstructed asthma	Decreased	Yes	Yes	Yes	Yes	Yes
Persistent asthma (current asthma)	Near normal	Yes	Yes	Yes	Yes	Yes
Episodic asthma	Normal	No	Yes/No	Yes	Yes	Yes
Asthma in remission	Normal	Yes	Yes	Yes	No	No
Potential asthma	Normal	Yes	? Yes	No	No	No
Trivial wheeze	Normal	No	No	Yes	? Yes	No

AHR, airway hyperresponsiveness; direct stimuli, provocation with histamine or methacholine; indirect stimuli, provocation with exercise, hyperventilation or hypertonic saline.

Potential Asthma

This is said to be present when there is AHR, to direct or indirect stimuli, without symptoms, especially when the responses to the provocation indicate moderately severe hyperresponsiveness (e.g. curve in Fig. 1.1). This abnormality is usually only identified during population surveys. In atopic subjects, symptoms may develop at a later time.[11] It is known that atopy *per se* affects the airway wall[12] but it is not known what feature is responsible for the symptoms.

Trivial Asthma

Trivial asthma is characterized by episodes of wheezing or of dry cough that are intermittent or mild and do not require treatment. This abnormality usually occurs in infants and children who have normal airway

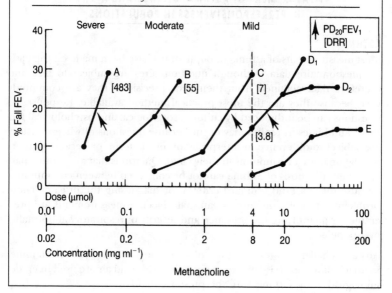

FIGURE 1.1: *Dose–response curves to methacholine, expressed either as doses (μmol) or concentration (mg ml^{-1}) plotted against percentage fall in the FEV$_1$. Curves A and B are from a severe asthmatic, C is from a moderate asthmatic and E is normal. Curve D is marginally abnormal and would be taken as normal if the PD$_{20}$FEV$_1$ was being calculated in an epidemiological study where the highest dose given is 3.9 μmol. Unadjusted values for dose–response ratios (DRR) calculated at the point of the greatest fall in FEV$_1$ are shown in brackets. In an epidemiological study the DRR for curve D would have been 3.8.*

responsiveness, normal spirometric function and it probably does not progress to one of the other forms of asthma.

EXTRINSIC AND INTRINSIC ASTHMA

In some studies asthma has been classified as "extrinsic" or "intrinsic" according to its association with allergy. However, no differences in the histology of the airways or in response to treatment with corticosteroids have been described between these two forms of asthma, and some workers suggest that all asthma may, in fact, be extrinsic.[13]

Extrinsic Asthma

Asthma that is present in an atopic subject is called extrinsic asthma. Such subjects can have asthma of varying severities and may have symptoms that are produced by a variety of provoking agents other than allergens. In random samples of all age groups, the majority of asthmatics can be classified as extrinsic because sensitivity to common allergens can be demonstrated by skin-prick tests.[14–16]

Intrinsic Asthma

Asthma that is present in a person in whom no evidence of atopy can be demonstrated is called intrinsic asthma. This form of the disease appears to start in adult life. Although a small proportion of asthma may be genuinely "intrinsic", an epidemiological study by Sears et al. found that all children with AHR had an elevated serum IgE level suggesting that some form of allergic sensitization may be present in all subjects who have AHR.[17]

MEASUREMENT OF ASTHMA, ALLERGY AND AIRWAY HYPERRESPONSIVENESS IN POPULATIONS

ASTHMA

Most measurements of asthma in populations have been made on the basis of questionnaire data. Although questionnaires are subject to bias and therefore data obtained from them lack precision,[8] they are commonly used because they are the most practical method available. Responses to questions can be influenced by cultural, sociological and psychological factors[18] and biases in replies may occur because questions of wheeze history are subject to difference in interpretation of the term, or because parents may be unaware of symptoms in their child. Questions that ask about a past or present diagnosis of asthma cannot be compared between communities because there are no standard criteria for diagnosing the disease. These problems with questionnaires mean that objective measurements are preferable for quantifying the presence and severity of respiratory abnormality in a population.

Airway challenge tests with pharmacological agents (histamine, methacholine), exercise or hyperventilation with cold air are used in epidemiological studies to measure the presence of AHR.

Usually histamine or methacholine are administered, using a dosimeter or a nebulizer, in increasing doses or concentrations and the lung function response at each dose step is measured (see Chapter 8). The response, in terms of a percentage fall in lung function, can be plotted as a dose–concentration response curve as shown in Fig. 1.1. The position of the curve can be defined by the dose or concentration that causes a 20% fall in the FEV_1 ($PD_{20}FEV_1$ or $PC_{20}FEV_1$) or as the "dose–response ratio" (DRR), which is the percentage fall in FEV_1 divided by the total dose that has been administered.[19] The DRR, which is often termed the "two-point slope", can be obtained for all individuals regardless of the severity of their response, whereas $PD_{20}FEV_1$ can be obtained only for subjects who experience a fall in FEV_1 of 20% or greater. The measurement of DRR is particularly useful for comparing the severity of hyperresponsiveness between different populations, or between different groups within a population, because a measurement can be obtained for all subjects and the measurement is log-normally distributed so that standard parametric statistics can be used to compare groups.[20]

Histamine and methacholine are approximately equipotent,[21] so that, provided a standardized cut-off point is used to define abnormality, valid comparisons between studies can be made. However, comparisons between the results from studies that have used airway provocation with pharmacological agents and those that have used challenge with an exercise test may be less valid because the two challenges are thought to measure different aspects of airway wall function.[22]

In population studies,[15,23,24] AHR has been defined quite arbitrarily as a 20% fall in FEV_1 after the cumulative administration of 3.9 μmol (8 mg ml^{-1}) of histamine or methacholine.[25] In populations, the expression of responsiveness as a continuous measure of DRR for pharmacological challenges or as a percentage fall in FEV_1 following 6 min of exercise allows the more statistically rigorous calculation of an abnormal value as 1.96 standard deviations from the mean in the normal group of non-atopic, lifelong, asymptomatic subjects. Using this method, a DRR of greater than 6 (percentage fall in FEV_1/micromoles histamine) represents an abnormal value for histamine challenge in children or adults[20,26] and a 13% fall in FEV_1 following exercise indicates abnormal responsiveness to this challenge when used in children.[22]

ALLERGY

For epidemiological studies atopy is usually measured by skin-prick tests to a battery of common allergens using lancets or allergen-coated Phazets. Measurements of serum IgE levels are not a good guide to increased levels of specific IgE because total levels are affected by other allergic reactions including those to parasites, which are irrelevant to asthma. When comparing populations, it is important that allergens are standardized between studies and that comparable dilutions are used. The skin wheal size that is associated with respiratory illness has been shown to be 2 mm for infants, 3 mm for children and 4 mm for adults.[27]

RELATIONSHIP BETWEEN SYMPTOMS, AHR AND ALLERGY

The relationship between symptoms of asthma and AHR is not well defined. Some clinical studies have found that subjects with the most responsive airways may experience less respiratory distress than subjects with the least responsive airways[28] and it has been suggested that the mechanisms that lead to wheeze and to AHR are separate and unrelated.[29,30] However, epidemiological studies of children invariably find an overlap between the conditions of AHR and of asthmatic symptoms that is much larger than might be expected by chance.[31,32] In recent Australian studies of children, the prevalence of symptoms without AHR is approximately 12–15%, asymptomatic AHR is approximately 5–7% and "current asthma" (presence of both AHR and symptoms) occurs in 8–11%.[33]

The relationship between atopy and AHR is less complex because most subjects with AHR are atopic; however only about one-third to one-half of atopic subjects have AHR. In general, between 40 and 50% of adult populations are atopic as judged by skin tests[34–36] but usually less than 10% have current asthma. In most population studies between 85 and 90% of adults and children with well-documented asthma are atopic and the association between atopy and more severe AHR is particularly strong.[14–16,37] Burrows and his co-workers have suggested that all asthma may be atopic because, after adjusting for age, the prevalence of asthma increases with increasing levels of IgE and asthma does not occur in subjects with low serum IgE levels.[13] This relationship was confirmed in a study of New Zealand children by Sears et al.[17] The factors that determine which atopic subjects develop AHR and/or asthma have not been identified.

PREVALENCE AND MORTALITY

INTERNATIONAL COMPARISONS OF PREVALENCE RATES

Collaborative studies are now underway to obtain worldwide data from adults about symptoms, AHR and atopy using standard methods.[18] However, at present few data exist that can be compared. Table 1.2 shows the results of studies of children in whom AHR and "current asthma" have been measured. The same table also gives values for "diagnosed asthma" obtained from questionnaires.

There is a large difference in the prevalence of asthma between countries. The prevalence in Australia, New Zealand and the UK is high by comparison with populations in the Asian–Pacific region. Although there are no data available for the prevalence of AHR in children in the USA, questionnaire data suggest that rates of asthma in that country are not as high as in other countries that have a similarly affluent life-style.

TABLE 1.2: *Prevalence of current asthma, diagnosed asthma, wheeze, airway hyperresponsiveness and atopy in populations of children*

Country	Study year	Number	Age (years)	Current asthma (%)	Asthma ever diagnosed (%)	Wheeze ever (%)	AHR (%)	Atopy (%) (SPT)c	Reference
Australia	1982	1487	8–10	5.4	11.0	21.7	10.1 (H)	29.3	38
	1986	1217	8–11	6.7	17.3	26.5	10.0 (H)	31.9	39
	1991	1339	8–11	11.0	23.5	33.4	17.2 (H)	42.4	40
New Zealand	1981	813	9	11.1a	27.0		22 (M)		32
	1988	1084	6–11	9.1	14.2	27.2	20 (H)		41
	1989	873	12	8.1a	16.8	26.6	12 (E)		42
England	1980	1613	7	8.0a		14.8b	? (H)		43
Wales	1989	965	12	5.3a	12	22.3	8 (E)		42
Germany	1990	5768	9–11	4.2a	7.9		? (C)	?	44
Denmark	1987	527	7–16	5.3			16 (H)	31	45
Indonesia	1981	406	7–15	1.2	2.3	14.5	2.2 (H)	24.1	46
China	1988	3067	11–17	1.9	2.4	6.3	4.1 (H)	30	24
Papua New Guinea	1985	257	6–20	0	0	1.7	1.0 (H)	17	47
Australian indigenous	1991	215	7–12	0.1	0	1.4	2.8 (H)	20.5	48

a Calculated from published data.
b Since starting school.
c SPT, skin-prick test.
AHR, airway hyperresponsiveness; Australian indigenous, aborigines; C, cold air hyperventilation; current asthma, AHR + wheeze in last 12 months; E, exercise; H, histamine; M, methacholine.

Childhood asthma appears to be increasing in all countries of the world where it has been measured. Table 1.3 shows published studies that have used the same questionnaires at an interval of 8 or more years to study populations of roughly the same age. In Australia, the increase in prevalence has occurred steadily over 20 years and cannot be entirely explained by changes in diagnostic labelling practices because AHR has also increased (Table 1.2). This rapid increase, which appears to be a worldwide phenomenon, suggests that a ubiquitous environmental factor or several factors are responsible. Although changes in diet, increased allergen load and changed treatment methods have been suggested, there is no evidence to date that any of these factors are actually involved in the increasing prevalence of asthma. Only carefully conducted epidemiological studies that measure environmental factors including allergen levels with precision are likely to help elucidate the factors that are responsible.

MORTALITY RATES

Because they lack some of the complications in labelling that may occur for deaths in older or younger age groups, mortality statistics for the 5–34 year age group are probably most reliable. These values give some estimation of the amount of severe disease in the community. The mortality rates for asthma in 5–34 year olds in the USA, Canada, England and Wales, Australia, New Zealand and France are shown in Fig. 1.2. From this figure, two epidemics are evident. The first occurred in the 1960s in England and Wales, Australia, New Zealand (and several other countries), while the second occurred in the 1980s in New Zealand. The second epidemic led to studies that strongly suggested that the regular, long-term use of high doses of fenoterol is associated with an increased risk of death.[56] This finding has led to the suggestion that the 1960s epidemic was associated with the regular use of isoprenaline forte.[57] A recent study in Canada suggested that the use of salbutamol as well as fenoterol may increase the risk of death.[58] However, the data are, in part, circumstantial and the death rate is now decreasing in Australia and New Zealand where salbutamol is used regularly by a large number of asthmatics. Mortality data are useful in alerting countries to epidemics and thus influence management. It is of interest that the rates in 1992 are similar for all countries.

RISK FACTORS

The risk factors for asthma fall into three separate categories: genetic factors, i.e. an inherited predisposition to develop atopy or AHR; environmental factors, which induce and increase the prevalence of the disease; and trigger factors, such as exercise, irritating substances and episodes of atmospheric pollution, which bring on episodes of symptoms in those who already have asthma. The most important are the environmental factors because they are potentially preventable.

TABLE 1.3: *Changes in prevalence of asthma or symptoms in same population studied with same method on two occasions*

Country	Study year	Number	Age (years)	Current asthma (%)	Asthma ever diagnosed (%)	Reference
Australia	1982	769	8–11		12.9	38
	1992	795	8–11		19.3	49
New Zealand	1975		12–18		26.2[a]	50
	1989		12–18		34.0[a]	50
Wales	1973	?	12		6.0	51
	1988	965	12		12.0	42
USA	1971–74	Large	6–11		4.8	52
	1976–80	27 275	6–11		7.6	52
Finland	1961	38 000	19	0.1		53
	1989	38 000	19	0.8		53
France	1968	8 140	21		3.3	54
	1982	10 559	21		5.4	54
Tahiti	1979	3 870	16		11.5	54
	1984	6 731	13		14.3	55

[a] Cumulative prevalence of asthma and/or wheeze.

FIGURE 1.2: *Mortality per 100 000 people for 5–34 year olds for six countries from 1960 to 1992. The epidemics of deaths in the 1960s and in New Zealand in the 1980s can be seen. Rates in Australia and New Zealand have fallen in the last few years so that values are now similar in all countries. ■, England and Wales; ⊙, Australia; ▲, New Zealand; □, USA; ○, Canada; ●, France.*

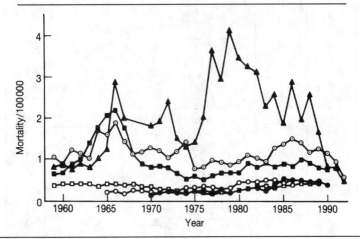

GENETIC FACTORS

There is good evidence from both clinical and epidemiological studies that the ability to become atopic is, in part, inherited and that genetic factors play a major role in the regulation of IgE production.[59] Studies of twins suggest that a genetic factor confers susceptibility to asthma because the concordance of asthma in monozygotic twins is significantly greater than in dizygotic twins,[60] but the relatively low concordance in monozygotic twins suggests that environmental factors make important contributions to the development of asthma. It is not yet known if there are separately inherited components of asthma, one gene (or genes) leading to the development of atopy and others predisposing to asthma. The Oxford research group[61] have recently suggested that the tendency to IgE responses is conferred by an "atopy locus" on chromosome 11q, although other research groups dispute this.[62,63] Studies in twins which have adjusted for atopic status do not show that AHR has a strong genetic component.[64,65] Although relatives of children with asthma have increased airway lability to exercise, the significance is difficult to interpret because the study did not control for atopy.[66]

Figure 1.3 shows the magnitude of risk (adjusted odds ratios) of children having AHR in the presence of factors that are associated with childhood

FIGURE 1.3: *Odds ratios for the risk factors for airway hyperresponsiveness (AHR) in Australian school children, ages 8–11 years, living in Sydney. ERI, early respiratory illness (a respiratory illness before the age of 2 years that required treatment by a doctor).*

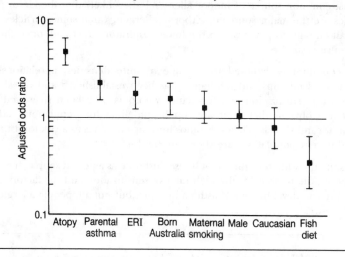

asthma in Australia.[25] The data points in the figure are adjusted odds ratios, so that each estimate takes account of the effect of the other risk factors. If either parent has asthma then the child has approximately twice the risk of having asthma compared with a child whose parents are non-asthmatic. The relative contribution of genetic and environmental factors to this risk is difficult to measure because environmental exposures that are common to both children and parents are usually present.

ALLERGEN EXPOSURE

In 1984, Cockcroft and co-workers studied a random population sample of young adults and showed a relationship between the severity of asthma and the degree of atopy.[14] Sensitization to allergens is now known to be the most important risk factor for asthma in both childhood and adulthood.[25,67,68] In Fig. 1.3, atopy is clearly the most important factor associated with childhood AHR. However, a perfect concordance between sensitization to allergens and asthma symptoms has not been found. Although most asthmatics are sensitized to recognized allergens, the majority of sensitized subjects do not develop asthma.

House-dust Mite Allergens

The allergens of house-dust mites *Dermatophagoides pteronyssinus* and *Dermatophagoides farinae* appear to be among the most potent of the common aeroallergens. In regions where the humidity is greater than 55% for most of the year and where skin scales accumulate as a source of food, these allergens are ubiquitous and there is evidence that they are probably the most common source of indoor allergen.[69] It is likely that the faecal particles are the major source of airborne allergen,[70] that some particles are small enough to penetrate to the lower respiratory tract and, once there, dissolve easily.[69]

In communities exposed to a range of mite densities, a relationship between symptoms and infestation has been established[33] and threshold levels for sensitization and for acute symptoms have been suggested[71,72] but it is obvious that these are rough guidelines for populations rather than for individuals. The odds ratios for atopy to mites as a risk for asthma in different populations are shown in Fig. 1.4.[33,67,73]

Despite the wide recognition of house-dust mite as a potent source of sensitization, the reasons for the high rates of sensitization and the factors that lead to the development of asthma in some, but not all, people allergic to

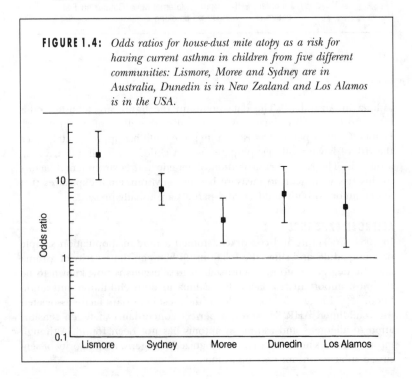

FIGURE 1.4: *Odds ratios for house-dust mite atopy as a risk for having current asthma in children from five different communities: Lismore, Moree and Sydney are in Australia, Dunedin is in New Zealand and Los Alamos is in the USA.*

house-dust mite are not known. There is evidence that the numbers of house-dust mites are increasing in Australia. This increase may be at least in part responsible for the increasing prevalence of AHR in sensitized children.[50,74]

RESPIRATORY INFECTIONS

Early respiratory illness is defined as a respiratory illness before the age of 2 years, severe enough to have required treatment by a doctor or at a hospital. It is a risk factor for AHR in Australian children (Fig. 1.3). However, the extent to which such illness represents acute infections or early attacks of asthma is not known. In contrast, respiratory infections in late childhood or adult life have not been shown to be a risk factor for the development of the disease. Although asthma is more common in children who have had croup[75] or other lower respiratory illnesses in early life,[76-78] there is only anecdotal evidence that early childhood infection actually precipitates the first attack of asthma. In non-affluent populations where asthma is exceedingly rare (Table 1.2), viral respiratory infections are known to be as common as in other populations so that it seems likely that viral infections in the absence of atopy are not a risk factor of importance for the development of asthma. Nevertheless, viral infections remain important triggers of attacks, especially in atopic infants.[79]

RACE

There is evidence that some racial groups are more prone to develop asthma than others. For instance, it appears that Maoris have a high prevalence of asthma and Australian Aborigines a low prevalence (Table 1.2). Asthma is extremely rare in many non-affluent countries.[80-82] This may or may not be due to race, because lack of exposure to environmental aeroallergens and diets that are associated with affluent living conditions may protect some populations from the disease. In Xhosa children, the prevalence of asthma in those living in the Transkei was only 0.15% compared with 3.2% in those living in townships near Capetown[81] and a study by Waite et al. found that Tokelaun children living on the islands had a lower prevalence of asthma than Tokelaun children living on the New Zealand mainland,[83] suggesting that environmental factors and not race are responsible for the low prevalence in village populations.

GENDER

Asthma symptoms are more common in boys than in girls.[1] Figure 1.3 shows that gender is not an important risk factor for AHR in Australian children after other important factors, such as atopy, have been taken into account. However, it is clear that atopy develops more commonly in boys[25,84] and that boys have a smaller airway calibre in infancy.[85] This suggests that variations in the prevalence of symptoms that are normally assigned to gender are a secondary result of factors such as atopy, the increased ability to produce IgE in response to common allergens or airway calibre, which do have a clear gender difference.

DIET

Although diet may be responsible for some of the differences in the prevalence rates of asthma between countries, the extent of the effect is not known. Breast-feeding is often cited as being a protective factor although the evidence is contradictory. Epidemiological studies in England and Wales have suggested that both morbidity and mortality from asthma may be related to sodium intake.[86] Figure 1.3 shows that, in Australia, a regular fish diet appears to reduce the risk of AHR in children. There are theoretical reasons why fish oils could alter the course of asthma via the types of metabolites produced from arachidonic acid[81] but no studies have yet been undertaken to investigate whether changes in intake of fish alter the course of asthma in children. This area has been well reviewed[88] and it seems likely that diet will prove to play a role in making some children susceptible to allergens.

PASSIVE SMOKING

There is increasing evidence that passive smoking is involved, to a small extent, in the aetiology of childhood asthma. Although maternal smoking was not a risk in the study shown in Fig. 1.3, other studies have shown that parental smoking is a small, but consistent, risk factor for children having increased respiratory infections, which, as discussed above, are in themselves a risk factor for later asthma, and increased symptoms of wheeze. Children with mothers who smoke are at an increased risk of having elevated cord IgE levels at birth,[89] which may have an effect on the later development of atopy. These children also have reduced birthweight and perhaps reduced airway size.[90] The risk conferred by passive smoking is higher in children of a lower socio-economic status.[91] The possibility that passive smoking is involved is important because positive interventions are possible that may help to reduce the prevalence of the disease in future generations.

OUTDOOR AIR POLLUTANTS

At high concentrations, sulphur dioxide, and to a lesser extent nitrogen dioxide and ozone, act as respiratory irritants and may be powerful trigger factors for acute episodes of symptoms. Whilst it is tempting to attribute a high prevalence of asthma in some urban populations to the presence of air pollution, there is no evidence that air pollutants (in concentrations found in cities) induce asthma or AHR. In a recent study of children living in two regions of Germany, there was a higher prevalence of bronchitis and a lower prevalence of allergic disorders in the eastern region (with high levels of sulphur dioxide and total suspended particles (TSP) air pollutants) compared with the western part of the country.[92] Although causation could not be attributed, this suggests that air pollutants increase the prevalence of respiratory infections but that affluent living conditions are a more important risk factor for allergic illness. In Australia, the prevalence of asthma is equally high in urban and rural regions, suggesting that factors other than pollutants are responsible for the high rates of disease in this country.[93]

It is important to interpret the results of studies that investigate the role of air pollutants in respiratory illness very carefully because circumstantial evidence of an association is weak. Air pollutants may act synergistically with allergens by increasing allergic responses, implying that air pollutants may have an indirect role in causing AHR.[94] A study in Japan found that diesel exhaust particles potentiated the IgE production in mice.[95] These data, although often quoted, have not been corroborated by large epidemiological studies in which the severity of asthma is well characterized.

PREVENTING ASTHMA

In terms of preventing asthma, the epidemiological evidence shows consistently that asthma is a disease caused largely by environmental, and therefore preventable, factors. By far the most important are the commonly occurring aeroallergens. Although asthma is still perceived as easy to treat and impossible to prevent, better methods of allergen avoidance are becoming available and, in public health terms, are likely to provide much greater benefits than treatment with medications. Furthermore, allergen avoidance from birth, particularly for infants who are most at risk, may have the potential to prevent asthma from developing.

A good model of effective prevention was demonstrated by studies of epidemics of acute symptoms and consequent hospitalizations in Barcelona.[96] These epidemics occurred on days when soya beans were being unloaded from ships into a silo without an adequate filter, which allowed the release of soya dust into the atmosphere. During the epidemics, those who required hospitalization were already allergic to the dust, suggesting that the allergen was potent enough to cause prior sensitization at relatively low atmospheric concentrations. In addition, on symptom days people living many kilometres away from the silo had symptoms. It is of interest that the problem appeared only to affect adults, perhaps because prolonged exposure was needed to build sensitization. Since the silo has been modified, so that the dust cannot become airborne, no further epidemics have occurred.

In essence, the only available options for improving the severity of asthma are long-term treatment with inhaled corticosteroids and allergen reduction or avoidance. Epidemiological studies need to present overviews that enable physicians in different communities to predict, in a given child, the likelihood of wheeze having an important outcome. It is not yet possible to do this, but some of the factors that increase the risk to the individual child are known. In particular, babies who are small for their age or premature, who have a family history of asthma or of atopy, who are exposed to tobacco smoke because their mothers smoked during or after pregnancy, and who are exposed to perennially high levels of domestic allergens have high risk of developing asthma. Interventions that address these problems are likely to be effective in both preventing and reducing the severity of asthma in children.

REFERENCES

1 Gregg I. Epidemiological aspects. In: Clark TJH, Godfrey S (eds) *Asthma*. London: Chapman and Hall, 1983: 242–84.

2 Woolcock AJ. Asthma. In: Murray JF, Nadel J (eds) *Textbook of Respiratory Medicine*. Philadelphia: Saunders, 1994: 1288-330.

3 American Thoracic Society. Standards for the diagnosis and care of patients with chronic obstructive pulmonary disease (COPD) and asthma. Am Rev Respir Dis 1987; 136: 225–44.

4 Toelle BG, Peat JK, Salome CM, Mellis CM, Woolcock AJ. Towards a definition of asthma for epidemiology. Am Rev Respir Dis 1992; 146: 633–7.

5 Laitinen LA, Heino M, Laitinen A, Kava T, Haahtela T. Damage of the airway epithelium and bronchial reactivity in patients with asthma. Am Rev Respir Dis 1985; 131: 599–606.

6 Ollerenshaw S, Woolcock AJ. Characteristics of the inflammation in biopsies from large airways of subjects with asthma and subjects with chronic airflow limitation. Am Rev Respir Dis 1992; 145: 922–7.

7 Townley RG, Ryo UY, Kolotkin BM, Kang B. Bronchial sensitivity to methacholine in current and former asthmatic and allergic rhinitis patients and control subjects. J Allergy Clin Immunol 1975; 56: 429–42.

8 Peat JK, Toelle B, Salome CM, Woolcock AJ. Predictive nature of bronchial responsiveness and respiratory symptoms in a one year cohort study of Sydney schoolchildren. Eur Respir J 1993; 6: 662–9.

9 Chan YM, Lam S. Occupational asthma. Am Rev Respir Dis 1986; 133: 686–703.

10 Stanescu DC, Frans A. Bronchial asthma without increased airway reactivity. Eur J Respir Dis 1982; 63: 5–12.

11 Hopp RJ, Townley RG, Biven RE, Bewtra AK, Nair NM. The presence of airway reactivity before the development of asthma. Am Rev Respir Dis 1990; 141: 2–8.

12 Holgate S, Wilson J, Howarts P. New insights into airway inflammation by endobronchial biopsy. *Am Rev Respir Dis* 1992; 145: S2–S6.

13 Burrows B, Martinez FD, Halonen M, Barbee RA, Cline MG. Association of asthma with serum IgE levels and skin-test reactivity to allergens. *N Engl J Med* 1989; 320: 271–7.

14 Cockcroft DW, Murdock KY, Berscheid BA. Relationship between atopy and bronchial responsiveness to histamine in a random population. *Ann Allergy* 1984; 53: 26–9.

15 Burney PG, Britton JR, Chinn S *et al.* Descriptive epidemiology of bronchial reactivity in an adult population: results from a community study. *Thorax* 1987; 42: 38–44.

16 Woolcock AJ, Peat JK, Salome CM *et al.* Prevalence of bronchial hyperresponsiveness and asthma in a rural adult population. *Thorax* 1987; 42: 361–8.

17 Sears MR, Burrows B, Flannery EM, Herbison GP, Hewitt CJ, Hodaway MD. Relation between airway responsiveness and serum IgE in children with asthma and in apparently normal children. *N Engl J Med* 1991; 325: 1067–71.

18 Burney P, Detels R, Higgins M, Peckham C, Samet JM, Tager IB. Recommendations for research in the epidemiology of asthma. *Chest* 1987; 91: 194–5.

19 O'Connor G, Sparrow D, Taylor D, Segal M, Weiss S. Analysis of dose–response curves to methacholine; an approach suitable for population studies. *Am Rev Respir Dis* 1987; 136: 1412–17.

20 Peat JK, Salome CM, Berry G, Woolcock AJ. Relation of dose–response slope to respiratory symptoms in a population of Australian schoolchildren. *Am Rev Respir Dis* 1991; 144: 663–7.

21 Woolcock AJ. Tests of airway responsiveness in epidemiology. In: Hargreave FE, Woolcock AJ (eds) *Airway Responsiveness: Measurement and Interpretation.* Missassauga, Ontario: Astra, 1985: 136–40.

22 Haby MM, Anderson SD, Peat JK, Mellis CM, Toelle BG, Woolcock AJ. An exercise challenge protocol for epidemiological studies of asthma in children; comparison with histamine challenge. *Eur Respir J* 1994; 7:43–9.

23 Backer V, Dirksten A, Bach-Mortensen N, Hansen KK, Laursen EM, Wendelboe D. The distribution of bronchial responsiveness to histamine and exercise in 527 children and adolescents. *J Allergy Clin Immunol* 1991; 88: 68–76.

24 Zhong NS, Chen RC, O-Yang M, Wu JY, Fu WX, Shi LJ. Bronchial hyperresponsiveness in young students of southern China: relation to respiratory symptoms, diagnosed asthma, and risk factors. *Thorax* 1990; 45: 860–5.

25 Peat JK, Salome CM, Woolcock AJ. Factors associated with bronchial hyper-responsiveness in Australian adults and children. *Eur Respir J* 1992; 5: 921-9.

26 Peat JK, Salome CM, Berry G, Woolcock AJ. Relation of dose–response slope to respiratory symptoms and lung function in a population study of adults living in Busselton, Western Australia. *Am Rev Respir Dis* 1992; 146: 860-5.

27 Peat JK, Salome CM, Woolcock AJ. Longitudinal changes in atopy during a 4-year period: relation to bronchial hyperresponsiveness and respiratory symptoms in a population sample of Australian schoolchildren. *J Allergy Clin Immunol* 1990; 85: 65-74.

28 Brand PLP, Postma DS, Kerstjens HAM *et al.* Relationship of airway hyper-responsiveness to respiratory symptoms and diurnal peak flow variation in patients with obstructive lung disease. *Am Rev Respir Dis* 1991; 143: 916-21.

29 Stick SM, Turnbull S, Chua HI, Landau LI, Le Souef PN. Bronchial respon-siveness to histamine in infants and older children. *Am Rev Respir Dis* 1990; 142: 1143-6.

30 Josephs LK, Gregg I, Mullee WA, Holgate ST. Nonspecific bronchial reac-tivity and its relationship to the clinical expression of asthma. A longitudi-nal study. *Am Rev Respir Dis* 1989; 140: 350-7.

31 Salome CM, Peat JK, Britton WJ, Woolcock AJ. Bronchial hyperresponsive-ness in two populations of Australian schoolchildren. I. Relation to respir-atory symptoms and diagnosis. *Clin Allergy* 1987; 17: 271-81.

32 Sears MR, Jones DT, Holdaway MD *et al.* Prevalence of bronchial reactivity to inhaled methacholine in New Zealand children. *Thorax* 1986; 41: 283-9.

33 Peat JK, Tovey ER, Mellis CM, Leeder SR, Woolcock AJ. Importance of house dust mite and alternaria allergens in childhood asthma: an epidemi-ological study in two climatic regions of Australia. *Clin Exp Allergy* 1993; 23: 812-20.

34 Witt C, Stuckey MS, Woolcock AJ, Dawkins RL. Positive allergy prick tests associated with bronchial histamine responsiveness in an unselected popu-lation. *J Allergy Clin Immunol* 1986; 77: 698-702.

35 Haahtela T, Jokela H. Asthma and allergy in Finnish conscripts. *Allergy* 1979; 34: 413-20.

36 Barbee RA, Lebowitz MD, Thompson HC, Burrows B. Immediate skin-test reactivity in a general population sample. *Ann Intern Med* 1976; 84: 129-33.

37 Cockcroft DW, Killian DN, Mellon JJ, Hargreave FE. Bronchial reactivity to inhaled histamine: a method and clinical survey. *Clin Allergy* 1977; 7: 235-43.

38 Britton WJ, Woolcock AJ, Peat JK, Sedgwick CJ, Lloyd DM, Leeder SR. Prevalence of bronchial hyperresponsiveness in children: the relationship between asthma and skin reactivity to allergens in two communities. *Int J Epidemiol* 1986; 15: 202-9.

39 Hurry VM, Peat JK, Woolcock AJ. Prevalence of respiratory symptoms, bronchial hyperresponsiveness and atopy in schoolchildren living in the Villawood area of Sydney. *Aust NZ J Med* 1988; 18: 745–52.

40 Gray EJ, Peat JK, Mellis CM, Harrington J, Woolcock AJ. Asthma severity and morbidity in a population sample of Sydney schoolchildren Part 1 – Prevalence and effect of air pollutants in coastal regions. *Aust NZ J Med* 1994; 24: 168–75.

41 Pattemore PK, Asher MI, Harrison AC, Mitchell EA, Rea HH, Stewart AW. Ethnic differences in prevalence of asthma symptoms and bronchial hyper-responsiveness in New Zealand schoolchildren. *Thorax* 1989; 44: 168–76.

42 Barry DMJ, Burr ML, Limb ES. Prevalence of asthma among 12 year old children in New Zealand and South Wales: a comparative survey. *Thorax* 1991; 46: 405–9.

43 Lee DA, Winslow NR, Speight AN, Hey EN. Prevalence and spectrum of asthma in childhood. *BMJ* 1983; 286: 1256–8.

44 Nicolai T, von Mutius E, Reitmeir P, Wjst M. Reactivity to cold air hyperventilation in normal and asthmatic children in a survey of 5697 school children in Southern Bavaria. *Am Rev Respir Dis* 1993; 147: 565–72.

45 Backer V, Bach-Mortensen J, Dirksen A. Prevalence and predictors of bronchial hyperresponsiveness in children aged 7–16 years. *Allergy* 1989; 44: 214–19.

46 Woolcock AJ, Konthen PG, Sedgwick CJ. Allergic status of children in an Indonesian village. *Asian Pac J Allergy Immunol* 1984; 2: 7–12.

47 Turner KJ, Dowse GK, Stewart GA, Alpers MP. Studies on bronchial hyper-reactivity, allergic responsiveness, and asthma in rural and urban children of the highlands of Papua New Guinea. *J Allergy Clin Immunol* 1986; 77: 558–66.

48 Veale AJ, Peat JK, Salome CM, Woolcock AJ. Low prevalence of asthma in aboriginal children. *Thoracic Society of Australia and New Zealand, Annual Scientific Conference*, Canberra: 1992: 2.

49 Laird R, Chansin R, Neukirch F, Levallois M, Leproux P. Prevalence of asthma among teenagers attending school in Tahiti. *J Epidemiol Community Health* 1988; 2: 149–51.

50 Peat JK, van den Berg RH, Mellis CM, Leeder SR, Woolcock AJ. Changes in the prevalence of asthma and allergy in Australian children 1982–1992. *Am Rev Respir Dis* 1993; 147: A800.

51 Shaw RA, Crane J, O'Donnell TV, Porteous LE, Coleman ED. Increasing asthma prevalence in a rural New Zealand adolescent population: 1975–1989. *Arch Dis Child* 1990; 65: 1319–23.

52 Burr ML, Butland BK, King S, Vaughan WE. Changes in asthma prevalence: two surveys 15 years apart. *Arch Dis Child* 1989; 64: 1452–6.

53   Gergen PJ, Mullally DI, Evans R. National survey of prevalence of asthma among children in the United States, 1976 to 1980. *Pediatrics* 1988; 81: 1–7.

54   Haahtela T, Lindohlm H, Bjorksten F, Koskinen S, Laitinen LA. Prevalence of asthma in Finnish young men. *BMJ* 1990; 301: 266–8.

55   Perdrizet S, Neukirch F, Cooreman J, Liard R. Effects of long-term inhaled salbutamol therapy on the provocation of asthma by histamine. *Chest* 1987; 6: 104S–106S.

56   Crane J, Flatt A, Lackson R *et al.* Prescribed fenoterol and death from asthma in New Zealand, 1981–83: Case-controlled study. *Lancet* 1989; i: 917–22.

57   Beasley R, Pearce N, Crane J, Windom H, Burgess C. Asthma mortality and inhaled beta agonist therapy. *Aust NZ J Med* 1991; 21: 753–63.

58   Spitzer WO, Suissa S, Ernst P *et al.* The use of β-agonists and the risk of death and near death from asthma. *N Engl J Med* 1992; 326: 501–6.

59   Marsh DG, Bias WB, Ishizaka K. Genetic control of basal serum IgE level and its effect on specific reaginic sensitivity. *Proc Natl Acad Sci USA* 1974; 71: 3588–92.

60   Duffy DL, Martin NG, Battistutta D, Hopper JL, Mathews JD. Genetics of asthma and hay fever in Australian twins. *Am Rev Respir Dis* 1990; 142: 1351–8.

61   Cookson W, Sharp PA, Faux JA, Hopkin JM. Linkage between immunoglobulin E responses underlying asthma and rhinitis and chromosome 11q. *Lancet* 1989; 1: 1292–5.

62   Lympany P, Welsh KI, Cochrane GM, Kemeny DM, Lee TH. Genetic analysis of the linkage between chromosome 11q and atopy. *Clin Exp Allergy* 1992; 22: 1085–92.

63   Amelung PJ, Panhuysen CIM, Postma DS *et al.* Atopy and bronchial hyperresponsiveness: exclusion of linkage to markers on chromosomes 11q and 6p. *Clin Exp Allergy* 1992; 22: 1077–84.

64   Falliers CJ, de Cardoso RR, Bane HN, Coffey R, Middleton E. Discordant allergic manifestations in monozygotic twins: genetic identity versus clinical, physiologic, and biochemical differences. *J Allergy* 1971; 47: 207–19.

65   Zamel N, Leroux M, Vanderdoelen JL. Airway response to inhaled methacholine in healthy nonsmoking twins. *J Appl Physiol* 1984; 56: 936–9.

66   Konig P, Godfrey S. Prevalence of exercise-induced bronchial lability in families of children with asthma. *Arch Dis Child* 1973; 48: 513–18.

67   Sporik R, Chapman MD, Platts-Mills TAE. House dust mite exposure as a cause of asthma. *Clin Exp Allergy* 1992; 22: 897–906.

68   Kelly W, Hudson I, Phelan PD, Pain M, Olinsky A. Atopy in subjects with asthma followed to the age of 28 years. *J Allergy Clin Immunol* 1990; 85: 548–57.

69 Platts-Mills TAE, Mitchell EB, Tovey ER, Chapman MD, Wilkins SR. Airborne allergen exposure, allergen avoidance, and bronchial hyperreactivity. In: Kay AB, Austen KF, Lichtestein LM (eds) *Asthma, Physiology, Immunopharmacology and Treatment.* London: Academic Press, 1984: 297–414.

70 Tovey ER, Chapman MD, Platts MT. Mite faeces are a major source of house dust allergens. *Nature* 1981; 289: 592–3.

71 Korsgaard J, Iversen M. Epidemiology of house dust mite allergy. *Allergy* 1991; 46 (suppl 11): 14–18.

72 Platts-Mills TAE, de Weck AL. Dust-mite allergens and asthma – a world wide problem. Report of the International Workshop. *J Allergy Clin Immunol* 1989; 83: 416–27.

73 Sears MR, Herbison GP, Holdaway MD, Hewitt CJ, Flannery EM, Silva PA. The relative risks of sensitivity to grass pollen, house dust mite and cat dander in the development of childhood asthma. *Clin Exp Allergy* 1989; 19: 419–24.

74 Green W, Toelle B, Woolcock AJ. House dust mite increase in Wagga Wagga houses. *Aust NZ J Med* 1993; 23: 23.

75 Gurwitz D, Corey M, Levison H. Pulmonary function and bronchial reactivity in children after croup. *Am Rev Respir Dis* 1980; 122: 95–9.

76 Mok J, Simpson H. Outcome of acute lower respiratory tract infection in infants: preliminary report of seven-year follow-up study. *BMJ* 1982; 285: 333–7.

77 Rooney JC, Williams HE. The relationship between proved viral bronchiolitis and subsequent wheezing. *J Pediatr* 1971; 79: 744–7.

78 Zweiman B, Schoenwetter WF, Pappano JJ, Tempest B, Hildreth EA. Patterns of allergic respiratory disease in children with a past history of bronchiolitis. *J Allergy Clin Immunol* 1971; 48: 283–9.

79 Johnston SL, Bardin PG, Holgate ST. Viral infections in acute exacerbations of asthma: epidemiology and mechanisms. *Eur Respir J* 1992; 5: 429s.

80 Woolcock AJ, Green W, Alpers MP. Asthma in a rural highland area of Papua New Guinea. *Am Rev Respir Dis* 1981; 123: 565–7.

81 Van Niekerk CH, Weinberg EG, Shore SC, Heese HV, Van Schalkwyk J. Prevalence of asthma: a comparative study of urban and rural Xhosa children. *Clin Allergy* 1979; 9: 319–24.

82 Godfrey RC. Asthma and IgE levels in rural and urban communities of The Gambia. *Clin Allergy* 1975; 5: 201–7.

83 Waite DA, Eyles EF, Tonkin SL, O'Donnell TV. Asthma prevalence in Tokelauan children in two environments. *Clin Allergy* 1980; 10: 71–5.

84 Martinez FD, Antognoni G, Macri F *et al.* Parental smoking enhances bronchial responsiveness in nine-year old children. *Am Rev Respir Dis* 1988; 138: 518–23.

85 Martinez FD, Morgan WJ, Wright AL, Holberg CJ, Taussig LM. Diminished lung function as a predisposing factor to wheezing respiratory illness in infants. N Engl J Med 1988; 319: 1112–17.

86 Burney PG. Asthma mortality: England and Wales. J Allergy Clin Immunol 1987; 80: 379–82.

87 Thien FCK, Mencia-Huerta JM, Lee TH. Dietary fish oil effects on seasonal hay fever and asthma in pollen-sensitive subjects. Am Rev Respir Dis 1993; 147: 1138–43.

88 Seaton A, Godden DJ, Brown K. Increase in asthma: a more toxic environment or a more susceptible population? Thorax 1994; 49: 171–4.

89 Arshad SH, Twiselton R, Smith J, Hide DW. Influence of genetic and environmental factors on the level of IgE at birth. Pediatr Allergy Immunol 1992; 3: 79–83.

90 Sherrill DL, Martinez FD, Lebowitz MD et al. Longitudinal effects of passive smoking on pulmonary function in New Zealand children. Am Rev Respir Dis 1992; 145: 1136–41.

91 von Mutius E, Nicolai T, Martinez FD. Prematurity as a risk factor for asthma in preschool children. J Pediatr 1993; 123: 223–9.

92 von Mutius E, Fritsch C, Weiland SK, Roll G, Magnussen H. Prevalence of asthma and allergic disorders among children in united Germany: a descriptive comparison. BMJ 1992; 305: 1395–9.

93 Peat JK, van den Berg RH, Green WF, Mellis CM, Leeder SR, Woolcock AJ. Changing prevalence of asthma in Australian children. BMJ 1994; 308: 1591–6.

94 Bascom R, Naclerio RM, Fitzgerald TK, Kagey-Sobotka A, Proud D. Effect of ozone inhalation on the response of nasal challenge with antigen of allergic subjects. Am Rev Respir Dis 1990; 142: 594–601.

95 Takafuji S, Suzuki S, Koizumi K et al. Diesel-exhaust particulates inoculated by the intranasal route have an adjuvant activity for IgE production in mice. J Allergy Clin Immunol 1987; 79: 639–45.

96 Anto JM, Sunyer J. Epidemiologic studies of asthma epidemics in Barcelona. Chest 1990; 98 (suppl): 185S–190S.

KEY POINTS

1 Asthma is best classified into episodic and persistent forms. The former may remit but the latter appears to be an irreversible disease for which there is no cure.

2 Both forms of asthma are increasing in children while death rates in young people (5–34 years) have stabilized or decreased in the last 5 years, indicating improving management.

3 The risk factors for developing asthma are mostly defined making prevention, particularly of persistent disease, the most important approach to management in coming years.

2

NATURAL HISTORY

Charles E. Reed

INTRODUCTION

The course of asthma is variable. Thus the only accurate predictive statement about the natural history of asthma is that it will improve, get worse or stay the same. But this profound truism is of little use to patients or their families who want a reasonably accurate prognosis, or to physicians who want to plan a realistic individualized management programme that is not unnecessarily burdensome. The aim of this chapter is to review the available information about factors that affect the course of the disease. Because the natural history of asthma in children and teenagers is different from the natural history in older adults these age groups will be considered separately.

CHILDREN AND TEENAGERS

Asthma begins most often in early childhood, more commonly in boys than girls.[1-3] The age of onset is somewhat uncertain because of the difficulty in defining the diagnosis in infants. There are many infants with one or two episodes of wheezy bronchitis who never develop chronic asthma. But many infants do. In our population-based study of the incidence of asthma in Rochester, Minnesota, in which we were able to review the complete medical records of every physician visit and every inpatient and outpatient hospital visit that the patient ever made, we found the peak incidence rate of the first episode of wheezing to be in the first year of life, although the diagnosis of "asthma" was often not made for several years[4] (Fig. 2.1). Many infants with repeated episodes of wheezing during respiratory infections, particularly boys, do in fact "grow out of" asthma by school age. There has been considerable interest in identifying the factors that are associated with continued asthma throughout the childhood years. Perhaps the most important is the capacity to develop IgE antibody to allergens in the

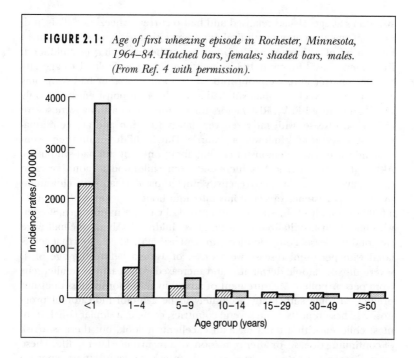

FIGURE 2.1: *Age of first wheezing episode in Rochester, Minnesota, 1964–84. Hatched bars, females; shaded bars, males. (From Ref. 4 with permission).*

environment. Development of asthma and allergy to house-dust mite correlates with the amount of mite allergen in the home.[5] Furthermore, the persistence of asthma, with episodes severe enough to require urgent treatment, is associated with exposure to mites, pets and cockroaches in the home.[6–10] Another important environmental factor, both for the initiation and persistence of asthma during childhood, is maternal cigarette smoking.[7,11–13]

In general, the prognosis of children with asthma as they mature to adulthood is quite good. A study of 688 patients with childhood asthma and followed for 20 years indicated that 26% were still having asthma, but that only in very few was the asthma considered severe.[14] Many subsequent studies have come to the same conclusion. In a population-based study, McNicol and Williams identified the 7-year-old children in Melbourne, Australia with asthma and followed them to age 14.[1,15,16] The factors that predicted persistence of asthma were onset before age 3 years, infantile eczema, and more severe disease. Subsequently Martin *et al.*[17,18] reported on the status of these children at age 20. About one-quarter were free of symptoms and had normal pulmonary function tests. One-half had occasional mild wheezing with exercise or respiratory infections. Only about 20% had frequent or persistent wheezing or reduced forced expiratory volume in 1 s (FEV_1). But by age 28, 30% of those who were free of symptoms at age 21 had relapsed and had recurrent wheezing.[19] This finding confirms the common clinical experience that patients who appear to have onset of asthma as adults often remember wheezing in childhood. Kokkonen et al.[20] followed 108 asthmatic children in Finland to age 20–24. One-quarter were symptom free, while another quarter had symptoms at least once a week; one-half still had airway hyperresponsiveness, but only 18% had reduced FEV_1. Risk factors for persistence of asthma were severe childhood disease, with impaired ventilatory function and atopic dermatitis. Gerritsen et al.[21] followed a group of Dutch children into their twenties and thirties and demonstrated that about one-half still had symptoms. Although skin test reactivity increased from childhood to adult years in this study, neither skin test reactivity nor atopic dermatitis in childhood predicted persistence of symptoms into adulthood. Jonsson et al. reported a follow-up study of the status as adults of 123 patients in northern Sweden who had been hospitalized for asthma as children.[22] About one-half were free of the disease. Four had died (three of asthma). The factors that correlated with persistent disease were onset of asthma before the age of 4, severe disease, atopic dermatitis, and increased skin reactivity to allergens from pets or pollen. Measurement of airway hyperresponsiveness does not predict outcome sufficiently accurately to be a useful indicator of prognosis.[23] These reports, from several countries, come to a similar conclusion: most children with asthma have an excellent outlook, but there is a risk of continuing disease, or after remission, of a recurrence later in life. These formal prospective studies were not able to evaluate continuing exposure to indoor allergens as a key factor in the persistence of the disease, but it almost certainly is. Not only does continued exposure cause continued allergic reaction in the airways, but also, once established, chronic asthma may persist indefinitely after exposure ceases (see Chapter 43). Risk factors for persisting or recurring asthma are summarized in Table 2.1. It should be pointed out that, although current asthma management reduces morbidity, it is not yet known whether treatment influences the long-term outcome.[24]

TABLE 2.1: *Risk factors for persistence of asthma from childhood into adult life*

Onset before 3 years, especially with repeated episodes in infancy
Infantile eczema or allergic rhinitis
Positive skin tests to airborne allergens
Severe disease in childhood
Continued exposure to allergens, especially indoor allergens
Female

ADULTS

Prospective population-based studies of the natural history of asthma in adults are few, and like the studies in children are limited by difficulties in defining the disease. It has been difficult to establish the distinction between asthma persisting into adult life from childhood, and asthma beginning later in life. Most of the patients whose asthma persists from childhood have allergy to various aeroallergens, but the new-onset asthmatics are rarely allergic unless they have developed occupational asthma. The prognosis of allergic and non-allergic (intrinsic) asthma may be quite different. Rackemann, who introduced the term intrinsic asthma, reported a 15–30 year follow-up of 272 patients with adult-onset, non-allergic asthma.[25] Most of these patients were treated before glucocorticoids were available. About 20% had a remission of symptoms, but one-third were unimproved and seven patients had died of asthma. Samter and Beers reported similar outcome for aspirin-sensitive asthmatics, most of whom had adult-onset non-allergic asthma.[26] Ulrick et al. reported on a 10-year follow-up of 170 adult hospitalized asthmatics.[27] Both the rate of decline in FEV_1 and mortality were greater in the non-allergic than in the allergic group. A higher degree of reversibility was associated with a greater decline in lung function in the non-allergic asthmatics, whereas a greater degree of obstruction and past need for glucocorticoid treatment was associated with a greater decline in the allergic patients (Table 2.2).[28]

Braman et al. reported that, although symptoms and need for medications were similar, patients with long-standing asthma had more severe obstruction than those whose disease was of recent onset.[29] It is common clinical experience that older asthmatic patients frequently develop a substantial degree of fixed airway obstruction, and the rate of decline in lung function is accelerated in asthma.[29–31] It is not yet known whether current therapy with aerosol glucocorticoids will prevent this accelerated decline. Nor is the anatomical histopathological basis for the development of fixed obstruction in asthma known. Chronic asthma is associated with hypertrophy of mucous glands and smooth muscle, but it is more likely that the

---

TABLE 2.2: *Risk factors for persistence of asthma in adults*

Severe disease with fixed airway obstruction
Onset after age 40 years and negative skin tests to common allergens
Continued exposure to allergens after asthma has developed
Continued exposure to occupational agents

major cause is permanent obstruction of small airways caused by contraction of the collagen deposited beneath their basement membrane. Obliterative bronchiolitis may also contribute.

Population-based studies indicate that the view of the prognosis of adult asthma gained from the perspective of specialty practice may be overly pessimistic. Asthma, particularly relatively mild allergic asthma, quite often goes into remission.[2,3] The Tuscon population-based study reported a 7-year follow-up of asthma in patients 65 years of age and older. Mild asthma often remitted, but severe disease tended to remain a disabling disorder.[32,33] Even so, the death rate for adults with asthma is not different from that of the population at large.[34,35]

OCCUPATIONAL ASTHMA

A priori one would assume that, once the diagnosis of occupational asthma is made and the patient's exposure terminated, the disease would rapidly improve and the patient would recover. Unhappily, this is not the case. Many patients with asthma from exposure to di-isocyanates, western red cedar and allergens from snow crabs had chronic asthma unchanged in severity 2 years or more after exposure had ceased.[36–38] The patients who had poorest prognosis were the ones with chronic airway obstruction poorly responsive to bronchodilators. Early diagnosis by careful surveillance of exposed workers would appear to be the most effective means of preventing chronic disease.

REFERENCES

1 Williams H, McNicol KN. Prevalence, natural history, and relationship of wheezy bronchitis and asthma in children. An epidemiologic study. *BMJ* 1969; 4: 321-5.

2 Broder I, Higgins MW, Mathews KP, Keller JB. Epidemiology of asthma and allergic rhinitis in a total community, Tecumseh, Michigan. IV. Natural history. *J Allergy Clin Immunol* 1974; 54: 100-10.

3 Dodge RR, Burrows B. The prevalence of asthma and asthma-like symptoms in a general population sample. *Am Rev Respir Dis* 1980; 122: 567-75.

4 Yunginger JW, Reed CE, O'Connell EJ, Melton LJ, O'Fallon WM, Silverstein MD. A community-based study of the epidemiology of asthma. Incidence rates, 1964–1983. *Am Rev Respir Dis* 1992; 146: 888-94.

5 Sporik R, Holgate ST, Platts-Mills TA, Cogswell JJ. Exposure to house-dust mite allergen (Der p I) and the development of asthma in childhood. A prospective study. N Engl J Med 1990; 323: 502–7.

6 Platts-Mills TA, Ward GW Jr, Sporik R, Gelber LE, Chapman MD, Heymann PW. Epidemiology of the relationship between exposure to indoor allergens and asthma. Int Arch Allergy Appl Immunol 1991; 94: 339–45.

7 Morgan WJ, Martinez FD. Risk factors for developing wheezing and asthma in childhood. Pediatr Clin North Am 1992; 39: 1185–203.

8 Call RS, Smith TF, Morris E, Chapman MD, Platts-Mills TA. Risk factors for asthma in inner city children. J Pediatr 1992; 121: 862–6.

9 Gelber LE, Seltzer LH, Bouzoukis JK, Pollart SM, Chapman MD, Platts-Mills TA. Sensitization and exposure to indoor allergens as risk factors for asthma among patients presenting to hospital. Am Rev Respir Dis 1993; 147: 573–8.

10 Brunekreef B, Groot B, Hoek G. Pets, allergy and respiratory symptoms in children. Int J Epidemiol 1992; 21: 338–42.

11 Jenkins MA, Hopper, JL, Flander LB, Carlin JB, Giles GG. The associations between childhood asthma and atopy, and parental asthma, hay fever and smoking. Paediatr Perinat Epidemiol 1993; 7: 67–76.

12 Toyoshima K, Hayashida M, Yasunami J, Takamatsu I, Niwa H, Muraoka T. Factors influencing the prognosis of wheezy infants. J Asthma 1987; 24: 267–70.

13 Tager IB. "Passive smoking" and respiratory health in children – sophistry or cause for concern? Am Rev Respir Dis 1986; 133: 959–63.

14 Rackemann FM. Asthma in children: follow-up study of 688 patients after interval of 20 years. N Engl J Med 1952; 246: 858–62.

15 McNicol KN, Williams H. Spectrum of asthma in children. I. Clinical and physiological components. BMJ 1973; 4: 7–11.

16 McNicol KN, Williams H. Asthma in children. II. Allergic components. BMJ 1973; 4: 12–16.

17 Martin AJ, McLennan LA, Landau LI, Phelan PD. The natural history of childhood asthma to adult life. BMJ 1980; 280: 1397–400.

18 Martin AJ, Landau LI, Phelan PD. Lung function of young adults who had asthma in childhood. Am Rev Respir Dis 1980; 122: 609–12.

19 Kelly WJW, Hudson I, Phelan PD, Pain MCF, Olinski A. Childhood asthma in adult life: a further study at 28 years of age. BMJ 1987; 294: 1059–62.

20 Kokkonen J, Linna O. The state of childhood asthma in young adulthood. Eur Respir J 1993; 6: 657–61.

21 Gerritsen J, Koëter G, de Monchy JG, Knol K. Allergy in subjects with asthma from childhood to adulthood. *J Allergy Clin Immunol* 1990; 85: 116–25.

22 Jonsson JA, Boe J, Berlin E. The long-term prognosis of childhood asthma in a predominantly rural Swedish county. *Acta Paediatr Scand* 1987; 76: 950–4.

23 Nelson HS. The natural history of asthma. *Ann Allergy* 1991; 66: 196–203.

24 de Benedictis FM, Canny GJ, Levison H. The progressive nature of childhood asthma. *Lung* 1990; 168 (suppl): 278–85.

25 Rackemann FM, Edwards MC. Is intrinsic asthma a reversible disease? *Allergy* 1958; 29: 528–36.

26 Samter M, Beers RF. Intolerance to aspirin. *Ann Intern Med* 1968; 68: 975–82.

27 Ulrik CS, Backer V, Dirksen A. Mortality and decline in lung function in 213 adults with bronchial asthma: a ten-year follow up. *J Asthma* 1992; 29: 29–38.

28 Ulrik CS, Backer V, Dirksen A. A 10 year follow-up of 180 adults with bronchial asthma: factors important for the decline in lung function. *Thorax* 1992; 47: 14–18.

29 Braman SS, Kaemmerlen JT, Davis SM. Asthma in the elderly: a comparison between patients with recently acquired and long standing disease. *Am Rev Respir Dis* 1991; 143: 336–40.

30 Finucane KE, Greville HW, Brown PJE. Irreversible airflow obstruction: evolution in asthma. *Med J Aust* 1985; 142: 602–4.

31 Peat JK, Woolcock AJ, Cullen K. Rate of decline of lung function in subjects with asthma. *Eur J Respir Dis* 1987; 70: 171–9.

32 Burrows B, Barbee RA, Cline MG, Knudson RJ, Lebowitz MD. Characteristics of asthma among elderly adults in a sample of the general population. *Chest* 1991; 100: 935–42.

33 Bronnimann S, Burrows B. A prospective study of the natural history of asthma: remission and relapse rates. *Chest* 1986; 90: 480–4.

34 Hunt LW Jr, Silverstein MD, Reed CE, O'Connell EJ, O'Fallon WM, Yunginger JW. Accuracy of the death certificate in a population-based study of asthmatic patients. *JAMA* 1993; 269: 1947–52.

35 Braman SS, Corrao WM, Kaemmerlen JT. The clinical outcome of asthma in the elderly: a 7-year follow-up study. *Ann N Y Acad Sci* 1991; 629: 449–50.

36 Fabbri LM, Saetta M, Picotti G, Mapp CE. Late asthmatic reactions, airway inflammation and chronic asthma in toluene-diisocyanate-sensitized subjects. *Respiration* 1991; 58 (suppl 1): 18–21.

37 Chan-Yeung M, MacLean L, Pagiaro PL. Follow-up study of 232 patients with occupational asthma caused by western red cedar (*Thuja plicata*). *J Allergy Clin Immunol* 1987; 79: 292–6.

Allard C, Cartier A, Ghezzo H, Malo J-L. Occupational asthma due to various agents. Absence of clinical and functional improvement at an interval of four or more years after cessation of exposure. *Chest* 1989; 96: 1046-9.

KEY POINTS

1   Asthma most often begins in early childhood, but may occur at any age.

2   75% of cases are mild, 20% moderate, and 5% severe. Death is rare.

3   Many mild cases remit; moderate and severe cases tend to persist.

4   Persistent cases, especially if severe, often develop irreversible obstruction.

5   Continued exposure to allergen often causes irreversible disease.

3
PATHOGENESIS

Paul M. O'Byrne

INTRODUCTION

Asthma is currently defined by the presence of characteristic symptoms and by reversible airway narrowing and airway hyperresponsiveness to a variety of inhaled bronchoconstrictor stimuli (Fig. 3.1). Airway hyperresponsiveness is present in virtually all asthmatics with current symptoms;[1] however, airway hyperresponsiveness is not specific for asthma, as it can be present in patients with other airway diseases.[2]

In 1892, William Osler published the medical textbook, *The Principles and Practice of Medicine*. In the chapter on asthma, Osler describes "bronchial asthma . . . in many cases is a special form of inflammation of the smaller bronchioles".[3] This reflected the then current descriptions of the pathology of the airways of patients dying of severe, fatal asthma. A more complete description of airway inflammation in patients dying of acute asthma was provided by Dunnill and colleagues[4] in the 1960s. Thus, while airway inflammation and its structural consequences had been recognized for more than 100 years, it was believed that inflammation was confined to the airways of asthmatic patients with very severe disease. More recently, the importance of airway inflammation in the pathogenesis of asthma, ranging in severity from mild to severe, or in transient asthma after exposure to an inflammatory stimulus, has been recognized.

DEFINING AIRWAY INFLAMMATION

Dorlands Medical Dictionary defines inflammation as the "condition into which tissues enter as a reaction to injury". A common manifestation of inflammation is the presence, at some time in the process, of activated inflammatory cells at the affected tissue site. The type of inflammatory cell varies with the type of inflammation. The most important inflammatory cell at sites of acute inflammation is the neutrophil. However, in other,

FIGURE 3.1: *Airway responses to a bronchoconstrictor agonist in a normal subject and subjects with mild and moderate asthma. Asthmatic airways are more sensitive to the agonist (a), have a steeper slope of the concentration–response curve (b), and have a greater maximal response (c).*

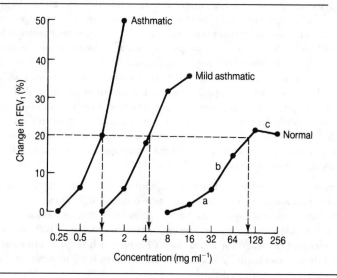

more chronic inflammatory conditions, eosinophils, lymphocytes or mast cells appear to be more prominent. For the purposes of this chapter, airway inflammation will be defined as the presence of activated inflammatory cells in the airways. While this definition is restrictive and excludes other important components of inflammatory events, such as oedema and vasodilatation, quantifying numbers, and occasionally state of activation, of inflammatory cells has been the most commonly used index of airway inflammation in studies of asthma.

TRANSIENT ASTHMA AND AIRWAY INFLAMMATION

The identification of stimuli that can cause transient asthma has proved to be important in studies of the pathogenesis of asthma. This is because the evidence that the presence of inflammatory cells is causally related to the development of airway hyperresponsiveness and transient asthma in human subjects initially depended on studies which examined numbers of cells and cellular differentials in bronchoalveolar lavage (BAL) fluid before and after inhalation of ozone,[5] the occupational sensitizing agent toluene diisocyanate (TDI)[6] and allergen,[7] all of which are known to cause airway hyperresponsiveness and transient asthma, or exacerbate persisting asthma. These studies have all demonstrated an acute inflammatory response in the airways associated with the development of variable airflow obstruction, airway hyperresponsiveness and asthma. In addition, the studies have suggested that the stimulus which initiates the airway hyperresponsiveness determines the type of cellular response. For example, a substantial increase in neutrophils and a smaller increase in eosinophils was described in BAL fluid from subjects with airway hyperresponsiveness following TDI.[6] In contrast, airway challenge with plicatic acid (responsible for western red cedar asthma, a different form of occupational asthma), caused increases in eosinophil numbers but not neutrophils in BAL fluid.[8] After allergen challenge, some studies describe increases in eosinophils,[7] or eosinophils and neutrophils,[9] or eosinophils, lymphocytes and basophils.[10] However, measurements in these studies have been carried out at different time points and with different challenge techniques, which might explain the varied results.

A more recent focus has been the examination of the state of activation of the inflammatory cells after allergen inhalation.[11] These studies have identified that eosinophils are activated, as indicated by positive staining for the marker for cleaved eosinophil cationic protein (EG2), as early as 3 hours and persisted for more than 24 hours in BAL fluid after allergen inhalation; this change preceded the increase in total number of eosinophils after allergen inhalation.

More recently, a less invasive method than bronchoscopy has been developed, using sputum induced by the inhalation of hypertonic saline, to quantify and characterize inflammatory cells in asthmatic airways. Studies using this method have demonstrated that eosinophils increase markedly in sputum samples of asthmatics undergoing a naturally occurring exacerbation of their asthma;[12] this increase also occurs 24 hours after allergen inhalation and persists for 3 days after allergen.[13]

PERSISTING ASTHMA AND INFLAMMATION

There have been a number of studies that have provided information on cell populations in BAL fluid in mild stable asthmatics with persistent airway hyperresponsiveness and asthma.[14-16] A common finding in all these studies, as well as in recent examinations of bronchial mucosal biopsies,[17,18] is the presence of increased numbers of inflammatory cells such as eosinophils, lymphocytes and mast cells compared with normal control subjects with normal airway responsiveness. The eosinophils show signs of activation, as indicated by increased levels of granular proteins, major basic protein (MBP)[15] and eosinophilic cationic protein (ECP).[16] In the bronchial mucosa the eosinophils show morphological features of activation, as indicated by the heterogeneity of the granular structure[17] or as eosinophil granules lying free in the mucosal interstitium.[17] Azzawi and colleagues[19] and Poston et al.[20] have also demonstrated increased numbers of EG2-positive cells, as well as significant increases in numbers of activated T-lymphocytes.[19] Mast cells in the airway mucosa exhibit various stages of degranulation[17] suggesting that mediator release is an ongoing process in the airways of stable asthmatics with persistent airway hyperresponsiveness.

Some studies have correlated numbers of inflammatory cells in BAL fluid with the severity of methacholine airway hyperresponsiveness in stable asthmatics. Kirby et al.[14] demonstrated close correlations between degree of airway hyperresponsiveness in subjects with mild asthma and number of mast cells and eosinophils respectively in lavage fluid. Kelly and co-workers[21] showed correlations between numbers of neutrophils and airway hyperresponsiveness. They also found that the activity of both neutrophils and alveolar macrophages, as indicated by luminol enhanced chemoluminescence, was increased in asthmatics compared with normal controls, demonstrating that these cells were metabolically active.

These studies can be summarized as demonstrating the presence of activated inflammatory cells, eosinophils, neutrophils, lymphocytes and mast cells, in the airways of asthmatics even at a time when they are considered stable and asymptomatic. The numbers of cells increase following a stimulus that causes airway hyperresponsiveness, as well as in natural exacerbations of asthma. However, the precise role of these different cells in causing airway hyperresponsiveness has not yet been clarified.

INFLAMMATORY MEDIATORS AND ASTHMA

Identifying a role for an inflammatory mediator in the pathogenesis of asthma has relied on the collection of various types of evidence. Generally, when the structure of the mediator is identified, and it is synthesized, the mediator is given (usually by inhalation) to asthmatics, to identify whether it can mimic some component of the asthmatic response. Subsequently, when assays for its measurement are available, efforts are made to measure the mediator or its metabolite during asthmatic responses. Then, when antagonists of the mediator or inhibitors of its synthesis are available, they are studied in clinical models of asthma. The final, and most difficult, hurdle is to determine whether the mediator antagonists or synthesis inhibitors are useful in treating asthmatic patients. A variety of mediators have been suggested to be important in the pathogenesis of asthma. These have included histamine, acetylcholine, prostaglandin (PG)D_2 and $PGF_{2\alpha}$, thromboxane, cysteinyl leukotrienes, platelet activating factor and, most recently, cytokines and growth factors.

HISTAMINE AND ACETYLCHOLINE

Histamine and acetylcholine have biological effects that are relevant to asthma: both are released in response to appropriate stimuli, acetylcholine from airway nerves and histamine from airway mast cells; and both are potent bronchoconstrictors. Histamine also causes vasodilatation and increased vascular permeability. In addition, H_1-receptor antagonists have been demonstrated to partially inhibit some asthmatic responses, such as exercise-induced bronchoconstriction.[22] However, even very potent and long-acting antihistamines are not effective bronchodilators, nor do they have a useful role in the management of asthma. Atropine and other anti-cholinergics, such as ipratropium bromide, are bronchodilators and have been used for many years to treat bronchoconstriction, and more recently to treat (together with inhaled β_2-agonists) acute severe asthma.[23] This suggests that acetylcholine is released from airway nerves in asthmatics and causes bronchoconstriction. However, anticholinergics do not modify any other important component of asthma, which indicates that acetylcholine release is not involved in the underlying pathogenesis of asthma.

THROMBOXANE

Thromboxane $(Tx)A_2$ is a potent constrictor of smooth muscle, as is its analogue, U46619 of human airways.[24] A recent study examining the effects of a thromboxane synthetase inhibitor on airway responses after allergen challenge demonstrated slight, but significant, inhibition of the allergen-induced early asthmatic responses by 20–25%, but no inhibition of aller-gen-induced late asthmatic responses nor allergen-induced histamine air-way hyperresponsiveness 24 hours after allergen.[25] This suggested that thromboxane may be released following allergen challenge and be partly responsible for the early asthmatic response, but is not important in caus-ing other allergen-induced responses. The TxA_2 synthetase inhibitor, OKY 046, administered orally, has been shown to improve acetylcholine airway hyperresponsiveness in stable asthmatic subjects.[26] However, these studies were uncontrolled, and need to be repeated in a placebo-controlled double-blind study before the results can be properly interpreted. There are no published studies on the clinical efficacy of thromboxane recep-tor antagonists or synthetase inhibitors in the management of asthma. However, the weak activity in protecting against allergen-induced asth-matic responses would suggest that these compounds are unlikely to have a major clinical effect.

PLATELET ACTIVATING FACTOR

Platelet activating factor (PAF) has a variety of actions, which include the recruitment and activation of inflammatory cells, particularly eosinophils and neutrophils.[27] Inhaled PAF has also been described as causing bron-choconstriction and airway hyperresponsiveness in normal subjects in some[28] but not other[29] studies. PAF has also been demonstrated to be released into the plasma following allergen inhalation in mild asthmatic subjects.[30] For these reasons, PAF has been sugegsted as being an important mediator in the development of allergen-induced late asthmatic responses and airway hyperresponsiveness, and to play an important role in the ongoing airway inflammation of asthma.

A variety of very potent and selective PAF receptor antagonists have become available for clinical study. Until recently, the "gold standard" compound has been the thieno-triazolodiazepine, WEB 2086. The compound has been used to characterize the PAF receptor, and has been shown to prevent PAF-induced bronchoconstriction in human subjects.[31] Recent studies have demonstrated that WEB 2086, or another very potent PAF antagonist, UK 74,505, were completely ineffective in inhibiting allergen-induced early or late asthmatic responses or allergen-induced airway hyper-responsiveness.[32,33] Thus, PAF does not appear to be important in the pathogenesis of allergen responses in asthma. It is very unlikely that oral PAF antagonists will have clinical efficacy in asthma, although high concentrations delivered topically by inhalation may be more effective.

CYSTEINYL LEUKOTRIENES

Leukotriene (LT)C_4 and LTD_4 are the most potent bronchoconstrictors yet studied in human subjects, being up to 10 000 times more potent than methacholine in some normal subjects,[34] and with a longer duration of action than inhaled histamine.[35] Also, increases in urinary levels of LTE_4, the metabolite of LTC_4 and LTD_4, have been demonstrated following allergen-induced early responses,[36,37] in patients presenting to hospital with acute severe asthma[37] and following exercise-induced bronchoconstriction.[38] Studies with potent and specific leukotriene antagonists have supported an important role for the leukotrienes in clinical models of asthma, such as exercise- [39] (Fig. 3.2), allergen- [40] and aspirin-induced asthma.[41] Also, leukotriene release is, in part, responsible for spontaneous broncho-constriction in asthma.[42] Recent studies have suggested that the cysteinyl leukotrienes can also cause the release of inhibitory prostaglandins in asthmatic airways, which is likely the cause of exercise refractoriness in asthmatic subjects.[43] Lastly, the initial studies of leukotriene antagonists and synthesis inhibitors have demonstrated clinical efficacy in asthma.[44] These results taken together indicate that the cysteinyl leukotrienes are important in the pathogenesis of asthma.

CYTOKINES

There are now more than 30 different protein mediators that are classed as cytokines. Some of these have been implicated in the pathogenesis of asthma, mainly because of the ability of some of these proteins to promote inflammatory cell growth and differentiation, or inflammatory cell migration and activation, or cause changes in the structural cells of the airways. The study of cytokines in asthma is not yet as developed as for the lipid mediators, mainly because of the lack of specific antagonists that can be studied in humans. However, the cytokines interleukin (IL)-3, IL-5 and granulocyte macrophage-colony stimulating factor (GM-CSF) may be

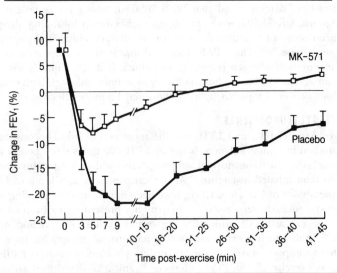

FIGURE 3.2: *The percentage change in FEV$_1$ (mean and SEM) over time post-exercise following treatment with placebo (■) or the leukotriene receptor antagonist MK-571 (□). Treatment with MK-571 significantly reduced the maximal fall in FEV$_1$ after exercise (P < 0.001) and shortened the recovery time (P < 0.001). (From Ref. 39 with permission).*

important because of their ability to promote eosinophil and mast cell differentiation, recruitment and activation into the airways, and prolong the survival of these cells once in the airways. All these cytokines, as well as IL-4, which is necessary for IgE production, are produced by one type of helper T cell, the TH$_2$ cell, which is present in asthmatic airways.[45] In addition, other airway cells may be responsible for the production of these cytokines. Increased amounts of GM-CSF, but not IL-3, are present in airway biopsies from mild asthmatics, and the levels increase after allergen challenge.[46,47] It would appear very likely that these, as well as other cytokines, are responsible for the presence of persisting activated eosinophils and mast cells in asthmatic airways; however, further studies with drugs that block the action of specific cytokines will be needed to precisely establish their role in asthma.

AIRWAY STRUCTURAL CHANGES IN ASTHMA

A number of structural changes have been described in asthmatic airways, which appear to be characteristic of the disease and which may also be responsible for the presence of persisting airway hyperresponsiveness in asthma. These changes include patchy desquamated epithelium; thickening of the reticular collagen layer below the basement membrane; and airway smooth muscle hypertrophy. Both epithelial damage and smooth muscle hypertrophy have been implicated in the pathogenesis of airway hyperresponsiveness in asthma.

AIRWAY EPITHELIAL DAMAGE

Epithelial damage and desquamation are present in airways of patients with asthma.[48] One hypothesis to explain epithelial damage and desquamation in asthmatic airways is that basic proteins released from activated eosinophils damage the epithelium. Levels of MBP have been shown to be increased in BAL fluid from asthmatic patients.[15] Using immunofluorescence, MBP has also been identified in tissue sections from airways of patients dying from severe asthma.[49] Even in sections where identifiable eosinophils could not be seen, evidence showed MBP to be present in epithelium and submucosa giving signs of tissue damage.

Several hypotheses have been proposed to explain how epithelial damage may result in airway hyperresponsiveness in asthma. These include increased permeability of the airway epithelium, loss of inhibitory mediators generated by the airway epithelium and loss of neutral endopeptidase. Several studies have compared the permeability of the respiratory epithelium in normal subjects, asthmatics and asymptomatic smokers. These studies demonstrated that the clearance of inhaled radiolabelled aerosols from the lung into the blood was much faster in the asymptomatic smokers with normal airway responsiveness than in either the normal subjects with normal airway responsiveness or the asthmatic subjects with airway hyperresponsiveness.[50] These results make it very unlikely that increase in airway epithelial permeability is the cause of airway hyperresponsiveness in asthma.

The epithelium has been reported to release a factor that reduces the airway smooth muscle contractile responses to agonists such as histamine and acetylcholine.[51] This mediator has been called epithelium-derived relaxing factor (EpDRF). The hypothesis that loss of an inhibitory EpDRF may be responsible for airway hyperresponsiveness in asthma has not been possible to test in human subjects. Studies in dogs have demonstrated that the function of EpDRF *in vitro*, as determined by the ability to reduce the contractile responses of the trachealis to acetylcholine, histamine or serotonin, was unaltered in dogs with airway hyperresponsiveness *in vivo*, when compared to control dogs.[52] It is unlikely, therefore, that loss of EpDRF is the cause of airway hyperresponsiveness, at least in this animal preparation.

Airway epithelial cells are known to release PGE_2,[53] which has potent inhibitory effects in the airways, such as presynaptic modulation and inhibition of acetylcholine release from muscarinic nerves.[54] In addition, PGE is able to reduce contractile responses to inhaled histamine, acetylcholine and methacholine,[55] and reduce bronchoconstrictor responses to exercise in asthmatics.[56] The airway epithelium also contains enzymes, neutral endopeptidases, capable of metabolizing tachykinins, such as substance P,[57] which are bronchoconstrictor and pro-inflammatory mediators. Loss of these inhibitory mediators may have important results in asthmatic airways; however, this hypothesis has not yet been tested in asthmatic subjects.

AIRWAY SMOOTH MUSCLE

Airway hyperresponsiveness in asthma is non-specific. This means that asthmatic airways are more responsive to all bronchoconstrictor mediators acting on airway smooth muscle receptors. One explanation for the lack of specificity is that the underlying abnormality in asthmatic airways resides in the smooth muscle. The responses of airway smooth muscle from human subjects with airway hyperresponsiveness *in vivo* have been studied by a number of different investigators.[58,59] No consistent increase in smooth muscle responsiveness *in vitro* has been associated with airway hyperresponsiveness *in vivo*. Very few studies have examined smooth muscle *in vitro* from subjects with airway hyperresponsiveness *and* asthma. A small number of studies of airway smooth muscle from asthmatic subjects suggest that the smooth muscle is hyperresponsive to agonists *in vitro*, when compared to airways from non-asthmatic subjects.[60,61] Thus, an inherent defect may exist in asthmatic airway smooth muscle, which would account for airway hyperresponsiveness.

Another possibility by which the increase in airway smooth muscle volume in asthmatics causes airway hyperresponsiveness is thickening of asthmatic airways. James *et al.*[62] have, by using modelling studies, demonstrated that a small increase in the thickness of the airway wall, which is not possible to demonstrate by changes in spirometric indices, could result in airway hyperresponsiveness in asthma.

CONCLUSIONS

Airway inflammation appears to be central to the pathogenesis of all the clinical manifestations of asthma. Many studies have now demonstrated the presence of activated eosinophils and of mast cells in the airway lumen and airway wall of patients with asthma, even those with mild disease. The presence and survival of these inflammatory cells may be promoted by the presence of increased levels of pro-inflammatory cytokines, such as GM-CSF, in asthmatic airways. These cells have the capacity to release potent bronchoconstrictor mediators such as the cysteinyl leukotrienes, which are responsible, in part at least, for airway narrowing in asthma and for allergen-, exercise- and aspirin-induced asthma. Other cells, such as a subset of T lymphocytes (TH_2), may also be important in maintaining the inflammatory cascade. Airway structural changes caused by the persisting inflammation, such as airway epithelial damage or altered smooth muscle function or volume, are likely important in the pathogenesis of stable long-standing airway hyperresponsiveness. Mediators released from the inflammatory cells may be responsible for these changes. Despite the great increase in knowledge about the importance of airway inflammation in the pathogenesis of asthma, the precise sequence of events that leads to the presence of persisting airway inflammatory cells, airway structural changes and airway hyperresponsiveness in asthma remains to be clarified.

REFERENCES

1 Cockcroft DW, Killian DN, Mellon JJA, Hargreave FE. Bronchial reactivity of inhaled histamine: a method and clinical survey. *Clin Allergy* 1977; 7: 235–43.

2 Ramsdale EH, Morris MM, Roberts RS, Hargreave FE. Bronchial responsiveness to methacholine in chronic bronchitis: relationship to airflow obstruction and cold air responsiveness. *Thorax* 1984; 39: 912–8.

3 Osler W. *The Principles and Practice of Medicine*. New York: Appleton and Co., 1892: 497.

4 Dunnill MS, Massarell GR, Anderson JA. A comparison of the quantitive anatomy of the bronchi in normal subjects, in status asthmaticus, in chronic bronchitis and in emphysema. *Thorax* 1969; 24: 176–9.

5 Stelzer J, Bigby BG, Stulbarg M *et al.* Ozone-induced changes in bronchial reactivity to methacholine and airway inflammation in humans. *J Appl Physiol* 1986; 60: 1231–6.

6 Fabbri LM, Boschetto P, Zocca E *et al.* Bronchoalveolar neutrophilia during late asthmatic reactions induced by toluene diisocyanate. *Am Rev Respir Dis* 1987; 136: 36–42.

7 DeMonchy JGR, Kauffman HF, Venge P *et al.* Bronchoalveolar eosinophilia during allergen-induced late asthmatic reaction. *Am Rev Respir Dis* 1985; 131: 373–6.

8 Lam S, Chan-Yeung M, Le Riche J, Kijek K, Phillip D. Cellular changes in bronchial lavage fluid following late asthmatic reactions in patients with red cedar asthma. *Am Rev Respir Dis* 1985; 131: 42A.

9 Metzger WJ, Zavala D, Richerson HB *et al.* Local allergen challenge and bronchoalveolar lavage of allergic asthmatic lungs. *Am Rev Respir Dis* 1987; 135: 433–40.

10 Diaz P, Gonzalez MC, Galleguillos FR *et al.* Leucocytes and mediators in bronchoalveolar lavage during allergen-induced late-phase asthmatic reactions. *Am Rev Respir Dis* 1989; 139: 1383–9.

11 Aalbers R, Kauffman HK, Vrugt B *et al.* Bronchial lavage and bronchoalveolar lavage in allergen-induced single early and dual asthmatic responses. *Am Rev Respir Dis* 1993; 147: 76–81.

12 Gibson PG, Girgis-Gabardo A, Hargreave FE *et al.* Cellular characteristics of sputum from patients with asthma and chronic bronchitis. *Thorax* 1989; 44: 693–9.

13 Pin I, Freitag AP, O'Byrne PM *et al.* Changes in the cellular profile of induced-sputum after allergen-induced asthmatic responses. *Am Rev Respir Dis* 1992; 145: 1265–9.

14 Kirby JG, Hargreave FE, Gleich GJ, O'Byrne PM. Bronchoalveolar cell profiles of asthmatic and nonasthmatic subjects. *Am Rev Respir Dis* 1987; 136: 379–83.

15 Wardlaw AJ, Dunnette S, Gleich GJ, Collins JV, Kay AB. Eosinophils and mast cells in bronchoalveolar lavage in subjects with mild asthma. *Am Rev Respir Dis* 1988; 137: 62–9.

16 Ädelroth E, Rosenhall L, Johansson SÅ, Linden M, Venge P. Inflammatory cells and eosinophilic activity in asthmatics investigated by bronchoalveolar lavage: the effects of anti-asthmatic treatment with budesonide or terbutaline. *Am Rev Respir Dis* 1990; 142: 91–9.

17 Beasley R, Roche WR, Roberts JA, Holgate ST. Cellular events in the bronchi in mild asthma and after bronchial provocation. *Am Rev Respir Dis* 1989; 139: 806–17.

18 Jeffery PK, Wardlaw AJ, Nelson F, Collins JV, Kay AB. Bronchial biopsies in asthma. An ultrastructural, quantitative study and correlation with hyperreactivity. *Am Rev Respir Dis* 1989; 140: 1745–53.

19 Azzawi M, Bradley B, Jeffery PK *et al.* Identification of activated T-lymphocytes and eosinophils in bronchial biopsies in stable atopic asthma. *Am Rev Respir Dis* 1990; 142: 1407–13.

20 Poston RN, Chanez P, Lacoste JY, Litchfield T, Lee TH, Bousquet J. Immunohistochemical characterization of the cellular infiltration in asthmatic bronchi. *Am Rev Respir Dis* 1992; 145: 918–21.

21 Kelly C, Ward C, Stenton CS, Bird G, Hendrick PJ, Walters EH. Number and activity of inflammatory cells in bronchoalveolar lavage fluid in asthma and their relation to airway hyperresponsiveness. *Thorax* 1988; 43: 684–92.

22 Hartley JPR, Nogrady SG. Effect of an inhaled antihistamine on exercise-induced asthma. *Thorax* 1980; 35: 675–9.

23 Rebuck AS, Chapman KR, Abboud R *et al.* Nebulized anticholinergic and sympathomimetic treatment of asthma and chronic obstructive airways disease in the emergency room. *Am J Med* 1987; 82: 59–64.

24 Jones GL, Saroea G, Watson RL, O'Byrne PM. The effect of an inhaled thromboxane mimetic (U46619) on airway function in human subjects. *Am Rev Respir Dis* 1992; 145: 1270–5.

25 Manning PJ, Stevens WH, Cockcroft DW, O'Byrne PM. The role of thromboxane in allergen-induced asthmatic responses. *Eur Respir J* 1991; 4: 667–72.

26 Fujimura M, Sasaki F, Nakatsumi Y *et al.* Effects of a thromboxane synthetase inhibitor (OKY-046) and a lipoxygenase inhibitor (AA-861) on bronchial responsiveness to acetylcholine in asthmatic subjects. *Thorax* 1986; 41: 955–9.

27 Barnes PJ, Chung KF, Page CP. Platelet activating factor as a mediator of allergic disease. *J Allergy Clin Immunol* 1987; 81: 919–34.

28 Cuss FM, Dixon CMS, Barnes PJ. Effects of inhaled platelet activating factor on pulmonary function and bronchial responsiveness in man. *Lancet* 1986; ii: 189–92.

29 Lai CK, Jenkins JR, Polosa R, Holgate ST. Inhaled PAF fails to induce airway hyperresponsiveness to methacholine in normal human subjects. *J Appl Physiol* 1990; 68: 919–26.

30 Chan-Yeung M, Lam S, Chan H, Tse KS, Salari H. The release of platelet-activating factor into plasma during allergen-induced bronchoconstriction. *J Allergy Clin Immunol* 1991; 87: 667–73.

31 Adamus WS, Heuer HO, Meade CJ, Schilling JC. Inhibitory effects of a new PAF acether antagonist WEB 2086 on pharmacologic changes induced by PAF inhalation in human beings. *Clin Pharmacol Ther* 1990; 47: 456–62.

32 Freitag A, Watson RW, Matsos G, Eastwood C, O'Byrne PM. The effect of a platelet activating factor antagonist, WEB 2086, on allergen-induced asthmatic responses. *Thorax* 1993; 48: 594–8.

33 Kuitert LM, Hui KP, Uthayarkumar S *et al.* Effect of a platelet activating factor antagonist, UK 74,505 on early and late responses to allergen. *Am Rev Respir Dis* 1993; 147: 82–6.

34 Adelroth E, Morris MM, Hargreave FE, O'Byrne PM. Airway responsiveness to leukotrienes C4 and D4 and to methacholine in patients with asthma and normal controls. *N Engl J Med* 1986; 315: 480–4.

35 Barnes NC, Piper PJ, Costello JF. Comparative effects of inhaled leukotriene C4, leukotriene D4 and histamine in normal human subjects. *Thorax* 1984; 39: 500–4.

36 Manning PJ, Rokach J, Malo JL *et al*. Urinary leukotriene E_4 levels during early and late asthmatic responses. *J Allergy Clin Immunol* 1990; 86: 211–20.

37 Taylor GW, Black P, Turner N *et al*. Urinary leukotriene E_4 after antigen challenge and in acute asthma and allergic rhinitis. *Lancet* 1989; i: 584–7.

38 Kikawa Y, Miyanomae T, Inoue Y *et al*. Urinary leukotriene E_4 after exercise challenge in children with asthma. *J Allergy Clin Immunol* 1992; 89: 1111–19.

39 Manning PJ, Watson RM, Margolskee DJ, Williams V, Schwartz JI, O'Byrne PM. Inhibition of exercise-induced bronchoconstriction by MK-571, a potent leukotriene D_4 receptor antagonist. *N Engl J Med* 1990; 323: 1736–9.

40 Taylor IK, O'Shaughnessy KM, Fuller RW, Dollery CT. Effect of a cysteinyl-leukotriene receptor antagonist, ICI 204-219 on allergen-induced broncho-constriction and airway hyperreactivity in atopic subjects. *Lancet* 1991; 337: 690–4.

41 Dahlen B, Kumlin M, Johannson H *et al*. The leukotriene-antagonist, MK-0679, improves baseline pulmonary function and blocks aspirin-induced airway obstruction in aspirin sensitive asthmatics. *Am Rev Respir Dis* 1992; 145: A15.

42 Gaddy J, Bush RK, Margolskee D, Williams VC, Busse W. The effects of a leukotriene D_4 (LTD_4) antagonist (MK-571) in mild to moderate asthma. *Am Rev Respir Dis* 1992; 146: 358–63.

43 Manning PJ, Watson RW, O'Byrne PM. Exercise-induced refractoriness in asthmatic subjects involves leukotriene and prostaglandin interdependent mechanisms. *Am Rev Respir Dis*: 1993; 148: 950–4.

44 Israel E, Rubin P, Kemp JP *et al*. The effect of inhibition of 5-lipoxygenase by Zileuton in mild-to-moderate asthma. *Ann Intern Med* 1993; 119: 1059–66.

45 Robinson DS, Hamid Q, Ying S *et al*. Predominant T_{H2}-like bronchoalveolar T-lymphocyte populations in atopic asthma. *N Engl J Med* 1992; 326: 298–304.

46 Woolley KL, Adelroth, E, Woolley MJ, Ellis R, Jordana M, O'Byrne PM. Granulocyte-macrophage colony-stimulating factor, eosinophils and eosinophil cationic protein in mild asthmatics and non-asthmatics. *Eur Respir J* 1994; 7: 1576–84.

47 Woolley KL, Adelroth E, Woolley MJ *et al*. Interleukin-3 in bronchial biopsies from non-asthmatics and patients with mild and allergen-induced asthma. *Am J Respir Crit Care Med* 1995; in press.

48 Laitinen LA, Heino M, Laitinen A, Kava T, Haahtela T. Damage of the airway epithelium and bronchial reactivity in patients with asthma. *Am Rev Respir Dis* 1985; 131: 599–606.

49 Gleich GJ, Frigas E, Loegering DA *et al*. Cytotoxic properties of the eosino-phil major basic protein. *J Immunol* 1979; 123: 2925–7.

50 O'Byrne PM, Dolovich M, Dirks R, Roberts RS, Newhouse MT. Lung epithelial permeability: relation to nonspecific airway responsiveness. *J Appl Physiol* 1984; 57: 77–84.

51 Flavahan NA, Aarhuus LL, Rimele TJ, Vanhoutte PM. Respiratory epithelium inhibits bronchial smooth muscle tone. *J Appl Physiol* 1985; 58: 834–8.

52 Jones G, Lane CG, O'Byrne PM. Release of epithelium-derived relaxation factor (EpDRF) after ozone inhalation in dogs. *J Appl Physiol* 1988; 65: 1238–43.

53 Leikauf GD, Ueki IF, Nadel JA, Widdicombe JH. Bradykinin stimulates Cl secretion and prostaglandin E_2 release by canine tracheal epithelium. *Am J Physiol* 1985; 248: F48–55.

54 Walters EH, O'Byrne PM, Fabbi LM, Graf PD, Holtzman MJ, Nadel JA. Control of neurotransmission by prostaglandins in canine trachealis smooth muscle. *J Appl Physiol* 1984; 57: 129–34.

55 Manning PJ, Lane CG, O'Byrne PM. The effect of oral prostaglandin E_1 on airway responsiveness in asthmatic subjects. *Pulmonary Pharmacol* 1989; 2: 121–4.

56 Melillo E, Woolley KL, Manning PJ, Watson RM, O'Byrne PM. Effect of inhaled PGE_2 on exercise-induced bronchoconstriction in asthmatic subjects. *Am J Respir Crit Care Med* 1994; 149: 1138–41.

57 Dusser DJ, Jacoby DB, Djokic TD, Rubinstein I, Borson DB, Nadel JA. Virus induces airway hyperresponsiveness to tachykinins: role of neutral endopeptidase. *J Appl Physiol* 1989; 67: 1504–11.

58 Vincenc CS, Black JL, Yan K *et al.* Comparison of *in vivo* and *in vitro* responses to histamine in human airways. *Am Rev Respir Dis* 1983; 128: 875–9.

59 Roberts JA, Raeburn D, Rodger IW, Thomson NC. Comparison of *in vivo* airway responsiveness and *in vitro* smooth muscle sensitivity to methacholine in man. *Thorax* 1984; 39: 837–43.

60 Schellenberg RR, Foster A. *In vitro* responses of human asthmatic airway and pulmonary vascular smooth muscle. *Int Arch Allergy Appl Immunol* 1984; 75: 237–41.

61 Bai TR. Abnormalities in airway smooth muscle in fatal asthma. *Am Rev Respir Dis* 1990; 141: 552–7.

62 James AI, Pare PD, Hogg JC. The mechanics of airway narrowing in asthma. *Am Rev Respir Dis* 1989; 139: 242–6.

KEY POINTS

1   Asthma is a disease characterized by:
- Variable airflow obstruction
- Airway hyperresponsiveness
- Airway inflammation

2

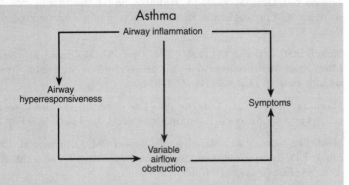

Airway inflammation is necessary for all the clinical manifestations of asthma.

Diagnosis and
Investigations of Asthma

4

TRIGGERS OF ASTHMA

Neil C. Thomson

INTRODUCTION

The diagnosis of asthma based on a history of episodic cough, wheezing, chest tightness or dyspnoea is usually not difficult to make but the clinical presentation may be less straightforward (see Chapters 5 and 6). Asthma attacks can be provoked by different trigger factors and each of these stimuli will be considered briefly in this chapter. The assessment and management of asthma induced by the more important of these triggers is reviewed in Chapters 14, 21 and 31–40.

CLASSIFICATION OF TRIGGER FACTORS

Asthma is now recognized to be a chronic inflammatory disorder of the airways (see Chapter 3). The asthmatic airway exhibits variable airflow obstruction and bronchial hyperreactivity to different stimuli (Fig. 4.1, Table 4.1). In susceptible individuals allergens, occupational agents and probably viruses can induce airway inflammation, bronchial hyperreactivity and symptoms of asthma (inducers of asthma) (see Chapter 3). Allergens, occupational agents and also non-steroidal anti-inflammatory drugs produce bronchoconstriction only in asthmatics "sensitized" to these agents and

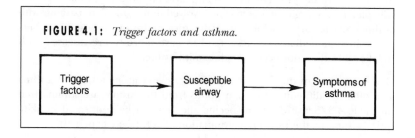

FIGURE 4.1: *Trigger factors and asthma.*

TABLE 4.1: *Triggers of asthma*

Infections[a]
Allergens[a]
Occupational agents[a]
Environmental pollutants[b]
Exercise
Cold air
Hyperventilation
Aerosols of distilled water or hypertonic solutions
Drugs
Foods
Psychological factors

[a] These stimuli can induce the asthmatic state as well as precipitating attacks of asthma.
[b] It is uncertain whether this stimulus can induce asthma in humans.

even high "doses" of these substances will not produce asthma in non-sensitive patients. Other triggers such as exercise or irritants (inciters of asthma) produce symptoms of asthma because the airways are inflamed and hyperreactive but these stimuli probably do not induce chronic airway inflammation. Asthma symptoms will occur in most if not all asthmatic patients provided a high enough "dose" of these latter stimuli is administered.

ALLERGENS

Inhaled, ingested or injected allergens can all precipitate asthma although the inhaled route is the commonest and most important[1,2] (Table 4.2) (see Chapter 14). Allergic factors may be involved in up to 75% of patients with asthma, particularly in children. Asthmatic children with larger numbers of positive immediate skin tests tend to have more severe disease.[3] This relationship does not occur in adults with asthma.[4]

The assessment of the possible role of allergy in causing attacks of asthma can often be difficult. The main points from the history are summarized in Table 4.3. Sensitivity to a specific allergen can be confirmed by skin-prick testing or the *in vitro* determination of IgE (see Chapter 9).

TABLE 4.2: *Inhaled allergens and asthma*

Allergen	Comments
Pollens	
Grass	Seasonal asthma (May–July)
Weeds (e.g. ragweed)	Seasonal asthma (Aug.–Oct.); important in North America
Tree	Seasonal asthma (Feb.–May); birch pollen important in Scandinavia
Fungi	
Aspergillus fumigatus	Causes allergic bronchopulmonary aspergillosis
Cladosporium sp., *Alternaria* sp.	Importance in causing asthma unclear; peak spore levels in late summer and early autumn
House-dust mite	
Dermatophagoides spp.	Commonest positive skin-prick test found in asthmatic patients in many countries
Animal danders	
Cats	Symptoms may be related to species,
Dogs	e.g. dogs. Siamese cats and other
Birds	cats: allergen may persist in
Horses	household furnishings and cause
Hamsters	asthma in sensitive subjects
Rabbits	
Mice	
Rats	
Gerbils	
Guinea-pigs	

SPECIFIC ALLERGENS CAUSING ASTHMA (Table 4.2)

Pollen Allergens

Pollens particularly from grasses, weeds and trees can cause seasonal symptoms of allergic rhinitis and/or conjunctivitis and asthma[5,6] (Table 4.2). Tree pollens usually cause symptoms in the spring months, grasses in the early and midsummer, and weeds in late summer and autumn. The importance of oil-seed rape in provoking asthma is uncertain.[7]

TABLE 4.3: *Assessment of the possible role of allergy in causing attacks of asthma: main points from the history*

Are asthma symptoms seasonal or perennial?

Is there an association between allergen exposure and environment, e.g. at home, at work, on holiday, etc.? It should be noted that symptoms may persist for several days after allergen exposure

Are there associated nasal, skin or eye symptoms after exposure to allergen?

Remember that sensitivity to allergens is commoner in children and young adults

Fungal Allergens

The most important fungus associated with asthma is *Aspergillus fumigatus.* The spores of this organism, which are 2–3 μm in diameter, are almost always found in the atmosphere and counts are highest in late autumn and winter. Allergic bronchopulmonary aspergillosis (ABPA) is characterized by the association of immunological sensitivity to *A. fumigatus*, although other fungi have been implicated,[8] and recurrent pulmonary eosinophilia. The majority of patients have asthma. In the UK and North America approximately 20% of asthmatic patients have positive skin-prick reactions to *A. fumigatus*. The exact percentage of these patients who have ABPA is unknown; estimates range between 2 and 8%. A non-asthmatic form of ABPA has been described in which patients present with non-wheezy dyspnoea often associated with low-grade fever and malaise.[9] The mechanisms by which colonization of the airways with *A. fumigatus* results in disease and the assessment and treatment of ABPA is discussed further in Chapter 33.

The importance of other airborne fungi such as *Cladosporium* sp. and *Alternaria* sp. in causing asthma is uncertain (see Chapter 14).

House-dust Mites

Allergy to the house-dust mites *Dermatophagoides pteronyssinus* or *Dermatophagoides farinae* is an important cause of asthma. *Dermatophagoides pteronyssinus* is the commonest allergen causing IgE-mediated sensitivity in asthma, particularly among asthmatic children. The assessment and treatment of house-dust mite allergy is discussed further in Chapter 14.

Animal and Insect Allergens

Household pets can cause asthma due to allergy not only to the animal's dander but also to its saliva, urine or faeces (Table 4.2). Cats are probably the most frequent pet to cause allergic symptoms (see Chapter 14 for more details). The cockroach allergen can cause asthma in sensitive individuals in warm climates and inner city areas in cooler climates[10] (see Chapter 14 for more details).

TYPES OF ASTHMATIC RESPONSE TO INHALED ALLERGEN

Two main types of asthmatic response occur after allergen exposure.[8] The early or immediate asthmatic response peaks at 10–30 min after allergen exposure and subsides by 1–2 hours. The late asthmatic response starts 3–4 hours after allergen exposure, and usually begins to resolve by 6–12 hours. The possible pathogenic mechanisms involved in allergen-induced asthma are reviewed elsewhere[8] (see Chapter 3).

INFECTIONS

Respiratory tract infections are thought frequently to precipitate attacks of asthma, particularly in children.[11] Infections are mainly viral, especially human rhinoviruses but also respiratory syncytial virus, adenoviruses, parainfluenza and influenza viruses.[12,13] The role of infection in provoking asthma attacks in adults is less certain.[11] Bacterial infections seem rarely to precipitate asthma.[14]

Viral respiratory infections are thought to be involved as "inducers" of asthma although this association is difficult to establish (see reference 12). Interestingly a history of a respiratory infection precedes the development of late-onset asthma in adults in up to 50% of cases. The mechanism by which viral infections might exacerbate asthma is unclear but may involve epithelial damage, stimulation of virus-specific IgE antibodies, airway inflammation and/or sensitization of sensory vagal nerve endings.[11,13] Respiratory tract infections can cause transient increases in bronchial reactivity to non-specific stimuli such as histamine, and this effect may last for 6 weeks after the infection.

OCCUPATIONAL AGENTS

Occupational asthma occurs when agents at work cause asthma.[15] It is thought to account for up to 5% of all cases of adult asthma. There are well over 200 reported cases of occupational asthma.[16] Some of the commoner causes are listed in Table 4.4. Atopic subjects are more likely to

TABLE 4.4: *Causes of occupational asthma*

Agent	Industries
Isocyanates	Plastics, polyurethane foam makers, paints, varnish, adhesives, printing
Grains and flour	Bakers, millers, farmers
Laboratory animals	Laboratory workers exposed to rats, mice, guinea-pigs, rabbits, locusts
Epoxy resins, e.g. phthalic anhydride, triethylene tetramine	Plastics, adhesives and paint workers
Colophony	Electronics
Platinum salts	Platinum metal refiners and in some laboratories
Crustaceans	Processing of crabs, prawns
Woods	Workers using various woods including western red cedar, oak, mahogany, iroka, walnut
Drugs	Manufacturers of pharmaceuticals including cimetidine, psyllium, penicillin, cephalosporins, tetracyclines, sulphathiazole, ispaghula
Ispaghula powder	Manufacture of bulk laxatives
Castor bean dust	Merchant seamen
Other chemicals, e.g.	
Formaldehyde	Plastics; medical staff
Azodicarbonamide	Plastics and rubber
Ethylenediamine	Photographic processors
Other metals, e.g.	
Cobalt	Hard metal industry
Nickel	Metal plating
Reactive dyes, e.g.	
Henna	Hairdressing
Proteolytic enzymes	Manufacture of washing powders, also in brewing, baking and leather industries

develop occupational asthma to high molecular weight agents such as animal products, but not to low molecular weight compounds such as isocyanates. Patients diagnosed late and with severe disease are more likely to have persistent asthma symptoms following removal from the offending occupational agent. Thus, early diagnosis and complete removal from the industrial agent is very important. The diagnosis and treatment of occupational asthma is discussed in Chapter 31. Occupational agents can induce airway inflammation, bronchial hyperreactivity and symptoms of asthma (see Chapter 3). This airway response should be differentiated from that caused by "inciters" of asthma that may be encountered at work, e.g. irritants or exercise. These stimuli produce symptoms of asthma because the airways are inflamed and hyperreactive but probably do not induce chronic airway inflammation.

DRUGS

Many drugs have been reported to lead to exacerbations of asthma[17,18] (Table 4.5). The drugs that most frequently provoke asthma are reviewed below.

ASPIRIN AND OTHER NON-STEROIDAL ANTI-INFLAMMATORY DRUGS

The true incidence of aspirin-induced asthma is unknown. It has been estimated that between 3 and 5% of adult asthmatic patients develop asthma after ingesting aspirin or other non-steroidal anti-inflammatory drugs (NSAIDs), but the incidence is higher when oral aspirin challenges are performed.[19] This condition is rarely seen in children.

Clinical features include acute severe bronchoconstriction that develops within minutes to several hours after ingestion of aspirin or other NSAIDs, such as indomethacin, naproxen, ibuprofen, flurbiprofen or mefenamic acid. The asthmatic symptoms may be associated with rhinorrhoea, flushing and loss of consciousness. Fatal attacks have been recorded. There is often a past history of chronic rhinitis and nasal polyps before asthma develops. These patients often have chronic severe perennial asthma requiring regular oral corticosteroid treatment. A small percentage of these patients also develop urticaria and angio-oedema after aspirin ingestion.

The possible mechanisms involved in aspirin and other NSAIDs-induced asthma are discussed in Chapter 32.

β-ADRENOCEPTOR ANTAGONISTS

Bronchoconstriction is more likely to occur with non-selective than selective β-adrenoceptor antagonists. Nevertheless severe asthma can occur with selective β-adrenoceptor antagonists such as atenolol or metaprolol and has also been reported with timolol eye drops when used to treat glaucoma.

TABLE 4.5: *Drug-induced asthma: some of the drugs reported to cause asthma in susceptible individuals*

ACTH
ACE inhibitors
Aminophylline (ethylenediamine)
Aspirin and other non-steroidal anti-inflammatory drugs
β-Adrenoceptor antagonists
Cholinergic drugs, e.g. pilocarpine
Cholinesterase inhibitors, e.g. pyridostigmine
Contrast media
Dextrans
Hydrocortisone
Inhaled agents, e.g.
   Short and long acting β₂ agonists
   Corticosteroids
   Hypotonic solutions
   Ipratropium bromide
   Local anaesthetics
   Pentamidine
   Sodium cromoglycate
Pancreozymin
Penicillin
Quinine
Sulphasalazine

Fatal attacks of asthma have been reported after the ingestion of β-adrenoceptor antagonists. All β-adrenoceptor antagonists should be avoided in patients with asthma. In the treatment of hypertension or ischaemic heart disease in a patient with asthma, calcium antagonists, nitrates, thiazides, can be used safely.

The possible mechanisms involved in β-blocker induced asthma are unknown. These drugs may block inhibitory presynaptic β receptors on vagal nerves resulting in increased vagal-induced bronchoconstriction.[19]

ANGIOTENSIN-CONVERTING ENZYME (ACE) INHIBITORS
ACE inhibitors can cause cough. Occasionally cases have been reported of worsening asthma due to these drugs.[20]

INHALED DRUGS
Cough and/or bronchospasm have been reported following the administration of nearly all types of inhaled drugs. Asthmatic patients may develop

bronchoconstriction with topical local anaesthetics administered during fibreoptic bronchoscopy[21] or with inhaled pentamidine when used prophylactically for *Pneumocystis carinii* pneumonia.[22] Bronchodilation treatment should be given to prevent these reactions occurring.

FOODS AND DRINKS

Foods and drinks are uncommon causes of asthma in adults and in the majority of children.[23] Asthma symptoms are often accompanied by other allergic symptoms, e.g. urticaria, rhinitis. Food allergy may be commoner in asthmatic children of Indian descent. The commonest foods and additives causing asthma include nuts, milk, eggs, tartrazine (yellow colouring agent), cola drinks, metabisulphite (preservative)[24] and possibly monosodium L-glutamate. Alcoholic drinks can cause bronchoconstriction in some patients, and this response is usually due to congeners but can be caused by ethanol itself. The diagnosis and treatment of food allergy is discussed in Chapter 40.

EXERCISE

After sufficient exercise most asthmatic patients develop exercise-induced asthma.[25–27] Exercise-induced asthma is often a problem in children and in adults involved in physical sports and may be the sole symptom in some patients with mild asthma. The maximum degree of bronchoconstriction occurs usually about 5–10 min after the cessation of exercise and symptoms subside within 15–30 min. There is often a refractory period of around 2 hours after the development of exercise-induced asthma. During this period repeated exercise does not cause bronchospasm. The diagnosis and management of exercise-induced asthma is discussed in Chapter 34.

Exercise-induced asthma is thought to be due to loss of water from the respiratory mucosa possibly also associated with cooling and drying of the airway.[25,27] The ventilation rate appears to be the critical factor causing these effects. The loss of water increases the osmolarity in the lining of the airway and this is thought to result in bronchoconstrictor mediator release from mast cells. Alternatively it has been suggested that bronchoconstriction is due to reactive hyperaemia of the bronchial circulation and associated airway oedema.[28]

HYPERVENTILATION

Voluntary isocapnic hyperventilation and aerosols of distilled or hypertonic solutions may produce bronchoconstriction through similar mechanisms to those of exercise.[27] Crying and laughing can both provoke symptoms of asthma.

ENVIRONMENTAL FACTORS

INDOOR IRRITANTS

The inhalation of irritants such as cigarette smoke, wood smoke and strong odours and sprays, e.g. perfume, household cleaning agents, fresh paint, can all precipitate attacks of asthma. The asthmatic children of mothers who smoke have more acute attacks, worse lung function and increased drug requirements than non-smoking mothers.[29,30] Maternal smoking is also associated with an increased incidence of asthma in children who live in the house.[31]

AIR POLLUTANTS

Outdoor pollutants have been implicated as inciters of asthma and as contributing to the rising prevalence of asthma. Ozone, produced by the effect of sunlight on traffic fumes, can cause reductions in lung function and bronchoconstriction in normal and asthmatic individuals taking exercise when atmospheric ozone concentrations are elevated, as can occur during hot summer months.[32] Asthmatic patients are not more likely to be sensitive to the airway effects of ozone than normal individuals. Those asthmatic patients sensitive to ozone, however, are likely to experience more severe respiratory symptoms. Asthmatic patients can experience acute respiratory symptoms including cough, chest tightness and wheeze when exposed to elevated atmospheric concentrations of sulphur dioxide.[33] Elevated concentrations of particulate air pollutants, which are emitted mainly from diesel vehicles, have been associated with acute attacks of asthma and with increased morbidity.[34,35] Nitrogen dioxide is thought to have limited direct effects on airway function in asthma.[36] However, recent studies have implicated nitrogen dioxide as contributing towards acute respiratory infections in children.[37]

ATMOSPHERIC TEMPERATURE

The inhalation of cold air can precipitate symptoms in asthmatic patients. Exercise-induced asthma is more likely to occur when an asthmatic patient is exercising in cold weather. Thunderstorms have been reported to be associated with sudden increases in asthma attacks.[38] Damp housing and mould have been related to increased respiratory symptoms in patients with asthma.[39,40]

NOCTURNAL ASTHMA

Patients with poorly controlled asthma frequently wheeze at night. The cause is not fully established but appears to involve the effects of increased vagal tone and reduced non-adrenergic non-cholinergic tone acting on a hyperreactive airway. In addition, airway inflammation is increased at night, which may contribute to airway narrowing[41,42] (see Fig. 35.2). The assessment and management of nocturnal asthma are discussed in Chapter 35.

PSYCHOLOGICAL FACTORS

Adverse psychological factors may contribute to poor asthma control, but do not cause asthma. In susceptible individuals increased anti-asthma treatment usually results in a reduction in the adverse effects of stress but specific psychological treatments may on occasions also be helpful.[43]

An increased mortality from asthma is associated with depression, recent family loss, recent unemployment, schizophrenia and alcohol abuse.[44,45] Asthma can cause psychological symptoms including panic attacks and low self-esteem.

PREGNANCY AND PRE-MENSES

Approximately 40% of asthmatic patients require more anti-asthma medication during pregnancy and 20% require less therapy.[46] In an individual asthmatic patient the effect of pregnancy on asthma control may differ in successive pregnancies. Asthma control deteriorates in approximately one-third of female asthmatic patients before menses.[47] The management of asthma in pregnancy and premenstrual asthma are discussed in Chapter 36.

THYROID DISEASE

The development of hyperthyroidism may result in a worsening of asthma control, with subsequent improvement after treatment of the thyrotoxicosis.[48-50] Conversely the occurrence of hypothyroidism has been reported to be associated with improvement in asthma control.[50] Several possible mechanisms may account for the relationship between asthma and thyroid disease and these include alterations in β-adrenergic function, airway reactivity, arachidonic acid metabolism, hydrocortisone metabolism or respiratory muscle function.[51]

GASTRO-OESOPHAGEAL REFLUX

Gastro-oesophageal reflux can trigger attacks of asthma although the incidence is unclear. The mechanism is unknown; possibilities include aspiration or an oesophago-bronchial reflex triggered by acid irritation of the oesophageal mucosa. Xanthines relax the lower oesophageal sphincter and may precipitate reflux by this mechanism. The management of gastro-oesophageal reflux and asthma is discussed in Chapter 38.

REFERENCES

1. Platts-Mills TAE, de Weck AI. Dust mite allergens and asthma – a worldwide problem. J Allergy Clin Immunol 1989; 83: 416–27.

2. Sporik R, Holgate ST, Platts-Mills TAE, Cogswell JJ. Exposure to housedust mite allergen and the development of asthma in childhood: a prospective study. N Engl J Med 1990; 323: 502–7.

3. Zimmerman B, Feanny S, Reisman J et al. Allergy in asthma. I. The dose relationship of allergy to severity of childhood asthma. J Allergy Clin Immunol 1988; 81: 63–77.

4. Innouye T, Tarlo S, Broder I et al. Severity of asthma in skin test-negative and skin test-positive patients. J Allergy Clin Immunol 1985; 75: 313–19.

5. Boulet L-P, Cartier A, Thomson NC et al. Asthma and increases in non-allergic bronchial responsiveness from seasonal pollen exposure. J Allergy Clin Immunol 1983; 71: 399–406.

6. Reid MJ, Moss RB, Hsu Y-P. Seasonal asthma in Northern California: allergy causes and efficacy of immunotherapy. J Allergy Clin Immunol 1986; 78: 590–600.

7. McSharry C. New aeroallergens in agricultural and related practice. Clin Exp Allergy 1992; 22: 423–6.

8. Cockcroft DW. Allergens. In: Barnes PJ, Rodger IW, Thomson NC (eds) Asthma: Basic Mechanisms and Clinical Management, 2nd edn. London: Academic Press, 1992: 413–33.

9. Berkin KE, Vernon DRH, Kerr JW. Lung collapse caused by allergic bronchopulmonary aspergillosis in non-asthmatic patients. BMJ 1982; 285: 552–3.

10. Lan J-L, Lee D-T, Wu C-H et al. Cockroach hypersensitivity: preliminary study of allergic cockroach asthma in Taiwan. J Allergy Clin Immunol 188; 82: 736–40.

11 Busse WW, Calhoun WJ. Infections. In: Barnes PJ, Rodger IW, Thomson NC (eds) *Asthma: Basic Mechanisms and Clinical Management*, 2nd edn. London: Academic Press, 1992: 452–71.

12 Pattemore PK, Johnston SL, Bardin PG. Viruses as precipitants of asthma. I. Epidemiology. *Clin Exp Allergy* 1992; 22: 325–6.

13 Bardin PG, Johnston SL, Pattemore PK. Viruses as precipitants of asthma symptoms. II. Physiology and mechanisms. *Clin Exp Allergy* 1992; 22: 809–22.

14 Berman SZ, Mathison DA, Stevenson DD, Tan EM, Vaughan JH. Trans-tracheal aspiration studies in asthmatic patients in relapse with "infective" asthma and in subjects without respiratory disease. *J Allergy Clin Immunol* 1975; 56: 206–14.

15 Newman-Taylor AJ. Occupational asthma. In: Barnes PJ, Rodger IW, Thomson NC (eds) *Asthma: Basic Mechanisms and Clinical Management*, 2nd edn. London: Academic Press, 1992: 435–49.

16 Chan-Yeung M, Lam S. Occupational asthma. *Am Rev Respir Dis* 1986; 133: 686–703.

17 Israel-Biet D, Labrune S, Huchon GJ. Drug-induced lung disease: 1990 review. *Eur Respir J* 1991; 4: 465–78.

18 Meeker DP, Wiedemann HP. Drug-induced bronchospasm. *Clin Chest Med* 1990; 11: 163–75.

19 Barnes PJ, Thomson NC. Drug-induced asthma. In: Barnes PJ, Rodger IW, Thomson NC (eds) *Asthma: Basic Mechanisms and Clinical Management*, 2nd edn. London: Academic Press, 1992: 499–513.

20 Lunde H, Hedner T, Samuelsson O *et al.* Dyspnoea, asthma and broncho-spasm in relation to treatment with angiotensin converting enzyme inhibi-tors. *BMJ*, 1994; 308: 18–21.

21 McAlpine LG, Thomson NC. Lidocaine-induced bronchoconstriction in asthmatic patients. Relation to histamine airway responsiveness and effect of preservative. *Chest* 1989; 96: 1012–15.

22 Conte JE Jr, Hollander H, Golden JA. Inhaled or reduced dose intravenous pentamidine for *Pneumocystis carinii* pneumonia. *Ann Intern Med* 1987; 107: 495–8.

23 Metcalfe DD, Sampson HA. Workshop on experimental methodology for clinical studies of adverse reactions to foods and food additives. *J Allergy Clin Immunol* 1990; 86: 421–42.

24 Bush RK, Taylor SL, Busse W. A critical evaluation of clinical trials in reac-tions to sulfites. *J Allergy Clin Immunol* 1986; 78: 191–202.

25 Godfrey S, Bar-Yishay E. Exercise-induced asthma revisited. *Respir Med* 1993; 87: 331–44.

26 McFadden ER, Gilbert IA. Exercise-induced asthma. *N Engl J Med* 1994; 330: 1362-7.

27 Anderson SD. Asthma provoked by exercise, hyperventilation and the inhalation of non-isotonic aerosols. In: Barnes PJ, Rodger IW, Thomson NC (eds) *Asthma: Basic Mechanisms and Clinical Management*, 2nd edn. London: Academic Press, 1992: 473-90.

28 McFadden ER. Hypothesis: exercise-induced asthma as a vascular phenomenon. *Lancet* 1990; 335: 880-2.

29 Evans D, Levison MJ, Feldman CH *et al*. The impact of passive smoking on emergency room visits of urban children with asthma. *Am Rev Respir Dis* 1987; 135: 567-72.

30 Murray AB, Morrison BJ. Passive smoking and the seasonal difference of severity of asthma in children. *Chest* 1988; 94: 701-8.

31 Gortmaker SL, Walker DK, Jacobs FH, Ruch-Ross H. Parental smoking and the risk of childhood asthma. *Am J Public Health* 1982; 72: 574-9.

32 Ozone. Advisory group on medical aspects of air pollution exposure. London: HMSO, 1991.

33 Sulphur dioxide, acid aerosols and particulates. Advisory group on medical aspects of air pollution exposure. London: HMSO, 1992.

34 Swartz J, Slater D, Larson TV, Pierson WE, Koenig JQ. Particulate air pollution and hospital emergency room visits for asthma in Seattle. *Am Rev Respir Dis* 1993; 147: 826-31.

35 Roemer W, Hoek G, Brunekreef B. Effect of ambient winter air pollution on respiratory health of children with chronic respiratory symptoms. *Am Rev Respir Dis* 1993; 147: 118-24.

36 Oxides of nitrogen. Advisory group on medical aspects of pollution exposure. London: HMSO, 1993.

37 Samet JM, Lambert WE, Skipper BJ *et al*. Nitrogen dioxide and respiratory illness in infants. *Am Rev Respir Dis* 1993; 148: 1258-65.

38 Packe GE, Ayres JG. Asthma outbreak during a thunderstorm. *Lancet* 1985; 11: 199.

39 Strachan DP. Damp housing and childhood asthma: validation of reporting of symptoms. *BMJ* 1988; 297: 1223-6.

40 Dales RE, Burnett R, Zevonenburg H. Adverse health effects among adults exposed to home dampness and moulds. *Am Rev Respir Dis* 1991; 143: 505-9.

41 Douglas NJ. Nocturnal asthma. *Thorax* 1993; 48: 100-2.

42 Martin RJ. Nocturnal asthma: circadian rhythms and therapeutic interventions. *Am Rev Respir Dis* 1993; 147: 525–8.

43 Lask B. Psychological treatments of asthma. *Clin Exp Allergy* 1991; 21: 625–6.

44 Miller BD. Depression and asthma: a potentially lethal mixture. *J Allergy Clin Immunol* 1987; 80: 481–6.

45 Struck RC. Identification of the fatality-prone subjects with asthma. *J Allergy Clin Immunol* 1989; 83: 477–85.

46 Schatz M, Harden KM, Forsythe A *et al.* The course of asthma during pregnancy, post partum, and with successive pregnancies: a prospective analysis. *J Allergy Clin Immunol* 1988; 81: 509–17.

47 Gibbs CJ, Coutts II, Lock R, Finnegan OC, White RJ. Premenstrual exacerbation of asthma. *Thorax* 1984; 39: 833–6.

48 Ayres J, Clark TJH. Asthma and the thyroid. *Lancet* 1981; ii: 110–11.

49 Lipworth BJ, Dhillon DP, Clark RA, Newton RW. Problems with asthma following treatment of thyrotoxicosis. *Br J Dis Chest* 1988; 82: 310–14.

50 Bush RK, Ehrlick EN, Reed CE. Thyroid disease and asthma. *J Allergy Clin Immunol* 1977; 59: 398–401.

51 Barnes PJ, Thomson NC. Neural and humoral control. In: Barnes PJ, Rodger IW, Thomson NC (eds) *Asthma: Basic Mechanisms and Clinical Management*, 2nd edn. London: Academic Press, 1992: 343–57.

KEY POINTS

1   In susceptible individuals allergens, occupational agents and probably viruses can induce airway inflammation, bronchial hyperreactivity and symptoms of asthma. These are called **inducers** of asthma.

2   Other triggers such as exercise or irritants produce symptoms of asthma because the airways are inflamed and hyperreactive but these stimuli probably do not induce chronic airway inflammation. These are called **inciters** of asthma.

5

DIAGNOSIS IN CHILDREN

Barry Zimmerman

INTRODUCTION

Asthma is the most common chronic illness in childhood.[1] Asthma is currently defined as a disease of variable airflow obstruction associated with inflammation in the airways and the symptoms of cough, wheeze and dyspnoea.[2] This definition applies to childhood asthma; however the diagnosis of asthma in children can be difficult to make. Many children are too young to do the tests that objectively measure airflow obstruction. The clinical diagnosis of cough, wheeze and shortness of breath can also be difficult in children who do not have classical wheeze and are too young to describe shortness of breath. As a result many studies have suggested that there is a significant underdiagnosis and ultimately undertreatment of childhood asthma.[3–6] Furthermore there are very little data to support the concept of airway inflammation in childhood asthma, especially very young children.[7,8]

This underdiagnosis has been partly attributed to the unwillingness of doctors to diagnose asthma in young children and the tendency to use terms such as wheezy bronchitis and asthmatic bronchitis. Clinically, physicians have felt that young children often "outgrow" intermittent and mild wheezing illnesses and are reluctant to label the child asthmatic. This reluctance may lead to treatment with cough suppressants and antibiotics even when the child has had several episodes of wheezing.[3,4,6] If asthma in childhood commonly begins before age 5 years,[9–12] and if early management of the inflammation in the airways can ameliorate the disease, then it becomes important to make the diagnosis early and treat aggressively. If, on the other hand, there is a large group of infantile wheezers with a self-limiting condition that is "outgrown", then aggressive management to prevent entrenchment of the illness may not be necessary. In some instances this might avoid side-effects from the medication. Clearly the importance of this issue relates to the choice of treatment for these patients.

DEFINING THE DISEASE

The long-term Melbourne studies[13–17] originally suggested that wheezy bronchitis and asthma were the same disease. Other studies suggested that the children fared much better if the distinction was not made between wheezy bronchitis and asthma. It was suggested that the condition should be called asthma, managed with asthma medication and the parents should be informed that the child had asthma.[3,4] Yet even in the Melbourne studies there were indications that patients diagnosed as having "wheezy bronchitis" were different from patients diagnosed as having asthma.[16] The former patients had peripheral eosinophil counts that were higher than non-wheezing controls but significantly lower than those in patients with asthma.[15]

ROLE OF ATOPY IN ASTHMA

Recent data seem to be providing a resolution to these conflicting opinions. Studies in adults have suggested that the eosinophil is a hallmark of the inflammation in asthmatic airways[18–21] and that permanent airway reactivity may result from inflammation and eosinophil activation in the airways. Atopy, especially in childhood, seems to be a major source of this inflammation, which then results in non-specific airway reactivity.[22–24] In older children with asthma, the majority are atopic while infants who wheeze with viral infections are commonly non-atopic.[11,24–26] In young wheezing children, atopy has been found to be associated with higher peripheral eosinophilia and higher levels of serum eosinophil cationic protein (ECP), a marker for eosinophilic activation,[27] than non-atopy. It seems likely that there is a group of young infants, more commonly male, who are at risk of wheezing with viral illness, possibly based on abnormal lung anatomy,[25,28–30] but who are not atopic. In this wheezing, eosinophils and perhaps other cellular components of inflammation are not mobilized to the same degree as in "true" asthma. These children are at different risk for continuation of the wheezing. As yet it is not clear whether they are at risk of recurrence later in life, perhaps with a later onset of sensitization to allergens or other environmental factors.[24] Sporik et al.[11] studied a cohort of children born to atopic parents. In this group of children who were followed from birth to age 11 years, there was a bimodal distribution of wheezing with a peak before the age of 2 years and a gradual increase thereafter. Most of the children who wheezed before age 2 years never wheezed again, while the majority who wheezed after age 2 years were still wheezing at age 11 years. The children who had transient wheezing at age 2 years were usually non-atopic at age 11 years, while those who had later onset and persistence of wheeze were usually atopic.

POST-INFECTIOUS WHEEZE

A number of studies have documented that following respiratory syncytial virus (RSV)-induced bronchiolitis, a percentage of the children continue to have recurrent wheeze with subsequent respiratory tract infections.[31-37] There has been much discussion as to whether the RSV infection induces airway hyperresponsiveness or simply selects children who are predisposed to asthma. Yet most of them have only mild symptoms, occurring primarily with viral infections, for a period of a few years after the original RSV infection.[35] The severity and persistence of these symptoms may depend in part on whether or not the syndrome occurs in an atopic individual[37] who has a greater propensity to eosinophilic inflammation.[27] Welliver suggested that wheezing with RSV infection was associated with IgE antibody to RSV.[38] This work was extended by Garofolo et al.[39] who demonstrated activation of eosinophils during RSV infection. This would suggest that post-RSV wheezing resembles asthma in the nature of the inflammation in the airways but the addition of atopy results in a more pronounced and persistent eosinophilic inflammation and therefore increased likelihood of asthma. In our own studies we found that symptomatic episodes of wheezing were associated with elevation in serum ECP in both non-atopic and atopic individuals but the levels were higher in the atopic patients.[27] The data suggest that the outcome between post-infectious wheezing and asthma has to do with the presence or absence of atopy. An atopic immune system in childhood can lead to greater eosinophilic inflammation resulting in airway reactivity and the possibility of a more persistent chronic asthma. Children inherit the tendency to wheeze and it first presents with viral respiratory infections. The addition of an atopic immune system may lead to an increase in severity and chronicity.[26] Nevertheless the management strategies for post-infectious wheezing and asthma should be similar, differing only in degree. Post-bronchiolitic wheezing has been reported to respond to steroid.[40,41]

POST-INFECTIOUS COUGH

Similar considerations apply to the diagnosis of asthma presenting with cough in the absence of wheeze. Several studies beginning with that of McFadden in adults called attention to the fact that cough could be the sole manifestation of asthma.[42] This observation has been confirmed in children.[43-45] Yet persistent cough in childhood is associated with a positive methacholine or histamine challenge test in only about 50% of children.[46] Similarly, cough is associated with less atopy and, by inference, less eosinophil mobilization and activation.[9,45] This implies that persistent cough may not always represent asthma and might signal a post-infectious phenomenon that has a different outcome from asthma, as suggested in the study by Sporik et al.[11] The distinction between post-infectious cough and asthma-variant cough may prove to be important in the long-term outcome of the illness, rather than suggesting a need for a different treatment regimen. For example, there is now evidence that treatment of croup (acute laryngotracheobronchitis) is benefited by the administration of glucocorticoid therapy,[47-51] including two studies that used a single dose of inhaled nebulized budesonide.[50,51]

Children who cough for 10–14 days or longer with each viral illness are often ill through much of the winter, with repeated viral illness leading to a cough that does not clear completely. If the viral infections occur close together some of these children have the potential to become quite ill as the symptoms snowball. Yet in the warmer months, when these children develop fewer viral illnesses, they are completely free of symptoms and require no medication. These children tend to be non-atopic and not surprisingly lack evidence for airway hyperresponsiveness.

Pertussis and pertussis-like syndromes, with paroxysmal cough leading to vomiting or an inspiratory whoop, are common in childhood. These pertussis-like syndromes can result from infection with several different organisms including RSV, parapertussis, *Mycoplasma*, etc. These organisms can trigger a syndrome of persistent post-infectious cough often termed the "100-day" cough. Experience suggests that children who tend to cough with each viral infection are most at risk of the post-infectious "100-day" cough. At the height of the paroxysmal coughing none of the medications for treatment of asthma yields improvement in symptoms. However the persistent cough seems to respond to steroid therapy.

For purposes of this discussion the term asthma will encompass the entire range from mild, self-limited post-viral wheezing (wheezy bronchitis) to chronic persistent asthma.

DIAGNOSING ASTHMA IN PRE-SCHOOL CHILDREN

A consensus statement on paediatric asthma published in 1989[52] attempted to divide the history and physical examination into: (1) features suggestive of asthma, (2) indeterminate features, and (3) features suggestive of alternative diagnoses.

Features suggestive of asthma were considered to be: (1) wheeze plus cough especially episodic, nocturnal, or early morning or exertional; (2) personal atopic features; and (3) family history of asthma and/or atopy.

Features considered to be indeterminate were: (1) productive cough and (2) recurrent infection. Since these symptoms are likely to occur with recurrent viral, rather than bacterial, infection, a trial of asthma therapy could be initiated and investigation might be started. Failure to respond to the trial of asthma medication would lead to re-evaluation.

Features suggestive of alternative diagnosis included: (1) neonatal onset, (2) failure to thrive, (3) chronic infection, (4) vomiting or reflux, (5) history of choking, cyanotic episodes, and (6) focal lung or cardiovascular signs. If these features were associated with wheezing, a trial of asthma therapy could be undertaken but investigation for alternative diagnoses would be warranted at the outset.[52]

Cough, wheeze and rattly chest are extremely common in pre-school children. In an epidemiological study in the Toronto area we found that 10% of children aged 0–5 years had had wheezing in the year prior to the study and a further 8–10% had had significant cough.[6] Other investigators have reported similar prevalences and an increase over the last 10 years.[53] These children have lower respiratory tract symptoms for a week or more with each viral infection. Children of this age can have six to eight viral respiratory tract infections per year.[54]

CLINICAL HISTORY

These children have cough with or without wheeze during the acute viral illness but then may fail to clear the symptoms completely. They are left with residual coughing, especially in the morning when they arise or with exercise or other forms of exertion. These symptoms are especially prominent when the child resides in a household with a smoker(s).[55–59] As discussed previously, many of these young children prove to be non-atopic and the youngest wheezers will outgrow the problem.[11,25] As the children get older they tend to develop fewer viral respiratory tract infections and improve. However, those children who are atopic at this time increasingly exhibit inflammation caused by the immune response to environmental allergens.

ATOPIC STATUS

Since atopy seems to predict the likelihood of persistent asthma this history must be carefully sought. A strong family history of atopy or asthma might identify the wheezing toddler more at risk of persistent asthma. A history of an immediate reaction to a food such as egg and/or the presence of significant atopic dermatitis will suggest the presence of an atopic immune system and identify children at risk for persistent asthma. Studies on the formation of IgE antibody in infancy suggest that when children are allergic in the first few years of life, they react to a food protein, commonly milk, egg or peanut.[60–62] This may be associated with a clinical reaction even at the first introduction of the food.[63] Later at around age 3 years the children may convert to airborne allergen sensitivity[60–62] and it is this sensitivity, especially to the perennial allergens such as house-dust mite and animal dander, that seems to be more important in the development of asthma.[64,65] Even prior to the development of IgE antibody to the airborne allergens, there might be developing sensitization at the cellular level, for example the subset of T lymphocytes necessary for the production of IgE antibody by B lymphocytes.[66] These T cells could be capable of producing the cytokines responsible for activating eosinophils in the airways.[67] Sporik et al.[68] have studied the development of asthma and found that those children with asthma at age 11 years had lived in houses with the highest levels of house-dust mite in their first year of life. Although these investigators did not comment on the immune status of the children in infancy, it seems likely that sensitivity to house-dust mite was having an effect before these children could easily be recognized as allergic.

DIFFERENTIAL DIAGNOSES

Children who have recurrent lower respiratory tract symptoms with each viral illness are common in the pre-school age. Asthma is by far the commonest cause of these symptoms while alternative diagnoses are far less common and can usually be excluded by history. Cystic fibrosis occurs in approximately 1 in 2000 children[69] compared to asthma in 1 in 10 children.[6] Other diagnoses such as an immune system problem, gastro-oesophageal reflux and recurrent aspiration, aspiration of a foreign body, tracheobronchiomalacia, bronchial stenosis and congenital heart disease are also less common than asthma. A history of failure to thrive, recurrent bacterial infections, significant vomiting or reflux, choking cyanotic episodes, sudden onset of symptoms after possible aspiration with no indication of a viral illness would suggest the need for further investigation. Physical examination revealing localized chest or cardiovascular abnormalities would also indicate the need for further investigation. Investigation should begin with a simple chest X-ray, but could include a sweat test, immune function tests, primarily quantitative immunoglobulins including IgG subsets, reflux studies and other more specific tests.

TRIAL OF ASTHMA THERAPY

A trial of therapy is often initiated as part of the diagnostic evaluation. In the very young, this can mean a trial of steroids, since inhaled steroids can be administered even to the youngest children. Failure to respond to an adequate dose of inhaled steroids within 3–4 weeks would suggest the need to re-evaluate the diagnosis. Failure could result from three general possibilities: (1) poor parental compliance with administration of medication either for philosophical or technical reasons; (2) a diagnosis other than asthma; or (3) more significant asthma than first appreciated or an intercurrent respiratory tract infection exacerbating the asthma. Whatever the cause, it is not unreasonable to initiate investigation beginning with a chest X-ray and a review of the history and physical examination in order to seek alternative diagnoses.

In summary, there are no tests in the pre-school age group that are definitive for the diagnosis of asthma. A chest X-ray should be done in any severe or unusual case to exclude foreign body or congenital anomaly. Selected allergy testing might help to assess aetiology and prognosis. Properly done skin tests are valid even in infants[70,71] and can help to identify atopic asthma. Even when the tests are negative but the asthma proves to be moderate in severity, atopy should be considered to be present and preventive measures instituted.

DIAGNOSING ASTHMA IN SCHOOL-AGE CHILDREN

At this age children are able to perform simple spirometry and the diagnosis can be supported with more formal evaluation. Moreover the majority of asthmatic children in this age group, especially those with significant asthma, are atopic[9] and allergy skin tests should be done.

CLINICAL HISTORY

The diagnosis of asthma will be suggested from a characteristic history of recurrent wheeze with or without cough or recurrent cough by itself. The child often has a prior history of cough and/or wheeze with each viral illness and a history of similar symptoms on exercise. There may also be symptoms occurring between respiratory tract infections at night or in the morning on rising. Children with a history of night or morning cough due to asthma may also have symptoms with exercise or in cold air.

Even in this age group a persistent cough may follow an infectious episode, particularly if the episode was associated with paroxysmal coughing. This persistent cough is more likely to be asthma if the child has had a prior history of symptoms with each viral respiratory tract infection, or if the child is allergic. If there is a family history of atopy and/or asthma, there is greater likelihood for expression of asthma with the viral illness. In the presence of these prognostic features, the chances for recurrent symptoms increases, while in their absence recurrent asthma becomes less likely.

PULMONARY FUNCTION TESTS

The pathophysiology of a simple post-infectious cough is not known and therefore it is not clear whether there is a resemblance to asthma.[5] Clinical experience suggests the cough might respond to treatment with inhaled steroids. A positive methacholine or histamine challenge test would increase the possibility that the cough represents asthma. Similarly, the diagnosis would be more likely if variability of forced expiratory volume in 1 s (FEV_1) or peak flows can be documented (e.g. a 15–20% response to inhaled β_2 agonist). Excessive variability in home peak flow monitoring, either a diurnal variation of 20% or more or day-to-day variation of 20% or more, would suggest the diagnosis of asthma. However the recognition of this variability may require that the maximum peak flow reading be established for each individual child, usually by a period of treatment with steroids, oral or inhaled.

Home peak flow monitoring can also be helpful in suggesting whether symptoms occurring only with exercise are due to asthma. Once the individual child's maximum has been established, readings can be examined after exercise in order to look for a fall of 20%, which suggests reversible airway obstruction. Similar strategies can be used to help distinguish between hyperventilation syndrome and asthma.

ATOPIC STATUS

The presence of an atopic immune system in a child with recurrent respiratory symptoms suggests the possibility of asthma. An elevated serum IgE[72] or elevated peripheral eosinophil count (in asthma the elevation is often in the high normal range)[73] might suggest the possibility of asthma. A history suggestive of allergy can be sought. Significant eczema in infancy or an immediate reaction (e.g. hives or swelling) to a food, commonly milk, egg, peanut, nut or fish, would suggest the presence of atopy. Symptoms exhibited in the presence of animals (dog, cat, horse, etc.), including rhinitis, conjunctivitis, asthma, hives or symptoms of allergic rhinitis especially with a seasonal variation, would suggest atopy, which in turn heightens the risk of asthma.[9]

DIFFERENTIAL DIAGNOSES

In this age group, asthma is by far the commonest diagnostic possibility for cough and wheeze. Alternative diagnoses might be suggested by physical examination. A chest X-ray, sinus X-ray and possibly a sweat test could be done. At least one-third of sinus X-rays will be abnormal in simple uncomplicated asthma, and the significance of these abnormalities is a matter of some controversy.[74,75] The abnormal X-rays are generally not associated with symptoms of sinusitis and may result from the same inflammation occurring in both the upper and lower respiratory tract.[75] Symptomatic sinusitis should be treated and recurrent bacterial infections of sinuses and elsewhere would suggest the need for an immunological work-up, particularly looking for an IgG subset deficiency.[76–78] IgG subset deficiency is uncommon but can present in very young children beginning with recurrent otitis media, sinusitis and cough. Recurrent or persistent symptomatic sinusitis, nasal discharge and cough might also suggest the need for nasal ciliary studies to rule out dysmotile cilia syndrome. A history of heartburn and reflux would suggest the need for more sophisticated studies of reflux with a pH probe. A trial of therapy for reflux would be warranted if the diagnosis can be entertained from the history. Occasionally a Mantoux test might be indicated.

TRIAL OF THERAPY

Because asthma is by far the commonest diagnosis, a trial of therapy should always be undertaken if a work-up for alternative diagnoses is negative. The therapy should include inhaled steroids and home peak flow monitoring along with a symptom diary card. This trial should be undertaken aggressively for a 3–4 week period, since most childhood asthma would be expected to show some response to inhaled steroids within that time.

CONCLUSION

At any age the diagnosis of asthma includes a wide range of severity from mild intermittent symptoms to continuous and severe. Even in older children there is no one test that will determine the severity of an individual patient's asthma. It is possible that in future tests that reflect airway inflammation, e.g. sputum eosinophil measurements[79,80] or measurement of granular proteins from blood eosinophils such as serum ECP levels,[73,81] might help to distinguish subtypes of asthma, but at present patients must be managed according to their clinical status.[82-84]

REFERENCES

1 Dodge RR, Burrows B. The prevalence and incidence of asthma and asthma-like symptoms in a general population sample. *Am Rev Respir Dis* 1980; 122: 567-75.

2 Sears MR. The definition and diagnosis of asthma. *Allergy* 1993; 48: 12-6.

3 Speight ANP, Lee DA, Hey EN. Underdiagnosis and undertreatment of asthma in childhood. *BMJ* 1983; 286: 1253-6.

4 Anderson HR, Bailey PA, Cooper JS, Palmer JC. Influence of morbidity, illness label, and social, family and health service factors on drug treatment of childhood asthma. *Lancet* 1981; ii: 1030-2.

5 Clifford RD, Radford M, Howell JB, Holgate ST. Prevalence of respiratory symptoms among 7 and 11 year old school children and association with asthma. *Arch Dis Child* 1989; 64: 1118-25.

6 Kirshner B, Gold M, Zimmerman B. Comparison between the prevalence and treatment of wheezing and coughing in Brampton and Mississauga children. *J Clin Epidemiol* 1990; 43: 765-71.

7 Gemou-Engesaeth V, Kay AB, Bush A, Corrigan CJ. Activated peripheral blood CD4 and CD8 T-lymphocytes in child asthma: correlation with eosinophilia and disease severity. *Pediatr Allergy Immunol* 1994; 5: 170-7.

8 Ferguson AC, Wong FW. Bronchial hyperresponsiveness in asthmatic children. Correlation with macrophages and eosinophils in broncholavage fluid. *Chest* 1989; 96: 988-91.

9 Zimmerman B, Feanny S, Reisman J *et al.* Allergy in asthma 1. The dose relationship of allergy to severity of childhood asthma. *J Allergy Clin Immunol* 1988; 81: 61-70.

10 Godfrey S. Childhood asthma. In: Clark TJH, Godfrey S (eds) *Asthma*, 2nd edn. London: Chapman and Hall, 1983: 415-56.

11 Sporik R, Holgate ST, Cogswell JJ. Natural history of asthma in childhood – a birth cohort study. *Arch Dis Child* 1991; 66: 1050-3.

12 Croner S, Kjellman NIM. Natural history of bronchial asthma in childhood. A prospective study from birth up to 12–14 years of age. *Allergy* 1992; 47: 150-7.

13 Williams HE, McNichol KN. Prevalence, natural history and relationship of wheezy bronchitis and asthma in children. An epidemiological study. *BMJ* 1969; 4: 321–5.

14 McNichol KN, Williams HE. Spectrum of asthma in children – I, Clinical and physiological components. *BMJ* 1973; 4: 7–11.

15 McNichol KN, Williams HE. Spectrum of asthma in children – II, Allergic components. *BMJ* 1973; 4: 12–6.

16 Martin AJ, Landau LI, Phelan PD. Predicting the course of asthma in children. *Aust Paediatr J* 1982; 18: 84–7.

17 Kelly WJW, Hudson I, Raven J, Phelan PD, Pain MCF, Olinsky A. Childhood asthma and adult lung function. *Am Rev Respir Dis* 1988; 138: 26–30.

18 Holgate ST. Mediator and cellular mechanisms in asthma. *J R Coll Physicians Lond* 1990; 24: 304–12.

19 Filley WV, Holley KE, Kephart GM, Gleich GJ. Identification by immunofluorescence of eosinophilic granule major basic protein in lung tissues of patients with bronchial asthma. *Lancet* 1982; ii: 11–6.

20 Venge P, Dahl R, Fredens K, Peterson CGB. Epithelial injury by human eosinophils. *Am Rev Respir Dis* 1988; 138: 54–7.

21 Kay AB. Eosinophils as effector cells in immunity and hypersensitivity disorders. *Clin Exp Immunol* 1985; 62: 1–12.

22 Cockcroft DW, Murdock KY, Berscheid BA. Relationship between atopy and bronchial responsiveness to histamine in a random population. *Ann Allergy* 1984; 53: 26–9.

23 Sears MR, Burrows B, Flannery EM, Herbison GP, Hewitt CJ, Holdaway MD. Relation between airway responsiveness and serum IgE in children with asthma and in apparently normal children. *N Engl J Med* 1991; 325: 1067–71.

24 Van Asperen PP, Kemp AS, Mukhi A. Atopy in infancy predicts the severity of bronchial hyperresponsiveness in later childhood. *J Allergy Clin Immunol* 1990; 85: 790–5.

25 Morgan WJ, Martinez FD. Risk factors for developing wheezing and asthma in childhood. *Pediatr Clin North Am* 1992; 39: 1185–203.

26 Zimmerman B, Chambers C, Forsyth S. Allergy in asthma II. The highly atopic infant and chronic asthma. *J Allergy Clin Immunol* 1988; 81: 71–6.

27 Zimmerman B, Enander I, Zimmerman R, Ahlstedt S. Asthma in children less than 5 years of age: eosinophils and serum levels of the eosinophil proteins ECP and EPX in relation to atopy and symptoms. *Clin Exp Allergy* 1994; 24: 149–55.

28 Martinez FD, Morgan WJ, Wright AL, Holberg C, Taussig LM. Initial airway function is a risk factor for recurrent wheezing respiratory illnesses during the first three years of life. *Am Rev Respir Dis* 1991; 143: 312–6.

29 Martinez FD, Morgan WJ, Wright AL, Holberg CJ, Taussig LM. Diminished lung function as a predisposing factor for wheezing respiratory illness in infants. *N Engl J Med* 1988; 319: 1112–7.

30 Young S, Arnott J, Le Souef PN, Landau LI. Flow limitation during tidal expiration in symptom-free infants and the subsequent development of asthma. *J Pediatr* 1994; 124: 681–8.

31 Kattan M, Keens T, Lapierre JG *et al.* Pulmonary function abnormalities in symptom-free children after bronchiolitis. *Pediatrics* 1977; 59: 683–8.

32 Gurwitz D, Mindorff C, Levison H. Increased incidence of bronchial reactivity in children with a history of bronchiolitis. *J Pediatr* 1981; 98: 551–5.

33 Sims DG, Downham MA, Gardner PS, Webb JK, Weightman D. Study of 8 year old children with a history of respiratory syncytial virus bronchiolitis in infancy. *BMJ* 1978; 1: 11–4.

34 Mok JY, Simpson H. Outcome of acute lower respiratory tract infection in infants: Preliminary report of seven year follow-up study. *BMJ* 1982; 285: 333–7.

35 Pullan CR, Hey E. Wheezing, asthma and pulmonary dysfunction 10 years after infection with respiratory syncytial virus in infancy. *BMJ* 1982; 284: 1665–9.

36 Sims D, Gardner PS, Weightman D, Turner MW, Soothill JF. Atopy does not predispose to RSV bronchiolitis or post-bronchiolitic wheezing. *BMJ* 1981; 282: 2086–8.

37 Laing I, Riedel F, Yap PL, Simpson H. Atopy predisposing to acute bronchiolitis during an epidemic of respiratory syncytial virus. *BMJ* 1982; 284: 1070–2.

38 Welliver RC, Wong DT, Sun M *et al.* The development of respiratory syncytial virus-specific IgE and the release of histamine in nasopharyngeal secretions after infection. *N Engl J Med* 1981; 305: 841–6.

39 Garofolo R, Kimpen JL, Welliver RC, Ogra PL. Eosinophilic degranulation in the respiratory tract during naturally acquired respiratory syncytial virus infection. *J Pediatr* 1992; 120: 28–32.

40 Bisgaard H, Munck S, Nielsen J *et al.* Inhaled budesonide for treatment of recurrent wheezing in early childhood. *Lancet* 1990; 336: 649–51.

41 Mayaan C, Itzhaki T, Bar-Yishay E *et al.* The functional response of infants with persistent wheezing to nebulized inhaled beclomethasone dipropionate. *Pediatr Pulmonol* 1986; 2: 9–14.

42 McFadden ER. Exertional dyspnoea and cough as preludes to acute attacks of bronchial asthma. *N Engl J Med* 1975; 292: 555–9.

43 Cloutier MM, Loughlin GM. Chronic cough in children: a manifestation of airway hyperreactivity. *Paediatrics* 1981; 67: 6–12.

44 Konig P. Hidden asthma in childhood. *Am J Dis Child* 1981; 135: 1053–5.

45 Hannaway PJ, Hopper GDK. Cough variant asthma in children. *JAMA* 1982; 247: 206–8.

46 Clifford RD, Howell JB, Radford M, Holgate ST. Association between respiratory symptoms, bronchial response to methacholine, and atopy in two age groups of schoolchildren. *Arch Dis Child* 1989; 64: 1133–9.

47 Kuusela AL, Vesikari T. A randomized double-blind placebo controlled trial of dexamethasone and racemic epinephrine in the treatment of croup. *Acta Pediatr Scand* 1988; 77: 99–104.

48 Super DM, Cartelli NA, Brooks LJ, Lembo RM, Kumar ML. A prospective randomized double-blind study to evaluate the effect of dexamethasone in acute laryngotracheitis. *J Pediatr* 1989; 115: 323–9.

49 Tibballs J, Shann FA, Landau LI. Placebo-controlled trial of prednisolone in children intubated for croup. *Lancet* 1992; 340: 745–8.

50 Husby S, Agertoft L, Mortensen S, Pedersen S. Treatment of croup with nebulized steroid (budesonide): a double blind placebo controlled study. *Arch Dis Child* 1993; 68: 352–5.

51 Klassen TP, Feldman ME, Watters LK, Sutcliffe T, Rowe PC. Nebulized budesonide for children with mild to moderate croup. *N Engl J Med* 1994; 331: 285–9.

52 Warner JO, Gotz M, Landau LI *et al.* Management of asthma: a consensus statement. *Arch Dis Child* 1989; 64: 1065–79.

53 Wright AL, Taussig L, Ray CG, Harrison HR, Holberg CJ. The Tucson children's respiratory study: II. Lower respiratory tract illness in the first year of life. *Am J Epidemiol* 1989; 129: 1232–46.

54 Welliver RC. Upper respiratory tract infections in asthma. *J Allergy Clin Immunol* 1983; 72: 341–6.

55 Coley J, Holland W, Corkhill R. Influence of passive smoking and parental phlegm on pneumonia and bronchitis in early childhood. *Lancet* 1974; ii: 1031–4.

56 Fergusson DM, Horwood LJ, Shannon FT. Parental smoking and respiratory illness in infancy. *Arch Dis Child* 1980; 55: 358–61.

57 Bland M, Bewley BR, Pollard V, Banks MH. Effect of children's and parents' smoking on respiratory symptoms. *Arch Dis Child* 1978; 53: 100–5.

58 Murray AB, Morrison BJ. The effect of smoke from the mother on the bronchial responsiveness and severity of symptoms in children with asthma. *J Allergy Clin Immunol* 1986; 76: 575–81.

59 Foratiere F, Agabiti N, Corbo GM *et al.* Passive smoking as a determinant of bronchial responsiveness in children. *Am J Respir Crit Care Med* 1994; 149: 365–70.

60 Foucard T. A follow-up study of children with asthmatoid bronchitis. I. Skin test reactions and IgE antibodies to common allergens. *Acta Paediatr Scand* 1973; 62: 633–44.

61 Zimmerman B, Forsyth S. Diagnosis of allergy in infants: Use of mixed allergen RAST disks, Phadiatop and Pediatric mix. *Clin Allergy* 1988; 18: 581–7.

62 Zeiger RS, Heller S, Mellon M, O'Connor R, Hamburger RN. Effectiveness of dietary manipulation in the prevention of food allergy in infants. *J Allergy Clin Immunol* 1986; 78: 224–38.

63 Zimmerman B, Forsyth S, Gold M. Highly atopic children: Formation of IgE antibodies to food protein especially peanut. *J Allergy Clin Immunol* 1989; 83: 764–8.

64 Platt-Mills TAE, Tovey ER, Mitchell EB, Moszoro H, Nock P, Wilkins P. Reduction of bronchial hyperreactivity during prolonged allergen avoidance. *Lancet* 1982; ii: 675–8.

65 Sears MR, Herbison GP, Holdaway MD, Hewitt CJ, Flannery EM, Silva PA. The relative risks of sensitivity to grass pollen, house dust mite and cat dander in the development of childhood asthma. *Clin Exp Allergy* 1989; 19: 419–24.

66 Leung DJM, Geha RS. Regulation of the human IgE antibody response. *Int Rev Immunol* 1987; 2: 75–91.

67 Walker C, Virchow J-C, Bruijnzeel PLB, Blaser K. T cell subsets and their soluble products regulate eosinophilia in allergic and non-allergic asthma. *J Immunol* 1991; 146: 1829–35.

68 Sporik R, Holgate ST, Platt-Mills TAE, Cogswell JJ. House dust mite allergen (Der p I) exposure and the development of sensitization and asthma in childhood; a prospective study. *N Engl J Med* 1990; 323: 502–7.

69 Cotton EK. Cystic fibrosis. In: Cherniak RM (ed) *Current Therapy of Respiratory Diseases.* Toronto: B.C. Decker, 1989: 184–9.

70 Van Asperen PP, Kemp AS, Mellis CM. Skin test reactivity and clinical allergen sensitivity in infancy. *J Allergy Clin Immunol* 1984; 73: 381–6.

71 Menardo JL, Bousquet J, Rodiere M, Astruc J, Michel F-B. Skin test reactivity in infancy. *J Allergy Clin Immunol* 1985; 75: 646–51.

72 Sears MR, Burrows B, Flannery EM, Herbison GP, Hewitt CJ, Holdaway MD. Relation between airway responsiveness and serum IgE in children with asthma and in apparently normal children. *N Engl J Med* 1991; 325: 1067–71.

73 Zimmerman B, Lanner A, Enander I, Zimmerman RS, Peterson CGB, Ahlstedt S. Total blood eosinophils, serum eosinophil cationic protein and eosinophil protein X in childhood asthma: relation to disease status and therapy. *Clin Exp Allergy* 1993; 23: 564–70.

74 Zimmerman B, Stringer D, Feanny S *et al.* Prevalence of abnormalities found by sinus X-rays in childhood asthma: lack of relation to severity of asthma. *J Allergy Clin Immunol* 1987; 80: 268–73.

75 Zimmerman B, Gold M. Role of sinusitis in asthma. *Pediatrician* 1991; 18: 312–6.

76 Smith TF, Morris EC, Bain RP. IgG subclasses in nonallergic children with chronic chest symptoms. *J Pediatr* 1984; 105: 896–900.

77 Bjorkander J, Bake B, Oxelius V-A, Hanseon LA. Impaired lung function in patients with IgA deficiency and low levels of IgG2 or IgG3. *N Engl J Med* 1985; 313: 720–4.

78 Umetsu DT, Ambrosino DM, Quinti I, Siber GR, Geha RS. Recurrent sino-pulmonary infection and impaired antibody response to bacterial capsular polysaccharide antigen in children with selective IgG-subclass deficiency. *N Engl J Med* 1985; 313: 1247–51.

79 Gibson PG, Dolovich J, Denburg J, Ramsdale EH, Hargreave FE. Chronic cough: eosinophilic bronchitis without asthma. *Lancet* 1989; i: 1346–8.

80 Gibson PG, Girgis-Gabardo A, Morris MM *et al.* Cellular characteristics of sputum from patients with asthma and chronic bronchitis. *Thorax* 1989; 44: 693–9.

81 Dahl R. Monitoring bronchial asthma in the blood. *Allergy* 1993; 48: 77–80.

82 Hargreave FE, Dolovich J, Newhouse MT (eds). The assessment and treatment of asthma: A conference report. *J Allergy Clin Immunol* 1990; 85: 1098–111.

83 Asthma: a follow up statement from an international paediatric asthma consensus group. *Arch Dis Child* 1992; 67: 240–8.

84 Guidelines for the diagnosis and management of asthma. National Heart, Lung, and Blood Institute National asthma education program expert panel report. *J Allergy Clin Immunol* 1991; 88: 425–534.

KEY POINTS

1   *Asthma in infants and toddlers:*
  - Wheezing and persistent cough is common in this age group.
  - Asthma and post-viral wheeze or cough is by far the commonest cause of these symptoms.
  - A trial of asthma therapy is warranted.
  - A history of failure to thrive; recurrent bacterial infections; significant vomiting or reflux; choking, cyanotic episodes; sudden onset of symptoms after possible aspiration suggest the need for further investigation.

2   *Asthma in school-age children:*
  - History can be supported by more formal evaluation with spirometry, peak flow measurements or, in some instances, tests for non-specific airway reactivity (methacholine or histamine challenge).
  - Personal history of allergy supports the diagnosis and should be sought.
  - In this age group asthma (including post-viral wheezing or coughing) is the most common cause of recurrent cough and wheeze by far.

6

DIAGNOSIS IN ADULTS

L.M. Fabbri, A.L. Cogo, P. Cosma, A. Guidoboni and A. Ciaccia

INTRODUCTION

The "Global Strategy for Asthma Management" prepared by an expert panel convened by the National Institute of Health and the World Health Organization[1,2] reports the following definition of asthma:

> Asthma is a chronic inflammatory disorder of the airways, in which many cells play a role, in particular eosinophils, mast cells, and T lymphocytes. In susceptible individuals this inflammation causes recurrent episodes of wheezing, breathlessness, chest tightness and cough, particularly at night and in the early morning. These symptoms are usually associated with widespread but variable airflow limitation that is at least partly reversible, either spontaneously or with treatment. The airway inflammation also causes an associated increase in airway responsiveness to a variety of stimuli.

If one accepts this definition, any lung disease that manifests itself with these symptoms and which is associated with (1) airway inflammation, (2) reversible airflow limitation, and (3) airway hyperresponsiveness may be labelled as asthma. Unfortunately, airway inflammation is not easy to measure with simple, clinically relevant methods, and airway hyperresponsiveness, which can be measured with standardized methods,[3] is not present at all times in all asthmatics,[4] may not accurately reflect the severity of the disease,[5] may be present in asymptomatic subjects,[6] and thus is not pathognomonic of asthma. The only reliable, simple objective method to confirm the diagnosis of asthma in a subject with symptoms of asthma (see below) is the assessment of reversible airflow limitation. While the spontaneous reversibility of airflow limitation may be assessed by monitoring the peak expiratory flow (PEF), the reversibility of airflow limitation induced by treatment may be assessed either by measuring PEF or forced expiratory volume in 1 s (FEV_1) before and after a single dose of a bronchodilator, or before and after a short course of full anti-asthma treatment including systemic steroids.

MINIMAL REQUIREMENTS TO ESTABLISH THE DIAGNOSIS OF ASTHMA

The diagnosis of asthma is based on careful medical history and monitoring of peak expiratory flows.

HISTORY

The characteristic symptoms of asthma are recurrent episodes of breathlessness and wheezing, often associated with cough, which are partially or completely relieved by bronchodilators. Other typical symptoms of asthma include non-productive cough, chest tightness and exercise intolerance. Cough induced by thermal stimuli, such as exposure to cold, dry air or fog, or by emotional responses (fear, crying, laughing) or an extended period of talking is a sign of bronchial lability and should also be investigated. Some patients, particularly children, complain only of a persistent, non-productive cough[7] with no wheezing or dyspnoea, while other patients have no symptoms until the airways are severely narrowed. Thus, breathlessness and wheezing cannot be the only subjective diagnostic criteria, since the individual tolerance to a given degree of dyspnoea is variable.

The onset, duration and frequency of symptoms should be carefully investigated. It is important to know the age of first attack and the patterns of symptoms, whether they have a seasonal or perennial appearance, or a day–night variation (i.e. symptoms at night or early in the morning), whether they worsen outdoors or indoors, at home or in the workplace. Several attempts have been made to find the most valid symptoms-based questions to diagnose asthma, particularly for epidemiological studies. A postal questionnaire suitable for epidemiological studies of asthma exists.[8,9] Five simple questions are included in the questionnaire developed by the International Union Against Tuberculosis and Lung Diseases, which could be used also in the single patient.

(1) Have you had wheezing or whistling in your chest at any time?

(2) Have you had an attack of shortness of breath that came on following strenuous activity at any time?

(3) Have you woken up with an attack of wheezing at any time?

(4) Have you woken up with an attack of cough at any time?

(5) Have you had an attack of shortness of breath that came on during the day when you were at rest at any time?

The sensitivity and specificity of any questionnaire should be tested. Self-reported asthma from a questionnaire has a sensitivity of 36% and a specificity of 94% if one uses airway hyperresponsiveness as the gold standard of asthma. The sensitivity increases to 68% and the specificity to 94% if one uses the clinical diagnosis as the gold standard of asthma.[10]

The relationship between the answers to a questionnaire and airway hyper-responsiveness has been reported recently.[11,12] The questions which more strongly predict the presence of airway hyperresponsiveness regard the appearance of symptoms in response to exercise or dusty environment, and/or development of symptoms at night or early in the morning. This questionnaire has a good sensitivity (65–91%) and specificity (85–96%). Even if these questionnaires have been designed for epidemiological research, the use of some questions on current respiratory symptoms can be useful to assess the diagnosis of asthma in the single individual.

Various scores have been developed to quantify the symptoms.[13] Interestingly if a questionnaire is properly used, it may help to follow single patients and to detect the deterioration of asthma before any change in PEF.[14]

Precipitating factors or aggravating factors should also be investigated carefully in order to establish the causes or trigger factors of asthma.

MEASURES OF AIRFLOW LIMITATION

The degree of airflow limitation may be assessed by physical examination, spirometry, or peak flow meters.

Physical Examination

Tachypnoea, hyperinflation of the chest, prolonged expiration, use of accessory respiratory muscles, hyperresonance of percussion note, wheezing, inspiratory and/or expiratory rhonchi reflect airflow limitation. Although physical examination remains quite an important diagnostic tool in the diagnosis and assessment of the severity of asthma exacerbations, it is of little help in the diagnosis of intermittent and mild asthma.

Spirometry and Peak Flow Monitoring (see also Chapter 7)

Lung volumes and flow can be measured with spirometers.[15,16] Vital capacity (VC) is the maximum volume of air that can be inhaled or exhaled from the lung. VC may be affected by parenchymal diseases, by chest wall diseases, by voluntary effort, and by significant airway diseases. To determine whether the reduction in VC is due to restriction or airway obstruction, measurements of flow are obtained. The most common indices of forced expiratory flow are FEV_1, the maximum volume of air expired in 1 s from full inspiration, and PEF, the maximum flow rate that can be generated during a forced expiratory manoeuvre. Although the FEV_1 is the single best measure for assessing severity of airflow obstruction, the PEF is a simple, reproducible measure of airway obstruction that correlates quite well with the FEV_1.[17] The FEV_1/VC ratio provides an early and sensitive indication of airflow obstruction. The FEV_1/VC ratio is increasingly used as a measure for diagnosis because it distinguishes between restrictive and obstructive disease.[15]

The degree of airflow limitation may be measured by spirometry or by a single set of PEF measurements. The reversibility of PEF after treatment and the variability of PEF are considered critical in establishing the diagnosis of asthma and an accurate evaluation of the severity of asthma.[1,2]

Spirometry is recommended in the initial assessment of most patients with suspected asthma, and periodically in selected patients to confirm home PEF measurements made with a peak flow meter, but subsequent measurements of PEF are sufficient to follow most adult patients in assessing the severity of symptoms and making therapeutic decisions. However, particularly in children, PEF may underestimate the severity of asthma exacerbations[18] and most peak flow meters are inaccurate.[19] Consequently, patients should be advised of these potential biases and spirometry should be performed in all subjects in whom PEF values do not fit with the clinical severity of asthma.

Peak Expiratory Flow Records

PEF is the highest flow obtained during a forced expiration starting immediately after a deep inspiration at total lung capacity. PEF can be measured with inexpensive and portable peak flow meters and in most subjects it correlates well with FEV_1. Daily monitoring of PEF over a period of time is a simple and inexpensive objective lung function test that establishes the diagnosis of asthma.[19–21] PEF measurements have some limitations. PEF is effort dependent, and proper training is required to obtain the best and most reproducible measurements from the individual. Also, PEF mainly reflects the calibre of large airways and it may therefore underestimate the degree of airflow limitation present in peripheral airways. Predicted values of PEF are related to gender, race, age and height, and normal values as well as normal limits of diurnal variability are available in the literature.[19,20]

Predicted values are useful in assessing individual measurements. However, because of the wide inter-individual variability, some subjects have PEF values that are very different from the average value of subjects with the same demographic characteristics, and some subjects with long-lasting asthma or other chronic obstructive pulmonary diseases may develop irreversible airflow limitation. For these two reasons, in addition to reference to predicted values, it is quite useful to establish the best personal PEF for each patient during a period of monitoring while the patient is under effective anti-asthma treatment. One should then refer to the personal-best PEF and the average diurnal variability identified during this period of effective treatment to assess the long-term changes and the daily variability of PEF. In other words, in clinical practice it is preferable to refer to each patient's personal best and daily variability rather than to a predicted percentage, particularly for patients with chronically impaired lung function.

To assess asthma, PEF should be measured at least twice a day, in the morning on awakening, and again in the evening hours. Further measurements should be recommended when symptoms develop, or to investigate specific allergen or workplace exposure.

Monitoring PEF provides an easy assessment of daily variability of respiratory function and activity of asthma. Diurnal variability is calculated in the following way:

$$\frac{PEF_{max} - PEF_{min}}{PEF_{max} + PEF_{min}/2} \times 100$$

In asthmatic subjects the diurnal variability of PEF is higher than in normal subjects.[17,19,20] An arbitrary limit of 20% in diurnal variability is conventionally assumed as normal.[2]

Asthma is a variable condition, and thus even a normal diurnal variation over a short period of time does not exclude asthma. In these cases it might be useful to calculate the diurnal variability from the maximum PEF measured after use of a bronchodilator. The diurnal variability of PEF measured in this way correlates with the degree of airway hyperresponsiveness to histamine.[22]

In addition to establishing the diagnosis, the monitoring of PEF is useful for adjusting the therapy and assessing its effect, for detecting early signs of deterioration and thus for determining when and how management should be revised. In some patients, an objective measurement with a PEF meter may help to distinguish whether the symptoms are caused by airflow limitation or by other factors.

REVERSIBILITY OF AIRFLOW LIMITATION INDUCED BY A SINGLE DOSE OF A SHORT-ACTING BRONCHODILATOR

In subjects with reduced lung function (e.g. PEF and/or FEV_1 less than 80% predicted), the response to a single dose of bronchodilator (e.g. two puffs of salbutamol, equivalent to 200 μg salbutamol) should be measured. Lung function measurements are usually repeated 15–30 min after the inhalation of a β-adrenergic agonist. A 12–15% increase in FEV_1 is usually assumed to be evidence of reversible airflow limitation.[15] In some patients, and particularly young patients and athletes with a history of symptoms, a reversibility test is recommended even when baseline lung function is normal, because their normal lung function might be significantly higher than the predicted value. In these cases, a marked improvement in lung function might reveal airflow limitation even if the observed PEF or FEV_1 are within normal limits.

ADDITIONAL CONFIRMATORY TESTS

In subjects with atypical history and symptoms, normal diurnal variability of PEF and/or airflow limitation not reversible by a single dose of bronchodilator, additional confirmatory tests are recommended, including the measurement of airway responsiveness to bronchoconstrictor stimuli and the reversibility of airflow limitation after a short course of steroids.

MEASUREMENT OF AIRWAY RESPONSIVENESS (see also Chapter 8)

Airway hyperresponsiveness is an exaggerated response to a large variety of physical, chemical and pharmacological bronchoconstrictor stimuli.[3] In other words airways narrow too easily and too much to a large variety of stimuli.[23]

Because, both in asthmatic and non-asthmatic subjects, airflow limitation may by itself be the cause of an exaggerated response to bronchoconstrictor stimuli, the measurement of airway hyperresponsiveness for the diagnosis of asthma is usually restricted to subjects with near-normal lung function.

The degree of airway responsiveness can be measured in the laboratory using various stimuli and methods. Because the airways respond to a variety of stimuli that, at variance with allergens and sensitizing agents, may cause airflow limitation even in normal subjects, airway hyperresponsiveness is sometimes referred to as non-specific. However, even non-specific stimuli act through very specific mechanisms and some of these stimuli (e.g. exercise, ultrasonically nebulized distilled water) cause airflow limitation only in asthmatics; thus the term "non-specific" should be avoided. Airway responsiveness should be referred to the stimulus used to measure it.

Bronchoconstrictor stimuli may be classified as causing airflow limitation *directly* by stimulating airway smooth muscles (e.g. methacholine and histamine) or *indirectly* by releasing pharmacologically active mediators (e.g. exercise, nebulized hypotonic or hypertonic solutions) or stimulating sensory nerves (e.g. metabisulphite, bradykinin), or a combination of both mechanisms.

Unlike inhalation challenges with indirect stimuli, those with histamine and methacholine have been properly standardized and validated in patients with asthma and are safe, and thus should be preferred in the clinical evaluation of patients.[3] Airway responsiveness is usually expressed as the amount of bronchoconstrictor stimulus able to change expiratory flows, i.e. the concentration (PC) or dose (PD) of the bronchoconstrictor agent that causes a certain decrease (e.g. 20%) of FEV_1 ($PC_{20}FEV_1$ or $PD_{20}FEV_1$). A $PC_{20}FEV_1$ methacholine or histamine greater than $16 \, mg \, ml^{-1}$, or a $PD_{20}FEV_1$ methacholine or histamine greater than $16 \, \mu mol$ or $1.4 \, mg^4$ are usually considered to be normal.

Airway hyperresponsiveness is present in the great majority of asthmatics, thus a negative inhalation challenge with methacholine or histamine does exclude the diagnosis of current asthma, except in subjects with occupational asthma.[4] However, in a follow-up study 33 (9%) of 334 subjects with suspected asthma but normal airway responsiveness developed asthma within 10 years. Age, a positive family history of allergy, and FEV_1 values appear to be the best predictors of future development of asthma.[24]

By contrast, up to 10% of normal asymptomatic subjects have an increased response to bronchoconstrictor stimuli and no evidence of asthma.[3,6] In a 2-year follow-up study, up to 45% of asymptomatic subjects with clear-cut hyperresponsiveness to methacholine (PD_{20} <3.2 μmol) developed asthma within 2 years, suggesting that airway hyperresponsiveness, in addition to being a feature of asthma, might be a risk factor for the development of asthma.[25] The need to treat asymptomatic airway hyperresponsiveness in order to prevent the subsequent development of asthma remains to be investigated.

REVERSIBILITY OF AIRFLOW LIMITATION INDUCED BY A COURSE OF STEROIDS

In patients with airflow limitation not relieved by a single dose of a short-acting bronchodilator, the improvement after 2 weeks of treatment with bronchodilators and steroids should be studied.[26,27]

Corticosteroids may be administered orally (e.g. 40 mg daily prednisolone), by aerosol (e.g. 2 mg daily beclomethasone) or both. Due to their efficacy and infrequent adverse events, inhaled corticosteroids are increasingly used as first-choice therapy to investigate the reversibility of airflow limitation.[28,29] Some patients with moderate or severe asthma, and up to 20% of patients with chronic obstructive pulmonary diseases, show a significant improvement in airflow limitation that confirms the presence of asthma.[27,30]

EVALUATION OF RISK FACTORS

Once the diagnosis of asthma is established, all the potential risk factors should be investigated. The major risk factors for asthma are atopy and allergen exposure.

HISTORY (see also Chapter 4)

The presence of asthma or other allergic disorders in family medical history should be investigated. History provides also important information about the life-style and the occupation, both influencing exposure to allergens, sensitizing agents and irritants, the time and the factors possibly involved in the onset of asthma, the frequency of asthmatic attacks, the exacerbation of asthmatic symptoms in relation to exposure to allergens or irritants, to physical exercise and to respiratory infections, and the evolution of asthma during the years.

The relationship should be established between exposure to one or more allergens and the occurrence of asthma symptoms and/or ocular and/or nasal symptoms. Also, the relationship should be assessed with certain months of the year (seasonal pollen asthma), with the presence in the house of pets or during certain operations of housecleaning, or at work.

The identification of possible causative risk factors (e.g. specific allergens) is important for the diagnosis and subsequent management of asthma in relation to the first step of treatment, represented, whenever possible, by allergen avoidance. Also the identification of triggers of asthma (e.g. exercise, cold air, emotions) is of paramount importance for the management of asthma, because it provides the necessary information for prevention[31] and/or pharmacological prophylaxis (e.g. pre-treatment with cromones or β_2 agonists before exercise).[2]

Allergens are the most important risk factor for asthma. House-dust mite, pollens, animal hair and dander, moulds and, in some countries, cockroaches are the allergens most frequently involved in asthma. The role of food allergy remains undetermined, but nonetheless needs to be investigated.

IN VIVO AND IN VITRO TESTS FOR ALLERGY (see also Chapter 9)
The choice of the most appropriate test to perform in a patient with suspected allergic asthma depends upon the kind of sensitization and on the nature of the allergen to be tested. No test for allergy can by itself prove that one or more allergens is/are the cause of asthma. Only the combination of history, skin tests and, in a few cases, in vitro measurement of allergen-specific IgE antibodies by radioimmunoassay or immunoenzymatic assay provides the necessary information to establish the importance of a given allergen in the development and maintenance of asthma.

Skin Tests
Skin tests with all relevant allergens to be found in the geographical area of the patient represent the first choice test in diagnosis of allergy, because they are simple, easy and rapid to perform, and are highly sensitive and specific. The method most frequently used is represented by the skin-prick test, performed by pricking the skin of the patient through a drop of the allergen extract. Skin-prick tests are reproducible and very seldom provoke systemic reactions. Although more variable and risky, intradermal tests may be used with low-potency allergen extracts.[32]

In Vitro Tests
The in vitro measurements of allergen-specific IgE antibodies by radioimmunoassay (RAST) or immunoenzymatic assay (ELISA) is much more expensive than skin-prick tests. They should be used only when skin-prick

tests cannot be performed. *In vitro* tests are specific, but not as sensitive as the *in vivo* tests. The measurement of total IgE as well as of other immunoglobulins (e.g. IgG_4) provides no additional information.[33,34]

INHALATION CHALLENGES WITH ALLERGEN, DRUGS AND CHEMICAL SENSITIZERS (see also Chapter 8)

Inhalation challenges with allergens are sometimes required to establish the relevance of single allergens for asthma. Because these tests are risky and demand skilful interpretation, they should be performed only in specialized centres.[3] Atopic individuals with airway hyperresponsiveness to methacholine or histamine often respond also to allergens to which they are skin-prick positive, but that may not be relevant for their asthma, and thus the real value of allergen provocation in the management of the single patient remains unclear. In general, because these tests are risky and do not provide real useful information on single patients, they should *not* be used in clinical practice.

By contrast, inhalation challenges with sensitizing agents such as drugs (e.g. aspirin) or small molecular weight chemical sensitizers (e.g. isocyanates), which cause asthma through a non-IgE-mediated mechanism (and thus cannot be used for skin or *in vitro* tests), may provide the only method that objectively confirms occupational asthma (see Chapter 31). The cost–benefit ratio of performing inhalation tests with allergens or other sensitizing agents should be carefully examined in each single patient, taking into account the high cost and the potential risk involved.[3,35]

ANCILLARY TESTS (see also Chapters 10 and 13)

CELLULAR AND BIOCHEMICAL MARKERS OF INFLAMMATION

Cell counts and mediators in peripheral blood and sputum may provide useful information in asthma. The numbers of eosinophils in peripheral blood[36] and sputum[37] are significantly correlated with the degree of airway hyperresponsiveness, and they decrease after treatment with steroids,[38] reflecting an improvement in asthma. Inflammatory mediators such as eosinophil cationic protein (ECP) and myeloperoxidase (MPO) are increased in the serum, bronchoalveolar lavage fluid and sputum[36] of asthmatics, particularly during asthma exacerbations. Similarly, urinary leukotriene metabolites increase during an asthma attack, and during asthma exacerbations.

Although these markers of inflammation may provide quite useful information when used in controlled clinical studies, they are at present of no value in clinical practice because they rarely provide information specific to asthma, and it is still unclear what they may add to history and measurement of lung function. In particular, apart from a few exceptions where a differential diagnosis needs to be established, bronchoscopy and related techniques (bronchial biopsies, bronchoalveolar lavage) have no clinical indications in asthma. By contrast, induced sputum may provide a simple, non-invasive method of assessing airway inflammation in asthma.[37]

DIFFERENTIAL DIAGNOSIS

On a patient's admission to hospital, an asthma attack is usually easily identified. However, in a few cases a differential diagnosis with other pathological conditions that manifest themselves with wheezing and dyspnoea needs to be established.

Upper airway obstruction due to laryngeal oedema, vocal cord dysfunction, laryngeal or tracheal stenosis or malacia, primary or secondary neoplasm and foreign bodies should always be considered. In addition to a suggestive history, patients present with stridor, and physical examination reveals harsh respiratory sounds in the area of the trachea. Laryngoscopy or bronchoscopy may sometimes be useful. Also, glottic dysfunction is a rather rare disorder that may cause asthma-like symptoms. Bronchial stenosis, neoplasm or aspiration of foreign body may all mimic asthma. The patients usually complain of paroxysms of cough, and continuous wheezing is heard in a localized area.

Patients with chronic obstructive pulmonary diseases, i.e. subjects with chronic irreversible airflow limitation, may have a transient reversibility of airflow limitation, and may develop acute airflow limitations during exacerbations. A history of chronic cough and sputum production is suggestive of chronic bronchitis, and physical and radiological signs of irreversible hyperinflation are suggestive of emphysema. When asthma and/or chronic bronchitis, and/or emphysema, occur in the same patient, they should be recognized and treated appropriately. Congestive heart failure in patients with chronic obstructive pulmonary disease is usually recognizable from signs of left ventricular failure, including basilar rales, gallop rhythms and jugular congestion.

Pulmonary infiltrations with tissue and blood eosinophilia occur in eosinophilic pneumonia, pulmonary parasitic infections, allergic bronchopulmonary aspergillosis and some pulmonary vasculitis syndromes. In some patients, pulmonary eosinophilic infiltrations may be associated with asthma, and therefore they should be properly investigated.

Pulmonary microembolism or recurrent episodes of pulmonary embolism may mimic asthma attacks because of the sudden development of dyspnoea. The development of dyspnoea is usually unexpected, is not associated with acute airflow limitation and occurs in patients at risk of pulmonary embolism (venous thrombosis at the extremities, surgery).

Radioisotope lung scans and sometimes pulmonary angiography may be necessary to exclude pulmonary embolism in patients at risk. Pneumothorax may also cause acute breathlessness, but it is accompanied by acute chest pain, the absence of airflow limitation and, ultimately, a chest radiograph will provide the diagnosis.

Cardiogenic pulmonary hypertension may both mimic asthma in non-asthmatic cardiopathic subjects and trigger asthma attacks in cardiopathic asthmatic subjects. History, physical and radiological signs of cardiomegaly and/or valvular disease, or additional cardiological examination may be required for the differential diagnosis.

Bronchial carcinoid tumours may mimic asthma symptoms. Patients with carcinoid may develop the carcinoid syndrome, i.e. flushing of the face and other portions of the body, hyperperistalsis of the gut with diarrhoea, hypotension and tachycardia sometimes associated with wheezing. Facial rash and diarrhoea, in addition to the increase of urinary 5-hydroxyindole-acetic acid, are usually guidelines for a correct diagnosis.[39]

MINIMAL REQUIREMENTS TO ESTABLISH THE SEVERITY OF ASTHMA AND ASTHMA EXACERBATIONS
(see also Chapters 11–13)

The assessment of severity is based on history, assessment of symptom score, repeated measurement of spirometry and/or PEF and the amount of medication required to keep asthma under control.

SEVERITY OF ASTHMA: INTERMITTENT, MILD, MODERATE AND SEVERE ASTHMA

In clinical practice it is most important to define the severity of asthma, as the physician's decisions on short-term and long-term management depend almost entirely on severity.[2] In addition, a classification of a patient's asthma based on disease severity over the preceding year[40] has been shown to relate to pathological indices of airway inflammation.

The descriptions of levels of disease severity based on a combination of symptoms and treatment requirements, as well as objective measurements of lung function, differ little between the guidelines produced in various countries. The most recent classification scheme is presented in Fig. 6.1, and it includes the categories mild persistent, moderate persistent, and severe persistent.[2] The severity of asthma exacerbations is also based on symptoms, lung function and response to treatment (Fig. 6.1), but must also take into account the time-course and frequency of the exacerbations, which are predictors of outcome.

FIGURE 6.1: *Classification of asthma severity. The presence of one of the features of severity is sufficient to place a patient in that category. (From Ref. 2 with permission.)*

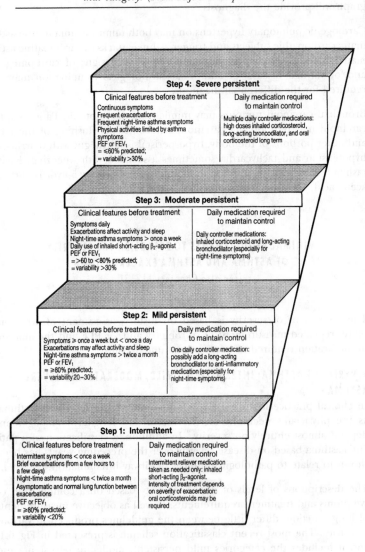

Step 4: Severe persistent

Clinical features before treatment	Daily medication required to maintain control
Continuous symptoms Frequent exacerbations Frequent night-time asthma symptoms Physical activities limited by asthma symptoms PEF or FEV_1 = ≤60% predicted; = variability >30%	Multiple daily controller medications: high doses inhaled corticosteroid, long-acting broncodilator, and oral corticosteroid long term

Step 3: Moderate persistent

Clinical features before treatment	Daily medication required to maintain control
Symptoms daily Exacerbations affect activity and sleep Night-time asthma symptoms > once a week Daily use of inhaled short-acting β_2-agonist PEF or FEV_1 = >60 to <80% predicted; = variability >30%	Daily controller medications: inhaled corticosteroid and long-acting bronchodilator (especially for night-time symptoms)

Step 2: Mild persistent

Clinical features before treatment	Daily medication required to maintain control
Symptoms ≥ once a week but < once a day Exacerbations may affect activity and sleep Night-time asthma symptoms > twice a month PEF or FEV_1 = ≥80% predicted; = variability 20–30%	One daily controller medication: possibly add a long-acting bronchodilator to anti-inflammatory medication (especially for night-time symptoms)

Step 1: Intermittent

Clinical features before treatment	Daily medication required to maintain control
Intermittent symptoms < once a week Brief exacerbations (from a few hours to a few days) Night-time asthma symptoms < twice a month Asymptomatic and normal lung function between exacerbations PEF or FEV_1 = ≥80% predicted; = variability <20%	Intermittent reliever medication taken as needed only: inhaled short-acting β_2-agonist. Intensity of treatment depends on severity of exacerbation: oral corticosteroids may be required

These categories are purely arbitrary; studies to validate them will be important, both as regards their relationship to quality of life and prognosis and, more importantly, as regards the effect of the recommended stepwise approach to treatment.

Interestingly, because of the specific features of asthma, which is a syndrome manifesting itself recurrently with asymptomatic periods during which lung volumes might be normal, guidelines have recently been issued that take into account both symptoms and baseline lung function, but also the degree of airway hyperresponsiveness and the amount of medication required to keep the disease under control.[41]

SEVERITY OF ASTHMA EXACERBATIONS

Exacerbations of asthma are episodes of worsening shortness of breath, cough, wheezing or chest tightness, or some combination of these symptoms. Exacerbations are usually associated with acute airflow limitation that can be measured with physical examination, spirometry and/or measurements of PEF. Exacerbations usually reflect either a failure in long-term management or exposure to a precipitating stimulus. The severity of asthma exacerbations may range from mild to life threatening. The deterioration usually progresses over hours or days, but may occasionally occur precipitously over some minutes. Assessment of the patient's pulse, respiratory rate and current symptoms also guides treatment decisions, but objective measures of lung function are critical.

Previous hospital admission for asthma, especially in an emergency department, must be carefully investigated. Hospital admission in the previous 12 months is reported to be the strongest marker of subsequent risk of asthma deaths, and the risk increases with the number of previous admissions.[42]

Thus, patients with a history of current use of, or recent withdrawal from, systemic corticosteroids, hospitalization for asthma and/or emergency treatment for asthma in the past year, prior intubation for asthma, psychiatric disease or psychosocial problems and non-compliance with an asthma medication plan are at high risk of asthma-related death. While symptoms may be a sensitive indicator of mild asthma exacerbations, symptoms and physical signs alone cannot be considered accurate indicators of severe airflow limitation.

The severity of the exacerbation determines the treatment administered. Table 6.1 provides a guide to the severity of an exacerbation of asthma at the time the examination is made. Since these are guidelines only, all features in a category need not be present. A more severe grading should be given if the patient has a lack of response to initial treatment, if the attack has progressed quickly or if the patient is at high risk historically as just defined.

Indices of severity, particularly PEF (in patients over 5 years old), pulse and respiratory rate should also be monitored during treatment. Any

TABLE 6.1: *Severity of asthma exacerbations. (From Ref. 2 with permission).*

	Mild	Moderate	Severe	Respiratory arrest imminent
Breathless	Walking Can lie down	Talking Infant: softer shorter cry; difficulty feeding Prefers sitting	At rest Infant: stops feeding Hunched forward	
Talks in	Sentences	Phrases	Words	
Alertness	May be agitated	Usually agitated	Usually agitated	Drowsy or confused
Respiratory rate	Increased	Increased	Often $>30 \ min^{-1}$	

Guide to rates of breathing associated with respiratory distress in awake children:

Age	Normal rate
<2 months	$<60 \ min^{-1}$
2–12 months	$<50 \ min^{-1}$
1–5 years	$<40 \ min^{-1}$
6–8 years	$<30 \ min^{-1}$

	Mild	Moderate	Severe	Respiratory arrest imminent
Accessory muscles and suprasternal retractions	Usually not	Usually	Usually	Paradoxical thoraco-abdominal movement

	Moderate, often only end expiratory	Loud	Usually loud	Absence of wheeze
Wheeze	Moderate, often only end expiratory	Loud	Usually loud	Absence of wheeze
Pulse (min^{-1})	<100	100–120	>120	Bradycardia
Guide to limits of normal pulse rate in children: Infants: 2–12 months Normal rate <160 min^{-1}; Pre-school: 1–2 years <120 min^{-1}; School age: 2–8 years <110 min^{-1}				
Pulsus paradoxus	Absent <10 mmHg	May be present 10–25 mmHg	Often present >25 mmHg (adult) 20–40 mmHg (child)	Absence suggests respiratory muscle fatigue
PEF after initial bronchodilator % predicted or % personal best	Over 80%	Approx. 60–80%	<60% predicted or personal best (<100 l min^{-1} adults) or response lasts <2 hours	
P_aO_2 (on air)	Normal. Test not usually necessary	>60 mmHg	<60 mmHg Possible cyanosis	
and/or P_aCO_2	<45 mmHg	<45 mmHg	>45 mmHg Possible respiratory failure (see text)	
S_aO_2 (on air)	>95%	91–95%	<90%	

Hypercapnia (hypoventilation) develops more readily in young children than in adults and adolescents deterioration may require prompt intervention. Initiation of anti-asthma therapy at the earliest possible sign of deteriorating control of asthma is important in the successful management of asthma exacerbations. Home PEF determinations are an integral part of home management strategies. Ideally, all patients should have a written action plan that outlines how to recognize signs of deterioration, how to start treatment and how to get medical care.

The assessment of the severity of asthma exacerbations in the hospital requires, in addition to a brief history to document the time-course and severity of symptoms, information about potential triggering events, all current medication and prior hospitalizations and emergency department visits for asthma. The physical examination will assess severity of exacerbation (Table 6.1), the presence of complications (e.g. pneumonia, atelectasis, pneumothorax or pneumomediastinum). PEF and/or FEV_1 should be measured at least hourly, with initial measurement made before treatment, if possible.

Arterial blood gas measurement provides important information for assessing the severity of asthma exacerbations, particularly of severe asthma exacerbations, e.g. when FEV_1 or PEF <40% predicted or best personal value, and/or oxygen saturation is decreased, and/or PEF do not increase after the initial treatment. Gas exchange abnormalities, as reflected by arterial hypoxaemia, are common in asthma patients during a severe exacerbation.[43] The degree of ventilation–perfusion mismatching correlates poorly with clinical findings and indices of airflow obstruction (FEV_1 or FEF_{25-75}), and thus alterations of arterial blood gases may be present even when symptoms are mild and/or spirometric indices are normal or borderline. During a mild asthma attack, the usual pattern consists of a normal P_aO_2, associated with hypocapnia and slight respiratory alkalosis due to compensatory hyperventilation. Normocapnia or hypercapnia associated with normoxaemia or hypoxaemia are poor prognostic evidence of a severe attack. Respiratory failure with hypoxaemia, hypercapnia and respiratory acidosis occurs in a minority of patients.

Pulse oximetry provides measurement of oxygen saturation that can help monitor a patient's response to acute therapy. The more extensive information obtained from blood gas determinations may be important, particularly if pulse oximetry is normal in the presence of other indications of severe exacerbations. Once initial treatment has been established, other clinical examinations may be advisable, e.g. complete blood count and microbiological examinations in patients with purulent sputum or fever, and chest X-ray if complicating cardiopulmonary process is suspected.

ACKNOWLEDGEMENTS

Supported by the Italian Ministry of University and Research, the Italian National Research Council, a special Grant from ENEL-CNR, and the European Community for Coal and Steel.

REFERENCES

1　Sheffer AL (ed). International Consensus Report on Diagnosis and Management of Asthma. National Institutes of Health. NIH Publication No. 92-3091. March 1992. Eur Respir J 1992; 5: 601–41.

2　Sheffer AL (ed). Global Strategy for Asthma Management. World Health Organization and National Institutes of Health. WHO Technical Series, 1995, in press.

3　Sterk PJ, Fabbri LM, Quanjer Ph et al. Airway responsiveness. Standardized challenge testing with pharmacological, physiological, and sensitizing stimuli. Eur Respir J 1993; 6 (suppl 16): 53–83.

4　Mapp CE, Dal Vecchio L, Boschetto P, De Marzo N, Fabbri LM. Toluene diisocyanate-induced asthma without airway hyperresponsiveness. Eur J Respir Dis 1986; 68: 89–95.

5　Josephs LK, Gregg I, Mullee MA, Holgate ST. Non-specific bronchial reactivity and its relationship to the clinical expression of asthma. A longitudinal study. Am Rev Respir Dis 1989; 140: 350–7.

6　Cockcroft DW. Airway hyperresponsiveness. Relevance of random population data to clinical usefulness. Am Rev Respir Dis 1990; 142: 497–500.

7　Doan T, Patterson R, Greenberger PA. Cough variant asthma: usefulness of a diagnostic–therapeutic trial with prednisone. Ann Allergy 1992; 69: 505–9.

8　Burney PGJ et al. What symptoms predict the bronchial response to histamine? Evaluation in a community survey of the bronchial symptom questionnaire (1984) of the International Unit Against Tuberculosis and Lung Diseases. Int J Epidemiol 1989; 18: 165–73.

9　Burney PGJ, Laitinen LA, Perdrizet S et al. Validity of the IUATLD (1984) bronchial symptoms questionnaire: an international comparison. Eur Respir J 1989; 2: 940–2.

10　Toren K, Brisman J, Jarvholm B. Asthma and asthma-like symptoms in adults assessed by questionnaires. A literature review. Chest 1993; 104: 600–8.

11 Shaw RA, Crane J, Pearce N *et al.* Comparison of a video questionnaire with the IUATLD written questionnaire for measuring asthma prevalence. *Clin Exp Allergy* 1992; 22: 561–8.

12 Venables KM, Farrer N, Sharp L, Graneek BJ, Newman Taylor AJ. Respiratory symptoms questionnaire for asthma epidemiology: validity and reproducibility. *Thorax* 1993; 48: 214–9.

13 Marks GB, Dunn SM, Woolcock AJ. An evaluation of an asthma quality of life questionnaire as a measure of changes in adults with asthma. *J Clin Epidemiol* 1993; 46: 166–74.

14 Gibson PG, Wong BJ, Hepperle MJ *et al.* A research method to induce and examine a mild exacerbation of asthma by withdrawal of inhaled corticosteroids. *Clin Exp Allergy* 1992; 22: 525–32.

15 American Thoracic Society. Lung function testing: selection of reference values and interpretative strategies. *Am Rev Respir Dis* 1991; 144: 1202–18.

16 Quanjer PhH (ed). Standardized Lung Function Testing. *Eur Respir J* 1993; 6 (suppl 16).

17 Lebowitz MJ. The use of peak expiratory flow rate measurements in respiratory diseases. *Pediatr Pulmonol* 1991; 11: 166–74.

18 Sly P, Cahill P, Willet K, Burton P. Accuracy of mini peak flow meters in indicating changes in lung function in children with asthma. *BMJ* 1994; 308: 572–5.

19 Quanjer PhH, Lebowitz MB, Gregg I. Peak expiratory flow. Draft, conclusions and recommendations of a Working Party of the European Respiratory Society. *Eur Respir J* 1994.

20 Quackenboss JJ, Lebowitz MD, Krzyzanowski M. The normal range of diurnal changes in peak expiratory flow rates: Relationship to symptoms and respiratory diseases. *Am Rev Respir Dis* 1991; 143: 323–30.

21 Cotè J, Kennedy S, Chan-Yeung M. Quantitative versus qualitative analysis of peak expiratory flow in occupational asthma. *Thorax* 1993; 48: 48–51.

22 Ryan G, Latimer KM, Dolovich J, Hargreave FE. Bronchial responsiveness to histamine: Relationship to diurnal variations of peak flow rate, improvement after bronchodilator, and airway caliber. *Thorax* 1982; 37: 423–9.

23 Woolcock AJ. Asthma. In: Murray JF, Nadel JA (eds) *Textbook of Respiratory Medicine*, 2nd edn. Philadelphia: W.B. Saunders, 1994, pp. 1288–330.

24 Puolijoki H, Impivaara O, Liippo K, Tala E. Later development of asthma in patients with a negative methacholine inhalation challenge examined for suspected asthma. *Lung* 1992; 170: 235–41.

25 Zhong NS, Chen RC, Yang MO *et al.* Is asymptomatic bronchial hyperresponsiveness an indication of potential asthma? *Chest* 1992; 102: 1014–9.

26 Shenfield GM, Hodson ME, Clarke SW, Paterson JW. Interaction of corticosteroids and catecholamines in the treatment of asthma. *Thorax* 1975; 30: 430–5.

27 Callahan CM, Dittus RS, Katz BP. Oral corticosteroid therapy for patients
with stable chronic obstructive pulmonary disease. *Ann Intern Med* 1991; 114:
216–23.

28 Harding SM, Freeman S. A comparison of oral and inhaled steroids in
patients with chronic airways obstruction: features determining the
response. *Thorax* 1978; 33: 214–8.

29 Kerstjens HAM, Overbeek SE, Schouten JP *et al.* Airways hyper- responsiveness, bronchodilator response, allergy, and smoking predict improvement
in FEV_1 during long-term inhaled corticosteroid treat- ment. *Eur Respir J* 1993;
6: 868–76.

30 Mandella LA, Manfreda J, Warren CPW, Anthonisen NR. Steroid response
in stable chronic obstructive pulmonary diseases. *Ann Intern Med* 1982; 96: 17–21.

31 Bessot JC, de Blay F, Pauli G. From allergen sources to reduction of allergen exposure. *Eur Respir J* 1994; 7: 392–7.

32 Dreborg S, Frew A. Allergen standardization and skin tests. *Allergy* 1993; 48
(suppl): 55–62.

33 Klink M, Cline HG, Halonen M. Problems in defining normal limits for
serum IgE. *J Allergy Clin Immunol* 1990; 85: 440–4.

34 Homburger HA, Mauer K, Sachs MI. Serum IgG4 antibodies compared in
adults and children with asthma and non allergic subjects. *J Allergy Clin Immunol*
1986; 77: 427–32.

35 Fish JE. Bronchial challenge testing. In: Middleton E *et al.* (eds) *Allergy.
Principles and Practice*, 5th edn. St Louis: C.V. Mosby Co., 1983: 613–27.

36 Venge P. Soluble markers of allergic inflammation. *Allergy* 1994; 49: 1–8.

37 Hargreave FE, Popov T, Kidney J, Dolovich J. Sputum measurement to
assess airway inflammation in asthma. *Allergy* 1993; 48 (suppl 17): 81–3.

38 Baigelman W, Chodhos S, Pizzuto D *et al.* Sputum and blood eosinophilia
during corticosteroid treatment in acute exacerbations of asthma. *Am J Med*
1983; 75: 929–33.

39 Creutzfeldt W, Stockmann F. Carcinoid and carcinoid syndromes. *Am J Med*
1987; 82: 4–11.

40 Bousquet J, Chanez P, Lacoste JY *et al.* Eosinophilic inflammation in
asthma. *N Engl J Med* 1990; 323: 1033–9.

41 American Thoracic Society. Guidelines for the evaluation of impairment/disability in patients with asthma. *Am Rev Respir Dis* 1993; 147: 1056–61.

42 Crane J, Pearce N, Burgess C *et al.* Markers of risk of asthma death or readmission in the 12 months following a hospital admission for asthma. *Int J Epidemiol* 1992; 21: 737–44.

43 Rodriguez-Roisin R, Roca J. Contribution of multiple inert gas elimination technique to pulmonary medicine – 3. Bronchial asthma. *Thorax* 1994; 49: 1027–33.

KEY POINTS

1 The minimal requirements for establishing the diagnosis of asthma in adults are history, peak expiratory flow records, and/or reversibility tests with a single dose of a short-acting bronchodilator

2 Assessment of airway hyperresponsiveness to methacholine or histamine or reversibility of airflow limitation after a short course of steroids may be required to confirm the diagnosis in doubtful cases

3 Allergy skin tests and/or measurements should be used to diagnose atopy and to identify the allergen(s), if any, involved in asthma exacerbations

4 A differential diagnosis from other conditions mimicking asthma may require other investigations (e.g. chest X-rays, ECG, bronchoscopy)

7

PULMONARY FUNCTION TESTS

K.J. Killian

INTRODUCTION

Asthma originates with airway inflammation, which results in pathological processes that interact with normal physiological processes and ultimately culminates in symptoms. The aim of this chapter is to provide an understanding of pulmonary function testing within this context.

STRUCTURE AND FUNCTION

STRUCTURE

Some of the characteristic manifestations of asthma can be recognized from early medical literature.[1] The reliable identification of asthma was impossible until recent times because understanding of its pathophysiology was simply inadequate. *The Seats and Causes of Disease investigated by Anatomy* by Morgagni (1682–1771) provided a turning point.[2] Thereafter, the structural changes underlying human diseases were matched to the anatomical changes found following death. Using this approach, Laennec (1781–1826) characterized the presence of dyspnoea in life by association with its morbid anatomical appearances following death, introducing the terms "cardiac dyspnoea", "respiratory dyspnoea", and "renal dyspnoea".[3] Methodical physical examination, coupled with knowledge of the underlying morbid anatomy allowed the recognition of cardiac and respiratory disorders from physical symptoms and signs. Bronchial asthma was discriminated from cardiac asthma by the absence of cardiac and other respiratory pathological changes, but otherwise remained an enigma because the structural features were subtle.

FUNCTION

Despite these advances in the knowledge of structure, their functional counterparts remained obscure. The discovery of the circulation and the chemistry of the respiratory gases, and the recognition that respiration was the combustion of carbohydrate, fat and protein in cells, and that breathing was dependent on neural activity in the medulla oblongata, provided an appreciation of the sequence of functional processes over which homeostatic control mechanisms presided. P_aO_2, P_aCO_2 and hydrogen ion concentration were held constant in arterial blood despite the varying metabolic demands of life at rest and during exercise. This sequence of functional processes provided the framework for understanding the clinical features of cardiorespiratory disease and the structural changes found on morbid anatomy.

THE ORIGINS OF PULMONARY FUNCTION TESTING

VITAL CAPACITY AND RESPIRATORY MUSCLE CAPACITY

In the middle of the last century, Hutchinson measured the volume of air that could be displaced between a maximal inspiration and maximal expiration using a spirometer, and measured the pressures generated against an occluded airway following maximal voluntary activation of the inspiratory and expiratory muscles using a water manometer.[4,5] These measurements are known today as vital capacity (VC), maximal inspiratory pressure (MIP) and maximal expiratory pressure (MEP). A reduced VC implied muscle weakness, the presence of a space-occupying lesion in the chest (e.g. pleural effusion, masses, etc.), or a hindrance to breathing due to stiff lungs or obstructed airways.

PULMONARY MECHANICS

The respiratory muscles generate the forces required to expand and contract the lungs and chest cage. Rohrer studied the mechanical function of the respiratory system using the laws of motion introduced by Newton in the 1600s.[6–8] The relationship between pressure, volume and time at any moment during breathing was expressed by the following equation:

$$\text{Pressure} = (\text{volume} \times \text{elastance}) + (\text{flow} \times \text{resistance}) + (\text{acceleration} \times \text{inertance})$$

where elastance is the relationship of pressure to volume under static conditions (elastance = pressure/volume), resistance is the relationship between pressure and the rate of change of volume per unit time (resistance = pressure/flow), and inertance is the relationship between pressure and the rate of change of flow per unit time (inertance = pressure/acceleration).

Measurement of the Elastance of the Total Respiratory System

The pressures required to expand the total ventilatory system were described by Rohrer.[7] Inspiratory activity is required to increase lung volume from functional residual capacity (FRC) to total lung capacity (TLC).

If the subject relaxes against an occluded airway at any volume above FRC, the combined recoil pressure of the lung and chest cage can be measured at the mouth. Expiratory activity is required to decrease lung volume from FRC to residual volume (RV). If the subject relaxes, the expiratory muscles against an occluded airway below FRC, the chest cage rebounds, creating a negative recoil pressure that can also be measured at the mouth. The recoil pressure of the total respiratory system at lung volumes ranging from RV to TLC is illustrated in Fig. 7.1.

The pressure–volume relationship of the lung is also illustrated in Fig. 7.1. It takes 5 cmH$_2$O to half inflate the lung, a further 5 cmH$_2$O to half inflate

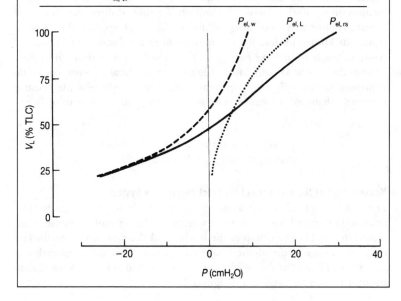

FIGURE 7.1: *Lung volume expressed as a percentage of total lung capacity is plotted against pressure in cmH$_2$O. The occlusion pressure measured at the mouth following relaxation of the inspiratory muscles is positive and falls to the right of the zero line; the occlusion pressure following relaxation of the expiratory muscles is negative and falls to the left of the zero line; the solid line represents the elastic characteristics of the respiratory system lung. The dotted line to the right of the zero line represents the recoil pressure of the lung and is positive at all lung volumes P$_{el,\,L}$. The dashed line represents the recoil pressure of the chest wall where P$_{el,\,w}$ = P$_{el,\,rs}$ − P$_{el,\,L}$.*

it again from 50% to 75% TLC; and so on. The relationship is close to exponential with a half-inflation pressure of 5 cmH$_2$O and a maximal inflation pressure of 30 cmH$_2$O.[9] The recoil pressure of the chest cage as shown in Fig. 7.1 is found by subtracting the recoil pressure of the lung from the recoil pressure of the total respiratory system. With inflation, the chest cage becomes more compliant, while the lung becomes stiffer. With deflation, the lungs become more compliant while the chest cage becomes stiffer (Fig. 7.1). As a result the elastance of the total respiratory system remains relatively constant at approximately 12 cmH$_2$O l^{-1} over the operating range of 30–80% of TLC (Fig. 7.1).[10]

Despite the utility of this approach in advancing our knowledge of respiratory mechanics, this technique did not become a routine pulmonary function measurement because many people cannot relax the respiratory muscles appropriately, making the measurement unreliable for general use.

Measurement of the Resistance of the Total Respiratory System

Alveolar pressure (P_{alv}) determines airflow up and down the airways because mouth pressure is always constant at atmospheric pressure. No airflow takes place when the pressure at the mouth and P_{alv} are the same. During inspiration, P_{alv} drops below atmospheric pressure resulting in movement of air down the airway. During expiration, the lung recoils and generates a positive P_{alv} that drives air out of the lungs. When ventilation is substantial the positive recoil of the chest cage and activation of the expiratory muscles also act to increase P_{alv}. In early years, the direct measurement of P_{alv} was not technically feasible. Rohrer measured the length, calibre and branching of the airways, and applied the physical equations known to describe the movement of a substance of known viscosity through branching passages.[8] The resistive pressure in the upper (above the trachea) and lower (below the trachea) airways could be expressed by the following polynomial relationship, whereby the resistive pressure calculated increased in an accelerating pattern relative to flow:

$$P(\mathrm{cmH_2O}) = 0.43 * \dot{V} + 0.73 * \dot{V}^2 \text{ and}$$
$$P(\mathrm{cmH_2O}) = 0.36 * \dot{V} + 0.09 * \dot{V}^2$$

Measurement of the Inertance of the Total Respiratory System

Pressure is required to accelerate the air from a state of rest to the velocities seen during inspiration and expiration. The air molecules are accelerated to very high velocities in the trachea but the mass is very small. The lung, chest cage and abdomen have a large mass, but the acceleration is very small. Hence, in the respiratory system inertance is a very small contributor to pressure and can be ignored.

Measurement of the Pressure Required to Drive the Total Respiratory System

Given the measurements of tidal volumes and flow rates under resting and exercising conditions, the pressures required to breathe can be approximated by adding the elastic and resistive pressures:

$$P = (\text{volume} \times \text{elastance}) + ((K_1 \times \text{flow}) + (K_2 \times \text{flow}^2))$$

Normal elastance is $12\,\text{cmH}_2\text{O}\,\text{l}^{-1}$, K_1 is $1.9\,\text{cmH}_2\text{O}\,\text{l}^{-1}\,\text{s}^{-1}$ and K_2 is $0.52\,\text{cmH}_2\text{O}\,\text{l}^{-1}\,\text{s}^{-1}$.[10]

Pleural Pressure (P_{pl})

By applying mechanical principles to the respiratory system, Rohrer recognized the following fundamental equation:[6]

$$P_{pl} = P_{alv} - P_{el\ lung} = P_{mus} + P_{el\ thorax}$$

where $P_{el\ lung}$ is the elastance of the lung measured in $\text{cmH}_2\text{O}\,\text{l}^{-1}$, P_{mus} is the pressure developed by the respiratory muscles, and $P_{el\ thorax}$ is the elastance of the total respiratory system minus the elastance of the lung.

At the end of a normal expiration when the respiratory muscles are inactive, P_{pl} is equal and opposite to the recoil pressure of the lungs, and equal to the recoil pressure of the chest cage. The elastance and resistance of the lung could now be isolated given the simultaneous measurements of volume, time and P_{pl}. Rohrer applied the technique successfully in rabbits, but his untimely death prevented him from applying the technique to human subjects; his colleagues, von Neergard and Wirz, went on to do this.[11,12] This approach did not progress further because of the need for the induction of a pneumothorax, and the timely introduction of the Fleisch pneumotachograph, which allowed measurement of airflow at the mouth. If the airway could be transiently occluded, the mouth and alveolar pressure would quickly equilibrate yielding the P_{alv}. P_{alv} could then be divided by the flow rate (flow) prior to occlusion, yielding airways resistance (airway resistance = P_{alv}/flow).[13] The interrupter technique was used in asthmatic subjects confirming the suspected increase in resistance. The early drop in pressure at the mouth following airway occlusion approximated the resistive pressure calculated later using oesophageal pressure. The pressure following occlusion continues to drop to a terminal pressure, which approximates the elastic pressure. The pressure drop between the early and terminal pressure is a combination of resistive and elastic pressures, due to equilibration throughout the lung following occlusion. Today a complete mechanical analysis can be performed with airway occlusion during ventilation, and is currently enjoying a resurgence of interest in the critical care community.

Oesophageal Pressure

Following the recognition that changes in oesophageal pressure closely mirror the changes in P_{pl} during breathing, and the rediscovery of Rohrer's approach by Otis, Rahn and Fenn in 1946,[14-16] mechanical analysis became widely available. The simultaneous measurement of oesophageal pressure, volume and flow allowed the derivation of pulmonary elastance and resistance.

Measurement of the Pressure Relative to Capacity

The value of mechanical analysis is optimized when the pressure actually generated during breathing is expressed relative to the capacity of the muscles to generate pressure. The patient becomes more compromised as the pressure generated encroaches on capacity. While MIP and MEP provide an indication of capacity under static conditions at optimum length of the relevant muscle groups, the actual capacity to generate pressure under conditions of usage are considerably less. The ability to generate inspiratory pressure declines with inspiration due to the shortened inspiratory muscle length; declines as lung volume increases due to the increasing curvature of the diaphragm with inspiration ($P = 2 \times$ tension/radius; Laplace's law); declines as the velocity of contraction increases with flow rate at all muscle lengths (force–velocity relationship); and declines with prolonged high-intensity activity due to fatigue. The oesophageal pressures generated at various work loads to maximal working capacity during exercise are illustrated in Fig. 7.2.[17,18] The capacity to generate pressure under both static and dynamic conditions is also illustrated. As can be seen in Fig. 7.2, the capacity to generate pressure is approached but not reached. Exertional discomfort related to the inspiratory muscles manifested as dyspnoea becomes intolerable before capacity is reached.

PULMONARY MECHANICS AND ASTHMA

Resistance, oesophageal pressure and the end-expiratory lung volume increase with bronchoconstriction. This can be illustrated when methacholine is inhaled in asthmatic subjects (Fig. 7.3).[19] Dyspnoea becomes "just noticeable" as resistance increases without appreciable increases in pressure. This is because an added resistance of as little as $0.6 \, \text{cmH}_2\text{O} \, \text{l}^{-1} \, \text{s}$ or a change in resistance, approximating 20% of the baseline resistance, is just noticeably detected by normal and asthmatic subjects.[20] The intensity of dyspnoea increases thereafter as the magnitude of inspiratory pressure increases. This is because exertional discomfort associated with any voluntary muscle intensifies in a positively accelerating manner as power output increases. Voluntary muscular activity is terminated when discomfort becomes "severe". Tolerance for exertional discomfort varies from person to person, with some individuals stopping when the discomfort reaches

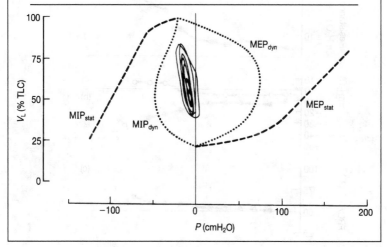

FIGURE 7.2: *Lung volume expressed as a percentage of total lung capacity is plotted against pressure in cmH₂O. The pressure–volume loops represent the oesophageal pressure at rest and at increasing levels of work to maximal capacity without a mouthpiece or unidirectional valve. The maximal inspiratory and expiratory oesophageal pressures are shown when the mouth is occluded at all lung volumes (MIP_stat and MEP_stat) and during a maximal inspiratory and expiratory flow manoeuvre (MIP_dyn and MEP_dyn). Note that the pressure developed in the pleura at maximal work performance is submaximal.*

"moderate" intensity, while others continue activity until exertional discomfort reaches "very, very severe".

In the asthmatic patient, the inspiratory pressure required to generate a given ventilation increases as resistance and elastance increase. Other factors act in an interactive manner, e.g. inspiratory flow rate is dependent on expiratory obstruction, inhomogeneous lungs increase dynamic elastance. Ventilation may increase because of hypoxic, hypercapnic or behavioural drive arising due to anxiety. The net result is that inspiratory pressure and the power output of the inspiratory muscles increase, and exertional discomfort intensifies. Inspiratory muscle capacity is also adversely affected in asthmatic subjects. Functional inspiratory muscle weakness arises due to hyperinflation, which shortens the operating muscle length and increases

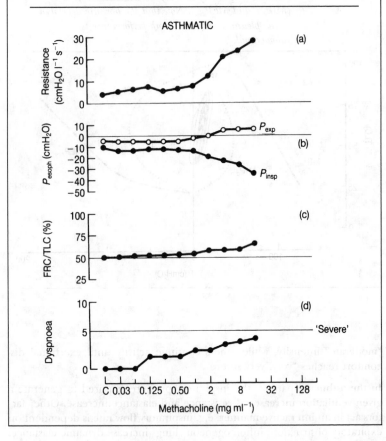

FIGURE 7.3: *(a) Measurement of inspiratory resistance, (b) peak oesophageal pressure, (c) functional residual capacity (end-expiratory lung volume), expressed as a percentage of TLC, following incrementally induced bronchoconstriction in an asthmatic subject. The intensity of dyspnoea experienced is shown in (d) where 5 is "severe", 4 is "somewhat severe", 3 is "moderate", 2 is "slight", 1 is "very slight" and 0.5 is "just noticeable".*

the curvature of the diaphragm. As the asthmatic state is prolonged, inspiratory muscle fatigue may also ensue. Inspiratory effort increases as the inspiratory pressure increases and the capacity to generate pressure decreases.

PULMONARY FUNCTION TESTING

Quite independent and parallel to the advances in pulmonary mechanics, Means, Hermannsen, Knipper and Anthony popularized the idea that ventilatory capacity was a generic measurement that was sensitive to neuro-muscular abnormalities, space-occupying diseases in the chest, stiff lungs and obstructed airways.[21–24] As breathing encroached on capacity, either at rest or during exercise, and breathing reserve decreased, dyspnoea was tacitly assumed to intensify. Cournand and Richards[25] formalized the measurement of cardiorespiratory function aimed at discriminating between ventilatory insufficiency, respiratory insufficiency and cardiocirculatory insufficiency.

(1) Ventilatory insufficiency was concerned with impairments in the mechanical movement of air in and out of the lungs, with its characteristic result being the symptom of dyspnoea.

(2) Respiratory insufficiency was concerned with impairments in gas exchange, with its characteristic result being anoxaemia.

(3) Cardiocirculatory insufficiency was concerned with impairments in perfusion, with its characteristic result being congestive failure and shock.

VENTILATORY INSUFFICIENCY

The maximal voluntary ventilation (MVV) proposed by Hermannsen was adopted whereby the patient breathed with a maximal respiratory effort for 12–15 s.[22] The breathing reserve (BR) was derived by subtracting the ventilation at rest (or during exercise) from the MVV and expressing it as a percentage of MVV (BR/MVV%). Dyspnoea was not expected with a BR/MVV% greater than 90%, but became more prevalent as the BR/MVV% decreased. The simpler expression of ventilation ($\dot{V}_E$) expressed as a percentage of MVV ($\dot{V}_E$/MVV), known as the ventilatory index, has now replaced the breathing reserve.

The nature of the ventilatory impairment was also addressed and subdivided into restrictive and obstructive. Prior to 1950, the measurement of airflow obstruction centred on the reduced MVV, the inspiratory drift during the MVV manoeuvre (high RV/TLC ratio with a high residual nitrogen) suggesting emphysema. In the presence of airflow limitation, the spirometer trace was noted to drift during the MVV manoeuvre, with a loss in spirometer volume as more air was trapped in the lungs. In contrast, the spirometer trace remained unchanged with restrictive disorders. Other indices of airflow obstruction were an RV greater than 35% of the TLC, and the nitrogen washout technique of measuring lung volume. A nitrogen fractional concentration greater than 2.5% at the end of 7 min of breathing 100% oxygen was considered evidence of inhomogeneous mixing. The higher the percentage of nitrogen, the greater was the likelihood that air-flow obstruction was due to emphysema.

RESPIRATORY INSUFFICIENCY

Respiratory insufficiency was concerned with disturbance in gas exchange. The dominant approach was the measurement of arterial blood gases, particularly arterial oxyhaemoglobin saturation. Desaturation was attributed to low $\dot{V}/\dot{Q}$, impaired diffusion, low cardiac output, and shunt. The conceptual importance of these factors has changed little over the years.

CARDIOCIRCULATORY INSUFFICIENCY

Cournand and Richards saw the heart, lungs and circulation as integrated and regarded the assessment of cardiorespiratory function incomplete without consideration of the heart and circulation. To identify cardiocirculatory insufficiency central venous pressure was measured. Pressure of less than $10\,cmH_2O$, which remained less than $10\,cmH_2O$ following the infusion of 1500 ml of saline (Caughey challenge), was considered normal. Decrease of >8% in the VC following 1500 ml saline infusion was taken as evidence of pulmonary congestion. The time taken following the infusion of calcium gluconate in the antecubital vein to first taste was used as an index of cardiac output (circulation time). An alternative was the injection "NaCn" in the antecubital vein and the time to carotid sinus-induced hyperventilation. The circulation time was normally <18 s.

TIME-BASED SPIROMETRY

The measurement of VC before and after challenge with acetylcholine, and before and after adrenaline inhalation, emerged in the 1940s. Tiffeneau noted that asthmatic subjects developed an asthma-like state following the inhalation of acetylcholine, and that asthmatic subjects experienced a sense of relief following the inhalation of adrenaline.[26,27] Tiffeneau went on to replace VC with the forced expiratory volume (FEV), whereby volume was now assessed relative to the expired time, yielding the $FEV_{0.5}$, FEV_1, FEV_2. He also introduced the expression of FEV_1 as a proportion of VC, which became known as the Tiffeneau index. Thereafter, the assessment of airflow obstruction changed to timed manoeuvres, with the FEV_1 emerging as the standard, coupled with a reduction in the FEV_1/VC ratio.

The $FEV_1 \times 35$–40 approximated the measured MVV with sufficient accuracy that the measurement of FEV_1 became the most popular index of ventilatory capacity, virtually replacing the measurement of MVV.[28] A reduced FEV_1 with an FEV_1/VC ratio of <75% became synonymous with airflow limitation.

CHRONIC NON-SPECIFIC LUNG DISEASE

Success in the treatment of pneumococcal pneumonia and tuberculosis resulted in the recognition of the magnitude of the problem of asthma, chronic bronchitis and emphysema. In the 1950s confusion abounded as to their interrelationships. The term "chronic non-specific lung disease" emerged in 1958 and evolved to chronic obstructive lung disease. For all practical purposes, the functional consequences of these disorders replaced the structural criteria in the recognition, identification and discrimination between these disorders. Use of the term "emphysema" receded in favour of "chronic obstructive pulmonary disease" (COPD). Airflow obstruction with impaired diffusion capacity was seen to reflect alveolar destruction and emphysema. Airflow obstruction with a normal diffusion capacity was seen to represent asthma and/or obstructive bronchitis. Strict criteria did not evolve. The gold standard for staging the severity of emphysema was the visual analysis of thin sections of the fixed inflated lungs. This was of limited value in life. The radiograph proved disappointing in that it had limited sensitivity and did not allow a reliable index of severity.

FLOW-VOLUME RELATIONSHIPS

The emergence of the measurement of flow relative to volume unravelled the mechanics of airflow obstruction.[29–32] Peak expiratory flow rate at high lung volume was modestly reduced, expiratory flow at lower lung volumes was dramatically reduced and inspiratory flow rate was only modestly reduced. Obstruction was recognized to be predominantly expiratory. The lung behaved like a Starling resistor, with expiratory resistance increasing as expiratory effort increased. Frequency dependence of compliance, flow–volume curves with and without helium oxygen mixtures, and closing volume amplified the sensitivity with which the consequences of airway resistance in large and small airways could be detected. The consequences of airway resistance in large and small airways became essential and the measurement of resistance was performed infrequently.

The measurement of flow rates at 75%, 50% and 25% of VC, maximal mid-expiratory flow rates and closing volume became broadly available as technical advances in equipment design improved. Nonetheless the FEV_1 was seen to be more closely related to disability and handicap even though it was less sensitive. The FEV_1 continues to enjoy enormous clinical appeal.

PULMONARY FUNCTION ASSESSMENT IN ASTHMA

A large number of tests can be used to diagnose, manage, study mechanisms and provide further understanding of the pathophysiology associated with asthma.

DIAGNOSIS (see also Chapters 5 and 6)

The fundamental abnormality in asthma is not currently known. The diagnosis depends on the demonstration of variable airflow limitation, airway hyperresponsiveness and eosinophils and metachromatic cells in the airways; atopic immune status is common. Functional tests are required for the first two criteria. The recognition of airflow limitation is relatively straightforward, and a reduction in FEV_1 with a reduced FEV_1/VC ratio is generally sufficient. The recognition of variability is also straightforward when there is substantial improvement in the FEV_1 following an inhaled β-adrenergic agent. The specificity of this response is high but its sensitivity is poor. When airflow limitation is absent the demonstration of airway hyperresponsiveness is the easiest approach to identifying the presence of asthma. This test is addressed in Chapter 8.

When airflow obstruction is present, variability of the FEV_1 over time or in response to treatment is required for diagnosis. Problems are encountered in interpreting function tests when the FEV_1 is low because asthma may coexist with other diseases of the lungs and airways. There are no perfect criteria for the recognition of asthma in the presence of other disorders. The recognition of variable airflow limitation remains deeply rooted in demonstrating a 15–20% variability in FEV_1. However, there are considerable problems with this approach, because when the FEV_1 is low the variability in the measurement is considerable. With a baseline value FEV_1 20% of predicted normal, 20% improvement in FEV_1 results in an increase to 24% predicted normal. The FEV_1 is always less than the VC and any mechanical factor reducing the VC and varying over time will result in a variable FEV_1. Patients often experience a sense of well-being following systemic steroid therapy and any inflammatory condition of the lungs may mechanically improve with systemic steroid therapy. This may result in the needless use of long-term steroids with considerable economic cost and undesirable side-effects. Response to inhaled steroids is less likely to result in these changes and may be preferable to systemic steroids in trials of treatment. Management strategies used in asthmatic patients minimize impairment, disability and handicap in some patients with other diagnostic labels such as COPD. Although certainty can be pursued, it is often not achieved, and clinical judgement continues to be required.

MANAGEMENT

The aim of management is to minimize symptoms, reduce airway inflammation, improve airway responsiveness and normalize ventilatory capacity. Routine surveillance of airway responsiveness is not common practice as yet. Surveillance remains deeply rooted in the measurement of the FEV_1 with the aim of maintaining a normal value or minimizing its reduction. A complete inspiration followed by a complete expiration is required for a reliable measurement. Failure to make a complete inspiration and expiration results in poor reproducibility and can be recognized in the spirogram trace by an experienced observer.

Common problems are encountered in the interpretation of spirometry in asthmatics. A low FEV_1 with a high FEV_1/VC ratio is occasionally seen in patients suspected to have airflow obstruction. When airways become totally obstructed, the FEV_1/VC ratio increases, and an obstructive disorder can be mistaken for a restrictive disorder. In this setting, flow–volume analysis will show a marked reduction in flow rates and measurement of lung volume will show a high total lung volume and a high RV/TLC ratio. Another common problem is the attribution of airflow obstruction to asthma and/or COPD. There is no infallible answer to this question. Low DL_{CO}* in older patients is generally helpful in identifying emphysema, but it does not exclude the possibility that asthma may coexist with COPD/emphysema. However, aggressive management to reverse airflow limitation should be attempted if the DL_{CO} is high.

Because of the simplicity of the equipment, the ease of measurement and the ability to measure flow rates outside a clinical laboratory at home and in the work place, peak flow rates are popular in the management of asthma. Peak flow rates are less reliable than the FEV_1 in the estimation of severity of airflow obstruction. With increasing obstruction, peak flow rates are better maintained than the decline in flow rates at lower lung volumes. In our laboratory, peak flow rates (expressed as a percentage of normal predicted) are on average 20% higher than the FEV_1 (expressed as a percentage of normal predicted) in patients with airflow obstruction. Experience with flow–volume relationships over the past 30 years have disclosed that peak flow rates are better preserved than the flow rates at lower lung volumes. Furthermore they are influenced to a large extent by the peak expiratory pressure, and there is a wide variability in expiratory muscle strength in the population. Submaximal activation of the expiratory muscles is also possible and this is less a problem with the FEV_1 where dynamic collapse of the airways prevents increases in flow rates with greater effort.

MECHANICS
Mechanical measurements of oesophageal pressure, lung volumes and respiratory pressures are useful in providing understanding. While these

---

*The carbon monoxide diffusing capacity (DL_{CO}) is a measure of the amount of CO transferred from alveolar gas to the pulmonary capillary blood per unit for each mmHg driving pressure of CO. Its units are ml of CO (STPD)/min/mmHg (CO).

measurements are not routine, they are useful in exploring how broncho-constriction contributes to dyspnoea. Mechanical measurements and the rating of dyspnoea can be conducted simultaneously during incrementally induced bronchoconstriction in patients with disproportionate dyspnoea. This approach is useful in some patients in the recognition of factitious asthma where patients will not perform maximal manoeuvres or where they are disproportionately dyspnoeic.

EXERCISE

The measurement of FEV_1, before and 10 min following a standard incremental exercise test in a laboratory environment, is relatively insensitive in detecting exercise-induced bronchoconstriction. Vigorous exercise, breathing dry air for a duration of 6 min, increases sensitivity; the addition of cold dry air further increases the sensitivity. Prolonged exercise may also increase the sensitivity but this approach is not usually feasible in a laboratory setting. The absence of exercise-induced bronchoconstriction in a laboratory environment does not exclude exercise-induced bronchoconstriction in more extreme circumstances in a natural setting.

REFERENCES

1. Brewis R. *Classic Papers in Asthma*, vol. 1. London: Science Press Ltd, 1990.

2. Morgagni G. The seats and causes of disease investigated by anatomy. (De Sedibus et Causis Morborum per Anatomen Indagatis). In: Nuland SB (ed) *Excerpts in Doctors, the Biography of Medicine*. New York: A.A. Knopf, 1989: 145–70.

3. Laennec R. *A Treatise on the Diseases of the Chest*. London: Hafner Publishing Co., 1962.

4. Hutchinson J. On the capacity of the lungs and on the respiratory movements with the view of establishing a precise and easy method of detecting disease by the spirometer. *Lancet* 1846; i: 630–2.

5. Hutchinson J. Pneumatic apparatus for valuing the respiratory powers. *Lancet* 1844; i: 390–1.

6. Rohrer F. The physiology of respiratory movements. In: Bethe ATJ *et al.* (eds) *Physiologie der Atembewegung. Handbuch der Normalen und Path. Physiol.*, vol. 2. Berlin: Springer, 1925: 70–127. Reprinted in: West JB (ed) *Translations in Respiratory Physiology*. Stroudsburg, Pennsylvania: Dowden, Hutchinson & Ross, Inc., 1975: 93–170.

7. Rohrer F. The correlation of respiratory forces and their dependence upon the state of expansion of the respiratory organs. (Der Zusammenhang der

Atemkräfte und ihre Abhängigkeit vom Dehnungszustand der Atmungsorgane). *Pflugers Arch Ges Physiol* 1916; 165: 419-44. Reprinted in: West JB (ed) *Translations in Respiratory Physiology*. Stroudsburg, Pennsylvania: Dowden, Hutchinson & Ross, Inc., 1975: 67-88.

8   Rohrer F. Flow resistance in the human air passages and the effect of irregular branching of the bronchial system on the respiratory process in various regions of the lungs. *Pflugers Arch Ges Physiol* 1915; 162: 225-99.

9   Pengelly LD. Curve-fitting analysis of pressure–volume characteristics of the lungs. *J Appl Physiol* 1977; 42: 111-6.

10 D'Angelo E, Calderini E, Torri G, Robatto F, Bono D, Milic-Emili J. Respiratory mechanics in anesthetized paralyzed humans: effects of flow, volume, and time. *J Appl Physiol* 1989; 67: 2556-64.

11 Wirz K. Changes in the pleural pressure during respiration, and causes of its variability. (Das Verhalten des Druckes in Pleuraraum bei der Atmung und die Ursachen seiner Veränderlichkeit). *Pflugers Arch Ges Physiol* 1923; 199: 1-56. Reprinted in: West JB (ed) *Translations in Respiratory Physiology*. Stroudsburg, Pennsylvania: Dowden, Hutchinson & Ross, Inc., 1975: 174-226.

12 Von Neergaard K, Wirz K. Method for measuring lung elasticity in living human subjects, especially in emphysema. (Über eine Methode zur Messung der Lungenelastizität am lebenden Menschen, insbesondere Emphysem). *Z Klin Med* 1927; 105: 35-50. Reprinted in West JB (ed) *Translations in Respiratory Physiology*. Stroudsburg, Pennsylvania: Dowden, Hutchinson & Ross, Inc., 1975: 227-69.

13 Von Neergaard K. New interpretations of basic concepts of respiratory mechanics. Correlation of pulmonary recoil force with surface tension in the alveoli. *Z Gesamte Exp Med* 1929; 66: 373-94.

14 Otis AB, Fenn WO, Rahn H. Mechanics of breathing in man. *J Appl Physiol* 1950; 2: 592-607.

15 Buytendijk HJ. *Oesophagusdruck en Longelasticiteit*. Dissertatie, Univ. Groningen, Netherlands, 1949.

16 Milic-Emili J, Mead J, Turner JM, Glauser EM. Improved technique for estimating pleural pressure from esophageal balloons. *J Appl Physiol* 1964; 19: 217-23.

17 Leblanc P, Summers E, Inman MD, Jones NL, Campbell EJM, Killian KJ. Inspiratory muscles during exercise: a problem of supply and demand. *J Appl Physiol* 1988; 64: 2482-9.

18 Inman MD. *The Role of Expiratory Muscle Activity in Ventilation During Exercise*. PhD Thesis, McMaster University, Hamilton, Ontario, 1992.

19 Hamielec CM, Summers E, O'Byrne PM, Killian KJ. Factors contributing to breathlessness during asthma (abstract). *Am Rev Respir Dis* 1988; 137: 242.

20 Zechman FW Jr, Wiley RL. Afferent inputs to breathing: respiratory sensation. In: Geiger SR, Widdicombe JG, Cherniack NS, Fishman AP (eds) *Handbook of Physiology, Section 3: The Respiratory System, Vol II, Part I.* Bethesda, Maryland: American Physiological Society, Williams & Wilkins, 1986: 449–74.

21 Means JH. Dyspnoea. *Medicine Monograph* 1924; 5: 309–416.

22 Hermannsen J. Untersuchungen über die maximale Ventilationsgrösse. (Atemgrenzwert). *Z Gesamte Exp Med* 1933; 90: 130.

23 Knipping HW, Lewis W, Moncrieff A. Über die Dyspnoe. *Beitr z Klin d Tuberk* 1933; 82: 133–52.

24 Anthony AJ. Untersuchungen über Lungen Volumina und Lungenventilation. *Deutsche Arch Klin Med* 1930; 167: 129.

25 Cournand A, Richards DW. Pulmonary insufficiency. I. Discussion of a physiological classification and presentation of clinical test. *Am Rev Tuberculosis* 1941; 44: 26–41.

26 Tiffeneau R, Beauvallet M. A synopsis of bronchoconstriction and bronchodilatation test using aerosols: detection, measurement and control in chronic respiratory insufficiency. *Bull Acad Natl Med* 1945; 129: 165–8.

27 Tiffeneau R, Pinelli A. Regulation bronchique de la ventilation pulmonaire. *J Fr Med Chir Thorac* 1948; 2: 221–44.

28 Gandevia B, Jones PH. Terminology for measurements of ventilatory capacity. *Thorax* 1957; 12: 290–3.

29 Hyatt RE, Schilder DP, Fry DL. Relationship between maximum expiratory flow and degree of lung inflation. *J Appl Physiol* 1958; 13: 331–6.

30 Hyatt RE. The interrelationships of pressure, flow and volume during various respiratory maneuvers in normal and emphysematous subjects. *Am Rev Respir Dis* 1961; 83: 676–83.

31 Hyatt RE. Forced expiration. In: Macklem PT, Mead J (eds) *Handbook of Physiology, Section 3, Vol 3: Mechanics of Breathing.* Bethesda, Maryland: American Physiological Society, 1986: 295–314.

32 Fry DL, Hyatt RE. Pulmonary mechanics. A unified analysis of the relationship between pressure, volume and gas flow in the lungs of normal and diseased human subjects. *Am J Med* 1960; 29: 672–89.

KEY POINTS

1 There is a wide variety of pulmonary function measurements that can be used to assess the asthmatic patient. All are best used in accordance with the sentiments expressed in the following quotation: "No natural phenomena can be adequately studied in itself alone, but to be understood must be considered as it stands connected with all of nature" (Sir Francis Bacon, 1561–1626).

8

PROVOCATION TESTS

D.W. Cockcroft

INTRODUCTION

Bronchoprovocation tests[1–16] have provided great insight into the patho-physiology and pharmacology of asthma.[17,18] Bronchoconstrictor stimuli can be either non-selective (affecting all asthmatics) or selective (affecting only certain asthmatics) (Table 8.1). Selective stimuli can be either sensitizers (allergens and chemical sensitizers) or non-sensitizers (acetylsalicylic acid (ASA), non-steroidal anti-inflammatory drugs (NSAIDs), additives, etc.). Histamine and methacholine (direct-acting, non-selective stimuli) inhalation tests are widely used as a diagnostic aid in asthma. The clinical role of provocation with indirect non-selective stimuli is currently uncertain. Bronchoprovocation with selective stimuli, e.g. chemical sensitizers, ASA and additives, can occasionally be of value in pinpointing aetiologic agents. Allergen inhalations are primarily a research tool.

NON-SELECTIVE STIMULI

Non-selective stimuli are either chemical (natural or synthetic) or physical (Table 8.1). An alternate, possibly more clinically relevant classification, is direct and indirect.[19] Direct stimuli act primarily on specific smooth muscle receptors to cause bronchoconstriction; histamine, cholinergic agonists and some other naturally occurring mediators are examples. Indirect stimuli act through intermediate (e.g. neurological reflexes, mediator release, etc.) and often incompletely understood pathways to provoke broncho-constriction; the physical stimuli, adenosine monophosphate (AMP) and probably β-adrenergic blockers are examples.[19] Naturally occurring bron-choconstriction in asthma occurs through "indirect" pathways. Therefore, it is possible that responses to indirect stimuli might be more specific for asthma and have more clinical relevance.[19] There are some data to support this, particularly in differentiating asthma from chronic airflow limitation.[20,21] This remains an incompletely studied area. Most clinical studies have used the direct stimuli, histamine and methacholine.

TABLE 8.1: *Stimuli used for provocation tests*

Non-selective	Selective
Chemical	*Sensitizers*
Autonomic nervous system	Allergens (inhaled)
Cholinergic agonists	Low molecular weight
β-Adrenergic antagonists	chemicals
α-Adrenergic agonists	Foods
Nicotinic (ganglionic) agonists	
Amines	
Histamine	
5-HT, etc.	*Non-sensitizers*
Lipid metabolites	ASA/NSAIDs
$PGF_{2\alpha}$	Sulphite/metabisulphite
Leukotrienes	Other food additives
PAF	Foods
Peptides	
Bradykinin	
Tachykinins	
AMP, adenosine	
Non-mediator	
SO_2	
KCl, etc.	
Physical	
Exercise/cold air/hyperventilation	
Non-isotonic aerosols	
"Inert" dusts	

AMP, adenosine monophosphate; ASA, acetylsalicylic acid; 5-HT, 5-hydroxytryptamine; NSAIDs, non-steroidal anti-inflammatory drugs; PAF, platelet activating factor; $PGF_{2\alpha}$, prostaglandin $F_{2\alpha}$.

HISTAMINE AND METHACHOLINE INHALATION TESTS

Methods

Histamine and methacholine inhalation tests, introduced as early as the 1940s,[22,23] are now widely used for measurement of "non-allergic airway hyperresponsiveness" or simply airway hyperresponsiveness.[18] Several methods are widely used, including timed tidal breathing from a continuous output nebulizer,[1,2] and counted inspiratory capacity breaths from either a handheld squeeze-bulb nebulizer[3] or a breath-activated dosimeter.[4] Results are comparable when tests are appropriately standardized. Technical factors requiring regulation are nebulizer type, output, flow rate, particle size, etc. Non-technical (subject) factors must also be controlled; these include medications (both bronchodilators and specific antagonists, e.g. H_1 blockers), recent respiratory infection, recent allergen exposure and airway calibre. Diluent is inhaled initially, followed by doubling amounts of the agent, at 1–5-min intervals. Expiratory flow, generally forced expiratory volume in 1 s (FEV_1), is measured initially and 0.5–3 min following each inhalation. Tests are continued until the top dose is administered or until the FEV_1 has fallen by $\geq 20\%$. Results are expressed from either the cumulative or non-cumulative dose–response curve as the provocation concentration or dose required to produce a 20% FEV_1 fall, the PC_{20} (mg ml^{-1}) or PD_{20} (μmol). Other information from the dose–response curve, including the slope[24] and the plateau,[25] are infrequently used clinically, but may be useful in epidemiological studies; future studies may identify important clinical correlates of these additional features.

Interpretation

A number of features noted below are important when interpreting tests of airway responsiveness. Many of these have been recognized recently and are not always appreciated.

Unimodal distribution Values of PC_{20} are continuously[26] distributed in a random population probably in a log-normal fashion.[27]

Imprecision Histamine and methacholine tests, even with the best of standardization, are not very precise. Tests are repeatable to within ± 1–1.6 doubling dilutions.[28,29] This is primarily a measurement imprecision rather than true variability in airway responsiveness.

Cutpoint Cutpoints used to define airway hyperresponsiveness are arbitrary, and generally selected to have a high sensitivity (i.e. identifying virtually all asthmatics). In a random population, a highly sensitive cutpoint has a fair specificity, but positive predictive value for current asthma symptoms is $<50\%$.[30] Positive tests in subjects denying symptoms occur for several reasons, including failure to encounter natural stimuli potent enough to provoke bronchoconstriction, failure to recognize bronchoconstriction as abnormal, failure to perceive bronchoconstriction and perhaps true false-positive tests.

Borderline area Because of the measurement imprecision, and the continuous distribution, there is a "grey zone" of borderline values of PC_{20}; the range is about two doubling concentrations.[31]

Variability Airway hyperresponsiveness is variable over time and often absent in asthmatics not exposed to a sensitizer.[1,30,32] Therefore, interpretation of these tests *vis-à-vis* a diagnosis of asthma requires the test be done when symptoms/exposures are current, i.e. within the past several days.

Airway calibre Subjects with non-asthmatic chronic airflow limitation demonstrate histamine or methacholine airway hyperresponsiveness that is highly correlated to the degree of airflow obstruction.[20,21,33–35] Thus, it is difficult if not impossible to interpret histamine and methacholine tests unless the baseline expiratory flow rates are normal.

Sensitizers Subjects with normal airway responsiveness can develop bronchoconstriction on exposure to either a chemical sensitizer[36,37] or an allergen[38,39] to which they are highly sensitized, either under natural conditions[36,38] or in the laboratory.[37,39] Therefore, a negative histamine or methacholine inhalation test does not completely exclude naturally occurring asthma due to high-dose exposure to a sensitizer, especially in highly sensitized individuals.

Clinical Uses

Diagnosis Histamine and methacholine inhalation tests are widely recommended as a diagnostic test for asthma. In the absence of variable airflow obstruction, there is no "gold standard" to validate the diagnosis. Therefore, it is impossible to critically assess the diagnostic performance of these tests. Since there is a low positive predictive value (in a random population), the presence of both airway hyperresponsiveness and symptoms cannot prove cause and effect. However, a positive challenge does provide a rationale for a trial of treatment. The high sensitivity and negative predictive value indicate that these tests are particularly useful in *ruling out* current asthma, keeping in mind the interpretive caveats noted above.

Cough-variant asthma Asthma presenting with cough alone and normal lung function is common.[40] Some have relied heavily on a positive methacholine challenge to make this diagnosis.[41] However, corticosteroid-responsive cough-variant asthma (or the equivalent) can exist without airway hyperresponsiveness.[42] Therefore, a trial of inhaled corticosteroids might be the preferred diagnostic test, regardless of the results of methacholine challenges.[43]

Occupational asthma Measurements of airway responsiveness have several uses in occupational asthma. Firstly, in this condition, it is particularly important to objectively confirm variable airflow obstruction. Secondly, serial measurements of PC_{20} can be used to infer presence to a sensitizer.[44] Thirdly, the tests can be useful in follow-up to assess adequacy of environmental control, and as an objective guide to determining impairment and disability.

Asthma severity In populations, the degree of airway hyperresponsiveness correlates strongly with asthma severity.[1,45,46] However, the scatter in the data precludes relying on this in an individual as an independent measure of severity.

Monitoring treatment Improvement in airway responsiveness can be used to monitor treatment with anti-inflammatory therapies.[47,48] It is not clear that this has any advantages over routine clinical assessment and thus this is currently a research tool. If it can be shown that treating airway hyperresponsiveness (rather than symptoms) improves outcome, monitoring of airway (hyper)responsiveness may become a useful clinical tool.

OTHER MEDIATORS

Inhalation tests with other mediators, e.g. serotonin, bradykinin, leukotrienes, prostaglandins, β blockers, α agonists, AMP, tachykinins, etc., performed with similar methods, are currently research procedures.

EXERCISE, COLD AIR, HYPERVENTILATION (see Chapter 34)

NON-ISOTONIC AEROSOLS

Background

Hypotonic and hypertonic aerosols are indirect bronchoconstrictors likely causing bronchoconstriction via the release of mediators from effector cells.

Methods

Non-isotonic aerosol inhalation tests[8,9] require high output (≥ 2 ml min^{-1}) ultrasonic nebulizers. A dose–response curve is obtained by inhaling distilled water or 4.5% saline for increasing times (0.5, 1, 2, 4 and 8 min). An alternative protocol for hypertonic saline inhalation is to use 2-min inhalations of doubling concentrations of saline up to a top concentration of 14.4%, or up to 4.5% followed by doubling inhalation times to 8 min. Spirometry is measured before and 1–5 min after each inhalation, and the results are expressed similarly to the methacholine challenge with a PD_{15} or PD_{20} expressed in millilitres.

Indications

Non-isotonic aerosol inhalation tests are an alternative way to measure airway responsiveness. Like exercise, cold air and hyperventilation, they are more specific and less sensitive than methacholine challenges. Many subjects develop significant cough, which causes both discomfort and difficulty measuring spirometry. The clinical value of these tests is being actively researched; currently, there are no clear-cut indications to prefer non-isotonic aerosol inhalations over a methacholine challenge.

SELECTIVE STIMULI

ALLERGEN INHALATION TESTS

Background

The airway response to allergens (and chemical sensitizers) is much more complex than to the bronchoconstrictors noted above.[49] The early asthmatic response (EAR) is an episode of bronchoconstriction maximal between 20 and 30 min after exposure and resolving within 90–120 min. The late asthmatic response (LAR) is an episode of airway obstruction, involving both bronchoconstriction and airway inflammation, and occurring between 3 and 8 hours after exposure. Approximately one-half of positive allergen challenges are isolated EARs, one-half EAR followed by LAR, and a small percentage isolated LARs. Increased airway responsiveness to methacholine can be seen between 3 hours[50] and several days[39] after allergen challenge usually with an LAR.[39] This is likely an indirect indicator of airway inflammation and is generally expressed as the Δ log methacholine PC_{20}.

Methods

Carefully standardized allergen inhalation tests[10,49] require measurement of EAR, LAR and Δ log PC_{20}. Subjects must be off all asthma medication and have an $FEV_1 \geq 70\%$ predicted.[49] On a control day, diluent is inhaled by any standardized method three times at 10–15-min intervals, and spirometry is then monitored for 7 hours. This allows the EAR to be differentiatedfrom an irritant response and the LAR to be differentiated from spontaneous fluctuations in FEV_1. On a second day, doubling concentrations of allergen, starting four or more concentrations below that predicted by skin test end-point and methacholine PC_{20},[10] are inhaled in similar fashion at 10–15-min intervals, until FEV_1 has fallen $\geq 15\%$. The FEV_1 is then measured every 10–15 min for the first hour, and hourly for the next 6 hours. The Δ log PC_{20} is assessed by comparing methacholine PC_{20} (or PD_{20}) from the day before to the day after allergen challenge, although some have found it more convenient to assess this at 3 hours.[50] The time commitment for a single allergen challenge is almost 20 hours. Unlike the very safe methacholine inhalation tests, allergen inhalation tests pose significant risks to the patient. Tests should be done in hospital with immediate access to bronchodilators and cardiopulmonary resuscitation (CPR) equipment. Continuous personal attendance of a physician trained in both the challenge procedure and CPR is mandatory throughout the inhalation and the EAR. Precautions must be taken to prevent exposure of laboratory personnel to allergen aerosol.

Indications

Clinical indications for allergen inhalation tests are controversial. The most common indication is to determine "clinical relevance" of allergens in the polyallergic asthmatic.[51] Other potential indications include a substitute for skin tests when these cannot be performed, and a method to convince patients of a cause-and-effect relationship.[51] However, the EAR can be predicted from simpler, shorter and safer tests.[10] Because of chronic treatment requirements, the LAR is impossible to assess in severe asthmatics, i.e. those in whom the issue of clinical relevance is most important. Most investigators thus feel there is no role for allergen inhalation tests in the clinical assessment of asthmatic patients.[49] Their research use is undisputed; these tests have proved important for investigating the pathophysiology and pharmacology of asthma and are necessary for the conclusive reporting of new allergens. Some investigators, however, maintain that it is important to characterize the complete allergen response in every allergic asthmatic subject.[52]

CHEMICAL SENSITIZERS (see Chapter 31)

ASA/NSAIDs

Background
A variable (depending on patient selection), significant proportion (likely about 5%) of adult asthmatic patients have the aspirin sensitivity–nasal polyp–asthma triad. The mechanism is uncertain; immunological sensitivity is unlikely.

Methods
ASA (or other NSAID) challenges[13] are done by ingesting increasing doses at 3-hour intervals. Sensitivity is often exquisite; the starting dose should be as low as 3 mg. Challenges must be appropriately controlled (as per above challenges) and in some circumstances blinded (either single or double).

Indications
The diagnosis of ASA/NSAID sensitivity is often clinically obvious. Prophylactic NSAID avoidance, particularly in asthmatics who are non-atopic and have severe rhinitis or nasal polyps, is often advised. NSAID challenges thus have relatively infrequent clinical application and are done only in selected centres where there is a special interest.

SULPHITE/METABISULPHITE

Background
Sulphites and metabisulphites (antioxidants added to beer, wine, vegetables, fruits, potatoes, etc.) are the commonest food additives that provoke bronchoconstriction. The mechanism likely involves inhaled SO_2 released in the mouth or stomach. Since SO_2 should provoke symptoms in all asthmatics, the selective nature of this stimulus may relate to breathing pattern during chewing, swallowing or eructing.

Methods

Although ingested capsules of potassium metabisulphite can be used, the most efficient method of controlled dose–response challenge involves drinking a citric fruit beverage in which the chemical is dissolved.[14] Single- or double-blinding may be useful.

Indications

Challenges are not routinely done; however, it may prove useful to clarify what otherwise appears to be single or multiple food sensitivities.

OTHER FOOD ADDITIVES

Other food or drug additives, such as monosodium glutamate, tartrazine, benzoate, etc., may infrequently provoke asthma. Methods for challenge, done in selected centres, are similar to that for ASA.[15]

REFERENCES

1 Cockcroft DW, Killian DN, Mellon JJA, Hargreave FE. Bronchial reactivity to inhaled histamine: a method and clinical survey. *Clin Allergy* 1977; 7: 235–43.

2 Juniper EF, Cockcroft DW, Hargreave FE. *Histamine and Methacholine Inhalation Tests: Tidal Breathing Method. Laboratory Procedure and Standardisation.* Lund, Sweden: A.B. Draco, 1991.

3 Yan K, Salome C, Woolcock AJ. Rapid method for measurement of bronchial responsiveness. *Thorax* 1983; 38: 760–5.

4 Fabbri LM, Mapp CE, Hendrick DJ. Standardization of the dosimeter method for measurement of airway responsiveness in man. In: Hargreave FE, Woolcock AJ (eds) *Airway Responsiveness: Measurement and Interpretation.* Astra Pharmaceuticals Canada Ltd, Mississauga, Ontario, 1985: 29–34.

5 Anderton RC, Cuff MT, Frith PA *et al.* Bronchial responsiveness to inhaled histamine and exercise. *J Allergy Clin Immunol* 1979; 63: 315–20.

6 Anderson SD, Schoeffel RE. Standardization of exercise testing in the asthmatic patient: a challenge in itself. In: Hargreave FE, Woolcock AJ (eds) *Airway Responsiveness: Measurement and Interpretation.* Astra Pharmaceuticals Canada Ltd, Mississauga, Ontario, 1985: 51–9.

7 O'Byrne PM, Ryan G, Morris M *et al.* Asthma induced by cold air and its relation to nonspecific bronchial responsiveness to methacholine. *Am Rev Respir Dis* 1982; 125: 281–5.

8 Boulet LP, Legris C, Thibault L, Turcotte H. Comparative bronchial responses to hyperosmolar saline and methacholine in asthma. *Thorax* 1987; 42: 953–8.

9 Smith CM, Anderson SD. Inhalation provocation tests using non-isotonic aerosols. *J Allergy Clin Immunol* 1989; 84: 781–90.

10 Cockcroft DW, Murdock KY, Kirby J, Hargreave FE. Prediction of airway responsiveness to allergen from skin sensitivity to allergen and airway responsiveness to histamine. *Am Rev Respir Dis* 1987; 135: 264–7.

11 Pepys J, Hutchcroft BJ. Bronchial provocation tests in etiologic diagnosis and analysis of asthma. *Am Rev Respir Dis* 1975; 112: 829–59.

12 Cartier A, Bernstein IL, Sherwood Burge P *et al.* Guidelines for broncho-provocation on the investigation of occupational asthma. Report on the Subcommittee on bronchoprovocation for occupational asthma. *J Allergy Clin Immunol* 1989; 84: 823–9.

13 Stevenson DD. Diagnosis, prevention, and treatment of adverse reactions to aspirin and nonsteroidal anti-inflammatory drugs. *J Allergy Clin Immunol* 1984; 74: 617–22.

14 Bush RK, Taylor SL, Busse W. A critical evaluation of clinical trials in reactions to sulfites. *J Allergy Clin Immunol* 1986; 78: 191–202.

15 Metcalfe DD, Sampson HA. Workshop on experimental methodology for clinical studies of adverse reactions to foods and food additives. *J Allergy Clin Immunol* 1990; 86: 421–42.

16 Bock SA, Sampson HG, Atkins FM *et al.* Double-blind, placebo-controlled food challenge (DBPCFC) as an office procedure: a manual. *J Allergy Clin Immunol* 1988; 82: 986.

17 Cockcroft DW, Murdock KY. Comparative effects of inhaled salbutamol, sodium cromoglycate and beclomethasone dipropionate on allergen-induced early asthmatic responses, late asthmatic responses and increased bronchial responsiveness to histamine. *J Allergy Clin Immunol* 1987; 79: 734–40.

18 Cockcroft DW, Hargreave FE. Airway hyperresponsiveness: definition, measurement, and clinical relevance. In: Kaliner MA, Barnes PJ, Persson CG (eds) *Asthma: Its Pathology and Treatment.* New York: Marcel Dekker, 1991: 51–72.

19 Pauwels R, Joos G, van der Straeten M. Bronchial hyperresponsiveness is not bronchial hyperresponsiveness is not bronchial asthma. *Clin Allergy* 1988; 18: 317–21.

20 Ramsdale EH, Roberts RS, Morris MM, Hargreave FE. Differences in responsiveness to hyperventilation and methacholine in asthma and chronic bronchitis. *Thorax* 1985; 40: 422–6.

21 Du Toit JI, Woolcock AJ, Salome CM, Sundrum R, Black JL. Characteristics of bronchial responsiveness in smokers with chronic airflow limitation. *Am Rev Respir Dis* 1986; 134: 498–501.

22 Dautrebande L, Philippot E. Crise d'asthme experimental par aerosis de carbaminoylcholine cher l'homme. *Presse Med* 1941; 49: 942–6.

23 Curry JJ. The action of histamine on the respiratory tract in normal and asthmatic subjects. *J Clin Invest* 1946; 25: 785–91.

24 Peat JK, Salome CM, Bauman A, Toelle BG, Wachinger SL, Woolcock AJ. Repeatability of histamine bronchial challenge and comparability with methacholine bronchial challenge in a population of Australian school-children. *Am Rev Respir Dis* 1991; 144: 338–43.

25 Woolcock AJ, Salome CM, Yan K. The shape of the dose–response curve to histamine in asthmatic and normal subjects. *Am Rev Respir Dis* 1984; 130: 71–5.

26 Woolcock AJ, Peat JK, Salome CM *et al.* Prevalence of bronchial hyperresponsiveness and asthma in a rural adult population. *Thorax* 1987; 42: 361–8.

27 Cockcroft DW, Berscheid BA, Murdock KY. Unimodal distribution of bronchial responsiveness to inhaled histamine in a random human population. *Chest* 1983; 83: 751–4.

28 Cockcroft DW. Measurement of airway responsiveness to inhaled histamine or methacholine: Method of continuous aerosol generation and tidal breathing inhalation. In: Hargreave FE, Woolcock AJ (eds) *Airway Responsiveness: Measurement and Interpretation.* Astra Pharmaceuticals Canada Ltd., Mississauga, Ontario, 1985: 22–8.

29 Dehaut P, Rachiele A, Martin RR, Malo JL. Histamine dose–response curves in asthma: reproducibility and sensitivity of different indices to assess response. *Thorax* 1983; 38: 516–22.

30 Cockcroft DW, Berscheid BA, Murdock KY, Gore BP. Sensitivity and specificity of histamine PC_{20} measurements in a random selection of young college students. *J Allergy Clin Immunol* 1992; 89: 23–30.

31 Woolcock AJ. Expression of results of airway hyperresponsiveness. In: Hargreave FE, Woolcock AJ (eds) *Airway Responsiveness: Measurement and Interpretation.* Astra Pharmaceuticals Canada Ltd, Mississauga, Ontario, 1985: 80–5.

32 Lam S, Wong R, Yeung M. Nonspecific bronchial reactivity in occupational asthma. *J Allergy Clin Immunol* 1979; 63: 28–34.

33 Ramsdale EH, Morris MM, Roberts RS, Hargreave FE. Bronchial responsiveness to methacholine in chronic bronchitis: relationship to airflow obstruction and cold air responsiveness. *Thorax* 1984; 39: 912–8.

34 Verma VK, Cockcroft DW, Dosman JA. Airway hyperresponsiveness to inhaled histamine in chronic obstructive airways disease: chronic bronchitis vs. emphysema. *Chest* 1988; 94: 456–61.

35 Bahous J, Cartier A, Ouimet G, Pineau L, Malo JL. Nonallergic bronchial hyperexcitability in chronic bronchitis. *Am Rev Respir Dis* 1984; 129: 216–20.

36 Hargreave FE, Ramsdale EH, Pugsley SO. Occupational asthma without bronchial hyperresponsiveness. *Am Rev Respir Dis* 1984; 130: 513–5.

37 Cockcroft DW, Mink JT. Isocyanate-induced asthma in an automobile spray painter. *Can Med Assoc J* 1979; 121: 602–4.

38 Boulet LP, Cartier A, Thomson NC, Roberts RS, Dolovich J, Hargreave FE. Asthma and increases in nonallergic bronchial responsiveness from seasonal pollen exposure. *J Allergy Clin Immunol* 1983; 71: 399–406.

39 Cockcroft DW, Ruffin RE, Dolovich J, Hargreave FE. Allergen-induced increase in nonallergic bronchial reactivity. *Clin Allergy* 1977; 7: 503–13.

40 McFadden ER Jr. Exertional dyspnea and cough as preludes to acute attacks of bronchial asthma. *N Engl J Med* 1975; 292: 555–9.

41 Irwin RS, Curley FJ, French CL. Chronic cough: the spectrum and frequency of causes, key components of the diagnostic evaluation, and outcome of specific therapy. *Am Rev Respir Dis* 1990; 141: 640–7.

42 Gibson PG, Dolovich J, Denburg J, Ramsdale EH, Hargreave FE. Chronic cough: eosinophilic bronchitis without asthma. *Lancet* 1989; i: 1346–8.

43 Cockcroft DW, Hargreave FE. Airway hyperresponsiveness: relevance of random population data to clinical usefulness. *Am Rev Respir Dis* 1990; 142: 497–500.

44 Cartier A, Pineau L, Malo JL. Monitoring of maximum expiratory peak flow rates and histamine inhalation tests in the investigation of occupational asthma. *Clin Allergy* 1984; 14: 193–6.

45 Juniper EF, Frith PA, Hargreave FE. Airways responsiveness to histamine and methacholine: relationship to minimum treatment to control symptoms of asthma. *Thorax* 1981; 36: 575–9.

46 Murray AB, Ferguson AC, Morrison B. Airway responsiveness to histamine as a test for overall severity of asthma in children. *J Allergy Clin Immunol* 1981; 68: 119–24.

47 Woolcock AJ, Yan K, Salome CM. Effect of therapy on bronchial hyperresponsiveness in the long-term management of asthma. *Clin Allergy* 1988; 18: 165–76.

48 Cockcroft DW. Therapy for airway inflammation in asthma. *J Allergy Clin Immunol* 1991; 87: 914–19.

49 Cockcroft DW. Bronchial inhalation tests II. *Ann Allergy* 1987; 59: 89–99.

50 Durham SR, Craddock CF, Cookson WO, Benson MK. Increases in airway responsiveness to histamine precede allergen-induced late asthmatic responses. *J Allergy Clin Immunol* 1988; 82: 764–70.

51 Spector SL. Bronchial inhalation challenges with antigens. In: Spector SL (ed) *Provocative Challenge Procedures: Bronchial, Oral, Nasal, and Exercise*, vol. I. Boca Raton, Florida: CRC Press, 1983: 97–112.

52 Pelikan Z, Pelikan-Filipek M. The late asthmatic response to allergen challenge – Part I. Ann Allergy 1986; 56: 414–20.

KEY POINTS

1   Provocation with direct-acting non-selective stimuli (histamine/methacholine) are safe, simple and widely used as a diagnostic aid in clinical asthma.

2   Provocation with indirect-acting non-selective stimuli (exercise/hypertonic saline) are more specific but less sensitive than histamine or methacholine (*vis-à-vis* a diagnosis of asthma).

3   Provocation with allergen remains an important research tool with little or no role in routine clinical assessment of asthma.

9

INVESTIGATIONS OF ALLERGY

Allan B. Becker

RATIONALE FOR ALLERGY INVESTIGATION

While allergy is usually considered to play an important role in childhood asthma, this has not been generally thought to be true of adults with asthma. However, studies suggest that a "dose–response" relationship exists between allergy and disease severity.[1,2] In a recent multicentre study of patients with moderate to severe asthma a large proportion of adults with asthma were found to be atopic.[3] Therefore, age and severity of disease are important considerations in deciding whether allergy investigations ought to be initiated.

Most national and international guidelines for the treatment of asthma note the importance of control of the environment before introduction of pharmacotherapy. Environmental control measures are without risk to the patient, although when considering the role of animals in asthma pathophysiology, appropriate consideration must be given to emotionally charged personal and family issues. Critical to this issue is the correct diagnosis of the role of allergy for each individual.

GENERAL CONSIDERATIONS

Allergens represent a spectrum of complex antigenic materials. Beginning in 1980, international committees began to agree on international standards for various allergens. Some allergens have proved to be relatively simple with one or two major antigenic proteins, whereas others have proved to be extremely complex with multiple proteins and multiple allergens (for example, various moulds).

A standardized allergen nomenclature has been applied wherein the first three letters of the genus are italicized, followed by a space, followed by the first letter of the species name (italicized), then a space and a roman numeral.[4] For example, *Der p* I refers to *Dermatophagoides pteronyssinus* P_1. Many of these allergens have been sequenced and some cloned materials are available for research purposes.

Better understanding of allergens has allowed us to define their source and their location in our environment. For example, the clinically important allergen in cat (*Fel d* I) occurs in hair follicles and is also secreted into saliva and subsequently deposited on cat hair by licking. This material disseminates as an aerosol, tenaciously clinging to surfaces and subsequently widely transferred throughout the environment on clothing.[5] On the other hand, the primary house-dust mite allergens (*Der p* I and *Der f* I) are highly concentrated in house-dust mite faeces, are large particles and do not disseminate widely from their source (primarily bedding, mattresses and carpets).

For asthma, it is generally considered that inhalant aeroallergens are relevant whereas food allergens seldom play an important role. However, food allergens may be important for some infants and in a very few older patients.[6] In general, there are a limited number of groups of important aeroallergens to which patients are exposed. For outdoor aeroallergens, environmental exposure to tree pollens, grass pollens and weed pollens must be considered. Also, mould spores are a concern and specific moulds have a seasonal prevalence in many areas.[7,8] Indoors, perennial aeroallergens also include mould spores as well as house-dust mites, cats and dogs. Cockroach is an increasingly important aeroallergen, particularly in inner city areas. Occupational (or recreational) exposure to other mammals (such as horses, cattle and rodents) and to a number of other allergenic occupational materials will be considered in Chapter 31. Therefore, in general, to assess the role of allergy for any individual patient it is necessary only to consider a limited number of allergens; specifically, mixtures of tree pollens, grass pollens and weed pollens indigenous to the area, plus mixtures of common indoor and outdoor mould spores, in addition to cats, dogs, house-dust mites and possibly cockroach, plus other specific allergens of major local importance. More complete assessment of sensitization to individual pollens or moulds should only be performed if consideration is being given to immunotherapy. There is no rationale to test for aeroallergens to which the patient is not exposed.

PRACTICAL APPROACH TO INVESTIGATION

GENERAL INVESTIGATION

Some consideration may be given to defining, in general, a patient's "degree of atopy". For this purpose, a complete blood count with differential white blood cell count to determine the number of peripheral blood eosinophils and the concentration of total serum IgE may be considered.

However, these tests tend to be of more value for epidemiological studies than for practical purposes with an individual patient. Assessment of the presence of eosinophils in airway secretions may be helpful.

SPECIFIC ALLERGY TESTING

In vivo Testing

Skin testing, specifically epicutaneous (prick/puncture) testing, for inhalant aeroallergens remains the gold standard test of choice. This technique has been used since the beginning of the century.

Allergen extracts Well-standardized extracts, stabilized in 50% glycerol, should be used for epicutaneous tests. If consideration is given to intradermal testing, extracts should contain no more than 2% glycerol.[9] Extracts should be stored at 4 °C.

Positive and negative controls Positive control solutions are used to ensure that a patient exhibits a wheal in response to either histamine (usually histamine hydrochloride 1 mg ml^{-1}) or to a mast cell-activating compound such as codeine (codeine phosphate 30–60 mg ml^{-1}). The rationale for use of the opiate derivatives is to assess the rather more broad response of ensuring the ability of mast cells to become activated; however, this is seldom a specific problem and histamine is most commonly used as the positive control.

The negative control may be the diluent used to preserve the allergen or, more commonly, normal saline is used to assess the impact of the prick/puncture itself. Patients with marked dermatographism will develop wheal and flare reactions from the negative control and this must be carefully defined.

EPICUTANEOUS TESTING (Table 9.1)

Interruption of cutaneous integrity will allow for a small amount of fluid applied to the surface to penetrate to the site of cutaneous mast cells. Various techniques have been used, including scratch testing, which is relatively traumatic and highly variable, and prick or puncture tests. The prick/puncture tests are the most commonly used and have the most consistency from test to test in the hands of a well-trained individual.[10] A variety of tools have been proposed to puncture the skin. These include a disposable hypodermic needle (ranging from 18 to 26 gauge) and the standardized Morrow Brown needle.[11] A lancet produced by Pharmacia (the Phazet) was dipped in standardized allergen and allowed to dry. This method was convenient and reproducible[12] albeit somewhat expensive, but is no longer commercially available. Our device of choice is a no. 9 sewing needle, which is inexpensive and can be pre-packaged and sterilized so that it is easily accessible for use. A new needle should be used for each test to avoid any potential "carry-over" of antigen; however, many investigators choose to thoroughly clean a single needle or other puncture device between antigens.

TABLE 9.1: *Important considerations for epicutaneous testing*

Antigens
Use good-quality, well-defined, standardized antigens wherever possible

Controls
Always use positive and negative controls

Technique
Place tests 2 cm or more apart
Puncture skin cleanly to avoid traumatic testing
Use separate needle for each test
Blot, do not wipe, excess antigen

The skin of the forearm or upper back is most convenient for use for testing. We prefer the forearm in that it allows the patient the opportunity to observe the testing and the subsequent response. The skin is cleaned with alcohol and dried, and a mark indicating the site for each allergen extract is placed at intervals of no less than 2 cm. A small drop of each allergen extract is placed beside an indicator mark. A positive and negative control are also applied. The needle is passed through the drop and inserted just into the epidermal surface at approximately a 45 ° angle. The tip is then lifted upward and withdrawn. After all tests have been performed the allergen extracts may be blotted away with a tissue paper (do not wipe).

INTERPRETATION

The maximal wheal response to histamine is between 5 and 10 min and between 10 and 15 min for opiates. The maximal wheal response to allergen occurs between 15 and 20 min.[13] Practical assessment of the skin test is made in a semi-quantitative fashion by assessing the wheal response.

Wheal Response

The wheal may be outlined at the time of its maximal response as may the surrounding flare response. A permanent record of this response may be made using "invisible" tape to transfer the ink outline to paper. The mean wheal diameter may be recorded as a quantitative measure of the response. Commonly, grading of the response is usually semi-quantitative which may relate to the histamine wheal size (+, larger than negative, but less than 50% of histamine wheal; ++, 50%; +++, 100%; and ++++, 200% of the histamine wheal area),[14] or may be referenced to the negative control (+, 1 mm greater; ++, 1–3 min greater; +++, 3–5 mm greater; and ++++, more than 5 mm greater than the negative control). Reactions generally regarded as indicative of clinical allergy are usually 3 mm or more in net mean wheal diameter.[15] This is usually equivalent to the size of the response produced by histamine or an appropriate concentration of opiate.

INTRADERMAL TESTING

In general, there is no need to proceed with intradermal testing for the assessment of clinically relevant allergy to inhalant aeroallergens in patients with asthma. Intradermal testing is considered the most sensitive method of skin testing, but is much more capable of producing false-positive reactions because of technique or material used. The additional sensitivity that can be achieved by intradermal testing is indicated for diagnosis of anaphylactic sensitivity to drugs and to stinging insects.

In vitro Testing

The prototype *in vitro* assay for antigen-specific IgE was the radioallergosorbent test (RAST)[16] initially commercialized by Pharmacia Laboratories. A variety of modified antigen-specific IgE *in vitro* assays are being widely marketed to primary care and specialist physicians for office use. A recent physicians statement by the American Academy of Allergy and Immunology[17] concludes that "In principle, *in vitro* tests for IgE constitute a technically valid method for detection of allergen-specific antibody in serum. When these tests are performed appropriately and interpreted in the light of clinical history and physical examination obtained personally by a physician properly trained in the diagnosis and treatment of allergic and immunologic diseases, *in vitro* tests for IgE can provide a satisfactory alternative to skin testing for confirmation of the diagnosis of most patients with clinical significant aeroallergen disease and IgE-dependent food allergy". *In vitro* tests for IgE are comparable in sensitivity to prick/puncture skin tests. However: "Currently, skin testing is more economical per test than *in vitro* IgE tests, and therefore, properly performed skin testing is the test of choice".[17]

Use of antigen-specific *in vitro* testing should be considered in patients under the following circumstances:

- extensive severe dermatitis,
- marked dermatographism,
- inability to withdraw medications with H_1-receptor antagonism,
- patient preference.

THE ENVIRONMENT

Since the early 1900s, clinicians have had the ability to assess sensitivity of patients to their environment. It is only in the past decade that the ability to measure the potential exposure of patients to aeroallergens in their environment has become available, using immunoassays to quantify concentrations of specific allergens such as *Der p* I, *Der f* I and *Fel d* I. With this has come improved understanding of the physical, chemical and immunological properties of allergens, particularly of those allergens from domestic animals and the house-dust mites. This, in turn, has allowed appropriate recommendations for environmental control to be provided and has allowed the assessment of the impact of these control measures on the patient's environment.

The seasonality of outdoor aeroallergens has been known for many years. Knowledge of the obvious tree, grass and weed pollen seasons has been helpful; however, exposure to outdoor mould spores has been poorly defined, yet may be critical to patients sensitized to those allergens.[7,8] Measurement of local area outdoor aeroallergens is becoming more common in many areas.

The importance of house-dust mites in allergy and asthma has been the increasing focus of research in recent years.[18,19] We have recently shown a relationship between exposure to house-dust mite allergen, skin test reactivity and asthma.[3] A number of laboratories have begun to offer assays to quantify indoor exposure to such allergens as cat (*Fel d* I), dog (*Can d* I) and house-dust mite (*Der p* I and *Der f* I). For the moment, issues of quality control in such commercial laboratories leave much to be desired.

The importance of aeroallergen exposure in both outdoor and indoor environments is just beginning to be understood in terms of primary sensitization issues and secondary triggering of symptoms. In the future it will be increasingly important to define not only an individual patient's sensitivities but also that patient's potential exposure to aeroallergens. Further, it will be critically important to define the impact of attempts at environmental control on the environment and on the individual patient.

REFERENCES

1 Burrows B, Martinez FD, Halonen M, Barbee RA, Cline MG. Association of asthma with serum IgE levels and skin-test reactivity to allergens. *N Engl J Med* 1989; 320: 271-7.

2 Zimmerman B, Feanny S, Reisman J *et al.* Allergy in asthma: The dose relationship of allergy to severity of childhood asthma. *J Clin Immunol* 1988; 81: 63-70.

3 Chan-Yeung M, Lam J, Ferguson A *et al.* Relationship between mite allergen levels in the homes, skin test reactivity and asthma. *Am Rev Respir Dis* 1993; 147: A459.

4 Marsh DG, Goodfriend L, King TP, Lowenstein H, Platts-Mills TAE. Allergen nomenclature. *J Allergy Clin Immunol* 1987; 80: 639–45.

5 Quirce S, Dimich-Ward H, Ferguson A, Becker A, Manfreda J, Simons E, Chan-Yeung M. Mite and cat allergens in the homes of asthmatics in two cities in Canada. *Am Rev Respir Dis* 1994; 149: A245.

6 Watson WTA, Simons FER, Roberts JR, Becker AB. Food hypersensitivity and changes in airway function. *J Allergy Clin Immunol* 1992; 89: 184.

7 O'Hollaren MT, Yunginger JW, Offord KP *et al.* Exposure to an aeroallergen as a possible precipitating factor in respiratory arrest in young patients with asthma. *N Engl J Med* 1991; 324: 359–63.

8 Watson WTA, Al-Malik SM, Lilley MK *et al.* The association of aeroallergens, precipitation, and environmental pollutants with emergency room visits and hospitalizations for asthma on the Canadian prairies. *J Allergy Clin Immunol* 1993; 91: 304.

9 Lindblad JH, Farr RS. The incidence of positive intradermal reactions and the demonstration of skin sensitizing antibody to extracts of ragweed and dust in humans without history of rhinitis or asthma. *J Allergy* 1961; 32: 392–401.

10 Demoly P, Bousquet J, Manderscheid J-C, Dreborg S, Dhivert H, Michel F-B. Precision of skin prick and puncture tests with nine methods. *J Allergy Clin Immunol* 1991; 88: 758–62.

11 Brown HM, Su S, Thantrey N. Prick testing for allergens standardized by using a precision needle. *Clin Allergy* 1981; 11: 95–8.

12 Kjellman N-IM, Dreborg S, Fälth-Magnusson K. Allergy screening including a comparison of prick test results with allergen-coated lancets (Phazet®) and liquid extracts. *Allergy* 1988; 43: 277–83.

13 Voorhorst R. Perfection of skin testing technique: a review. *Allergy* 1980; 35: 247–61.

14 Aas K, Belin L. Suggestions for biologic qualitative testing and standardizations of allergen extracts. *Acta Allergol* 1974; 29: 238–40.

15 Dreborg S. Skin tests used in type I allergy testing: Position paper. *Allergy* 1989; suppl 10: 1–59.

16 Wide L, Bennich H, Johansson SGO. Diagnosis of allergy by an *in-vitro* test for allergen antibodies. *Lancet* 1967; ii: 1105–7.

17 American Academy Executive Committee; The use of *in vitro* tests for IgE antibody in the specific diagnosis of IgE-mediated disorders and in the

formulation of allergen immunotherapy. Position statement, American Academy of Allergy and Immunology. *J Allergy Clin Immunol* 1992; 90: 263–7.

 18 Sporik R, Chapman MD, Platts-Mills TAE. House dust mite exposure as a cause of asthma. *Clin Exp Allergy* 1992; 22: 897–906.

19 Platts-Mills TAE, de Weck AL. Dust mite allergens and asthma – a world wide problem. *J Allergy Clin Immunol* 1989; 83: 416–27.

KEY POINTS

INVESTIGATIONS OF ALLERGY

Allergy plays an important role in asthma in both children and adults.

● Defining sensitivity to allergens is critical in recommending environmental control measures.

● Epicutaneous testing for inhalant aeroallergen sensitivity remains the gold standard test of choice.

● Assessment of aeroallergen exposure, both outdoors and indoors, will be increasingly important in the future.

10

OTHER INVESTIGATIONS: SPUTUM, BRONCHOALVEOLAR LAVAGE, BRONCHIAL BIOPSY, ENT, RADIOGRAPHY

P. Gibson and N. Saltos

INTRODUCTION

Airway inflammation has emerged as a major characteristic of asthma. Investigation of the mechanisms and features of airway inflammation has helped to define the pathogenesis of asthma, to determine treatment strategies and to indicate new directions for therapy.

These studies have been undertaken by directly sampling airway cells using sputum, bronchoalveolar lavage (BAL) and bronchial biopsy. The need for an objective marker of airway inflammation in asthma has never been greater. This chapter will detail the use of these techniques and their safety and utility for the investigation of asthma. The contribution of radiography will also be considered.

SPUTUM

Although sputum eosinophilia has been a hallmark of asthma for many years, the clinical application of sputum analysis has been limited. This may be due to technical problems, since sputum cannot be obtained spontaneously from all individuals, it is variably contaminated by saliva and there can be problems with the quantification of results. Recent improvements in methodology have renewed interest in the use of sputum to investigate airway disease. Analysis of sputum is now a useful technique for the investigation of asthma. Sputum can be induced from most individuals and gives reproducible results that correlate with clinical measures of disease severity.

SPUTUM INDUCTION

Increased mucous production is a cardinal feature of the inflammatory response in the airway.[1] Since bronchial mucus is often swallowed, sputum expectoration is not a constant feature in asthma. About one in five asthmatic patients report no sputum production at any time. Other asthmatic patients expectorate variably, either during an exacerbation or during recovery from an attack.[2] The analysis of spontaneous sputum is therefore limited by unpredictable sampling. This problem can be surmounted by the use of induced sputum.

Sputum can be induced from both normal and asthmatic subjects via the inhalation of hypertonic saline.[3] This technique can be applied to both adults and children (over 8 years), and can be performed on multiple occasions to follow disease progression.[4,5] Airway narrowing due to hypertonic saline is blocked by pretreatment with a β_2 agonist, which does not alter the cellular differential. An alternative technique is to combine sputum induction and bronchial provocation challenge using hypertonic saline.[6] This combined challenge provides a measure of both airway inflammation and airway responsiveness in a single test.[7,8] When performed in a controlled fashion the combined challenge technique does not lead to excessive bronchoconstriction or oxygen desaturation in asthmatic subjects.[7]

MECHANISM

Inhalation of hypertonic saline causes bronchoconstriction, cough and sputum expectoration. Hypertonic saline is a stimulus for mast cell degranulation. This is the probable mechanism for bronchoconstriction since pre-treatment with agents that block mast cell mediators also block airway narrowing due to hypertonic saline.[9] There is a close correlation between airway epithelial mast cells and sensitivity to hypertonic saline. The higher the number of airway mast cells, the lower the dose of 4.5% saline that is required to induce airway narrowing.[10] These studies suggest that hypertonic saline causes mast cell mediator release, which leads to smooth muscle contraction and airway narrowing. Cough occurs independent of bronchoconstriction[11] and may be due to stimulation of afferent nerves in the airway.

The mechanism of sputum production after hypertonic saline challenge is not established. Mast cell degranulation is unlikely to be the sole mechanism since β_2-agonist pre-treatment does not influence sputum results. The success of the technique may be related to a reduction in the viscosity of tracheobronchial mucus and increased mucociliary clearance or to increased mucus production. Hypertonic saline could reduce the viscosity of mucus by promoting an influx of water to the airway lumen along an osmotic gradient. Hypertonic saline may also lead to an increase in the volume of airway secretions by changing bronchoalveolar permeability leading to an influx of plasma protein.[12] These changes would improve mucus clearance and could lead to sputum expectoration.

SAMPLE COLLECTION AND ANALYSIS

Sputum is a variable mixture of tracheobronchial secretions and saliva. Analysis of tracheobronchial secretions can contribute to the investigation of asthma and airway diseases, whereas saliva is a contaminant that can confound the interpretation of sputum results. The two largest problems to overcome when using sputum for analysis are, firstly, how to deal with contaminating saliva and, secondly, how to quantify results.[13] Reliable results that reflect disease severity in asthma can be obtained when these sources of variability are controlled.[14]

Sample Analysis

Sputum is collected at a standardized time by expectoration into a sterile container, and held at 4 °C until processed. Salivary contamination at this stage can be minimized by mouth rinsing or using dental wads to block secretions from the salivary ducts. Microscopic selection of sputum plugs for analysis is an established method for minimizing the effects of salivary contamination.[13,14] A sputum plug can be chosen that is free of contaminating squamous epithelial cells and which contains macrophages. This confirms the lower respiratory origin of the sample.

Cells can be studied by direct smear, cytocentrifugation or flow cytometry. Each of these preparations is useful for cytochemistry and immunocyto-chemistry. The suitability of the samples for molecular biological techniques and cell culture remains to be determined. Eosinophils are easily recognized using carbol chromotrope 2R staining, and mast cells and basophils stain metachromatically with acidic toluidine blue. Mast cells and basophils from asthmatic subjects require fixation in Carnoy's fluid, as the use of formalin blocks any metachromatic staining.[14] The cell-free supernatant can be used for biochemical analysis of proteins and inflammatory mediators.[15]

An alternative method of dealing with salivary contamination is to collect and analyse both sputum and saliva.[15] The salivary results are subtracted from the sputum results to give a "corrected cell-count". This method assumes constant salivary contamination and does not provide confirmation of the lower respiratory origin of the sample at the time of collection. It may underestimate the concentration of eosinophils when compared with methods that analyse lower airway plugs.

Reproducibility

The reproducibility of sputum cell counts has been examined in two studies. Total and differential cell counts demonstrate good reproducibility within the same subject on consecutive days[14] and within a 1-week period.[3] The reproducibility of biochemical markers remains to be determined.

SPUTUM EOSINOPHILS

Sputum eosinophilia is a hallmark of asthma. Eosinophils were shown to be associated with asthma at the beginning of this century and recent work implicates the eosinophil as a major effector cell in asthma.[16] Eosinophils arise from a bone marrow-derived progenitor cell and circulate via the bloodstream to the airways[17] where they transmigrate across the endothelium to the airway lumen under the influence of cellular adhesion molecules and cytokines. Sputum eosinophils in asthma are in an activated state, expressing cleaved eosinophil cationic protein (ECP) and CD11b.[18] The cell adhesion molecules ICAM-1 and HLA-DR are present on sputum (but not blood) eosinophils to allow migration across endothelium and facilitate interaction with other immunocompetent cells such as T lymphocytes.[19]

The eosinophil has an important role in the pathogenesis of asthma. Eosinophil counts in sputum reflect disease severity[3] and change in a clinically meaningful way during asthma exacerbations that occur spontaneously[14,20] or after allergen inhalation.[4] These findings indicate that sputum eosinophil counts have potential as objective markers of airway inflammation in asthma. A marker of eosinophil degranulation such as ECP could also be helpful and future studies are needed to define the clinical utility of these markers.

CLINICAL CORRELATES

Several studies have examined sputum analysis in relation to clinical diagnosis in adults and children. Eosinophils[3,8,14,15] and the biochemical markers ECP, albumin and fibrinogen[15] are higher in sputum from asthmatic subjects than in sputum from normal subjects (Fig. 10.1). Similarly, asthmatic subjects have increased eosinophils compared to smokers with chronic bronchitis.[14] Children with methacholine airway hyperresponsiveness but no symptoms of current or past asthma do not have increased sputum eosinophils.[21] These studies indicate that eosinophils and their secretory products form the characteristic profile of airway inflammation in asthma.

Sputum eosinophilia may not be a constant feature of asthma but may reflect disease activity (Fig. 10.1). In controlled asthma, the degree of sputum eosinophilia tends to be no greater than normal,[3] whereas in asthma exacerbations high sputum eosinophil counts are observed.[14] Sputum eosinophilia increases several fold during exacerbations of asthma[5,17] and following allergen challenge.[4]

Sputum eosinophils correlate with objective markers of disease severity in asthma. High levels of induced sputum eosinophils and ECP are associated with greater airflow obstruction (forced expiratory volume in 1 s, FEV_1).[3,15,22] The same association holds in severe asthma, where sputum eosinophil counts correlate with the degree of airflow obstruction in

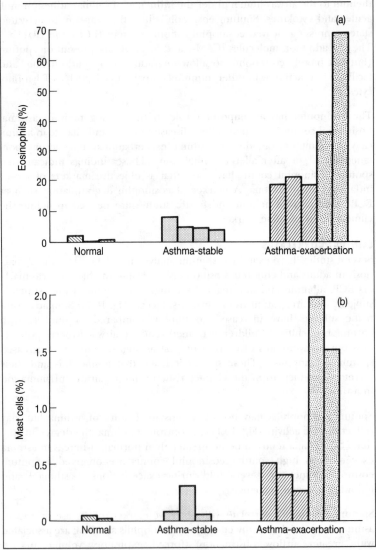

FIGURE 10.1: *Sputum eosinophils (a) and mast cells (b) from normal subjects, subjects with stable asthma and subjects with asthma in exacerbation. (Data from Refs 3–5, 14, 15, 17 and 21 for induced sputum and spontaneous sputum samples (last two bars only).)*

patients attending the emergency room with status asthmaticus.[23] Following allergen challenge, the increases in sputum eosinophils are correlated with the magnitude of the late response and with the allergen-induced changes in airway responsiveness.[4] These studies indicate a potential role for measuring eosinophils and their degranulation products in monitoring disease severity.

Perhaps one of the most useful and well-established roles for sputum eosinophil examination lies in the prediction of corticosteroid response. The presence of sputum eosinophils is associated with a good clinical response to corticosteroid, whereas their absence suggests a poor response. This has been demonstrated in patients with asthma[24] where corticosteroid treatment reduces sputum eosinophils in several days.[5,20] The association of eosinophilia and corticosteroid response also holds for patients in other airway diseases, e.g. chronic cough, where there is no airflow obstruction or airway hyperresponsiveness.[25] The short-term response to corticosteroid is poor when sputum eosinophilia is absent, such as in chronic bronchitis.[14,15]

In summary, sputum eosinophilia is a feature of current symptomatic asthma that can be used to predict short-term response to corticosteroid in airway diseases. There have been no studies relating sputum eosinophilia to long-term prognosis in asthma.

SPUTUM MAST CELLS

Both spontaneous and induced sputum samples demonstrate a 10-fold increase in mast cell counts from asthmatic subjects when compared with either normal subjects[3] or smokers with chronic bronchitis.[14] This increase occurs in the formalin-sensitive mast cell population.[14] Formalin-sensitive mast cells are commonly seen at mucosal sites, and stain positive for mast cell tryptase but not chymase. Mast cell counts are highest during exacerbations of asthma and increase after allergen challenge.[4] There does not appear to be a strong correlation between sputum mast cell counts and other markers of disease severity such as FEV_1 or methacholine airway responsiveness. The results with sputum mast cells differ from the results of BAL or bronchial brushings, where mast cell numbers do relate to airway responsiveness.[27,28]

Mast cell mediators such as tryptase and histamine can be detected in induced sputum, but may not differ between normal and asthmatic subjects.[15]

BRONCHOALVEOLAR LAVAGE

BAL is a useful research technique in asthma and has an established clinical role in the investigation of diffuse lung disease and infectious lung diseases. Whilst BAL has not yet gained a place in the diagnosis of asthma or for monitoring therapy, there is a need for further studies in these areas. The role of BAL in asthma to date has been to contribute to an understanding of disease mechanisms and treatment effects.[29] The major limitation of the technique is its invasive nature.

TECHNIQUE

BAL involves the instillation of saline via the fibreoptic bronchoscope into a segmental or subsegmental airway, and the subsequent recovery of diluted epithelial lining fluid containing cells and fluid-phase constituents. The first 60-ml aliquot of instilled saline samples predominantly the proximal airways, whereas subsequent aliquots sample distal airways and alveoli.[31] BAL produces a heterogeneous sample and therefore BAL fluid collection, processing and reporting need to be standardized in order to minimize variation in results. When this is done, normal values are available for cell counts,[3] but problems with dilution limit the quantitation of soluble substances. Albumin may be used as a suitable marker to standardize the expression of soluble substances in BAL fluid.[32]

Reproducibility

The reproducibility of BAL cell counts and soluble parameters has not been examined over time; however, interlobar variability has been assessed. BAL eosinophil and neutrophil counts are consistent between two lobes from the same individual, indicating that lavage of a single site provides values representative of the remainder of the lung.[33] However, there is poor agreement between soluble markers. Levels of the neutrophil product, myeloperoxidase, and the eosinophil marker, ECP, did not correlate in lavage fluids aspirated from two separate lobes.[33]

BAL AND ASTHMA PATHOGENESIS

BAL has played an important role in furthering the understanding of asthma in recent years. The importance of airways inflammation in even mild, stable asthma was demonstrated by finding increased eosinophils and mast cells in BAL fluid from such patients.[27] Further studies have identified that allergic and non-allergic asthmatic subjects have the same pattern of inflammation, with increased airway eosinophils and mast cells[28] (Fig. 10.2). This inflammatory response is considered to be mediated by locally produced cytokines and cell adhesion molecules. Interleukin-5 (IL-5) and granulocyte/macrophage-colony stimulating factor (GM-CSF) are produced by activated T_{H2} lymphocytes and eosinophils[34] in the airway. These cytokines potentiate the recruitment and activation of eosinophils leading to the persistent eosinophilic and mast cell inflammation that characterizes asthma.

BAL eosinophils correlate with asthma symptoms,[35] airflow obstruction[35] and airway responsiveness.[27] Allergen challenge causes an increase in BAL eosinophils[36] and in eosinophil activation. This is accompanied by increased gene transcription for those cytokines that control eosinophil

FIGURE 10.2: *Airway mast cells (a) and eosinophils (b) are increased in allergic and non-allergic asthma. Cell counts from BAL (solid bars) and bronchial brushings (hatched bars) in non-allergic non-asthmatic, allergic non-asthmatic, non-allergic asthmatic and allergic asthmatic subjects. (From Ref. 28 with permission.)*

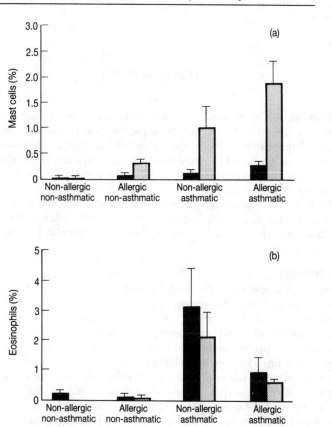

function, IL-5 and GM-CSF.[35] Prednisone treatment, on the other hand, reduces BAL eosinophils and IL-5 gene transcription, in concert with its improvement in airway responsiveness.[37]

BAL mast cells are increased as part of the inflammatory process in asthma, being present in both allergic, non-allergic and occupational asthma (Fig. 10.2). Mast cell numbers are correlated with methacholine hyperresponsiveness in atopic asthma.[27] Allergen exposure causes mast cell degranulation, with increases in BAL histamine, tryptase and other mediators.[36] Mast cell degranulation has a clear role in the early allergen response. The role of mast cells in persistent asthma remains to be defined.

In general, there is a correlation between the severity of airways responsiveness in asthma and the numbers of eosinophils, mast cells and their mediators in BAL. Allergen inhalation challenge leads to increases in these cells[29,33] and corticosteroid therapy reduces the level of airway inflammation.[37]

BRONCHIAL BIOPSY

Biopsy of the large airways has provided invaluable information on the pathogenesis of asthma. The typical pathological changes of asthma are easily demonstrated in biopsy specimens, leading some investigators to consider a role for biopsy in the diagnosis of difficult cases of asthma. Whilst cytological preparations (sputum, BAL) are superior to biopsy for demonstrating cellular detail and for quantifying cell concentrations, bronchial biopsy has other advantages. Bronchial biopsy allows definition of the structural changes that occur in asthma, such as subepithelial fibrosis, and enables the study of the relationship between inflammatory cells and airway structure.

TECHNIQUE

Bronchial biopsies can be obtained using either a rigid or a fibreoptic bronchoscope. Rigid bronchoscopy is superior in that it provides a sample that is larger in size and has less artefactual damage to the epithelium. However, because rigid bronchoscopy usually requires general anaesthesia to minimize patient discomfort, it carries added morbidity and mortality. Fibreoptic bronchoscopy and biopsy can be simply performed under local anaesthesia with minimal discomfort to the patient. It is the most frequently used technique. Adequate samples of the lamina propria are obtained by fibreoptic biopsy. Examination of the bronchial epithelium may be limited because of damage caused by the biopsy forceps.[38]

Biopsies are obtained at the level of bifurcation of lobar and segmental bronchi. There is acceptable agreement between biopsy findings at both levels.[39,40] Once a biopsy is taken, it is crucial to orient the sample correctly to assist with sample preparation. Some groups address this by having a pathologist present at the bronchoscopy to identify the luminal border of the biopsy sample. Subsequent handling of the sample is determined by the nature of the studies to be performed. In addition to conventional histological examination, biopsies can be frozen for immunohistochemistry and specially fixed for electron microscopy or *in situ* hybridization.

Quantification of cells or structures in biopsy samples requires care. Fixation can induce artefacts in the relative size of some structures. Computerized image analysis gives greater precision to quantitation as do newer developments in stereology.

CLINICAL RESULTS

Bronchial biopsy in asthma demonstrates an inflammatory cell infiltrate in the lamina propria as well as increased collagen deposition beneath the basement membrane (subepithelial fibrosis) and epithelial changes. The cell infiltrate comprises activated eosinophils, activated lymphocytes[40] and mast cells undergoing degranulation.[41] These changes occur in both allergic and non-allergic asthma[42] and correlate with symptom severity and methacholine airway responsiveness.[35,42,43] The lymphocyte population comprises activated T cells that transcribe potent pro-inflammatory cytokines (IL-3), IL-5 and GM-CSF, leading to the accumulation and activation of eosinophils. Inhaled corticosteroid therapy reduces airway eosinophils[44] and airway GM-CSF production,[45] leading to improved asthma control.

There are discrepancies in the literature as to whether mast cells are increased in biopsies of asthmatic subjects. This probably relates to the sampling methods used and the nature of the mast cell accumulation in asthma. In normal subjects, mast cells are present in the lamina propria but not usually in the airway epithelium[28] or airway lumen.[3] With the development of asthma, mast cells accumulate in the airway epithelium[28,41] and in the airway lumen[3,28] (Fig. 10.2). Numbers of lamina propria mast cells remain relatively unaltered in asthma. When the airway epithelium is sampled either by bronchial brushing or by rigid bronchoscopic biopsy, then the epithelial mast cell accumulation in asthma is apparent. Fibreoptic biopsy provides good samples of the lamina propria, but there is artefactual damage to the bronchial epithelium.[38] Hence, fibreoptic biopsies may fail to identify increased mast cells in asthma because of a sampling problem.

COMPARISON OF SPUTUM, BAL AND BIOPSY

SAFETY OF BAL AND BIOPSY IN ASTHMA

Bronchoscopy is, in general, a safe procedure in mild to moderate asthma. BAL and bronchial biopsy do, however, have adverse effects on oxygen saturation and lung function, which need to be considered when using the technique in asthma. The importance of careful subject selection, adequate pre-medication and the experience of the operator cannot be overstated. Guidelines are provided for the use of bronchoscopy in asthma[46] (Table 10.1) and these should be adhered to in order to minimize risk to the patient.

BAL causes a fall in oxygen saturation that is minimized by the use of supplemental oxygen and rarely requires cessation of the procedure.[47–49]

TABLE 10.1: *Summary of recommendations and guidelines for investigative bronchoscopy in subjects with asthma and other obstructive airway diseases. (From Ref. 46 with permission)*

Bronchoalveolar lavage, bronchial brushing and biopsy, and airway instrumentation can be safely performed in subjects with mild to moderate asthma

Subjects considered unsuitable	Those sensitive to local anaesthetics/other medications; individuals exhibiting extreme bronchial hyperresponsiveness and severe airflow obstruction; and those with uncorrected bleeding diatheses (biopsy)
Subjects at high risk from the procedures	Those with FEV_1 <60% predicted and/or coexisting cardiopulmonary diseases
Procedural limitations	Instillation of no more than 400 ml fluid; three to six 2-mm biopsies from a combination of the main carina and one or more segmental or subsegmental carinae in a single procedure; and brushing limited to two to four areas
Potential hazards	Acute airflow obstruction; laryngospasm; hypoxaemia; apnoea; bleeding; drug reactions; airway perforation (biopsy); fever; pulmonary infiltrates; infections
Pre-procedure evaluation	Complete medical history; physical examination; electrocardiogram; blood pressure; oximetry
Post-procedure monitoring	Gag reflex; pulmonary function; stable clinical status; post-discharge follow-up

FEV_1, forced expiratory volume in 1 s.

With large volume (300 ml) lavage, oxygen desaturation can persist for up to 60 min after the procedure.[47] A further decrease in oxygen saturation occurs with bronchial biopsy,[48,49] but this promptly reverses at the end of the procedure. Major oxygen desaturation is uncommon, but does occur. It cannot be predicted from baseline variables, and hence many centres routinely monitor oxygen saturation during bronchoscopy and administer oxygen via nasal cannulae. Fever and chest X-ray infiltrates occur in <5% of subjects after BAL and resolve spontaneously. BAL does not appear to alter methacholine airway responsiveness[50] or airway eosinophils in asthma,[51] though it may induce a short-lived BAL neutrophilia.

Airway obstruction may occur during or after bronchoscopy and responds readily to bronchodilators.[48,49] On average, FEV_1 falls only 25% after bronchoscopy, and the degree of fall is related to baseline airway responsiveness. Bronchoscopy in patients with baseline airway obstruction or severe airway hyperresponsiveness needs to be performed with caution.[49]

RELATIONSHIP BETWEEN THE SAMPLING METHODS

Biopsy and BAL

BAL has been compared with biopsy samples in several studies, and the two techniques appear to yield qualitatively similar results. One study has shown correlations between cellularity in BAL and in biopsy specimens from asthmatic subjects.[52] Correlations between "memory" (CD45RO+) T lymphocytes in BAL and biopsy samples were reported by Poulter et al.[53] This study did not find agreement between other cell types in biopsy and BAL samples; however, the sample size was small. Recently, Aalbers et al. have compared bronchial biopsy to bronchial lavage and BAL performed before and after allergen challenge.[38] Bronchial lavage specimens reflected the accumulation of activated eosinophils that occurred in the biopsy samples taken after allergen inhalation. Bronchial lavage appeared more sensitive to these changes than BAL. This study emphasized the dynamic nature of eosinophil recruitment, as eosinophils appeared first in the submucosa, followed by the airway lumen.

Biopsy and Autopsy

The distribution of inflammatory cells in asthmatic airways has recently been studied in post-mortem tissue.[39] There is fairly uniform distribution of eosinophils, with low variability between sampling sites. Whilst there has been no direct comparison of autopsy and bronchial biopsy results, this study suggests that proximal airway biopsy is representative of the tissue changes seen in the large airways in asthma. There have been no formal studies comparing sputum and bronchoscopic samples.

CLINICAL RELEVANCE OF BIOPSY AND BAL

The important role that BAL and biopsy play in studying the pathogenesis of asthma is not reflected by the clinical utility of these techniques. There have been no controlled studies to define a role for BAL or bronchial biopsy in the diagnosis of asthma.

Similarly, although bronchoscopic BAL findings correlate with disease severity and reflect treatment changes, there have been no studies demonstrating a role for BAL or biopsy in predicting or monitoring therapy. There is, nonetheless, a need for an objective test of inflammation in asthma. The invasive nature of bronchoscopic sampling will limit its use in disease monitoring, unless it can be demonstrated to provide substantially more information than clinical assessment with history and lung function. As treatment options for asthma increase and the value of identifying patient subgroups becomes clearer, a role for these procedures in clinical practice may emerge. Interesting reports of the benefits of BAL in the therapy of mucous impaction in severe refractory asthma await confirmation by controlled trials.[29]

SUMMARY

The results of the above studies indicate that whilst each of the sampling techniques provides a valid reflection of the inflammatory process in asthma, they are not identical and hence are not tightly correlated with each other. This is to be expected since each technique samples a different anatomical compartment: fibreoptic biopsy samples the lamina propria; bronchial brushings sample the epithelium; BAL samples the airway lumen and alveoli; and sputum samples the airway lumen. Inflammation in asthma is a dynamic process. Eosinophils traffic from the submucosal blood vessels, through the lamina propria and epithelium to the airway lumen. The variability between each of the sampling techniques can be used to investigate this dynamic process and assemble a meaningful picture of inflammation in asthma. The various sampling techniques are thus best reviewed as complementary. Sputum, BAL and biopsy each have good measurement properties (Table 10.2). The choice between techniques is determined by the research question under study.

NASAL CYTOLOGY

Cytologic examination of nasal secretions can be a helpful investigation in patients with upper respiratory symptoms. Nasal disease frequently coexists with asthma and requires appropriate treatment for symptom control. Some authors consider untreated upper airway inflammation a trigger for asthma symptoms.

Hansel described the use of nasal smears to differentiate allergic from infectious nasal disease.[54] Recent studies describe increased nasal eosinophils in both allergic rhinitis and non-allergic rhinitis, as well as in aspirin sensitivity and nasal polyposis.[55,56] The presence of nasal eosinophilia is

TABLE 10.2: *Measurement properties of airway sampling techniques*

	Sputum	BAL	Bronchial biopsy
Reproducibility			
Within sample	Good	Good	Good
Over time	Good	?	?
Responsiveness			
Does the sample reflect change in response to:			
Allergen inhalation	Yes	Yes	Yes
Asthma exacerbation	Yes	?	Yes
Corticosteroid therapy	Yes	Yes	Yes
Validity			
Relation to objective measures of lung function	Good	Good	Good
Adverse effects			
Fall in FEV_1	Yes	Yes	Yes
Fall in Sao_2	Yes	Yes	Yes
Subject discomfort	Minor	Moderate	Moderate
Costs			
Major equipment needs:			
To collect sample	Nebulizer Spirometer	Bronchoscope Spirometer Oximeter	Bronchoscope Forceps Spirometer Oximeter
To process sample	Haemocytometer Microscope	Centrifuge Haemocytometer Microscope	Microtome Embedding microscope

associated with a favourable response to topical corticosteroids, whereas increased neutrophils are seen with infection such as bacterial sinusitis or viral upper respiratory tract infection.[56]

TECHNIQUE

Nasal secretions may be obtained by nose blowing, nasal scraping with a cotton-tipped swab or plastic scoop, or by nasal lavage with saline. Semi-quantitative cellular differentials from stained smears are often used for clinical assessment, whereas nasal lavage provides increased precision for research purposes.

RADIOLOGY OF ASTHMA

Radiology finds its greatest utility in the investigation of acute asthma that is poorly responsive to therapy and in the detection of the complications of asthma. There is a spectrum of radiographic abnormalities in asthma, largely reflecting the spectrum of disease severity. In about 70% of cases the chest radiograph is normal. Abnormalities occur more frequently in children than in adults, and more often in severe persistent asthma than in episodic asthma. High-resolution computerized tomography (HRCT) of the thorax (Fig. 10.3) provides a superior image of the airways and is more sensitive to abnormalities in asthma than the plain chest radiograph. HRCT demonstrates abnormalities in up to 72% of unselected patients with asthma.[57]

Hyperinflation of the lungs is a frequent abnormality on the plain radiograph. It is recognized by finding an increase in the depth of the retrosternal space (>3.5 cm) on the lateral film, and low placement of the diaphragm below the anterior end of the sixth rib. Studies have reported hyperinflation in 27% of children with uncomplicated asthma[58] and in 19% of adults.[59] Although hyperinflation can reverse with therapy, it may become chronic, especially in children with severe persistent asthma.

The cardiac silhouette is normal in asthma, except in occasional cases of severe persistent asthma where extreme hyperinflation is accompanied by a long narrow heart shadow, as occurs with emphysema. Abnormalities of the vascular pattern have often been noted in asthma. Prominent hilar vessels with attenuation of mid-lung and peripheral vessels occurs in about 10% of patients, probably due to pulmonary arterial hypertension induced by hypoxia. Fraser *et al.* report "subpleural oligaemia", a relative paucity of vessels in the outer 2–4 cm of the lungs, as part of the reversible vascular changes seen in asthma.[60]

Bronchial wall thickening occurs in the segmental and subsegmental bronchi in asthma. It is probably due to airway wall inflammation and fibrosis, and manifests as ring shadows or tramline opacities on the plain radiograph. Bronchial wall thickening is related to the severity of asthma and

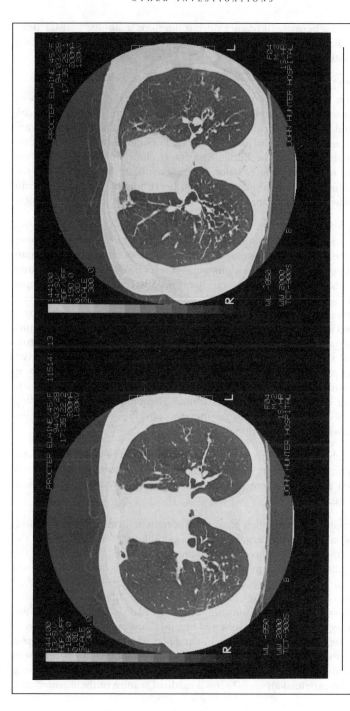

FIGURE 10.3: High-resolution CT scan of a patient with asthma and allergic bronchopulmonary aspergillosis demonstrating thickening and dilatation of proximal bronchi due to bronchiectasis.

tends to be a permanent feature once it develops in adults.[61] HRCT demonstrates bronchial wall thickening in more than 20% of cases of moderate-severity asthma.[57,62,63]

COMPLICATIONS

The chest radiograph is very useful in detecting the complications of asthma such as pneumothorax, pneumomediastinum, collapse, bronchiectasis and allergic bronchopulmonary aspergillosis.[64] These conditions are discussed more fully in Chapters 33 and 42. Pneumothorax may complicate acute asthma, and can be difficult to detect clinically because of diffuse wheezing and severe hyperinflation. Pneumomediastinum manifests on the chest radiograph as a line parallel to the heart border due to air beneath the mediastinal pleura and can be associated with subcutaneous emphysema.

Collapse may vary from subsegmental to lobar although rarely it may involve the whole lung. Lung collapse develops from either mucoid impaction of large airways or mucus plugging of several small airways, the latter probably being the commoner mechanism. HRCT demonstrates collapse in about 20% of moderate asthmatic patients and mucoid impaction in a similar number. These changes are reversible with corticosteroid therapy.[57] Abnormal dilatation of the bronchi has been noted in several HRCT studies of asthma in the absence of aspergillosis.[57,62,63] This may represent bronchial wall damage secondary to asthmatic airway inflammation; however, the exact pathological correlate requires further definition. Recent autopsy studies using quantitative morphometry demonstrate bronchial wall thickening but not bronchiectasis[65] in asthma. This interesting HRCT finding of increased bronchial diameter is therefore insufficient to diagnose cylindrical bronchiectasis in asthma.

In relatively stable patients, chest radiography should be considered where the diagnosis is not clear, when allergic bronchopulmonary aspergillosis is suspected and when there is suspicion of coexisting cardiac or pulmonary disease.

Radiographic abnormalities provide important information for the diagnosis of allergic bronchopulmonary aspergillosis. Sensitization to the fungus *Aspergillus fumigatus* causes intense eosinophilic inflammation of the lungs leading to asthma, pulmonary consolidation, atelectasis and proximal cylindrical bronchiectasis. Areas of consolidation are typically fleeting[64] and may clear, leaving the shadow of a bronchus filled with inspissated mucus forming a band shadow, or a shadow like the fingers of a glove. With expectoration of the inspissated mucus, damaged and distorted bronchi may be visible as ring shadows or parallel tramlines, depending upon whether they are viewed *en face* or tangentially. These changes represent areas of bronchiectasis typically seen in the upper zones and involving mainly the proximal airways. This is a cardinal feature of the disease[66] and is best demonstrated by HRCT (Fig. 10.3), which has largely replaced bronchography in the diagnosis of bronchiectasis. Parenchymal fibrosis associated with upper lobe contraction may develop as a long-term complication of allergic bronchopulmonary aspergillosis.

Osteoporosis is an important complication of corticosteroid therapy in asthma that can be detected and monitored using radiographic techniques.[67] Rib fractures and vertebral compression fractures seen on the plain radiograph suggest the presence of osteoporosis and the need for therapy. An assessment of bone mineralization using HRCT of the lumbar spine or dual photon absorptiometry is more sensitive and may detect osteoporosis before fractures occur. Vertebral fractures can occur in corticosteroid-treated asthmatic patients in the absence of detectable bony demineralization and this represents a limitation of these investigations.[67]

MAGNETIC RESONANCE IMAGING

There has been limited application of magnetic resonance imaging (MRI) to asthma. In other airway diseases, MRI can differentiate normal blood vessels from mucus plugging and peribronchial thickening in areas of the lung with increased linear markings.[68] Localized tracheal narrowing may simulate asthma in children and MRI is useful for the investigation of this problem.[69] MRI offers a potential advantage over CT in providing images of the trachea in both coronal and sagittal planes. Movement artefact may limit some applications.

CHEST RADIOGRAPHY IN ACUTE SEVERE ASTHMA

Chest X-ray has an important role in detecting the complications of acute severe asthma, such as pneumothorax, pneumomediastinum and lobar collapse. Clinical signs of these conditions may be masked by diffuse wheezing, and hence the early diagnosis of these complications requires a radiograph. Chest X-ray seems indicated in patients requiring admission to hospital, or where there is an inadequate response to therapy.

The place of chest X-ray in acute asthma is dependent upon the frequency of the complications. It is therefore necessary to select patients for investigation. If the patient responds to therapy, routine chest radiography is unnecessary since in this setting the yield is quite low.[70,71] However, in adults who fail to respond to bronchodilator therapy and who are admitted to hospital, the chest X-ray demonstrates abnormalities that alter management in up to 34% of cases.[71,72] Radiological assessment is almost always essential prior to mechanical ventilation of acute severe asthma.

REFERENCES

1. Florey H. Secretion of mucus in the inflammation of mucous membranes. In: Florey H (ed) *General Pathology*, 3rd edn. London: Lloyd Luke Medical Books, 1962: 167–96.

2. Openshaw PJ, Turner-Warwick M. Observations on sputum production in patients with variable airflow obstruction: implications for the diagnosis of asthma and chronic bronchitis. *Respir Med* 1989; 83: 25–31.

3. Pin I, Gibson PG, Kolendowicz R *et al.* Use of induced sputum cell counts to investigate airway inflammation in asthma. *Thorax* 1992; 47: 25–9.

4. Pin I, Freitag AP, O'Byrne PM *et al.* Changes in the cellular profile of induced sputum after allergen-induced asthmatic responses. *Am Rev Respir Dis* 1992; 145: 1265–9.

5. Wong BJO, Gibson PG, Hussack P *et al.* Early asthma exacerbation by steroid reduction – examination of inflammation and treatment with inhaled budesonide. *Am Rev Respir Dis* 1993; 147: A291.

6. Smith SM, Anderson SD. Inhalation provocation tests using non-isotonic aerosols. *J Allergy Clin Immunol* 1989; 84: 781–90.

7. Gibson PG, Hopkins YJ, Talbot P, Murree-Allen K. Combined hypertonic saline inhalation challenge: a single test to assess airway inflammation and airway responsiveness in asthma. *Abstracts of the Annual Scientific Meeting of the Thoracic Society of Australia and New Zealand, Sydney, 1993:* 2.

8. Iredale MJ, Wanklyn S, Phillips IP, Krausz T, Ind PW. Airway inflammation in asthma assessed by induced sputum. *Am Rev Respir Dis* 1992; A725.

9. Finney MJB, Anderson SD, Black JL. Terfenadine modifies airway narrowing induced by the inhalation of nonisotonic aerosols in subjects with asthma. *Am Rev Respir Dis* 1990; 141: 1151–7.

10. Gibson PG, Saltos N, Hopkins YJ *et al.* Repair of airway inflammation in asthma: the role of mast cells in persisting airway hyperresponsiveness. *Am Rev Respir Dis* 1992; 145: A19.

11. Eschenbacher WL, Boushey HA, Sheppard D. Alteration in osmolarity of inhaled aerosols cause bronchoconstriction and cough, but absence of a permanent anion causes cough alone. *Am Rev Respir Dis* 1984; 129: 211–5.

12. Umeno E, McDonald DM, Nadel JA. Hypertonic saline increases vascular permeability in the rat trachea by producing neurogenic inflammation. *J Clin Invest* 1990; 85: 1905–8.

13 Chodosh S, Zaccheo CV, Segal MS. The cytology and histochemistry of sputum cells. *Am Rev Respir Dis* 1962; 85: 635–48.

14 Gibson PG, Girgis-Gabardo A, Morris MM *et al.* Cellular characteristics of sputum from patients with asthma and chronic bronchitis. *Thorax* 1989; 44: 693–9.

15 Fahy JV, Liu J, Wong H, Boushey HA. Cellular and biochemical analysis of induced sputum from asthmatic and from healthy subjects. *Am Rev Respir Dis* 1993; 147: 1126–31.

16 Frigas E, Gleich GJ. The eosinophil and the pathophysiology of asthma. *J Allergy Clin Immunol* 1986; 77: 527–32.

17 Gibson PG, Wong BJ, Hepperle MJ *et al.* A research method to induce and examine a mild exacerbation of asthma by withdrawal of inhaled corticosteroid. *Clin Exp Allergy* 1992; 22: 525–32.

18 Walker C, Rihs S, Braun RK, Betz S, Bruijnzeal PL. Increased expression of CD11b and functional changes in eosinophils after migration across endothelial monolayers. *J Immunol* 1993; 150: 4061–71.

19 Hassall TT, Braunstein JB, Walker C *et al.* Sputum eosinophils from asthmatics express ICAM-1 and HLA-DR. *Clin Exp Immunol* 1991; 86: 271–7.

20 Baigelman W, Chodosh S, Pizzuto D, Cupples LA. Sputum and blood eosinophils during corticosteroid treatment of acute exacerbations of asthma. *Am J Med* 1983; 75: 929–36.

21 Pin I, Radford S, Kolendowicz R *et al.* Airway inflammation in symptomatic and asymptomatic children with methacholine hyperresponsiveness. *Eur Respir J* 1993; 6: 1249–56.

22 Virchow JG Jr, Holscher U, Virchow C Snr. Sputum ECP levels correlate with parameters of airflow obstruction. *Am Rev Respir Dis* 1992; 146: 604–6.

23 Alfaro C, Sharma OP, Navarro L, Glovsky MM. Inverse correlation of expiratory lung flows and sputum eosinophils in status asthmaticus. *Ann Allergy* 1989, 63: 251–4.

24 Brown HM. Corticosteroids in asthma. *Lancet* 1958; ii: 1245–7.

25 Gibson PG, Dolovich J, Denburg J, Ramsdale EH, Hargreave FE. Chronic cough: eosinophilic bronchitis without asthma. *Lancet* 1989; i: 1346–8.

26 Syed A, Hoeppner VH, Cockcroft DW. Prediction of a non-response to corticosteroids in stable chronic airflow limitation. *Clin Invest Med* 1991; 14: 28–34.

27 Kirby JG, Hargreave FE, Gleich GJ, O'Byrne PM. Bronchoalveolar cell profiles of asthmatic and non-asthmatic subjects. *Am Rev Respir Dis* 1987; 136: 379–83.

28 Gibson PG, Allen CJ, Yang JP *et al.* Intraepithelial mast cells in allergic and non-allergic asthma. *Am Rev Respir Dis* 1993; 148: 80–6.

29 Smith DL, Deshazo RD. Bronchoalveolar lavage in asthma. *Am Rev Respir Dis* 1993; 148: 523–32.

30 Kelly CA, Kotre CJ, Ward C, Hendrick DJ, Walters EH. Anatomical distribution of bronchoalveolar lavage fluid as assessed by digital subtraction radiography. *Thorax* 1987; 42: 624–8.

31 The BAL Cooperative Group Steering Committee. Bronchoalveolar lavage constituents in healthy individuals, idiopathic pulmonary fibrosis, and selected comparison groups. *Am Rev Respir Dis* 1990; 141: S169–S202.

32 Ward C, Duddridge M, Fenwick J *et al.* Evaluation of albumin as a reference marker of dilution in bronchoalveolar lavage fluid from asthmatics and controls. *Thorax* 1993; 48: 518–22.

33 Schmekel B, Blom-Bulow B, Hornblad Y, Laitinen LA, Linden M, Venge P. Granulocytes and their secretory products, myeloperoxidase and eosinophil cationic protein, in bronchoalveolar lavage fluids from two lung lobes in normal subjects. *Eur Respir J* 1991; 4: 867–71.

34 Broide DH, Paine MM, Firestein GS. Eosinophils express interleukin 5 and granulocyte/macrophage-colony stimulating factor mRNA at sites of allergic inflammation in asthmatics. *J Clin Invest* 1992; 90: 1414–24.

35 Bousquet J, Chanez P, Lacoste JY. Eosinophilic inflammation in asthma. *N Engl J Med* 1990; 323: 1033–9.

36 Wenzel SE, Fowler A III, Schwartz LB. Activation of pulmonary mast cells by bronchoalveolar allergen challenge. *In vivo* release of histamine and tryptase in atopic subjects with and without asthma. *Am Rev Respir Dis* 1986; 137: 1002–8.

37 Robinson D, Hamid Q, Ying S *et al.* Prednisolone treatment in asthma is associated with modulation of bronchoalveolar lavage cell interleukin-4, interleukin-5 and interferon-gamma cytokine gene expression. *Am Rev Respir Dis* 1993; 148: 401–6.

38 Aalbers R, de Monchy JGR, Kauffman HF *et al.* Dynamics of eosinophil infiltration in the bronchial mucosa before and after the late asthmatic reaction. *Eur Respir J* 1993; 6: 840–7.

39 Carroll N, Lehmann-Eastwood E, James A. The variability of airway morphometry and pathology using a stratified random sampling of the bronchial tree. *Abstracts of the Annual Scientific Meeting of the Thoracic Society of Australia and New Zealand,* Sydney 1993: 98.

40 Azzawi M, Bradley B, Jeffery PK *et al.* Identification of activated T lymphocytes and eosinophils in bronchial biopsies in stable atopic asthma. *Am Rev Respir Dis* 1990; 142: 1407–13.

41 Saetta M, Di Stefano A, Maestrelli P *et al.* Airway mucosal inflammation in occupational asthma induced by toluene diisocyanate. *Am Rev Respir Dis* 1992; 145: 160–8.

42 Bentley AM, Menz G, Storz G *et al.* Identification of T lymphocytes, macrophages, and activated eosinophils in the bronchial mucosa in intrinsic asthma. Relationship to symptoms and bronchial responsiveness. *Am Rev Respir Dis* 1992; 146: 500–6.

43 Woolley KL, Adelroth EZ, Woolley MJ, Ellis R, Jordana M, O'Byrne PM. Granulocyte/macrophage-colony stimulating factor and eosinophil cationic protein in bronchial biopsies: comparison between mild asthmatics and non-asthmatics. *Am Rev Respir Dis* 1993; 147: A783.

44 Laitinen LA, Laitinen A, Haahtela T. A comparative study of the effects of an inhaled corticosteroid, budesonide, and a β_2-agonist, terbutaline, on airway inflammation in newly diagnosed asthma: a randomised double-blind, parallel-group controlled trial. *J Allergy Clin Immunol* 1992; 90: 32–42.

45 Sousa AR, Poston RN, Lane SJ, Nakhosteen JA, Lee TH. Detection of GM-CSF in asthmatic bronchial epithelium and decrease by inhaled corticosteroids. *Am Rev Respir Dis* 1993, 147: 1557–61.

46 National Institutes of Health. Workshop summary and guidelines: investigative use of bronchoscopy, lavage, and bronchial biopsies in asthma and other airway diseases. *J Allergy Clin Immunol* 1991; 88: 808–14.

47 Gibson PG, Breit SN, Bryant DH. Hypoxia during bronchoalveolar lavage. *Aust N Z J Med* 1990; 20: 39–43.

48 van Vyve T, Chanez P, Bousquet J, Lacoste J, Michel F, Godard P. Safety of bronchoalveolar lavage and bronchial biopsies in patients with asthma of variable severity. *Am Rev Respir Dis* 1992; 146: 116–21.

49 Djukanovic F, Wilson RW, Lai CKW, Holgate ST, Howarth PH. The safety aspects of fibre-optic bronchoscopy, bronchoalveolar lavage and endobronchial biopsy in asthma. *Am Rev Respir Dis* 1991; 143: 772–7.

50 Kirby JG, O'Byrne PM, Hargreave FE. Bronchoalveolar lavage does not alter airway responsiveness in asthmatic subjects. *Am Rev Respir Dis* 1987; 135: 554–6.

51 Jarjour NN, Calhoun WJ. Bronchoalveolar lavage in stable asthmatics does not cause pulmonary inflammation. *Am Rev Respir Dis* 1990; 142: 100–3.

52 Foresi A, Bertorelli G, Pesci A, Chetta A, Olivieri D. Inflammatory markers in bronchoalveolar lavage and in bronchial biopsy in asthma during remission. *Chest* 1990; 98: 528–35.

53 Poulter LW, Norris A, Power C *et al.* T cell dominated inflammatory reactions in the bronchi of asthmatics are not reflected in matched bronchoalveolar lavage specimens. *Eur Respir J* 1992; 5: 182–9.

54 Hansel FK. Observations on the cytology of the secretions in allergy of the nose and paranasal sinuses. *J Allergy* 1934; 5: 357–66.

55 Lee HS, Majima Y, Sakakura Y, Shinogi J, Kawaguchi S, Kim BW. Quantitative cytology of nasal secretions under various conditions. *Laryngoscope* 1993; 103: 533–7.

56 Meltzer EO. Evaluating rhinitis: clinical, rhinomanometric and cytologic assessments. *J Allergy Clin Immunol* 1988; 82: 900–8.

57 Paganin F, Trussard N, Seneterre E *et al.* Chest radiography and high resolution computed tomography of the lungs in asthma. *Am Rev Respir Dis* 1992; 146: 1084–7.

58 Simon G, Connolly N, Littlejohns DW, McAllen M. Radiological abnormalities in children with asthma and their relations to the clinical findings and some respiratory function tests. *Thorax* 1973; 28; 115–23.

59 Hodson ME, Simon G, Batten JC. Radiology of uncomplicated asthma. *Thorax* 1974; 29: 269–303.

60 Fraser RG, Pare JAP, Pare PD, Fraser RS, Genereux GP (eds). Diseases of the airways. In: *Diagnosis of Diseases of the Chest*, 3rd edn. Sydney: W.B. Saunders, 1990: 2066–74.

61 Hodson ME, Trickey S. Bronchial wall thickening in asthma. *Radiology* 1960; 11: 183–91.

62 Neeld DA, Goodman LR, Gurney JW, Greenberger PA, Fink JN. Computerised tomography in the evaluation of allergic bronchopulmonary aspergillosis. *Am Rev Respir Dis* 1990; 142: 1200–5.

63 Lynch DA, Newell JS, Tschomper BA, Cink TM, Newman LS, Bethel R. Uncomplicated asthma in adults: comparison of CT appearance of the lungs in asthmatic and healthy subjects. *Radiology* 1993; 188: 829–33.

64 McCarthy DS, Simon G, Hargreave FE. The radiological apperances in allergic broncho-pulmonary aspergillosis. *Clin Radiol* 1970; 21: 366–75.

65 Carroll N, Elliott J, Morton A, James A. The structure of large and small airways in nonfatal and fatal asthma. *Am Rev Respir Dis* 1993; 147: 405–10.

66 Rosenburg M, Patterson R, Mintzer R, Cooper BJ, Roberts M, Harrish E. Clinical and immunologic criteria for the diagnosis of allergic bronchopulmonary aspergillosis. *Ann Intern Med* 1977; 86: 405–14.

67 Luengo M, Picardo C, Del Rio L, Guanabens N, Montserrat JM, Setoain J. Vertebral fractures in steroid dependent asthma and involutional osteoporosis: a comparative study. *Thorax* 1991; 46: 803–6.

68 Grum CM, Lynch JP 3rd. Chest radiographic findings in cystic fibrosis. *Semin Respir Infect* 1992; 7: 193–209.

69 Hofmann U, Hofmann S, Vogl T, Wilimzic C, Mantel K. MRI as a new diagnostic criterion pediatric airway obstruction. *Prog Pediatr Surg* 1991; 27: 221-30.

70 Zieverink SE, Harper AP, Holden RW, Klatte EL, Brittain H. Emergency room radiography of asthma: an efficacy study. *Radiology* 1982; 145: 27-9.

71 Aronson S, Gennis P, Kelly D, Landis R, Gallagher J. The value of routine admission chest radiographs in adult asthmatics. *Ann Emerg Med* 1989; 11: 1206-8.

72 White CS, Cole RP, Lubetsky HW, Austin JHM. Acute asthma – admission chest radiography in hospitalised adult patients. *Chest* 1991; 100: 14-6.

KEY POINTS

1 The need for an objective marker of airway inflammation in asthma has never been greater.

2 Eosinophil counts in sputum reflect disease severity and increase during asthma exacerbations or allergen challenge.

3 Sputum eosinophilia is a feature of current symptomatic asthma that can be used to predict short-term responses to corticosteroids in airway diseases.

4 Bronchoscopic biopsy and BAL have defined a role for cytokines in controlling the eosinophilic inflammation characteristic of asthma.

5 High-resolution CT of the thorax demonstrates abnormalities in up to 72% of unselected patients with asthma.

Assessment and Treatment of Asthma

11

ASSESSMENT OF ASTHMA CONTROL: SYMPTOMS, DRUG USE, PEFR

J.M. Corne, N. Chanarin and S.T. Holgate

The rising mortality from asthma has emphasized the need to monitor closely the state of patients' disease and their response, or lack of response, to treatment. Monitoring of patients has become the hallmark of both patient-directed and physician-directed care. Central to this is observation of the patient's symptoms but a number of studies have highlighted discrepancies between both the patient's and physician's perception of asthma and objective measurements of the state of the disease. Hence symptom monitoring needs to be backed up by more objective measurements of lung function, such as peak flow.

SYMPTOMS

Symptoms associated with asthma include wheeze, dyspnoea, cough and nocturnal waking. They all rely on accurate patient reporting and are difficult to quantify, as individual perception of each is highly subjective.

DYSPNOEA

This symptom is not a sensitive indicator of asthma severity and its nature remains poorly understood. Airflow obstruction in asthma is greater during expiration than inspiration, yet only 19% of patients perceive their dyspnoea to be expiratory.[1] During an exacerbation a characteristic feature is a sustained increase in inspiratory muscle activity[2] and it may be that it is this that provides the afferent stimulus interpreted centrally as dyspnoea. Therefore the sensation of dyspnoea probably reflects the effort of breathing rather than airflow obstruction itself.

WHEEZE

A wheeze is a high-pitched musical sound that may be present in inspiration or expiration and audible with or without a stethoscope. The noise is produced by air moving at a relatively high speed through an airway that is narrowed almost to the point of closure. The walls are thought to flutter so producing a high-pitched musical note.[3] Mathematical models lend support to this theory[3,4] and predict that wheeze is always accompanied by flow limitation but that flow limitation is not always accompanied by wheeze. This is borne out in clinical observation where it is well recognized that episodes of asthma do not always feature wheezing. Baughman and Loudon[5] studied a group of 33 patients in whom wheeze had not been observed and challenged them with histamine or allergen. Two-thirds of these patients showed no wheeze or dyspnoea despite developing marked airflow obstruction.

Patients are not always aware that wheeze is present. Shim and Williams[6] examined 93 patients on 320 occasions. During 165 occasions of patient-reported wheeze, auscultation also demonstrated wheezing on 95% of occasions. During 132 occasions when the patient was not aware of any wheezing, wheeze was heard by auscultation 28% of the time. The presence of wheeze, as determined by auscultation, was significantly associated with lower peak expiratory flow rate (PEFR), but the range of PEFR was great. The investigators noted that biphasic wheezing was associated with lower PEFR than expiratory wheeze alone. The proportion of the respiratory cycle occupied by wheeze correlates closely with forced expiratory volume in 1 s (FEV$_1$) ($r = 0.893$, $P < 0.001$),[5] but unfortunately this index is not accurately assessable by either the patient or clinician. It is the only sign that correlates with airflow obstruction but does not lend itself to subjective assessment.

COUGH

Cough is a defence mechanism that protects against aspiration. It is associated with bronchoconstriction and mucous secretion, which enhance its effectiveness. Nerve impulses that originate mainly in the proximal bronchial tree are carried by the vagus nerve.[7,8] The trigeminal, glossopharyngeal and phrenic nerves also carry afferent information. The efferent pathway is mainly autonomic and carried by the recurrent laryngeal, phrenic and spinal nerves. In human subjects with asthma, inhalation challenge produces both bronchoconstriction and cough.[9,10] The two mechanisms appear closely related and can potentiate each other but are not interdependent.[11] For instance, inhaled lignocaine blocks the cough induced by aerosolized water but not the associated bronchoconstriction, while sodium cromoglycate blocks bronchoconstriction but not the cough.[12]

Cough is a very common complaint and not specific to asthma. It has been described as the only symptom in so-called "cough variant asthma" where it is the sole manifestation of asthma.[13,14] This type of asthma is thought to be characterized by central airways narrowing, the site at which cough receptors are most abundant.[15]

Cough may indicate the presence of asthma but does not correlate with the severity of the underlying disease.

NOCTURNAL WAKING

It is well recognized that circadian rhythms affect pulmonary function in both normal and asthmatic subjects with a decline of pulmonary function being evident in the early hours of the morning. A sign of worsening asthma can be the appearance of symptoms during these hours, typically awakening the patient at night or being present on waking first thing in the morning. A full enquiry into asthma symptoms is not complete until details of night-time and early morning symptoms have been sought. Indeed, the presense of nocturnal asthma correlates strongly with disease activity.

PATIENTS' AND PHYSICIANS' PERCEPTIONS

Several studies have examined the accuracy of patients' perceptions of the severity of their asthma either by artificially changing airway resistance or by comparing patients' estimation of their peak flow with measured values. Rubinfield and Pain[16,17] induced bronchoconstriction through methacholine challenge in 19 asthmatic volunteers. Bronchoprovocation was undertaken to the point when tightness in the chest was just perceived and static lung volumes, spirometric FEV_1 and airway conductance measured and compared with baseline; 15 of the 19 subjects could detect changes of 25% or less in FEV_1 and four could detect changes of less than 10%. However, four subjects could only detect changes of between 25 and 50% in FEV_1. Changes in small airway resistance (R_{aw}) and lung volumes were perceived in a similar fashion but were proportionally greater than changes in FEV_1, with some subjects experiencing increases of more than 50% in static lung volumes with only a modest development of symptoms. The obvious conclusion was that whereas some asthmatic patients were able to detect changes in R_{aw} greater than 20% 4 of 19 subjects could not. Presumably this group are at particular risk from the development of unheralded attacks of asthma, making continual and objective measurements of lung function vital.

Other studies have asked asthmatic subjects to assess the severity of their asthma by predicting their PEFR. In a study of 255 patients 60% showed no correlation between visual analogue scores and simultaneous PEFR measurements. In a study of 75 patients Shim and Williams[18] demonstrated a closer correlation between estimated and measured PEFR, with 63% of estimates being within 20% of measured values. However, this study recruited from a hospital- rather than community-based population and the subjects were likely to have had more experience in measuring peak flows and more education about their asthma. Indeed all subjects had had previous experience of using a peak flow meter. An interesting feature of the Shim and Williams study was that 17 patients were examined by physicians whom were then asked to estimate a PEFR. Only 44% of estimates were within 20% of the measured value thus showing the difficulty, outside the acute attack, of predicting PEFR.

PEAK EXPIRATORY FLOW RATE

The nineteenth-century chest physician would conclude his examination by asking the patient to blow out a candle. Donald[19] pointed out that this was a crude means of assessing maximum respiratory velocity and suggested that a 'whistle like instrument' be developed to measure this objectively. In 1959 Wright[20] described the Wright peak flow meter (Fig. 11.1), a portable instrument that can be produced commercially and that measures the highest flow rate sustained for at least 10 ms during forced expiration thus providing a measure of large airways resistance. This has subsequently been demonstrated to be easily used and understood by patients.[21]

Several studies have examined the accuracy of peak flow measurements as recorded by the Wright peak flow meter. Meltzer et al.[22] questioned the use of PEFR as a surrogate measurement of FEV_1. They examined 23 stable, treated asthmatic children between 6 and 17 years of age and compared the percentage predicted value of PEFR with the percentage predicted value of FEV_1. Although as a group there was a good correlation between the two (Pearson correlation, coefficient 0.854–0.892) over one-half of patients demonstrated a 10% or greater difference in percentage predicted value between the two measurements and one-third a 20% or greater discrepancy. Miller et al.[23] looked at a variety of peak flow meters. Those based on the Wright principle had very similar error profiles with overreading of up to 80 l min^{-1} in the mid-flow range though, more importantly (see below), the readings were highly repeatable. Errors can be reduced by taking readings with the patient standing, avoiding squeezing the meter, and taking the best reading of three.

It is clear from these studies that peak flow meters give a less accurate measure of airway resistance than FEV_1 and should not be used as an alternative. However, they are valuable as a convenient way of monitoring the condition of an asthmatic subject. To do this one needs to look at the changes in PEFR with time.

DIURNAL VARIATION

PEFR has a circadian rhythm both in normal and asthmatic subjects. Hetzel et al.[24] demonstrated PEFR variability in 145 out of 221 normal subjects with a mean amplitude of variation of 8.3% of the mean PEFR. Quackenbass et al.[25] worked out normal limits for variation that were defined in

FIGURE 11.1: *Diagram of mini-Wright peak-flow meter. The cylindrical body (1) and one end of the instrument are moulded in one piece with a slot (2) down one side. The other end (3) carries a tapered socket (4) which accepts a sterilizable mouthpiece (5) or a disposable cardboard mouthpiece. It has a central hollow boss (6) which houses a tension spring (7). The mouthpiece end is held to the body by a knurled nut (8) screwed on to the threaded end of a central rod (9), the other end of which is secured in the fixed end of the body. Both ends are hexagonal in section to prevent the instrument from rolling and are pierced by a ring of six holes (10, 11) to allow free passage of air. A thin PTFE disc valve (12) is secured to the boss inside the mouthpiece end. The piston (13), which is a light plastic disc with a short sleeve, rides freely on the rod and just clear of the cylinder bore. The scale, which is read vertically, is marked in litres per minute from 60 to 800, but a scale in litres per second to conform with SI units will be available if required. The rider (14) is spring-loaded in the slot with sufficient friction to prevent it overshooting without appreciably affecting movement of the piston. The meter is 5.0 cm in diameter and 15 cm long, and weighs 75 g. (Reproduced with permission from Clement Clarke International Ltd, Harlow, Essex, UK).*

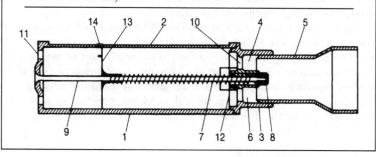

terms of amplitude/mean, this being the amplitude of variation as a percentage of the day's mean PEFR. These limits are shown in Table 11.1. An exaggeration of this diurnal variation is the hallmark of asthma. In the Hertzel study nearly 100% of asthmatic subjects showed diurnal variation with a mean variation of 50%. In the Quackenbass *et al.* study there was a very high sensitivity for diagnosed asthma if diurnal variation exceeded the quoted normal limits, with a sensitivity and specificity of 94.5% and 72%

TABLE 11.1: *Limits to diurnal changes in PEFR by age group for a reference population. (Adapted from Ref. 25)*

Age group (years)	Diurnal changes (%)	95% percentile	97.5% percentile	Median
6–14	Max./Min.	129.6	140.0	105.0
	Amp./Mean	31.0	37.7	8.2
15–34	Max./Min.	116.7	121.9	102.7
	Amp./Mean	19.0	26.8	5.0
35–65	Max./Min.	118.4	126.0	103.4
	Amp./Mean	19.1	28.8	4.9

respectively for those under 15 years and 70% and 56% for those over 15 years.

Increases in diurnal variation, usually expressed as amplitude of variation as a percentage of mean PEFR, are an important indication of poorly controlled disease. One-third of all patients admitted with asthma show a 50% or greater variation in PEFR. Hertzel et al.[26] studied cases of patients requiring ventilation or dying of their asthma. A feature common to all these patients was the presence of large diurnal swings in PEFR; eight out of the nine patients who sustained a respiratory arrest showed a greater than 50% diurnal variation in PEFR compared with 30% of the total asthma admissions. Interestingly, although the standard signs of worsening asthma (heart rate, respiratory rate and absolute PEFR) paralleled the severity of the attack, they were unhelpful in predicting its course. This stresses the need for measuring peak flows regularly as the best means of assessing the state of a patient's asthma and the only means of predicting its likely course, especially important in the subgroup of asthmatic subjects who experience sudden deteriorations and in whom increases in peak flow variability may be the only sign.

DRUG USE

The need for symptom-relieving bronchodilators by patients is a good indicator of the severity of their asthma. Several studies have shown a good correlation between drug use and risk of hospital admission or death; Rea et al.[27] showed that the use of three or more categories of drugs was associated with an increased risk of dying of asthma. Nowadays, with asthma management based on the regular use of inhaled steroids, with β_2 agonists reserved for symptomatic relief, the use of the latter, if accurately documented, should provide a reasonable assessment of the patient's clinical state.

PRACTICAL ASSESSMENT

The clinic assessment of the patient must begin with enquiry into symptoms of wheeze, cough, noctural awakening and dyspnoea; although not completely reliable, these symptoms will give a good indication of disease severity in many. Nocturnal awakening is a particularly important symptom to elicit.

Regular monitoring of peak flow for a period of at least 3 weeks is an essential part of the diagnosis of asthma and it should be continued if initial results suggest poor control, or suggest low peak flows with little in the way of associated symptoms. Admission to hospital with an asthma attack, recurrent need for oral steroids or persistent symptoms suggest a need for continual peak flow monitoring as an important part of patient assessment. In fact, all patients requiring regular inhaled steroids should undertake monitoring of peak flow since this is the basis of the asthma management plans outlined later. However, many patients find this inconvenient and, if they are asymptomatic, it is probably reasonable to periodically check 2-week periods of regular peak flows to confirm that their asthma is as well controlled as their symptoms suggest.

Peak flow needs to be checked twice daily if changes in diurnal variation are to be picked up. This is convenient for patients who can keep their peak flow meters by their beds and record readings first thing in the morning and last thing at night, preferably before taking their bronchodilators. The presence of the peak flow meter may also act as useful *aide-mémoire* for the taking of their twice-daily inhaled medication.

ASSESSMENT OF SEVERITY (see Chapter 6)

REFERENCES

1 Morris MJ. Asthma: expiratory dyspnoea? *BMJ* 1981; 283: 838–9.

2 Muller N, Bryan AC, Zamel N. Tonic inspiratory muscle activity as a cause of hyperventilation in asthma. *J Appl Physiol* 1981; 50: 279–82.

3 Loudon RG, Murphy RLH. Wheezing. In: Weiss EB, Stein M (eds) *Asthma: Mechanisms and Therapeutics*, 3rd edn. Boston: Little, Brown and Co., 1993: 650–4.

4 Grotberg JB, Davis SH. Fluid dynamic flapping of a collapsible channel: sound generation and flow limitation. *J Biomech* 1980; 13: 219–30.

5 Baughman RP, Loudon RG. Lung sound analysis for continuous evaluation of airflow obstruction in asthma. *Chest* 1985; 88: 364–8.

6 Shim CS, Williams HM. Relationship of wheezing to the severity of obstruction in asthma. *Arch Intern Med* 1983; 143: 890–2.

7 Widdicombe JG. Physiology of cough. In: Braga PC, Allegra L (eds) *Cough*. New York: Raven Press, 1989: 3–25.

8 Karlsson JA, Sant-Ambrogio G, Widdicombe J. Afferent neural pathways in cough and reflex bronchoconstriction. *J Appl Physiol* 1988; 65: 1007–23.

9 Chausow AM, Banner AS. Comparison of the tussive effects of histamine and methacholine in humans. *J Appl Physiol* 1983; 55: 541–6.

10 Simonsson BG, Jacobs FM, Nadel JA. Role of autonomic nervous system and the cough reflex in the increased responsiveness of airways in patients with obstructive airways disease. *J Clin Invest* 1967; 46: 1812–8.

11 Editorial. Cough and wheeze in asthma: are they interdependent? *Lancet* 1988; i: 447–8.

12 Sheppard D, Rizk NW, Boushey HA, Bethel RA. Mechanisms of cough and bronchoconstriction induced by distilled water aerosol. *Am Rev Respir Dis* 1983; 127: 691–4.

13 Corrao WM, Braman SS, Irwin RS. Chronic cough as the sole presenting manifestation of bronchial asthma. *N Engl J Med* 1979; 300: 633–7.

14 Johnson D, Osborn LM. Cough variant asthma: a review of the clinical literature. *J Asthma* 1991; 28: 85–90.

15 McFadden ER. Exertional dyspnoea and cough as preludes to attacks of bronchial asthma. *N Engl J Med* 1975; 292: 555–9.

16 Rubinfield AR. Relationship between bronchial reactivity, airways caliber and severity of asthma. *Am Rev Respir Dis* 1977; 115: 381.

17 Rubinfield AR, Pain MCF. Perception of asthma. *Lancet* 1976; ii: 822–4.

18 Shim CS, Williams MH. Evaluation of the severity of asthma: patients versus physicians. *Am J Med* 1980; 68: 11–3.

19 Donald KW. *BMJ* 1953; 1: 415.

20 Wright BM, McKerrow CB. Maximum forced expiratory flow rate as a measure of ventilatory capacity. *BMJ* 1959; 1041–7.

21 Hetzel MR, Williams IP, Shakespeare RM. Can patients keep their own peak flow records reliably? *Lancet* 1979; i: 597–8.

22 Meltzer A, Smolensky MH, D'Alenzo GE, Harrist RB, Scott PH. An assessment of peak expiratory flow as a surrogate measurement of FEV_1 in stable asthmatic children. *Chest* 1989; 96: 329–33.

23 Miller MR, Dickinson SA, Hitchings J. The accuracy of portable peak flow meters. *Thorax* 1992; 47: 904–9.

24 Hetzel MR, Clark TJH. Comparison of normal and asthmatic circadian rhythms in peak expiratory flow rate. *Thorax* 1980; 35: 732–8.

25 Quackenbass JJ, Lebowitz MD, Kryzanowski M. The normal range of diurnal changes in peak expiratory flow rates. *Am Rev Respir Dis* 1991; 143: 323–30.

26 Hetzel MR, Clark TJH, Branthwaite MA. Asthma: analysis of sudden deaths and ventilatory arrests in hospital. *BMJ* 1977; 1: 808–11.

27 Rea HR, Scragg R, Jackson R, Beaglehole R, Fenwick J, Sutherland DC. A case-control study of deaths from asthma. *Thorax* 1986; 41: 833–9.

KEY POINTS

1 Symptoms associated with worsening of asthma are dyspnoea, wheeze, cough and nocturnal wakening, though patients' perception of these are not always an accurate reflection of the state of their airways.

2 A small but important group of asthmatic subjects may develop severe airflow limitation without a marked change in symptoms.

3 *Changes* in peak flow are a convenient way of monitoring the severity of asthma but absolute peak flows are not as reliable as FEV_1.

4 Accurate documentation of medication use may provide useful early warning of an asthma attack.

12

ASSESSMENT OF ASTHMA CONTROL: QUALITY OF LIFE

Elizabeth F. Juniper

INTRODUCTION

Until fairly recently, health-related quality of life was rarely incorporated into the assessment of asthma. This was mainly because there were no suitable valid instruments and because there has tended to be the assumption that conventional clinical outcomes give an accurate reflection of how patients are feeling and how they are able to function physically, socially and emotionally in their day-to-day lives. Several recent studies have challenged this assumption by showing that correlations between conventional indices of clinical asthma severity and quality of life are only weak to moderate.[1-3] It can no longer be accepted that if there are improvements in the conventional indices of clinical asthma severity (such as airway calibre, symptoms and airway responsiveness), then the patient has benefited. Similarly, some patients may genuinely benefit from an intervention but this may not be captured by the conventional measures.[4] The recent development of scientifically sound quality-of-life instruments with strong measurement properties now allow assessment of quality of life to be incorporated very easily and quickly into clinical trials, surveys and clinical practice.

Having decided that it would be a good idea to measure quality of life, the intrepid investigator may become bewildered by the array of instruments. The aim of this chapter is to provide information that should help clinicians make appropriate choices. There is no "best" instrument; the choice has to be made according to the study question and design, the setting, the patients and time considerations.

TYPES OF INSTRUMENTS (Table 12.1)

GENERIC: HEALTH PROFILES
These questionnaires are designed to be applicable to all health states. The most commonly used are the MOS Short Form 36 (SF-36),[5] the Sickness

TABLE 12.1: *Types of health-related quality-of-life instruments*

Instrument type	Strengths	Weaknesses
Generic		
Health profiles	Comparison across conditions possible	Do not focus adequately on areas of interest
	Established reliability and validity	May not be responsive
Utilities	Single number representing quality of life	Do not allow examination of different aspects of quality of life
	Cost–utility analysis possible	May not be responsive
Disease specific	Clinically sensible More responsive	Comparison across conditions not possible

Impact Profile (SIP),[6] the Nottingham Health Profile[7] and the McMaster Health Index Questionnaire.[8] The main advantage of health profiles is that impairment can be compared across different medical conditions. Although each health profile attempts to measure all important aspects of quality of life, this is achieved in different ways. For instance, the SF-36 measures three major health attributes (functional status, well-being and overall evaluation of health) that are not combined into one overall score. In contrast, the SIP has two domains (physical and psychosocial) that can be combined into a total.

A limitation of health profiles is that they may not capture areas of specific interest. For instance, the SIP tends to focus on quite severe impairments (feeding, dressing, etc.) that are not applicable to most asthma patients.[1,9] In addition, health profiles may not be responsive to small but important changes when used in clinical trials.[2] Preliminary work suggests that the SF-36 may have good discriminative properties in asthma.[10]

GENERIC: UTILITIES

These instruments meet the criteria of utility theory and yield a single score from 0 (death) to 1 (perfect health). The best known are the Standard Gamble[11] and the Time Trade Off[11] from which data are used to generate

Quality-Adjusted-Life-Years (QALYs)[11] and Health-Years Equivalents (HYEs)[12] for health economic research and policy decision. Measurement properties of utilities in asthma have not yet been established.

DISEASE SPECIFIC

Recognition that the generic instruments are often insufficiently responsive or sensitive in specific conditions to detect changes or differences that are important has led to the development of disease-specific instruments. Currently, there are four that are applicable to patients with asthma (see below).

MEASUREMENT PROPERTIES OF QUALITY-OF-LIFE INSTRUMENTS (Table 12.2)

Questionnaires used in cross-sectional studies require different measurement properties from those used in longitudinal studies.[13,14] When choosing an instrument, it is important to make sure that it has the measurement properties suited to the task.

DISCRIMINATIVE INSTRUMENTS

These instruments are used to distinguish between individuals or groups of patients (e.g. mild, moderate, severe asthma) and are used for screening

TABLE 12.2: *Measurement properties necessary for evaluative and discriminative instruments*

	Discrimination	Evaluation
Signal	Between-subject differences	Within-subject differences related to true within-subject change
Noise	Within-subject differences	Within-subject differences unrelated to true within-subject change
Signal-to-noise ratio: descriptive term	Reliability	Responsiveness
Construct validity	Cross-sectional	Longitudinal

and in cross-sectional surveys. A simple way of deciding what measurement properties are necessary for any type of instrument is to consider the "signal" and the "noise". Discriminative instruments need to be able to detect differences between patients (signal). The noise that may mask this signal is the within-subject variance, in other words poor reproducibility. The statistic usually used to express the relationship of between-subject variance to within-subject variance is the intra-class correlation coefficient. (Cronbach's alpha, which measures internal consistency does not give an indication of this measurement property). The second measurement property that a discriminative instrument must possess is cross-sectional construct validity. When there is no gold standard against which to demonstrate that the instrument is actually measuring what it purports to measure, the developer puts forward hypotheses or constructs that, if they are met, provide evidence that the instrument is valid. One method of providing evidence that an instrument is valid in asthma might be to show that the new quality-of-life instrument correlates in a predicted manner with indices of clinical asthma and with other quality-of-life measures.

EVALUATIVE INSTRUMENTS

These instruments are designed to measure longitudinal change within an individual or group and are the type used in clinical trials. Evaluative instruments must be responsive to small but clinically important within-subject changes that occur either spontaneously or as the result of an intervention. The signal in evaluative instruments is true within-subject change over time and the noise is within-subject variance unrelated to true within-subject change. The relationship between the two demonstrates the responsiveness of the instrument.[15] The second measurement property essential for evaluative instruments is longitudinal construct validity. One way to establish this is to demonstrate that changes in the various domains of the new quality-of-life instrument are related in a predicted way to changes in other appropriate outcome measures.

ASTHMA-SPECIFIC QUALITY-OF-LIFE INSTRUMENTS

At present, there are four disease-specific quality-of-life questionnaires that may be used in asthma. Summarized below are the characteristics that a clinician or an investigator may need to take into consideration when selecting an instrument.

THE ASTHMA QUALITY-OF-LIFE QUESTIONNAIRE (Juniper)[1,16]
This is a 32-item instrument, designed specifically for use in clinical trials. The items, identified by asthma patients as being important, are in four domains (symptoms, emotions, exposure to environmental stimuli and activity limitation). Patients respond to each item on a seven-point scale. Five of the eleven items in the activity limitation domain are self-identified

by patients. The instrument is in both interviewer and self-administered format and takes approximately 10 min to complete at the first visit and 5 min at follow-up. In two validation studies, the instrument has demonstrated excellent responsiveness and longitudinal construct validity.[1,3] Although designed as an evaluative instrument, it also has good discriminative properties with an intra-class correlation coefficient of 0.92 and good cross-sectional construct validity.[1,17]

THE ASTHMA QUALITY-OF-LIFE QUESTIONNAIRE (AQLQ) (Marks)[2,18]

The AQLQ is a self-administered questionnaire containing 20 items in four domains (breathlessness and physical restrictions, mood disturbance, social disruption and concerns for health). Responses are given on a five-point scale. Items were selected using both patient importance and psychometric techniques. The instrument has been thoroughly tested for both discriminative and evaluative properties. It has an intra-class correlation coefficient of 0.80, is responsive to change and has good cross-sectional and longitudinal construct validity. The questionnaire takes approximately 5 min to complete.

THE LIVING WITH ASTHMA QUESTIONNAIRE (Hyland)[19,20]

This is a self-administered 68-item instrument with 11 domains (social/leisure, sport, holidays, sleep, work, colds, morbidity, effects on others, medication use, sex and dysphoric states and attitudes). Items, identified from patient focus group discussions, were selected for the questionnaire using psychometric techniques and factor analysis. Unlike the Juniper and Marks instruments, impairments experienced as a direct result of asthma symptoms are not included. Responses are given using a three-point scale, suggesting that it may have acceptable discriminative properties but be less responsive to within-patient changes. For discriminative purposes it has a test–retest $r = 0.9$ and shows moderate cross-sectional correlations with the SIP and peak flow rates. Although the Living with Asthma Questionnaire has been used in a clinical trial,[21] the evaluative properties of the instrument have not yet been reported. The time needed to complete the questionnaire has not been reported.

THE ST GEORGE'S RESPIRATORY QUESTIONNAIRE (Jones)[22]

This questionnaire is self-administered and contains 76 items in three domains (symptoms, activity and impacts (on daily life)). The questionnaire has been developed for patients with chronic airflow limitation, both chronic obstructive pulmonary disease and asthma. The methods used for the development have not yet been published and so the criteria for item selection are unclear. As a discriminative instrument, it has demonstrated good reliability with an intra-class correlation coefficient of 0.91 and very acceptable cross-sectional correlations with the SIP, anxiety, depression and the 6-min walk test, but correlations with airway calibre were very weak. Although patients were followed for over 1 year, their health state did not change and therefore it is difficult to determine whether the instrument is responsive to change and whether it has longitudinal construct validity. The length of time needed to complete the questionnaire has not been reported.

INTERPRETATION OF RESULTS

With sufficient subjects in a survey or a clinical trial, even the smallest differences can be shown to be statistically significant and therefore interpreting the magnitude of differences is very important. Most clinicians will have an intuitive feel for whether or not differences in objective outcomes, such as airway calibre or airway responsiveness, are also clinically important. For questionnaires, interpretation is often difficult. In fact, for most conventional symptom scores it is almost impossible to estimate whether changes are clinically important. Recent developments in questionnaire methodology allow this problem to be addressed and we have calculated that a clinically important difference for the Asthma Quality-of-Life Questionnaire is a change in score > 0.5 on a scale where 1 is worst and 7 best quality of life.[23] This applies to overall quality of life and to each of the domains; it also applies to improvements as well as deteriorations. Knowing the magnitude of the minimally important difference is important not only for interpreting results but also for calculating sample sizes for research studies. At present, it has only been determined for the Asthma Quality-of-Life Questionnaire;[1] it is hoped that similar data will soon be available for the other instruments.

QUALITY OF LIFE IN CHILDREN WITH ASTHMA

Problems that children with asthma and their parents experience as a result of the child's asthma have been evaluated[24] and the data used to construct the Paediatric Asthma Quality-of-Life Questionnaire and the Paediatric Asthma Caregiver's Quality-of-Life Questionnaire. In validation studies, both instruments have shown strong measurement properties and both longitudinal and cross-sectional construct validity.[25,26]

REFERENCES

1. Juniper EF, Guyatt GH, Ferrie PJ, Griffith LE. Measuring quality of life in asthma. *Am Rev Respir Dis* 1993; 147: 832–8.

2. Marks GB, Dunn SM, Woolcock AJ. An evaluation of an asthma quality of life questionnaire as a measure of change in adults with asthma. *J Clin Epidemiol* 1993; 46: 1103–11.

3. Rowe BH, Oxman AD. Performance of an asthma quality of life questionnaire in an outpatient setting. *Am Rev Respir Dis* 1993; 148: 675–81.

4. Juniper EF, Guyatt GH, Ferrie PJ, King DR. Sodium cromoglycate eye drops (opticrom): regular versus prn use in the treatment of seasonal allergic conjunctivitis. *J Allergy Clin Immunol* 1994; 94: 36–43.

5. Stewart AL, Hays R, Ware JE. The MOS short-form general health survey. Reliability and validity in a patient population. *Med Care* 1988; 26: 724–32.

6. Bergner M, Bobbitt RA, Carter WB, Gilson BS. The sickness impact profile; development and final revision of a health status measure. *Med Care* 1981; 19: 787–805.

7. Hunt SM, McKenna SP, McEwen J, Backett EM, Williams J, Papp E. A quantitative approach to perceived health status; a validation study. *J Epidemiol Community Health* 1980; 34: 281–6.

8. Sackett DL, Chambers LW, MacPherson AS, Goldsmith CH, McAuley RG. The development and application of indices of health; general methods and summary of results. *Am J Public Health* 1977; 67: 423–8.

9. Jones PW, Baveystock CM, Littlejohn P. Relationships between general health measured with the sickness impact profile and respiratory symptoms, physiological measures and mood in patients with chronic airflow limitation. *Am Rev Respir Dis* 1989; 140: 1538–43.

10. Bousquet J, Knani J, Dhivert H *et al.* Quality of life in asthma. 1. Internal consistency and validity of the SF-36 questionnaire. *Am J Respir Crit Care Med* 1994; 149: 371–5.

11. Torrance GW. Measurement of health state utilities for economic appraisal. *J Health Econom* 1986; 5: 1–30.

12. Mehrez A, Gafni A. The health-years equivalents: how to measure them using the standard gamble approach. *Med Decis Making* 1991; 11: 140–6.

13. Guyatt G, Kirshner B, Jaeschke R. Measuring health status: what are the necessary measurement properties? *J Clin Epidemiol* 1992; 45: 1341–5.

14 Fitzpatrick R, Fletcher A, Gore S, Jones D, Spiegelhalter D, Cox D. Quality of life measures in health care. 1: applications and issues in assessment. *BMJ* 1992; 305: 1074-7.

15 Guyatt G, Walter S, Norman G. Measuring change over time: assessing the usefulness of evaluative instruments. *J Chron Dis* 1987; 40: 171-8.

16 Juniper EF, Guyatt GH, Epstein RS, Ferrie PJ, Jaeschke R, Hiller TK. Evaluation of impairment of health-related quality of life in asthma: development of a questionnaire for use in clinical trials. *Thorax* 1992; 47: 76-83.

17 Malo JL, Boulet LP, Dewitte JD *et al.* Quality of life of subjects with occupational asthma. *J Allergy Clin Immunol* 1993; 91: 1121-7.

18 Marks GB, Dunn SM, Woolcock AJ. A scale for the measurement of quality of life in adults with asthma. *J Clin Epidemiol* 1992; 45: 461-72.

19 Hyland ME, Finnis S, Irvine SH. A scale for assessing quality of life in adult asthma sufferers. *J Psychom Res* 1991; 35: 99-110.

20 Hyland ME. The living with asthma questionnaire. *Respir Med* 1991; 85: 13-6.

21 Palmer JBD, Hyland ME. Salmeterol in clinical practice: comparator and safety studies, quality of life studies. *Eur Respir Rev* 1991; 1: 301-3.

22 Jones PW, Quirk FH, Baveystock CM, Littlejohns P. A self-complete measure of health status for chronic airflow limitation. *Am Rev Respir Dis* 1992; 145: 1321-7.

23 Juniper EF, Guyatt GH, Willan A, Griffith LE. Determining a minimal important change in a disease-specific quality of life questionnaire. *J Clin Epidemiol* 1994; 147: 81-7.

24 Townsend M, Feeny DH, Guyatt GH, Seip AE, Dolovich J. Evaluation of the burden of illness for pediatric asthmatic patients and their parents. *Ann Allergy* 1991; 67: 403-8.

25 Juniper EF, Guyatt GH, Feeny DH, Ferrie PJ, Griffith LE, Townsend M. Measuring quality of life in children with asthma. *J Allergy Clin Immunol* 1995; 95: 226.

26 Juniper EF, Guyatt G, Feeny DH, Ferrie PJ, Griffith LE, Townsend M. Measuring quality of life in the parents of children with asthma (manuscript in preparation).

KEY POINTS

1 Health-related quality-of-life assessment captures the aspects of asthma that are most important to the patient.

2   There are only weak to moderate correlations between asthma quality of life and the conventional clinical measures of asthma severity.

3   To ensure that the overall effect of interventions is evaluated, quality-of-life assessments should be included in clinical studies in conjunction with conventional clinical measures.

4   Disease-specific quality-of-life instruments for asthma with strong measurement properties and validity are now available. Most are short and simple and can easily be incorporated into clinical studies.

5   The choice of quality-of-life questionnaire should depend on the study question. Each instrument has different measurement characteristics and these should be matched to the needs of the study.

13

ASSESSMENT OF ASTHMA CONTROL: MARKERS OF INFLAMMATION

Per Venge

INTRODUCTION

One major cause of asthma is inflammation of the lung. Although most cellular components of inflammation, such as macrophages, mast cells, neutrophils and T lymphocytes, are found in the lungs of asthmatic patients, the characteristic feature of this inflammatory process is the presence of raised numbers of eosinophils. The role played by the eosinophil in the lung in asthma has been debated over the years and has included both the view of the eosinophil as a protective cell to the view that eosinophils are aggressive cells, which are responsible for many of the pathological findings in asthma. The current thinking of the role of the eosinophil favours the latter.[1,2] Basically, three facts support this view.

(1) The increasing knowledge of the potent biological properties of the secretory products of the eosinophil, which include among other things the cytotoxic potential of the granule proteins (Table 13.1).

(2) The demonstration by immunohistochemical and quantitative immunological techniques of the presence of activated eosinophils in lung tissues and their relationship to asthma severity.

TABLE 13.1: *Secretory granule proteins of human eosinophils*

Eosinophil cationic protein (ECP)
Eosinophil peroxidase (EPO)
Eosinophil protein X/eosinophil-derived neurotoxin (EPX/EDN)
Major basic protein (MBP)

---

(3) The close correlation between the reduction of eosinophil activity by anti-inflammatory treatment such as corticosteroids and the improvement of asthma symptoms.

In the assessment and monitoring of asthma, objective tools are needed to monitor the inflammatory component of asthma. In an attempt to achieve this, for a number of years we have been developing sensitive immunoassays for the measurement of secretory products of inflammatory cells in various biological fluids. These include assays for ECP, EPX/EDN and EPO as markers of eosinophil activity, myeloperoxidase (MPO), lactoferrin (LF) and human neutrophil lipocalin (HNL) as markers of neutrophil activity and lysozyme as a marker of primarily monocyte/macrophage activity.[3-5] In addition to these assays others have developed methods to measure tryptase as a marker of mast cell activity and the soluble interleukin-2 receptor as a marker of T-lymphocyte activity (Table 13.2). Common to these markers are their reasonably cellular specificity, which means that the detection of raised levels of either of these proteins in a biological fluid is a sign of increased activity and involvement of the respective cell. However, it is also likely that less cell-specific assays, such as assays for various cytokines and soluble adhesion molecules, will be of interest in the

TABLE 13.2: *Some inflammation markers of potential interest in the assessment of asthma control*

Cell source	Inflammation marker
Eosinophil	Eosinophil cationic protein (ECP)
	Eosinophil protein X (EPX)
	Eosinophil peroxidase (EPO)
Neutrophil	Elastase
	Lactoferrin (LF)
	Myeloperoxidase (MPO)
	Human neutrophil lipocalin (HNL)
Mast cell	Tryptase
Monocyte/macrophage	Lysozyme
T lymphocyte	Interleukin-2 receptor
Many	Interleukin-4
	Interleukin-5
	Interleukin-8
	Adhesion molecules (VCAM-1, ICAM-1, ELAM-1)

future. One of the obvious candidates in this regard is interleukin 5 (IL-5), which is the major eosinophil-activating cytokine (Table 13.2).

In this chapter I will focus on the use of markers for eosinophil activity in the assessment of the inflammatory component of asthma. One reason for this emphasis is the probably unique role of this cell in asthma, and another is that experience of using other markers in the assessment and monitoring of asthma is very limited and largely lacking.

METHODS AND MATERIAL COLLECTION

Assays for the eosinophil secretory proteins, ECP, EPX/EDN and EPO, are generally available as radioimmunoassays[6–8] or as fluorescent enzyme immunoassays using the CAP system (Pharmacia Diagnostics). The sensitivity of the assays is about $1 \mu g \, l^{-1}$ and they can be used to measure the levels in most biological fluids such as serum, EDTA-plasma, bronchoalveolar fluid and sputum, with the exception of ECP, which is not recommended to be assayed in EDTA-plasma.

In the preparation of any material it is important to realize that leakage from contaminating eosinophils may occur unless specific precautions are taken. These precautions should include the careful separation of the eosinophils from the fluid by centrifugation. It is recommended to centrifuge the material twice. If unspecific leakage is suspected the material (not blood for serum preparation; see below) should be kept at +4 °C before and during centrifugation.

When serum is used, strict standardization of the sampling procedure is required. This standardization has to take into account the tubes in which blood is sampled, the time allowed for clotting, the temperature at which clotting is allowed and the separation of eosinophils from the serum. The recommended procedure is to use vacuum tubes with or without silicone (SST-tubes, Becton-Dickinson). Clotting is allowed for 1 hour at room temperature, i.e. 22 °C, after which the cells are separated from the serum by centrifugation. When plain tubes are used, the serum should be re-centrifuged once to eliminate any remaining and contaminating eosinophils. When silicone-containing tubes are used one centrifugation is sufficient. The preparation of serum from silicone-containing tubes is less sensitive to clotting time, which means that such tubes may be left between 1 and 2 hours before centrifugation.

After separation of the eosinophils the proteins are stable and the material could be stored for several years at −20 °C. Frequent freezing and thawing, however, should be avoided.

When the recommended procedure is used, the normal adult levels of ECP in serum are $2–16 \mu g \, l^{-1}$, of EPX/EDN $8–38 \mu g \, l^{-1}$ and of EPO 0.3–

14 µg l^{-1}. However, it is recommended that reference ranges are established, since the handling of the blood is critical and may vary between laboratories.

CLINICAL EXPERIENCE

MEASUREMENTS IN LUNG LAVAGE FLUIDS (see also Chapter 10)

In several studies eosinophil granule proteins have been measured in bronchoalveolar lavage (BAL) or bronchial lavage fluids as indicators of the activity and involvement of the eosinophil in asthmatic inflammation. The first study[9] was published 1986 and showed raised levels of ECP in allergic asthmatic subjects during the late asthmatic reaction after allergen challenge. These results were interpreted to indicate the active attraction and activation of the eosinophils as a direct consequence of allergen exposure. Since the eosinophils were the only cellular elements that were changed in the patients who experienced a late asthmatic reaction (LAR), these data were also taken as an indication of the important role of eosinophils in the development of this reaction. Subsequent studies showed that low-dose inhaled corticosteroids prevented the development of LAR in parallel with the reduction of ECP in BAL, as the only other consequence of corticosteroid medication (J.G.R. De Monchy and P. Venge, unpublished data).

In chronic asthmatic subjects ECP levels were found to be raised and correlated with the severity of asthma as measured by Aas-score.[10] Such patients were also treated with low-dose inhaled corticosteroids and the activity of the eosinophils was found to be reduced, both measured as activated eosinophils in the tissue and as levels of ECP in BAL.[11]

These and other similar data strongly suggest a direct relationship between the activity of eosinophils in the lung and the mechanisms underlying asthma. The data also show that measurements of secreted products from the eosinophil, such as ECP, are relevant indicators of asthmatic inflammation. The question was therefore raised whether these reactions would be reflected in the blood. Indeed, significant correlations were found between ECP levels in BAL and in serum.[11]

MEASUREMENTS IN SPUTUM (see Chapter 10)

MEASUREMENTS IN SERUM

When measured in serum, levels of the eosinophil granule proteins mainly reflect the activity of the circulating pool of eosinophils. Thus, it is unlikely that appreciable amounts of these very basic proteins are derived from any compartment outside the blood compartment. The current interpretation of the significant correlations between BAL and serum levels of ECP is therefore that there is parallel activation of the eosinophils in the lung and in the blood. This activation may be the consequence of T-lymphocyte production of various cytokines such as IL-5.

In asthmatic subjects ECP levels in serum are related to the severity of asthma. This has been demonstrated in several clinical studies involving allergen challenge, exercise, lung function measurement, etc. (Table 13.3).[4,5,12] A few examples will be given below to support this statement.

A relationship between asthma severity and serum ECP levels was first demonstrated in a group of patients who were exposed to allergen challenge.[13,14] In this group some developed LAR and others did not. The propensity to develop LAR after allergen challenge is determined by the allergen load but is also related to disease activity. When levels of ECP were measured before challenge it was obvious that these were high in those patients who subsequently developed LAR. Thus the activity of the circulating eosinophils was predictive of the outcome of the challenge. A few hours after challenge ECP levels were very variable, reduced in some and raised in others. However, the day after challenge levels were almost invariably increased in those patients who had experienced LAR. Furthermore, levels were well correlated with the severity of LAR. A similar study was conducted on another group of asthmatic patients. In this study patients were subjected to exercise.[15] One-half of the patients developed an exercise-induced asthma (EIA). In these patients pre-exercise ECP levels were significantly higher than in those who did not respond with EIA. Furthermore there was a striking correlation between the extent of the response to exercise as measured by the fall in peak expiratory flow rate (PEFR) and pre-exercise ECP levels, with those having the highest ECP levels being those who had the greatest fall in PEFR after exercise.

During a birch pollen season, birch-sensitive asthmatic patients increase their sensitivity to histamine and metacholine. This increased sensitivity was largely prevented by specific immunotherapy.[16] During birch pollen exposure, the activity of eosinophils was raised as reflected by increased

---

TABLE 13.3: *The clinical experience of serum measurement of ECP in asthma*

Related to the propensity to develop late asthmatic reactions after allergen challenge
Related to the propensity to develop exercise-induced asthma
Related to lung function, PEFR, histamine PC_{20}, etc.
Useful in the monitoring of anti-inflammatory treatment
Useful in the monitoring of allergen exposure
Useful in the assessment of asthma inflammation

serum and BAL levels of ECP. In the group who had received immunotherapy, however, the rise in ECP was absent. In the whole group of patients there was a significant correlation between ECP and histamine PC_{20}. However, it was evident that this correlation was not linear. Thus raised ECP levels were found in the one-third of patients who had the highest sensitivity to histamine, i.e. a PC_{20} below 0.03 mg ml^{-1}.

A group of moderately to severe asthmatic children were followed closely and their optimal PEFR was recorded.[17] In those childen who subsequently had a tendency towards a reduction in their PEFR, in spite of treatment with a seemingly optimal dose of inhaled corticosteroids, i.e. a dose that subjectively made the patients symptom free, raised ECP levels were found. This was in contrast to those children who had unaltered PEFR, since they had near normal ECP levels. Overall there was a significant correlation between PEFR and serum ECP levels in this group of children.

As mentioned above ECP levels also increase as a response to allergen exposure. This has been demonstrated several times in studies conducted during the short birch pollen season in Sweden.[16,18] Interestingly the highest levels of ECP in serum are seen at the end of the season, i.e. after 2–3 weeks of exposure. ECP levels parallel the maximal alterations in histamine reactivity of the lungs, which also occur with a time lag of 2–3 weeks. This delay in the response of the eosinophils is not seen after allergen challenge in the laboratory. The reason for this could be explained by differences in exposure and doses of allergen. A similar observation was made in a group of asthmatic children who were allergic to mite allergen (A. Boner and P. Venge, unpublished data). In order to protect these children from mite exposure they went to school at a very high altitude in an environment free of mite. However, during school holidays they went back to their homes and to mite exposure. ECP levels in these children were very high after a prolonged exposure to mite, i.e. during the summer holiday, whereas during 2 weeks of Christmas holiday only a slight increment in eosinophil granule proteins was seen.

One of the most promising applications of serum ECP measurements is in relation to monitoring of therapy. Thus, the response of eosinophils to corticosteroid medication is a reduction in ECP secretion as evidenced by reduced serum levels. This effect of corticosteroids is dose and time dependent. Inhalation of 400 mg budesonide daily caused a clear reduction of ECP in BAL of adult asthmatic subjects[11] whereas serum levels were virtually unaffected even after 9 months of treatment (R. Dahl and P. Venge, unpublished data). After inhalation of 1000–1600 mg daily serum ECP levels were reduced after only 1 day.[13] The effect of low-dose treatment with inhaled budesonide had a profound effect on the development of the LAR after allergen challenge but only marginal effects on the reactivity to histamine and on lung function as measured by forced expiratory volume in 1 s (FEV_1). This is in contrast to the higher doses which, as expected, had profound effects on histamine reactivity and lung function. Thus,

FIGURE 13.1: *Variation of lung function as measured by peak expiratory flow rate (PEFR, □), blood eosinophil counts (○) and serum levels of eosinophil cationic protein (ECP, ●) and myeloperoxidase (MPO, ■) in a non-atopic patient with asthma. At admission the patient was on peroral prednisolone 5 mg every second day and 800 mg inhaled beclomethasone daily. At day 8 the inhaled steroids were raised to 1600 mg daily. ECP levels were promptly reduced as a response to this rise in inhaled steroids. ECP levels were raised again at day 20. This rise was paralleled by elevated MPO levels and explained by a verified bronchopneumonia. (From H. Formgren and P. Venge, unpublished data.)*

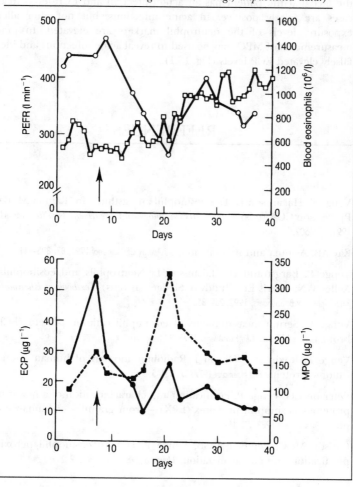

there is a striking correspondence between the effects on eosinophil activation and the effects on asthma symptoms. With low doses of inhaled corticosteroids only local effects on eosinophil activation are obtained. This gives rise to a certain degree of improvement of asthma symptoms. However, in order to achieve the full beneficial effects of inhaled corticosteroids it seems as if a systemic effect on eosinophil activation is required. Therefore, the interesting speculation is that serum ECP measurements reflect the systemic effects of inhaled corticosteroids.

Finally it has to be borne in mind that eosinophils are involved in acute infections. This is particularly evident in acute bacterial infections in which ECP levels are often elevated.[19] Elevated levels are also found in acute viral infections but at a lower level (P. Venge, unpublished data). Thus, in the monitoring of asthmatic patients raised ECP levels may be derived from the fact that the patient has an acute infection and ECP levels in these cases are falsely positive. In acute infections, but not after allergen exposure, levels of the neutrophil markers are elevated. In practice measurements of MPO may be used to reveal acute infections and identify falsely elevated ECP levels (Fig. 13.1).

REFERENCES

1. Venge P, Håkansson L. The eosinophil and asthma. In: Kaliner M, Barnes PJ, Persson CGA (eds) *Asthma. Its Pathology and Treatment.* New York: Marcel Dekker, 1991: 477–502.

2. Kay AB. Asthma and inflammation. *J Allergy Clin Immunol* 1991; 87: 893–911.

3. Venge P, Bergstrand H, Håkansson L. Neutrophils and eosinophils. In: Kelley WN, Harris ED, Ruddy S, Sledge CB (eds) *Textbook of Rheumatology.* Philadelphia: W.B. Saunders, 1992: 269–85.

4. Venge P. Serum measurements of eosinophil cationic protein (ECP) in bronchial asthma. *Clin Exp Allergy* 1993; 23 (suppl 2): 3–7.

5. Venge P, Roxin L-E, Olsson I. Radioimmunoassay of human eosinophil cationic protein. *Br J Haematol* 1977; 37: 331–5.

6. Peterson CG, Venge P. Purification and characterization of a new cationic protein – eosinophil protein-x (EPX) – from granules of human eosinophils. *Immunology* 1983; 50: 19–26.

7. Carlson MGC, Peterson CGB, Venge P. Human eosinophil peroxidase: purification and characterization. *J Immunol* 1985; 134: 1875–9.

8 Peterson CGB, Enander I, Nystrand J, Anderson AS, Nilsson L, Venge P. Radioimmunoassay of human eosinophil cationic protein (ECP) by an improved method. Establishment of normal levels in serum and turnover *in vivo*. Clin Exp Allergy 1991; 21: 561–7.

9 De Monchy JGR, Kauffman HF, Venge P, Koëter GH, De Vries K. Bronchoalveolar lavage and the late asthmatic reaction. In: Kay AB (ed) *Asthma. Clinical Pharmacology and Therapeutic Progress.* London: Blackwell Scientific Publications, 1986: 46–57.

10 Bousquet J, Chanez P, Lacoste JY *et al.* Eosinophilic inflammation in asthma. N Engl J Med 1990; 323: 1033–9.

11 Ädelroth E, Rosenhall L, Johansson S-Å, Linden M, Venge P. Inflammatory cells and eosinophilic activity in asthmatics investigated by bronchoalveolar lavage: The effects of antiasthmatic treatment with Budesonide or Terbutaline. Am Rev Respir Dis 1990; 142: 91–9.

12 Hällgren R, Venge P. The eosinophil in inflammation. In: Matsson P, Ahlstedt S, Venge P, Thorell J (eds) *Clinical Impact of the Monitoring of Allergic Inflammation.* London: Academic Press, 1991: 119–40.

13 Venge P, Dahl R, Peterson CG. Eosinophil granule proteins in serum after allergen challenge of asthmatic patients and the effects of anti-asthmatic medication. Int Arch Allergy Appl Immunol 1988; 87: 306–12.

14 Venge P, Dahl R. Are blood eosinophil number and activity important for the development of the late asthmatic reaction after allergen challenge? Eur J Respir Dis 1989; 2 (suppl 6): 430s–434s.

15 Venge P, Henriksen J, Dahl R. Eosinophils in exercise-induced asthma. J Allergy Clin Immunol 1991; 88: 699–704.

16 Rak S, Löwhagen O, Venge P. The effect of immunotherapy on bronchial hyperresponsiveness and eosinophil cationic protein in pollen-allergic patients. J Allergy Clin Immunol 1988; 82: 470–80.

17 Hedlin G, Ahlstedt S, Enander I, Håkansson L, Venge P. Eosinophil cationic protein (ECP), eosinophil chemotactic activity (ECA), neutrophil chemotactic activity (NCA) and tryptase in serum before and during bronchial challenge in cat-allergic children with asthma. Pediatr Allergy Immunol 1992; 3: 144–9.

18 Carlson M, Håkansson L, Kämpe M, Stålenheim G, Peterson C, Venge P. Degranulation of eosinophils from pollen-atopic patients with asthma is increased during pollen season. J Allergy Clin Immunol 1992; 89: 131–9.

19 Venge P, Strömberg A, Braconier JH, Roxin L-E, Olsson I. Neutrophil and eosinophil granulocytes in bacterial infection: Sequential studies of cellular and serum levels of granule proteins. Br J Haematol 1978; 38: 475–83.

KEY POINTS

1   Serum measurements of ECP (eosinophil cationic protein) may be used to monitor the asthmatic inflammation of the lungs.

2   Serum sampling for the measurements of ECP and other inflammation markers requires strict standardization as to time and temperature of clotting.

3   The combined assay of markers of several inflammatory cells provides further insight into the pathophysiology of the inflammatory process.

14

ALLERGEN AVOIDANCE MEASURES

Jennifer G. Wyman and Thomas A.E. Platts-Mills

INTRODUCTION

Eighty percent of asthmatic children and approximately 40–50% of asthmatic adults are "atopic".[1] Although many different antigens can give rise to immediate sensitivity, a large percentage of atopic individuals are sensitive to dust mite antigens or other indoor allergens on skin testing.[2–6] While pharmaceutical options for treating asthma have seemingly burgeoned, asthma has become more prevalent, more severe and with an overall increase in mortality. The factors that have contributed to the increase in prevalence or mortality are presently unclear, although an increase in maternal smoking, a gradual tendency to heat and then seal homes (thus increasing humidity), an increase in environmental ozone, a lack of access to timely primary care and even the asthma medications themselves have all been suggested.[2,3,7–14] Of these it is changes in temperature (increased) and ventilation rates (decreased) that appear to correlate temporally with increased asthma, and to provide improved conditions for growth of mites and/or fungi.

Studies in the last several years have demonstrated a marked inflammatory component with eosinophils and evidence for T-cell activation in the lungs of chronic asthmatic patients. Inflammatory responses of this kind can be reproduced in the lung following exposure to antigen in sensitized atopic individuals using bronchial challenge as well as in skin biopsies of atopic dermatitis patients.[15–18] Most asthmatic patients have airway hyperresponsiveness to exercise, cold air or challenge with a wide range of chemicals, e.g. histamine, methacholine and bradykinin. Bronchoalveolar lavage (BAL) in these patients reveals eosinophilia, sensitized lymphocytes, as well as markers for activation of CD4$^+$ T cells, including interleukin (IL)-4 and IL-5, which have been linked to the late allergic response.[15,19] A dose–response relationship between allergen exposure and clinical disease in susceptible atopic patients has been demonstrated and implies a causal relationship to the inflammation and airway hyperresponsiveness.[20,21] For these reasons, any patient with frequent symptoms requiring regular therapy to control their asthma, including anti-inflammatory medications, should be evaluated for the presence of specific IgE-mediated sensitivity and given advice on allergen avoidance.[20,22-24] In many cases, avoidance of the sensitizing agent(s) can produce relief in symptoms, decrease in medications and improved stability of airway and mucosal passages to non-specific stimuli.[25-30]

Indoor aeroallergens have been implicated as an increasingly important source of antigen exposure.[2,20,22,28,31] With the widespread use of wall-to-wall carpets, following the general introduction of vacuum cleaners in 1935, general use of central heating and tighter insulation, houses have changed dramatically over the last 30 years. As a result, household concentrations of airborne allergens have almost certainly increased. Exposure to this environment is repeated and prolonged, with the average person spending 97% of their time indoors with, more significantly, one-third of their time at home. Unlike seasonal exposures to pollens and grasses, chronic exposures are often insidious – not necessarily associated with acute conjunctivitis, or rapid onset of nasal symptoms, but more often chronic nasal congestion, and asthma.[31]

Measurement of allergens in house dust provides information about the reservoir from which allergens become airbone and also an archaeological record of organic and inorganic matter including accumulations of domestic pet, cockroach or mite allergens. Assays are also very important in assessing the success of avoidance measures. Specific antigens found on dust mite (*Der p* I, *Der f* I), cat (*Fel d* I) and cockroach (*Bla g* II) can be quantified using monoclonal antibody enzyme-linked immunosorbent assay (ELISA) systems that have recently been developed.[31-34] These monoclonal antibody assays measure a single protein derived from each source as a marker. This makes standardizations of the assays possible and simplifies analysis of the antigens, in that maintaining the large pools of human sera containing high levels of specific IgE for radioallergosorbent test (RAST) inhibition is not necessary.

DUST MITE

As previously stated, up to 80% of asthmatic children and young adults have positive skin-prick tests to *Dermatophagoides*. The major dust mites *Dermatophagoides farinae, D. pteronyssinus, Blomia tropicalis* and *Euroglyphus maynei* occur with varying distribution worldwide.[35-38] In the USA, *D. farinae* and *D. pteronyssinus* tend to dominate although *D. farinae* is favoured in climates that have a prolonged dry period and when the relative humidity remains at 60%, i.e. in air conditioned units.[39] *Blomia tropicalis* occurs in tropical and subtropical areas of the world including the USA, Europe,

Asia and South America. Presently its major specific antigens can be assayed with RAST inhibition assay or identified using crossed immunoelectrophoresis. Cross-reactivity with some *D. farinae* and *D. pteronyssinus* antigens has been reported.[40] *Euroglyphus* has been found predominantly in the southern USA and in Europe and has a 30% antigenic homology with *D. pteronyssinus*. Using polyclonal antisera for group I dust mite antigens, assays can detect *E. maynei* but probably underestimate the importance of this mite.[41] Two other methods for detecting mite exposure exist: mite counts, which are time consuming and require a worker trained in the morphological characteristics of mite species; and a guanine dipstick, which screens for the presence of guanine, the major nitrogenous waste product of arachnids.[40,42] Simple and sensitive, although presently not commercially available, guanine detection *per se* can overestimate mite prevalence due to other sources, but can be useful as a simple test for the presence of mites.[30,40,42]

The distribution of dust mite antigens is non-discriminatory, being equally present in urban and suburban homes. The highest concentrations are found in bedding and mattresses.[25,43] On the basis of multiple studies estimating exposure, it has been proposed that 2 μg *Der p* I per gram of house dust should be regarded as a threshold for sensitization to the mite, and that 10 μg g^{-1} dust is a level that both increases the risk of asthma and the tendency to develop symptoms earlier in life.[44] Avoidance measures that decrease exposure to < 1.0 μg g^{-1} dust have been shown to decrease airway hyperresponsiveness in asthmatic subjects.[25-27,44-46]

The source and structure of dust mite allergens has helped in understanding effective means of avoiding them. *Der p* I and *Der f* I are enzymes secreted by the gastrointestinal tract of mites. They are found in the mite faecal pellets, which are 10–20 μm in diameter.[31] While these particles become airborne with household disturbances such as fans, vacuuming, removing rugs and changing bedding, they settle rapidly, i.e. in less than 10 min.[31,46-48] More prolonged exposure is thought to occur while sleeping or resting on upholstered furniture, when the dust source is close to the mouth and inspiration of faecal particles is more likely with quiet respiration.[31,46]

CONTROL OF MITE ALLERGEN

Mite growth requires a humidity greater than 50% and is optimal at a relative humidity of 70–80%, temperatures of 25 °C (70–80 °F), and requires a supply of organic debris preferably skin scales.[38,49] Therefore mite allergen exposure can be reduced either by relocating to a high altitude and thus low-humidity areas, or by removing sites where mites can grow, or by creating unfavourable growing conditions.[50] While replacing bedding and mattresses will transiently reduce dust mite to near zero levels, avoidance must be maintained.[51] Mattresses can be inexpensively enclosed in impermeable plastic covers with the zipper taped shut, or with specially manufactured vapour-permeable covers that may be more comfortable and generally last longer.[29,52] Cotton bedding should be washed in hot water (55 °C, 130 °F) weekly. It has been shown that vacuuming and simply washing bedding and flooring alone is neither effective at decreasing mite counts nor improving pulmonary function.[53] While dry cleaning will kill mites, one report suggests that their antigens are left relatively intact.[54] Preliminary work suggests that the addition of benzylbenzoate (150–250 ml per 30 l wash) added to a cooler temperature wash is effective at killing mites and washing out the mite allergen.[55] Cool-water washing alone does not kill mites or remove them from bedding.[53,55] Benzylbenzoate as a 25% lotion has been safely used for years as a topical treatment for scabies.[57] Its major toxicity is its irritant effect on eyes or mucosa when used for these indications.[56–58] More work needs to be done to assess long-term toxicity before use of benzylbenzoate in washing can be routinely recommended.

Carpets are a major reservoir of mite antigen, as well as being an important site of mite growth.[28,29,56,58,59] For patients with moderate to severe asthma, e.g. inadequately controlled or on regular inhaled steroids, removing carpets and installing hardwood or vinyl floors followed by regular damp mopping weekly is essential, especially in the bedroom.[25,26,29] Probably less satisfactory is covering carpeted flooring with plastic vinyl sheeting; sealing the edges may also reduce exposure. This may be one of few options for the family restricted to a carpeted apartment. It is further recommended that bedroom curtains be washable fabric or venetian-type blinds and that clutter, including clothing, toys and curios be removed or kept in a closed closet. Upholstered furniture should be replaced with wooden, vinyl or leather, i.e. dust mite impermeable, washable surfaces.[28,29]

Other important areas where dust mites proliferate are in the family and living rooms. In these rooms, removing carpets and changing furniture is helpful but may not be possible. An attractive proposal has been to treat upholstered furniture and rugs with solutions of aqueous benzylbenzoate, tannic acid and benzyl derivatives.[56,58–60] While effective at lowering mite counts and allergens *in vitro*, success has been more varied when these chemicals have been used in homes, although they can reduce allergen levels in carpets when applied every 3 months.[56,58,59] However the ability of tannic acid to denature allergens is very dependent on the conditions, and the benzylbenzoate powder (Acarosan) requires repeated application. In addition, a white powder residue may continue to lift from the benzyl-benzoate-treated carpet after application.[56] There is also a report of a suffocating odour occurring after benzylbenzoate was placed on a carpet previously treated with water or an active cleaning substance in the preceding 8 months.[61] Carpets laid on an unventilated floor, e.g. cement or basement, can be very difficult to dry once exposed to moisture, and thus become a source of high mite levels. It is particularly important for the severely allergic patient not to live or work in such areas. Lifting rugs, mattresses and upholstered furniture and "beating" them with a rug beater, followed by vigorous vacuuming and airing in strong sunlight, are also effective measures to reduce antigen levels and kill mites.[62]

Reducing relative humidity to below 50% is an effective method for decreasing mite growth. While relative humidity is low during the winter in many areas of the world, during the summer expensive air conditioning may be required.[63,64] In some areas, increasing ventilation rates to one air change per hour for several hours per day is effective and may be accomplished by opening several windows.[64] Air conditioning individual rooms has been shown to decrease mite allergen and is indicated for severely allergic patients (Table 14.1).[39]

COCKROACH

Interest has recently developed in cockroach allergen, as it has become established that allergic patients living in infested areas have an increased incidence of skin-test positivity.[65-69] Cockroaches are tropical insects and are found wherever water, warmth and organic matter are present. Several studies have demonstrated a high prevalence of RAST or skin-test positivity to cockroach among inner-city, especially African American, asthmatic subjects. This is the population that has recently had a marked increase in asthma morbidity and mortality.[2,19,22] While sensitization is more likely to be seen in patients of deprived socio-economic status and those living in crowded conditions, it is worth noting that most of these patients are sensitized to dust mites and other aeroallergens as well.[2,19,22,70-72] As with dust mite and pollen aeroallergens, the prevalence of sensitivity is thought to correlate with exposure.[33,72,73] However the attempts to determine at what level sensitization occurs have not shown a close correlation between cockroach concentrations in individual's houses and the development of sensitization.[2] Whether this reflects changes in home environment in an ethnic community, such that there is general exposure to cockroach allergen, is uncertain. Therefore, while it is not clear at what level sensitization occurs or why some sensitized control subjects do not have asthma, exposure is an important factor in some asthmatic patients.[68,69,72]

Eliciting a history of cockroach exposure in patients should be done with tact. Questions could include: "Do you have a problem with insects in your house?", or "Have you ever seen a cockroach in your house?". Nonetheless, in approximately 20% of houses with high levels of cockroach allergen the families did not report cockroaches being present and the insects were not seen by the technician visiting the house.[33]

To quantify antigen exposure, sandwich ELISA to detect *Per a* I or *Bla g* I, produced by American (*Periplaneta americana*) and German (*Blatella germanica*) cockroaches respectively, have been developed. These assays

TABLE 14.1: *Summary of dust mite avoidance measures*

1. Enclose mattresses and pillows in a zippered, plastic cover or a special allergen-proof fabric. Tape the zipper; damp wipe the mattress cover every 2 weeks
2. Wash all bedding, including mattress pad, pillow cases and blankets in hot water (at least 55 °C, 130 °F) weekly. Replace comforters with Dacron or Orlon blankets, which are to be washed with the bedding. Alternatively, cover comforter with vapour-permeable, allergen-proof fabric
3. Remove small objects that accumulate dust from the room, or place in a closed closet or cabinet. Store clothing in drawers or in a closed closet. Store unused clothing away from the bedroom
4. Remove upholstered furniture and replace with leather, plastic or vinyl furniture
5. Remove carpets whenever possible, or vacuum weekly using a vacuum cleaner with an effective filter. The patient should avoid being in a room where vacuuming is occurring until at least 20 min after it has been completed. If the patient must vacuum, a mask should be worn during this time. Remove wall-to-wall carpets on cement slab and replace with area rugs, which are more easily treated or, optimally, install subflooring and hardwood floors
6. Treat carpets with acaricides, 3% tannic acid, or by airing in strong sunlight after mechanically removing dust
7. Replace drapes and curtains with washable curtains or venetian blinds. Clean and vacuum approximately every 2 weeks
8. Control humidity in the house either by increasing ventilation with fresh air when the outside air is dry, using air conditioning (central is best) or using a dehumidifier for very damp areas of the house such as the basement
9. Replace air filters on air conditioners, or wash with soap and water, approximately every 3 months to remove fungus and airborne debris. Electrostatic filters may also be useful on central air conditioning units for reducing allergens but will not affect the amount in, or produced by, reservoirs of dust mites

also cross-react with the Asian cockroach (*Blatella orientalis*) and the brown-banded cockroach (*Supella suspellectilium*), which are also common household pests.[74] However because this cross-reactivity is partial, the assays tend to underestimate exposure to other species.[74] Sensitive monoclonal antibody-based assays specific for *Bla g* I and *Bla g* II, antigens from the German cockroach, have been developed.[33] *Bla g* I has been associated with particles of 7–10 μm, which can be detected after air disturbance, but like mite faecal particles are thought to settle rapidly.[48,75] Environmental exposure has been assessed in a number of studies.[33,69,72] In paediatric patients with asthma presenting to an Atlanta emergency department, 9/35 had both cockroach-specific IgE antibodies greater than 50 units and exposure to *Bla g* II in two or more sites, whereas only 1/22 of control subjects had similar risk factors.[69]

CONTROL OF COCKROACH ALLERGEN

Studies of American house dust from Tampa, Florida, show levels of *Per a* I ranging from 7 to 200 000 ng *Per a* I equivalents per gram dust with many households having 10–10 000 ng *Per a* I equivalents per gram.[74] *Blatella* allergens are usually found in highest concentration in the kitchen, 50 times the amount elsewhere, with much less in the bedroom, bedding or living rooms of atopic asthmatic subjects. However, similar levels are found in the houses of non-atopic control subjects from the same neighbourhood.[33] Avoidance measures, in heavily infested areas, are difficult to maintain, especially in apartment dwellings where cockroaches notoriously avoid eradication by moving to surrounding apartments after pesticide applications, only to re-emerge at a later date. Nonetheless, extermination measures using organophosphates are effective to kill existing cockroaches and to reduce propagation.[76,77] It should be kept in mind that cockroaches often become resistant to any particular extermination method. Cleanliness is most important, by minimizing food or organic debris and careful vacuuming, which should be combined with using roach stations (or roach "motels").[76,77] In addition, what are sometimes referred to as "manic mechanical measures", such as careful caulking of all cracks may also be effective. Preliminary data indicate that these measures reduce cockroach antigens effectively, although the problem tends to reoccur within 3 months if stringent avoidance is not maintained (Table 14.2).[77]

CAT

Approximately 3% of the population are allergic to cats.[78] Household cats are present in approximately 28% of American families, and are owned by almost one-third of cat-allergic patients (i.e. approximately 2 million individuals). In emergency room studies, cat-specific IgE antibody has been strongly associated with treatment for asthma.[2,4,22,72] In two studies, the

TABLE 14.2: *Summary of cockroach avoidance measures*

1. Keep kitchen free of food debris and dirty dishes
2. Caulk all cracks near water sources, including bathrooms and kitchen, with special attention to areas around faucets, pipe fittings at walls, under sinks, around bathtub/shower
3. Vacuum or carefully sweep kitchen, dining room and other areas where food is consumed on a daily basis
4. Place roach stations in all food areas, concentrating especially on kitchen and bath; replace every 3 months
5. Spray with organophosphates or other insecticide on a monthly basis. Discard foods and wash dishes after being exposed to the sprays

prevalence of IgE antibody to cat allergen was 30/188 among patients with asthma and 1/202 among control subjects (odds ratio 38). It has been demonstrated that airborne cat allergen can precipitate asthma, in cat-sensitive patients, when 8–80 ng of cat allergen *Fel d* I is inhaled.[79] An epidemiological study suggesting that children can be sensitized by 8 μg *Fel d* I per gram house dust supports a causal relation between exposure and the expression of atopy.[63] The fact that many cat-allergic patients know within 15 min that they have entered a cat household suggests that significant quantities are airborne. This has been confirmed by studies of resting air in cat-containing homes.[20] *Fel d* I, the major cat allergen, is almost ubiquitous, but levels of > 8 μg g^{-1} in reservoir dust or 1–20 ng m^{-3} airborne have been found in almost all homes where cats are kept.[63,80]

Exposure may be quantified either by measuring *Fel d* I in dust, or with air sampling devices.[75,78,81] Airborne *Fel d* I, judged both by falling properties and by particle sizing, is carried on particles ranging from 1 to 20 μm.[31] This is quite unlike dust mite antigen, which becomes airborne on large particles > 8 μm in diameter. In addition, after disturbance of a room, airborne particles can reach concentrations of up to 100 ng m^{-3}. Inhaling these levels of allergen would take only 6 min for a sensitized asthmatic subject to inhale enough antigen to cause a significant drop in forced expiratory volume in 1 s (FEV$_1$).[75,81]

CONTROL OF CAT ALLERGEN

The main source of *Fel d* I is from the skin in the form of dander, with saliva being a relatively minor source; the main avoidance measure recommended is complete removal of the cat from the household. However, after removal of the cat, soft furniture, carpeting and even the walls are significant reservoirs of cat allergen (Fig. 14.1).[78] The allergen is easily disturbed by activities such as vacuuming, sweeping and even small fans.[31,81,82] Consequently, reduction of cat allergen after removal of the cat alone will take up to 12 weeks unless accompanied by vigorous cleaning and removal of the major reservoirs.[83]

If the patient or family decides not to remove the cat, allergen levels can be decreased in a number of ways. By washing the cat weekly with 1 l of water, cat dander and allergen can be reduced under specific circumstances (Fig. 14.2).[78] However, this may not be as simple as was originally thought, probably because the cat can reaccumulate allergen from reservoirs in its environment.[84] High efficiency particular air (HEPA) filters can reduce *Fel d* I by 90%, but only in non-carpeted rooms, as the air flow coming out of the filter can cause enough disturbance to increase airborne

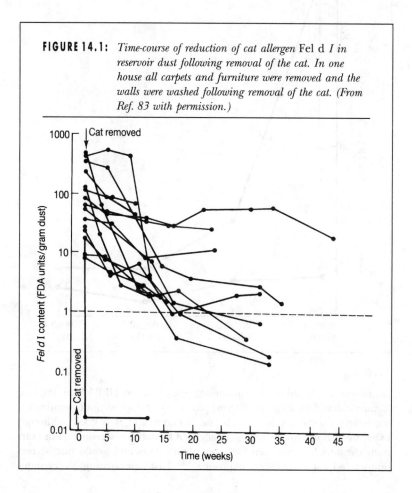

FIGURE 14.1: *Time-course of reduction of cat allergen* Fel d *I in reservoir dust following removal of the cat. In one house all carpets and furniture were removed and the walls were washed following removal of the cat. (From Ref. 83 with permission.)*

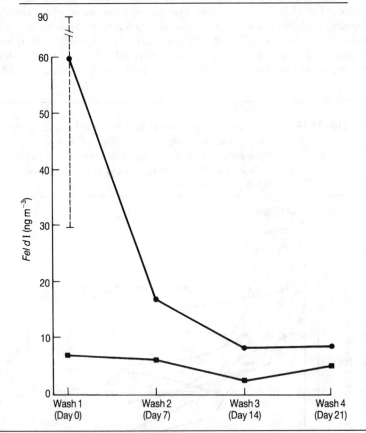

FIGURE 14.2: *Effect of washing the cat on airborne cat allergen. Airborne* Fel d *I concentrations measured immediately before the cat was washed (●) and during the 30 min after washing (■). The range of values for increase in airborne* Fel d *I when the cat entered a room is shown by the dotted bar. These results suggest that the allergen from the cat can be reduced for 1 week after washing.*

cat allergen.[78] In addition, vacuuming rugs with an HEPA-filter vacuum cleaner can reduce large (6–20 μm) particles of *Fel d* I, without significantly increasing overall levels of airborne allergen and is a good, although expensive, choice for reducing cat allergen from this reservoir.[81] Some vacuum cleaners leak allergen far more than others and would not be recommended for controlling exposure.[81,85] Lastly, increasing air changes from approximately 0.3 air changes per hour (ACH), a typical flow rate for a modern "tight" house, to 1–2.4 ACH using window or central fan units will help to reduce the < 2 μm particles, but has little effect on overall airborne cat allergen.[81] The clinical significance of this measure, i.e. changing the distribution of airborne particles, is presently unknown. Patients should be forewarned that reduction of airborne allergen to very low levels, e.g. < 2 ng m^{-3}, may still be associated with clinical symptoms of sneeze and congestion (Table 14.3).[86]

Due to limitations of space, dog allergen, *Can f* I, will only be briefly discussed. Essentially, as with cats, washing and other measures may be useful to decrease the amount of airborne allergen, but there is not a large body

---

TABLE 14.3: *Summary of cat allergen avoidance measures*

1. Remove cat from environment; replace upholstered furniture and carpets; steam clean walls

If cat remains:

2. Keep cat out of bedroom and other rooms where patient spends most of the time
3. Wash the cat in 1 l of water weekly. Kittens treated gently can tolerate this reasonably well; otherwise the veterinarian or pet-grooming service may be feasible to reduce trauma to both owner and cat
4. Reduce sources of reservoir cat allergen. Replace previously exposed upholstered furniture with leather, vinyl or plastic washable sources. Wash down weekly with water or equivalent
5. Remove carpets and replace with washable area rugs or hardwood floors. Clean regularly
6. Vacuum rugs with HEPA-filter vacuum cleaner to reduce large *Fel d* I particles; avoid water reservoir vacuum cleaners as these can disperse *Fel d* I
7. Increase ventilation rates with fans, air conditioning or by opening windows (1–2.4 ACH) to reduce small *Fel d* I particles
8. Clean air in bedroom or room where patient spends most of the time with use of HEPA-type air cleaner
9. Electrostatic filters on central air conditioning units may have limited value in face of significant exposure from cats and reservoirs but should otherwise be considered if other measures are instituted

---

of data to support this. The fact that fewer people keep dogs, and that they are often kept outside, thus contributing less to indoor aeroallergen load, is thought to be partially responsible for the lack of widespread sensitization and clinical symptoms attributed to dogs.[87]

MOULD

Using aerometric sampling devices, fungus spores are present in very large numbers in the outside air. However, the clinical relevance of these measurements is not clear for several reasons: the measurements show great variability from day to day, many of the spores are difficult to identify visually, while the results of cultures reflect viability rather than allergen content. In addition, house-dust samples reveal a combination of spores and mycelia and it is not clear what these elements contribute to allergen exposure.[88–90] However, it is clear that there is great variability in the optimal growing conditions of different moulds. Changes in growing conditions for a given species can trigger changes in expressed genes and therefore the pattern and distribution of specific allergens. In addition, the paucity of immunoassays for these allergens limits evaluation of exposure.[88,91]

There are four main groups of moulds: Phycomycetes, including *Rhizopus* and *Mucor* species; Basidiomycetes, including puffballs and gilled mushrooms such as *Amanita*; Ascomycetes; and the imperfect fungi, so called because they lack a sexual phase of reproduction. The latter includes most of the major fungi traditionally associated with allergy including *Cladosporium, Alternaria, Aspergillus, Helminthosporium* and *Penicillium*. Spores range from 2 to 17 μm in diameter. Fungi have traditionally been identified based on morphological characteristics and growth patterns.[92]

Mould seasons are not defined in the way that pollen seasons are, because most moulds can grow rapidly at any time, when adequate conditions are available. Spore release and distribution depends on wind speed and precipitation.[88] One species may be favoured over another, and this may vary both from one site to another, or with changes in the weather. Moulds such as *Aspergillus* enjoy warmth; basidiospores are dependent on free water; and *Cladosporium, Alternaria* and *Helminthosporium* are considered "dry spores" and are mobilized with dry windy conditions.[88] The substrate is important. While all moulds are saprophytic if not parasitic, some favour breads (the zygomycete *Rhizopus* and the ergot-producing ascomycete *Neurospora*). Damp foundations often harbour *Cladosporium*. Shower areas, air conditioners and humidifier units are important as sources of *Rhizopus, Mucor, Aspergillus* and *Penicillium*.[88,93] In Hawaii, air-conditioned homes are found to have fewer spores of outdoor fungi but markedly elevated levels of *Aspergillus*.[94] Several moulds are useful and essential for food processing and preparation (thus leaving traces in the food). For example, *Aspergillus* species are used in baking bread; and both *Aspergillus oryzae* and *Saccharomyces cerevisiae* are utilized in sake brewing. *Penicillium* species are used to make some cheeses.[88]

Classically the antigenic determinants of fungi have been detected using crossed-immunoelectropheresis (CIE). CIE has shown a wide variability of antigen quantity and quality, depending on growing and sampling conditions, as well as between the different commercial extracts available for skin testing.[88] While available, CIE is not presently used to standardize for the specific antigens and would probably not be feasible. Since some of the major spore and mycelial allergens are thought to have important carbohydrate components, characterizing them primarily by protein nitrogen units (PNU) is not accurate. These carbohydrate components also make protein purification difficult. Much of the work to date has focused on the major antigenic determinants of three organisms: *Aspergillus, Trichophyton* and *Alternaria*.[88,89,95–97] Two of these organisms, *Trichophyton* and *Aspergillus*, are important human pathogens. It is also important to remember that many fungi produce bioactive toxins during normal growth.[88,96]

An association between asthma and positive RAST and/or skin-prick test to several fungi including *Alternaria, Cladosporium* and *Aspergillus* has been demonstrated.[3,98] Bronchospasm can be induced by controlled inhalation of *Aspergillus* and *Trichophyton* fungal extracts in skin-prick-positive or RAST-positive asthmatic subjects but not in skin-prick-negative asthmatic or normal control subjects. Similar studies have documented nasal symptoms using *Alternaria* extracts.[99] In patients with positive bronchoprovocation to *Cladosporium*, symptoms and the use of medications have increased in parallel with increasing spore counts in Denmark, where up to one-third of atopic adults with respiratory allergic diseases are skin-prick positive to basidiomycete mycelia and/or spore extracts.[100]

Immunoassays using monoclonal antibodies are just becoming available to study the prevalence of specific fungal antigens in air and dust samples from the environment.[96,101] One of the best characterized fungal allergens is *Asp f* I from *Aspergillus fumigatus*. A monoclonal-based ELISA has been developed and used to compare levels of *Asp f* I in mycelial extracts, spores and culture media.[96] For example, *Asp f* I, a mycelial antigen, has been found to be absent in most house-dust extracts but present after culture indicating that spores are present.[102] It is readily detected by aerosampling during outdoor leaf disturbances. This antigen appears to be clinically relevant both in allergic bronchopulmonary aspergillosis (ABPA) and cystic fibrosis (CF). *Asp f* I IgG is found in 98% of CF patients by age 10, implying that *A. fumigatus* mycelia are growing in the bronchi of these patients. *Aspergillus fumigatus* has a very wide temperature tolerance and requires high relative humidity (about 80%). The mycelial forms of this organism have been found in pathology specimens and in BAL fluids from these patients.[103]

The genus *Trichophyton* includes a series of fungi that are responsible for chronic or severe cutaneous infections of the groin, feet or toenails in a large number of patients. What is less clear is how some of these patients become "allergic" to *Trichophyton*. It has been found that *Trichophyton*-sensitive patients, by RAST and skin test, have positive bronchoprovocation tests when challenged with extracts of *Trichophyton*.[99] It is assumed that these patients become sensitized from T cell-mediated reactions to their cutaneous infections, as specific IgE and IgG to *Trichophyton* have been measured.[97] Podiatrists have also been known to have *Trichophyton*-induced wheezing, but this was thought to be a result of sensitization from multiple exposures to airborne powders generated during grinding of toenails.[104]

Multiple fungi can occasionally be cultured from patients with allergic sinusitis, including *Aspergillus, Mucor, Candida* and *Rhizopus*.[88,105] While this is an uncommon cause of chronic sinusitis, most of these otherwise immunocompetent patients have a history of steroid or multiple antibiotic use. Increased specific IgG, eosinophilia and positive skin-prick test may be seen in these patients. The CT scans from these patients usually reveal sinusitis with or without boney erosions or radiographic invasion, findings which are confirmed on microscopy of pathology specimens.[24,105]

CONTROL OF MOULD EXPOSURE
There are three approaches to reducing exposure to mould antigens: (1) avoiding sites where exposure is high, i.e. basements, houses with active mould growth and outside sources; (2) reducing humidity in the house to discourage mould growth; (3) cleaning surfaces with bleach or comparable agents, e.g. shower curtains, refrigerator trays and sinks. However there are few published controlled trials to support many accepted practices of mould and fungus control.

All allergic patients, and particularly fungus-allergic patients, should avoid living or working in basements. Fungal growth is ubiquitous on basement walls and is very difficult to control. Houses with overt mould, particularly active mould in flooring, will cause severe problems to most mould-allergic patients. In addition, unventilated areas with a high fungus load may be the source of either allergens or toxins, especially during the air disturbance of cleaning or renovating.[94,96] While a mask will reduce the load of inhaled airborne mycelial fragments and spores, particles less than 5 μm are not effectively filtered by ordinary face masks. Other situations that represent high levels of mould exposure include lawn mowing, moving leaf mould, exposure to compost and rotting wood.[102]

Reducing humidity inside houses is important to control mite or mould growth. Controlling humidity involves reducing sources, and removing the humidity that naturally accumulates in houses.[63] Some sources such as clothes dryers or cooking equipment can be vented to the outside.[63,64] In addition, humidifiers and the watering of live plants can contribute to indoor humidity.[93] Reducing humidity can be achieved by opening windows, thus increasing the ventilation to two to three air changes per hour, but this is helpful only when the outside absolute humidity is $< 6\,\mathrm{g\,kg^{-1}}$. Alternatively, if the outside humidity is high, then using air conditioning or dehumidifiers is necessary.[64] Portable HEPA filters that reduce airborne particulates of $> 0.3\,\mu\mathrm{m}$ may also be helpful but have not been tested in relation to clinical symptoms.[106]

The primary method of controlling mould growth in the house is to keep surfaces, furniture, etc. dry. In addition, no organic matter, such as firewood, should be kept in the house. Surprisingly, household plants appear to be only a minor source of mould spores. Fungicidal cleaning agents, such as bleach in a dilution of 4–6 parts water to 1 part bleach, as well as commercially available fungicides, can be used to clean water-soaked areas in the bathroom and kitchen. Nebulizer tubing and humidifiers should be rinsed with a 1 : 3 parts diluted 5% acetic acid or one-half teaspoonful chlorine bleach in 1 pint (~ 0.5 l) of water to discourage fungal growth.

TABLE 14.4: *Summary of mycelial and spore avoidance measures*

1. Fungus-allergic patients should avoid sleeping or working for prolonged amounts of time in basements
2. Wear a mask when disturbing areas where there is high mould growth, e.g. when raking leaves, turning mulch, heavy cleaning of basements, etc. Maximize ventilation when working in these areas
3. Reduce sources of mould in house, keep houseplants free of dead leaves, avoid overwatering, bring in firewood for immediate use only
4. Reduce general humidity in house as outlined in Table 14.1 and vent kitchen and bathroom as well as any other rooms with water sources to the outside
5. Use kitchen fans when cooking
6. Keep doors closed while showering
7. Dry clothes outside or vent dryer to outside
8. Keep areas in kitchen and bathroom clean and dry; use fungicidal cleaners such as bleach diluted 1 : 4–6 parts water to eliminate growth on a weekly basis
9. Clean humidifiers with bleach solution and rinse out dehumidifiers daily. Reduce other collections of standing water
10. Allow nebulizer and other moist tubing to completely dry before storing. Rinse with vinegar or bleach solution

Paint additives, to inhibit mould growth, are also available and can be recommended for areas particularly susceptible to moisture (Table 14.4).

Compliance with avoidance measures has been studied and found to be especially difficult in patients from deprived socio-economic class. It has been shown that video-taped instructions are useful for understanding instructions, but a consistent theme has been that home visits by trained professionals have been very helpful to ensure that changes are implemented. Patients often report full compliance when only one or two of several measures have been instituted. Many times there is resistance from the spouse, or the importance of the measures in causing the disease is not realized.[107]

CONCLUSIONS

(1) Association between indoor allergens and asthma has been seen in all parts of the world and appears to be a major cause of the increasing prevalence of asthma.

(2) Measurement of exposure to some of the major indoor allergens is now possible and allows for specific monitoring of avoidance measures.

(3) Experimental exposure to allergens including mite, cat or cockroach can induce inflammatory changes in the lung, and it is exactly this form of inflammation that is the hallmark of naturally occurring asthma. Thus allergen avoidance is a logical first-line anti-inflammatory treatment for asthma.

(4) The detailed way in which avoidance should be incorporated into normal treatment needs more study. However, any patient who requires regular treatment or has had steroid courses should be evaluated for the role of allergens.

(5) Avoidance measures are allergen specific and it is not possible to give useful advice without knowing the specific sensitivity of the patient.

(6) Avoidance measures require education, encouragement and repeated reinforcement, as with any other form of chronic treatment.

REFERENCES

1   Weiss ST, Sparrow D, O'Connor GT. The interrelationship among allergy, airways responsiveness, and asthma. *J Asthma* 1993; 30: 329-49.

2   Lin RY, LaFrance J, Sauter D. Hypersensitivity to common indoor aeroallergens in asthmatic patients. *Ann Allergy* 1993; 71: 33-9.

3   O'Hollaren MT, Yunginger J, Offord KP *et al.* Exposure to an aeroallergen as a possible precipitating factor in respiratory arrest in young patients with asthma. *N Engl J Med* 1991; 324: 359-63.

4   Corbo GM, Forastiere F, Dell-Orco V, Pistelli R, Agabiti N, Perucci CA. Effects of environment on atopic status and respiratory disorders in children. *J Allergy Clin Immunol* 1993; 92: 616-23.

5   Canny GJ, Reisman J. Acute asthma: Observations regarding the management of a pediatric emergency room. *Pediatrics* 1989; 83: 507-12.

6   Sly MR, O'Donnell R. Regional distribution of deaths from asthma. *Ann Allergy* 1989; 62: 347-54.

7   Weiss KB, Wagener DK. Changing patterns of asthma mortality: Identifying target populations at high risk. *JAMA* 1990; 264: 1683-7.

8   Jackson R, Sears MR. International trends in asthma mortality 1970–1985. *Chest* 1988; 94: 914-8.

9   NHLBI – Asthma Mortality Institute. Asthma mortality. *J Allergy Clin Immunol* 1991; 88: 447-50.

10 Evans R, Mullally DI, Wilson RW *et al.* National trends in the morbidity and mortality of asthma in the U.S. *Chest* 1987; 91: 65S-74S.

11 Boulet L-P, Deschesnes F, Turcotte H, Gignac F. Near-fatal asthma: Clinical and physiologic features, perception of bronchoconstriction, and psychologic profile. *J Allergy Clin Immunol* 1991; 88: 838-46.

12 Chilmoncyzk BA, Salmun LM, Megathin KN, Neveux LM, Palomaki GE. Association between exposure to environmental tobacco smoke and exacerbations of asthma in children. *N Engl J Med* 1993; 326: 1665-9.

13 Gong H Jr. Health effects of air pollution. A review of clinical studies. *Clin Chest Med* 1992; 13: 201-14.

14 Warner JO, Price SA. Aero-allergen avoidance in the prevention and treatment of asthma. *Clin Exp Allergy* 1990; 20: 15-9.

15 Robinson D, Hamid Q, Bentley A, Ying S, Kay AB, Durham SR. Activation of CD4+ T cells, increased T_{H2}-type cytokine mRNA expression, and eosinophil recruitment in bronchoalveolar lavage after allergen inhalation challenge in patients with atopic asthma. *J Allergy Clin Immunol* 1993; 92: 313-24.

16 Platts-Mills TAE, Chapman MD, Mitchell B, Heymann PW, Deuell B. The role of inhalant allergens in atopic dermatitis. In: Ruzicka T, Ring J, Przybilla B (eds) *Handbook of Atopic Eczema*. Berlin: Springer-Verlag, 1991: 192–203.

17 Botey J, Gutierrez V, Pena JM, Eseverri JL, Marin A, Aulesa C. Specific IgE antibodies in nasal secretions: correlation with serum values and clinical tests. Ann Allergy 1993; 70: 26–9.

18 Sager N, Feldmann A, Schilling G, Kreitsch P, Neumann C. House dust mite-specific T cells in the skin of subjects with atopic dermatitis: Frequency and lymphokine profile in the allergen patch test. J Allergy Clin Immunol 1992; 89: 801–10.

19 Wasserman S, Olivenstein R, Renzi P, Xu L-J, Martin JG. The relationship between late asthmatic responses and antigen-specific immunoglobulin. J Allergy Clin Immunol 1992; 90: 661–9.

20 Platts-Mills TAE, Ward GW, Sporik R, Gelber LE, Chapman MD, Heymann PW. Epidemiology of the relationship between exposure to indoor allergens and asthma. Int Arch Allergy Appl Immunol 1991; 94: 339–45.

21 Wegner CD, Torcellini CA, Clarke CC, Letts LG, Gundel RH. Effects of single and multiple inhalations of antigen on airway responsiveness in monkeys. J Allergy Clin Immunol 1991; 87: 835–41.

22 Pollart SM, Chapman MD, Fiocco GP, Rose G, Platts-Mills TAE. Epidemiology of acute asthma: IgE antibodies to common inhalant allergens as a risk factor for emergency room visits. J Allergy Clin Immunol 1989; 83: 875–82.

23 Dodge R, Burrows B, Lebonitz MD. Antecedent features of children in whom asthma develops. J Allergy Clin Immunol 1993; 92: 744–9.

24 Newman LF, Platts-Mills TAE, Philips D, Hazen KC, Gross CW. Chronic sinusitis. J Allergy Clin Immunol 1994; 271: 363–7.

25 Murray AB, Ferguson AC. Dust-free bedrooms in the treatment of asthmatic children with house dust or house dust mite allergy: a controlled trial. Pediatrics 1983; 71: 418–22.

26 Platts-Mills TAE, Tovey ER, Mitchell EB, Moszoro H, Nock P, Wilkins SR. Reduction of bronchial hyperreactivity during prolonged allergen avoidance. Lancet 1982; ii: 675–8.

27 Dorward AJ, Colloff MJ, MacKay NS, McSharry C, Thomson NC. Effect of house dust mite avoidance measures on adult atopic asthma. Thorax 1988; 43: 98–105.

28 Korsgaard J. Mite asthma and residency. A case-control study on the impact of exposure to house-dust mites in dwellings. Am Rev Respir Dis 1983; 128: 231–5.

29 Walshaw MJ, Evans CC. Allergen avoidance in house-dust mite sensitive adult asthma. Q J Med 1986; 58: 199–215.

30 Sanda T, Yasue T, Oohashi M, Yasue A. Effectiveness of house-dust mite allergen avoidance through clean room therapy in patients with atopic dermatitis. J Allergy Clin Immunol 1992; 89: 653–7.

31 Platts-Mills TAE, Chapman MD, Pollart S, Luczynska GW, Ward GW Jr. Specific allergens evoking immune reactions in the lung: Relationship to asthma. *Eur Respir J* 1991; 4: 68s–77s.

32 Luczynska CM, Li Y, Chapman MD, Platts-Mills TAE. Airborne concentrations and particle size distribution of allergen derived from domestic cats (*Felis domesticus*): Measurements using cascade impactor, liquid impinger and a two site monoclonal antibody assay for *Fel d* I. *Am Rev Respir Dis* 1990; 141: 361–7.

33 Pollart S, Smith TF, Morris EC, Gelber LE, Platts-Mills TAE, Chapman MD. Environmental exposure to cockroach allergens: Analysis with monoclonal antibody-based enzyme immunoassays. *J Allergy Clin Immunol* 1991; 87: 505–10.

34 Chapman MD, Aalberse RC, Brown MJ, Platts-Mills TAE. Monoclonal antibodies to the major feline allergen *Fel d* I. II. Single step affinity purification of *Fel d* I, N-terminal sequence analysis, and development of a sensitive two-site immunoassay to assess *Fel d* I exposure. *J Immunol* 1988; 140: 812–8.

35 Llerena LP, Fernandez-Caldere ZE, Gracia LRC. Sensitization to *Blomia tropicalis* and *Lepidoglyphus destructor* in *Dermatophagoides* spp.-allergic individuals. *J Allergy Clin Immunol* 1991; 88: 943–50.

36 Platts-Mills TAE, Heymann PW, Chapman MD, Hayden ML, Wilkins SR. Cross-reacting and species-specific determinants on a major allergen from *Dermatophagoides pteronyssinus* and *D. farinae* development of a radioimmunoassay for antigen P1 equivalent in house dust and dust mite extracts. *J Allergy Clin Immunol* 1986; 78: 398–407.

37 Arruda K, Rizzo M, Chapman MD *et al.* Exposure and sensitization to dust mite allergens among asthmatic children in São Paulo, Brazil. *Clin Exp Allergy* 1991; 21: 433–9.

38 Kang C. Allergen exposure of inhaled arthropod material. *Clin Rev Allergy* 1985; 3: 363–75.

39 Linter TJ, Brame KA. The effects of season, climate and air conditioning on the prevalence of *Dermatophagoides* mite allergens in household dust. *J Allergy Clin Immunol* 1993; 91: 862–7.

40 Arlian LG, Vyszenski-Moher DL, Fernandez-Caldas E. Allergenicity of the mite, *Blomia tropicalis*. *J Allergy Clin Immunol* 1993; 91: 1042–50.

41 Arlian LG, Rapp CM, Fernandez-Caldas E. Allergenicity of *Euroglyphus maynei* and its cross reactivity with *Dermatophagoides* species. *J Allergy Clin Immunol* 1993; 91: 1051–8.

42 Chapman MD. Guanine – an adequate index of mite exposure? (editorial). *Allergy* 1993; 48: 301–2.

43 Rizzo MC, Arruda LK, Chapman MD *et al.* IgG and IgE antibody responses to dust mite allergens among children with asthma in Brazil. *Ann Allergy* 1993; 71: 152–8.

44 Sporik R, Holgate ST, Platts-Mills TAE, Cogswell J. Exposure to house dust mite allergen (*Der p* I) and the development of asthma in childhood: A prospective study. *N Engl J Med* 1990; 323: 502–7.

45 Price JA, Pollock J, Little SA, Longbottom JL, Warner JO. Measurements of airborne mite allergen in houses of asthmatic children. *Lancet* 1990; 336: 895–7.

46 Tovey ER, Chapman MD, Wells CW, Platts-Mills TAE. The distribution of dust mite allergen in the houses of patients with asthma. *Am Rev Respir Dis* 1981; 124: 630–5.

47 Platts-Mills TAE, Heymann PW, Longbottom JL, Wilkins SR. Airborne allergens associated with asthma: particle sizes carrying dust mite and rat allergens measured with a cascade impactor. *J Allergy Clin Immunol* 1986; 77: 850–7.

48 Swanson MA, Agarwal MK, Reed CE. An immunochemical approach to indoor aeroallergen quantitation with a new volumetric air sampler: studies with mite, roach, cat, mouse and guinea-pig antigens. *J Allergy Clin Immunol* 1987; 76: 724–9.

49 Sporik RB, Chapman MD, Platts-Mills TAE. House dust mite exposure as a cause of asthma (editorial). *Clin Exp Allergy* 1992; 22: 897–906.

50 Placentini GL, Martinati L, Formari A *et al.* Antigen avoidance in a mountain environment influence on basophil releasability in children with asthma. *J Allergy Clin Immunol* 1993; 92: 644–50.

51 Burr ML, Neale E. Effect of change to mite-free bedding. *Thorax* 1980; 35: 513–4.

52 Owen S, Morganstern M, Hepworth J, Woodcock A. Control of house dust mite antigen in bedding. *Lancet* 1990; 335: 396–7.

53 Burr ML, Dean BV, Merrett TG, Neale E, St Leger AS, Verrier-Jones ER. Effects of anti-mite measures on children with mite-sensitive asthma: a controlled trial. *Thorax* 1980; 35: 506–12.

54 MacDonald L, Tovey E. The role of water temperature and laundry procedures in reducing house dust mice populations and allergen content of bedding. *J Allergy Clin Immunol* 1992; 90: 599–608.

55 McDonald LG, Tovey E. The role of water temperature and laundry procedures in reducing HDM populations and allergen content of bedding. *J Allergy Clin Immunol* 1992; 90: 599–608.

56 Hayden ML, Rose G, Diduch KB *et al.* Benzyl benzoate moist powder: Investigation of acarical activity in cultures and reduction of dust mite allergens in carpets. *J Allergy Clin Immunol* 1992; 89: 536–45.

57 Goodman LS and Gillman A. *The Pharmacologic Basis of Therapeutics*, 6th edn. New York: Macmillan, 1980: 985.

58 Greene WF, Nicholas NR, Salome CM, Woolcock AJ. Reduction of house dust mite and mite allergens. *Clin Exp Allergy* 1989; 19: 203–7.

59 Kniest FM, Young E, Van Praag MCG *et al.* Clinical evaluation of a double-blind dust-mite avoidance trial with mite-allergic rhinitis patients. *Clin Exp Allergy* 1990; 21: 39–47.

60 Dietemann A, Bessof JC. A double-blind placebo controlled trial of solidified benzyl benzoate applied in dwellings of asthmatic patient sensitive to mites: clinical efficacy and effect on mite antigens. *J Allergy Clin Immunol* 1993; 91: 738–46.

61 Wolf ST. Suffocating odor and asthma after acarosan powder carpet treatment. *J Allergy Clin Immunol* 1992; 2: 637–8.

62 Tovey ER, Chapman MD, Platts-Mills TAE. Mite faeces are a major source of house dust allergens. *Nature* 1981; 289: 592–3.

63 Korsgaard J. House dust mites and absolute indoor humidity. *Allergy* 1983; 38: 85–92.

64 Korsgaard J. Preventive measures in house dust allergy. *Am Rev Respir Dis* 1982; 125: 80–4.

65 Kang B. Study on cockroach antigen as a probable causative agent in bronchial asthma. *J Allergy Clin Immunol* 1976; 58: 357–65.

66 Bernton HS, McMahon TF, Brown H. Cockroach asthma. *Br J Dis Chest* 1972; 66: 61–6.

67 Kang B, Sulit N. A comparative study of skin hypersensitivity to cockroach and house dust antigens. *Ann Allergy* 1978; 41: 333–6.

68 Kang B, Vellody D, Homburger H, Yunginger JW. Cockroach cause of allergic asthma. Its specificity and immunologic profile. *J Allergy Clin Immunol* 1979; 63: 80–6.

69 Call RS, Smith TF, Morris E, Chapman MD, Platts-Mills TAE. Risk factors for asthma in inner city children. *J Pediatr* 1992; 121: 862–6.

70 Fletcher-Bincent SA, Reece ER, Malveaux FJ. Reactivity to cockroach and other allergens in an inner city population with rhinitis and asthma. *J Allergy Clin Immunol* 1994; 93: 174.

71 Neffen HE, Jossen R, Aroaz I *et al.* Socioeconomic status and sensitization to cockroach allergens in asthmatic children in Santa Fe, Argentina. *J Allergy Clin Immunol* 1994; 93: 289.

72 Gelber LE, Seltzer LH, Bouzoukis JK, Pollart SM, Chapman MD, Platts-Mills TAE. Sensitization and exposure to indoor allergens as risk factors for asthma among patients presenting to hospital. *Am Rev Respir Dis* 1993; 147: 573–8.

73 Lau S, Falkenhorst G, Weber A *et al.* High mite-allergen exposure increases the risk of sensitization in atopic children and young adults. *J Allergy Clin Immunol* 1989; 84: 718–25.

74 Schou C, Fernandez-Caldas E, Lockey RF, Lowenstein H. Environmental assay for cockroach allergen. J Allergy Clin Immunol 1991; 87: 828-34.

75 De Blay F, Heymann PW, Chapman MD, Platts-Mills TAE. Airborne dust mite allergens: Comparison of Group II allergens with Group I mite allergen and cat allergen Fel d I. J Allergy Clin Immunol 1991; 88: 919-26.

76 Robinson WH, Zungoli PA. Integrated control program for German cockroaches (Dictyoptera: Blatella) in multiple-unit dwellings. J Econ Entomol 1985; 78: 595-8.

77 Sarpong SB, Wood RA, Eggleston PA. Cockroach allergen (Bla g II): Environmental control with extermination and cleaning. J Allergy Clin Immunol 1994; 93: 179.

78 De Blay F, Chapman MD, Platts-Mills TAE. Airborne cat allergen (Fel d I): Environmental control with the cat in situ. Am Rev Respir Dis 1991; 143: 1334-9.

79 Ohman JL, Findlay SR, Leitermann SB. Immunotherapy in cat-induced asthma. Double-blind trial with examination of in vivo and in vitro responses. J Allergy Clin Immunol 1984; 74: 230-9.

80 Enberg RN, Shamie SM, McCullough J, Ownby DR. Ubiquitous presence of cat allergen in cat-free buildings: probable dispersal from human clothing. Ann Allergy 1993; 70: 471-4.

81 Luczynska CM, Li Y, Chapman MD, Platts-Mills TAE. Airborne concentrations and particle size distribution of allergen derived from domestic cats (Felis domesticus): Measurements using cascade impactor, liquid impinger and a two site monoclonal antibody assay for Fel d I. Am Rev Respir Dis 1990; 141: 361-7.

82 Wood RA, Mudd KE, Eggleston PA. The distribution of cat and dust mite allergens on wall surfaces. J Allergy Clin Immunol 1992; 89: 126-30.

83 Wood RA, Chapman MD, Adkinson NF Jr, Eggleston PA. The effect of cat removal on allergen content in household-dust samples. J Allergy Clin Immunol 1989; 83: 730-4.

84 Klucka CV, Ownby DR, Green M. Cat washings, allerpet or acepromazine do not diminish Fel d I shedding. J Allergy Clin Immunol 1994; 93: 180.

85 Woodfolk JA, Luczynska CM, De Blay F, Chapman MD, Platts-Mills TAE. The effect of vacuum cleaners on the concentration and particle size distribution of airborne cat allergen. J Allergy Clin Immunol 1993; 91: 829-37.

86 Wood RA, Laheri AN, Eggleston PA. The aerodynamic characteristics of cat allergen. Clin Exp Allergy 1993; 23: 733-9.

87 Ingram JM, Sporik R, Rose G, Honsinger R, Chapman MD, Platts-Mills TAE. Quantitative assessment of exposure to dog (Can f I) and cat (Fel d I) allergens: relationship to sensitization and asthma among children living in Los Alamos, New Mexico. J Allergy Clin Immunol (in press).

88 Salvaggio J, Aukrust L. Postgraduate course presentations. Mold-induced asthma. *J Allergy Clin Immunol* 1981; 68: 327–46.

89 Paris S, Fitting C, Latge JP, Herman D, Guinnepain MT, David B. Comparison of conidial and mycelial allergens of *Alternaria alternata*. *Int Arch Allergy Appl Immunol* 1990; 92: 1–8.

90 Fadel R, David B, Paris S, Guesdon JI. *Alternaria* spore and mycelium sensitivity in allergic patients: *in vivo* and *in vitro* studies. *Ann Allergy* 1992; 69: 329–35.

91 Portnoy J, Pacheco F, Barnes C, Upadrashta B, Crenshaw R, Esch R. Selection of representative *Alternaria* strain groups on the basis of morphology, enzyme profile, and allergen content. *J Allergy Clin Immunol* 1993; 91: 773–82.

92 Al-Doory Y, Ramsey S. *Moulds and Health*. Springfield, IL: CC Thomas.

93 Solomon WR. Assessing fungus prevalence in domestic interiors. *J Allergy Clin Immunol* 1975; 56: 235.

94 Kodama AM, McGee RI. Airborne microbial contaminants in indoor environments. Naturally ventilated and air-conditioned homes. *Arch Environ Health* 1986; 41: 306–11.

95 Paris S, Debeaupuis JP, Prevost MC, Casotto M, Latge JP. The 31kd major allergen, *Alt a* I, of *Alternaria alternata*. *J Allergy Clin Immunol* 1991; 88: 902–8.

96 Arruda LK, Mann BJ, Chapman MD. Selective expression of a major allergen and cytotoxin, *Asp f* I, in *Aspergillus fumigatus*: Implications for the immunopathogenesis of *Aspergillus* related diseases. *J Immunol* 1992; 149: 3354–9.

97 Deuell BL, Arruda LK, Hayden ML, Chapman MD, Platts-Mills TAE. *Trichophyton tonsurans* allergen I (*Tri t* I): Characterization of a protein that causes immediate but not delayed hypersensitivity. *J Immunol* 1991; 147: 96–101.

98 Malling HF. Diagnosis and immunotherapy of mould allergy. *Allergy* 1986; 41: 342–50.

99 Ward GW Jr, Karlsson G, Rose G, Platts-Mills TAE. *Trichophyton* asthma: sensitisation of bronchi and upper airways to dermatophyte antigen. *Lancet* 1989; i: 859–62.

100 Lehrer SR, Lopez M, Butcher BT, Olson J, Reed M, Salvaggio JE. Basidiomycete mycelia and spore-allergen extracts: skin test reactivity in adults with symptoms of respiratory allergy. *J Allergy Clin Immunol* 1986; 78: 478–85.

101 Kleine-Tebbe J, Worm M, Jeep S, Matthiesen F, Lowenstein H, Kunkel G. Predominance of the major allergen (*Alt a* I) in *Alternaria* sensitized patients. *Clin Exp Allergy* 1992; 23: 211–8.

102 Sporik RB, Arruda LK, Woodfolk J, Chapman MD, Platts-Mills TAE. Environmental exposure to *Aspergillus fumigatus* (*Asp f* I). *Clin Exp Allergy* 1993; 23: 326–31.

103 El-dahr J, Fink R, Selden R, Arruda LK, Platts-Mills TAE, Heymann PW. Development of immune responses to *Aspergillus*, including allergen *Asp f* I, at an early age in children with cystic fibrosis. *Am J Resp Med Crit Care*, December 1994.

104 Goldstein MF, Dvorin DJ, Dunsky EH, Lesser RW, Heuman PJ, Loose JH. Allergic rhizomucor sinusitis. *J Allergy Clin Immunol* 1992; 90: 394–404.

105 Nagda NL, Rector HE, Koontz MD. *Guidelines for Monitoring Indoor Air Quality.* Washington: Hemisphere Pub. Co., 1987: 15–24.

106 Denson-Lino JM, Willies-Jacobo LJ, Rosas A, O'Connor RD, Wilson NW. Effect of economic status on the use of house dust mite avoidance measures in asthmatic children. *Ann Allergy* 1993; 71: 130–2.

107 Huss K, Rand CS, Buts AM *et al.* Home environmental risk factors in urban minority asthmatic children. *Ann Allergy* 1994; 72: 173–6.

KEY POINTS

1 Avoidance measures for dust-mite allergens should be prioritized and should focus first on the bedroom.

2 Mite avoidance is primarily achieved by physical measures such as encasing mattress and pillows as well as hot washing bedding.

3 Mite allergens become airborne during disturbance but fall rapidly afterwards, i.e. within 10 min. Cat allergen is also increased by disturbance but it remains airborne and is present even in undisturbed rooms.

4 Successful allergen avoidance can decrease not only symptoms but also non-specific airway hyperresponsiveness.

15

CORTICOSTEROIDS

Peter J. Barnes

INTRODUCTION

Glucocorticosteroids (also known as corticosteroids or steroids) are the most effective therapy in the treatment of asthma and indeed asthma may be clinically defined as airway obstruction that improves with steroids. Oral steroids are still very useful for the control of asthma exacerbations but their chronic use in the control of asthma has sharply declined with the introduction of inhaled steroids. Inhaled steroids give effective control of asthma and are largely free of the side-effects associated with maintenance treatment with oral steroids. Inhaled steroids have now become the mainstay of chronic asthma treatment in many countries. The recognition that airways inflammation is present even in the mildest of asthmatic patients has led to the introduction of inhaled steroids at a much earlier stage in therapy. Inhaled steroids are effective in all types of asthma and at all ages. The only limitation to their use is side-effects, but recent evidence suggests that this is not a problem for most patients.

This chapter discusses new advances in understanding the mechanism of action of steroids in asthma, the clinical use of oral and inhaled steroids in asthma and assessment of their side-effects.

MECHANISM OF ACTION

Although steroids are the most effective therapy known for asthma, their precise mechanism of action is not yet understood. Important advances have been made in elucidating some of the molecular and cellular actions of steroids that are relevant to their anti-asthma effects.[1,2]

MOLECULAR MECHANISMS

Inhaled steroids are highly lipophilic and rapidly enter target cells of the airway to bind to cytosolic glucocorticoid receptors (GR). In human airways there is a high level of GR expression in epithelial cells and in endothelial cells of bronchial vessels.[3] Binding of the corticosteroid to GR results in rapid localization to the nucleus, where GR binds to DNA at specific consensus sites termed glucocorticoid response elements (GRE) on the upstream promoter sequence of steroid-responsive genes.[4] This results in either increased or decreased transcription of a particular gene (Fig. 15.1).[5] It is likely that altered transcription of many different genes is involved in the anti-asthma effect of steroids and each cell is estimated to have between 10 and 100 steroid-responsive genes.[1] Perhaps their most important action is inhibition of transcription of the genes for all the cytokines implicated in asthmatic inflammation.[1]

Recently it has been demonstrated that GR may bind directly to certain transcription factors that are activated by cytokines. Thus pro-inflammatory cytokines activate the nuclear transcription factor activator protein-1 (AP-1). AP-1 when activated within the nucleus binds to response elements on

FIGURE 15.1: *Molecular mechanism of glucocorticosteroid (GCS) action. GCS binds to a cytosolic glucocorticoid receptor (GR) that is normally bound to two molecules of heat shock protein-90 (hsp90). The activated GR then moves rapidly into the nucleus where it binds to specific glucocorticoid response elements on the upstream regulatory region of genes which either inhibit (nGRE) or stimulate (+GRE) transcription of steroid-responsive genes. Several steroid-responsive genes that may be relevant in asthma therapy are shown.*

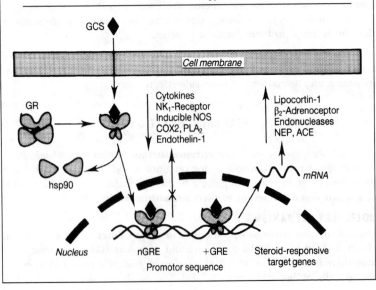

the promoter sequence and thus regulates the transcription of certain genes. AP-1 may also bind to the activated GR within the nucleus, and via this protein–protein interaction steroids may inhibit the cellular actions of cytokines.[1]

CELLULAR EFFECTS

Steroids may have directly inhibitory effects on many of the cells involved in asthmatic inflammation, including macrophages, T lymphocytes, eosinophils and epithelial cells (Fig. 15.2).[6] Steroids decrease cytokine-mediated survival of eosinophils in culture[7] by stimulating apoptosis and this may be

FIGURE 15.2: *Cellular effects of glucocorticosteroids in asthma therapy.*

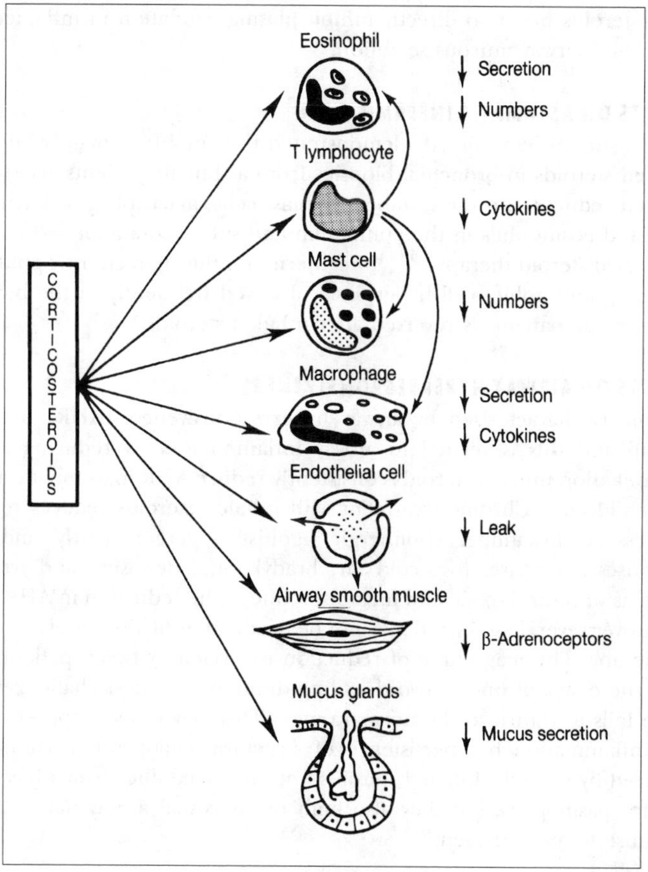

the basis for the marked reduction in numbers of eosinophils in the circulation and airways after steroid therapy.[8,9] Inhaled steroids also reduce the numbers of circulating eosinophils in asthmatic patients, and in particular the fraction of eosinophils with low density, indicating that inhibition of local cytokine production (interleukin-5 (IL-5), granulocyte-macrophage colony stimulating factor (GM-CSF)) in the airways.[10] Oral steroids have been shown to reduce mRNA for IL-4 and IL-5 in bronchoalveolar lavage cells from asthmatic patients[11] and inhaled steroids reduce the expression of GM-CSF in airway epithelial cells in asthma.[12] Although steroids may not have direct inhibitory effects on mast cell mediator release,[6] they reduce the numbers of mast cells within the airways,[8,9] which may be due to reduced synthesis of cytokines, such as IL-3 and stem cell factor, needed for mast cell survival.

In addition to the direct suppressive effects of steroids on inflammatory cells, steroids may also directly inhibit plasma exudation in inflamed airways[13] and airway mucous secretion.[14]

EFFECTS ON ASTHMATIC INFLAMMATION
Several studies have directly demonstrated the anti-inflammatory effect of inhaled steroids in bronchial biopsies from asthmatic patients. There is a marked reduction in the numbers of mast cells, macrophages, T lymphocytes and eosinophils in the epithelium and submucosa after 1–3 months of inhaled steroid therapy.[8,9,15,16] Furthermore, the characteristic epithelial shedding and goblet cell hyperplasia observed frequently in the biopsies of asthmatic patients is reversed after inhaled steroids.[8]

EFFECTS ON AIRWAY HYPERRESPONSIVENESS
Asthma is characterized by airway hyperresponsiveness (AHR) to many stimuli and this is related to airway inflammation. By reducing airway inflammation inhaled steroids consistently reduce AHR in asthmatic adults and children.[17] Chronic treatment with inhaled steroids reduces responsiveness to histamine, cholinergic agonists, allergen (early and late responses), exercise, fog, cold air, bradykinin, adenosine and irritants (such as sulphur dioxide and metabisulphite). The reduction in AHR takes place over several weeks and may not be maximal until after several months of therapy. The magnitude of reduction is variable between patients and is in the order of one to two doubling dilutions for most challenges and often fails to return to the normal range. This may reflect suppression of the inflammation but persistence of structural changes that cannot be reversed by steroids. Inhaled steroids not only make the airways less sensitive to spasmogens, but they also limit the maximal airway narrowing in response to a spasmogen.[18]

CLINICAL EFFICACY OF INHALED STEROIDS

Inhaled steroids are very effective in controlling asthma symptoms in asthmatic patients of all ages and severity.[19–21]

STUDIES IN ADULTS

Inhaled steroids were first introduced to reduce the requirement for oral steroids in patients with severe asthma and many studies have confirmed that the majority of patients can be weaned off oral steroids.[22] As experience has been gained with inhaled steroids they have been introduced in patients with milder asthma, with the recognition that inflammation is present even in patients with mild asthma.[23] Inhaled anti-inflammatory drugs have now become first-line therapy in any patient who needs to use a β_2-agonist inhaler more than once a day and this is reflected in national and international guidelines for the management of chronic asthma.[24–26] In patients with newly diagnosed asthma inhaled steroids (budesonide 600 μg twice daily) reduced symptoms and β_2-agonist inhaler usage and improved peak expiratory flows. These effects persisted over the 2 years of the study, whereas in a parallel group treated with inhaled β_2-agonists alone there was no significant change in symptoms or lung function.[27] In another study patients with mild asthma treated with a low dose of inhaled steroid (budesonide 200 μg twice daily) showed less symptoms and a progressive improvement in lung function over several months and many patients became completely asymptomatic.[28] Similarly inhaled beclomethasone dipropionate (BDP, 400 μg twice daily) improved asthma symptoms and lung function and this was maintained over the 2.5 years of the study.[29] There was also a significant reduction in the number of exacerbations. Although the effects of inhaled steroids on AHR may take several months to reach a plateau, the reduction in asthma symptoms occurs more rapidly.[30]

High-dose inhaled steroids have now been introduced in many countries for the control of more severe asthma. This markedly reduces the need for maintenance oral steroids and has revolutionized the management of more severe and unstable asthma.[31–33] Inhaled steroids are the treatment of choice in nocturnal asthma, which is a manifestation of inflamed airways,[34] reducing night-time awakening and the diurnal variation in airway function.[35,36]

Inhaled steroids effectively control asthmatic inflammation but must be taken regularly. When inhaled steroids are discontinued there is usually a gradual increase in symptoms and airway responsiveness back to pre-treatment values,[30] although in patients with mild asthma who have been treated with inhaled steroids for a long time symptoms may not recur in some patients.[37]

STUDIES IN CHILDREN

Inhaled steroids are equally effective in children. In an extensive study of children aged 7–17 years there was a significant improvement in symptoms, peak flow variability and lung function compared with a regular inhaled β_2-agonist that was maintained over the 22 months of the study,[38] but asthma deteriorated when the inhaled steroids were withdrawn.[39] There was a high proportion of drop-outs (45%) in the group treated with inhaled β_2-agonist alone. Inhaled steroids are also effective in younger children. Nebulized budesonide reduced the need for oral steroids and also improved lung function in children under the age of 3 years.[40] Inhaled steroids given via a large volume spacer improved asthma symptoms and reduced the number of exacerbations in pre-school children and in infants.[41,42]

PREVENTION OF IRREVERSIBLE CHANGES

Some patients with asthma develop an element of irreversible airflow obstruction, but the pathophysiological basis of these changes is not yet understood. It is likely that they are the result of chronic airway inflammation and that they may be prevented by treatment with inhaled steroids. There is some evidence that the annual decline in lung function may be slowed by the introduction of inhaled steroids.[43] Preliminary evidence also suggests that delay in starting inhaled steroids may result in less overall improvement in lung function in both adults and children.[44,45]

REDUCTION IN MORTALITY

Whether inhaled steroids may reduce the mortality from asthma is not yet established as prospective studies are almost impossible to conduct. In a retrospective review of the risk of mortality and prescribed anti-asthma medication, there was a significant apparent protection provided by regular inhaled BDP therapy (adjusted odds ratio of 0.1), although numbers were small.[46]

EFFECTS IN CHRONIC OBSTRUCTIVE PULMONARY DISEASE

Whilst the beneficial effects of inhaled steroids in asthma are now well documented, their role in the management of chronic obstructive pulmonary disease (COPD) are less clear. The failure of a short course (2–4 weeks) of an oral steroid to improve airway obstruction discriminates COPD from asthma. Inhaled steroids over 3 months fail to improve lung function or airway responsiveness in patients with mild to moderate COPD,[47] although with longer duration of treatment some beneficial effect may be apparent.[48] Larger studies of the effects of long-term treatment with inhaled steroids on the progression of airway obstruction in patients with COPD are currently underway.[49]

COMPARISON BETWEEN INHALED STEROIDS

Several inhaled steroids are currently prescribable in asthma, although their availability varies between countries (Fig. 15.3). There have been relatively few studies comparing efficacy of the different inhaled steroids, and

FIGURE 15.3: *Structure of currently available inhaled glucocorticosteroids.*

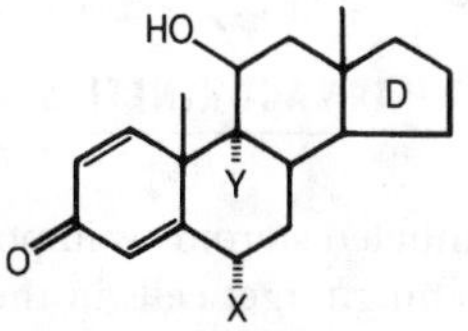

GCS	X	Y	D
Beclomethasone dipropionate	H	Cl	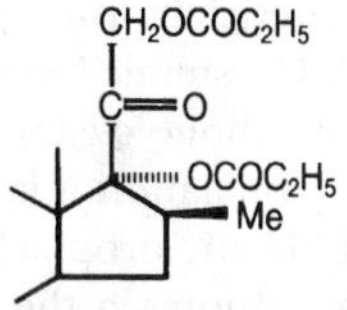 $CH_2OCOC_2H_5$, $C=O$, $OCOC_2H_5$, Me
Budesonide	H	H	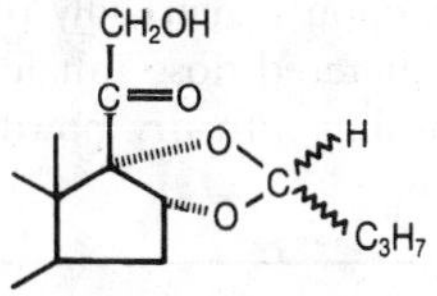 CH_2OH, $C=O$, $O-C-H$, $O-C_3H_7$
Flunisolide	F	H	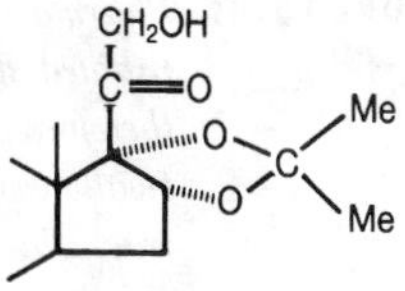 CH_2OH, $C=O$, $O-C-Me$, $O-C-Me$
Triamcinolone acetonide	H	F	— '' —
Fluticasone propionate	F	F	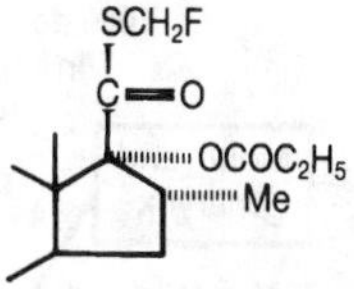 SCH_2F, $C=O$, $OCOC_2H_5$, Me

it is important to take into account the delivery system and the type of patient under investigation when such comparisons are made. In the UK BDP, betamethasone valerate, budesonide and fluticasone propionate are available, whereas in the USA BDP, flunisolide and triamcinolone are available. There are few studies comparing different doses of inhaled steroids in asthmatic patients. Budesonide has been compared with BDP and in adults and children appears to have comparable anti-asthma effects at equal doses.[50,51] However, there do appear to be some differences between inhaled steroids in terms of their systemic effects at comparable anti-asthma doses.

PHARMACOKINETICS

The pharmacokinetics of inhaled steroids is important in determining the concentration of drug reaching target cells in the airways and in the fraction of drug reaching the systemic circulation and therefore causing side-effects.[52] Beneficial properties in an inhaled steroid are a high topical potency, a low systemic bioavailability of the swallowed portion of the dose and rapid metabolic clearance of any steroid reaching the systemic circulation. After inhalation a large proportion of the inhaled dose (80–90%) is deposited on the oropharynx and is then swallowed and therefore available for absorption via the liver into the systemic circulation (Fig. 15.4). This fraction is markedly reduced by using a large volume spacer device with a metered dose inhaler (MDI) or by mouth-washing and discarding the washing with dry powder inhalers. Between 10 and 20% of inhaled

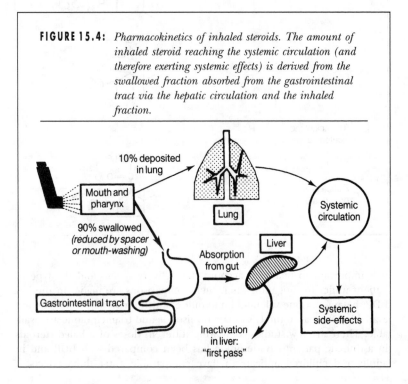

FIGURE 15.4: *Pharmacokinetics of inhaled steroids. The amount of inhaled steroid reaching the systemic circulation (and therefore exerting systemic effects) is derived from the swallowed fraction absorbed from the gastrointestinal tract via the hepatic circulation and the inhaled fraction.*

drug enters the respiratory tract, where it is deposited in the airways and this fraction is available for absorption into the systemic circulation. Most of the studies on the distribution of inhaled steroids have been conducted in healthy volunteers, and it is not certain what effect inflammatory disease, airway obstruction, age of the patient or concomitant medication may have on the disposition of the inhaled dose. There may be important differences in the metabolism of different inhaled steroids. BDP is metabolized to its more active metabolite beclomethasone monopropionate in many tissues including lung,[53] but there is no information about absorption or metabolism of this metabolite in humans. Flunisolide and budesonide are subject to extensive first-pass metabolism in the liver so that less reaches the systemic circulation.[54,55] Little is known about the distribution of triamcinolone.[56] Fluticasone propionate has a low oral bioavailability, which reduces systemic effects.[57]

FREQUENCY OF ADMINISTRATION

When inhaled steroids were first introduced it was recommended that they should be given four times daily, but several studies have now demonstrated that twice daily administration gives comparable control,[58,59] although four times daily administration may be preferable in patients with more severe asthma.[60] However, patients may find it difficult to comply with such frequent administration unless they have troublesome symptoms. For patients with mild asthma once daily therapy may be sufficient.[61]

SIDE-EFFECTS OF INHALED STEROIDS

The efficacy of inhaled steroids is now established in short- and long-term studies in adults and children, but there are still concerns about side-effects, particularly in children and when high inhaled doses are needed. Several side-effects have been recognized (Table 15.1).

LOCAL SIDE-EFFECTS

Side-effects due to the local deposition of the inhaled steroid in the oropharynx may occur with inhaled steroids, but the frequency of complaints depends on the dose and frequency of administration and on the delivery system used.

Dysphonia

The commonest complaint is of hoarseness of the voice (dysphonia) and may occur in over one-third of patients.[62] Dysphonia may be due to myopathy of laryngeal muscles and is reversible when treatment is withdrawn.[63] For most patients it is not troublesome but may be disabling in singers.

Oropharyngeal Candidiasis

Oropharyngeal candidiasis (thrush) may be a problem in some patients, particularly in the elderly, with concomitant oral steroids and more than

TABLE 15.1: *Side-effects of inhaled steroids*

Local side-effects
Dysphonia
Oropharyngeal candidiasis
Local irritation (cough, bronchoconstriction)

Systemic side-effects
Hypothalamic–pituitary–adrenal suppression
Increased bone turnover (increased breakdown, reduced
    formation, reduced density)
Impaired growth
Connective tissue effects (skin thinning, easy bruising)
Cataracts (postcapsular)
Metabolic disturbance (impaired insulin tolerance, increased
    glucose, hyperlipidaemia)
Haematological changes (decreased eosinophils, monocytes,
    increased neutrophils)
Psychiatric disturbance

twice daily administration.[62] Large volume spacer devices protect against this local side-effect by reducing the dose of inhaled steroid that is deposited in the oropharynx.

Other Local Complications
There is no evidence that inhaled steroids, even in high doses, increase the frequency of infections, including tuberculosis, in the lower respiratory tract.[64,65] There is no evidence for atrophy of the airway epithelium and even after 10 years of treatment with inhaled steroids there is no evidence for any structural changes in the epithelium.[66]

Cough and throat irritation, sometimes accompanied by reflex broncho-constriction, may occur when inhaled steroids are given via an MDI. These symptoms are likely to be due to surfactants in pressurized aerosols as they disappear after switching to a dry powder steroid inhaler device.[67]

SYSTEMIC SIDE-EFFECTS
The efficacy of inhaled steroids in the control of asthma is undisputed, but there are concerns about systemic effects of inhaled steroids, particularly as they are likely to be used over long periods and in children of all ages.[68–70] The safety of inhaled steroids has been extensively investigated since their introduction almost 30 years ago. One of the major problems is to decide

whether a measurable systemic effect has any significant clinical consequence and this will require careful long-term follow-up studies. As biochemical markers of systemic steroid effects become more sensitive, then systemic effects may be seen more often, but this does not mean that these effects are clinically relevant. There are several case reports of adverse systemic effects of inhaled steroids, and these are often idiosyncratic reactions, which may be due to abnormal pharmacokinetic handling of the inhaled steroid. The systemic effect of an inhaled steroid will depend on several factors, including the dose delivered to the patient, the site of delivery (gastrointestinal tract and lung), the delivery system used and individual differences in the patient's response to the steroid.

Effect of Delivery Systems

The systemic effect of an inhaled steroid is dependent on the amount of drug absorbed into the systemic circulation. As discussed above, approximately 90% of the inhaled dose from an MDI is deposited in the oropharynx and is swallowed and subsequently absorbed from the gastrointestinal tract. Use of a large volume spacer device markedly reduces the oropharyngeal deposition, and therefore the systemic effects of inhaled steroids.[71–73] For dry powder inhalers similar reductions in systemic effects may be achieved with mouth-washing and discarding the fluid.[73] All patients using a daily dose of 800 µg or more of an inhaled steroid should therefore use either a spacer or mouth-washing to reduce systemic absorption. Approximately 10% of an MDI enters the lung and this fraction (which presumably exerts therapeutic effect) may be absorbed into the systemic circulation. As the fraction of inhaled steroid deposited in the oropharynx is reduced, the proportion of the inhaled dose entering the lungs is increased. More efficient delivery to the lungs is therefore accompanied by increased systemic absorption, but this is offset by a reduction in the dose needed for optimal control of airway inflammation. For example, a multiple dry powder delivery system, the Turbuhaler, delivers approximately twice as much steroid to the lungs as other devices, and therefore has increased systemic effects. However this is compensated for by the fact that only half the dose is required.[74]

Hypothalamic-pituitary-adrenal Axis

Corticosteroids may cause hypothalamic–pituitary–adrenal (HPA) axis suppression by reducing corticotrophin (ACTH) production, which reduces cortisol secretion by the adrenal gland. The degree of HPA suppression is dependent on dose, duration, frequency and timing of steroid administration. The clinical significance of HPA axis suppression is two-fold. Firstly, prolonged adrenal suppression may lead to reduced adrenal response to stress. There is no evidence that cortisol responses to the stress of an asthma exacerbation or insulin-induced hypoglycaemia are impaired, even with high doses of inhaled steroids.[75] Secondly, measurement of HPA axis function provides evidence for systemic effects of an inhaled steroid. Basal adrenal cortisol secretion may be measured by a morning plasma cortisol, 24-hour urinary cortisol or by plasma cortisol profile over 24 hours.[76] Other tests measure the HPA response following stimulation with tetracosactrin (which measures adrenal reserve) or stimulation with metyrapone and insulin (which measure the response to stress).

There are many studies of HPA axis function in asthmatic patients with inhaled steroids, but the results are inconsistent as they have often been uncontrolled and patients have also been taking courses of oral steroids (which may affect the HPA axis for weeks).[20] Both BDP and budesonide at high doses by conventional MDI (> 1600 μg daily) give a dose-related decrease in morning serum cortisol levels and 24-hour urinary cortisol, although values still lie well within the normal range.[77,78] However, when a large volume spacer is used doses of 2000 μg daily of BDP or budesonide have no effect on 24-hour urinary cortisol excretion.[79] Studies with inhaled flunisolide and triamcinolone in children show no effect on 24-hour cortisol excretion at doses of up to 1000 μg daily.[80,81] Stimulation tests of HPA axis function show no consistent effects of doses of 1500 μg or less of inhaled steroid. At high doses (> 1500 μg daily) budesonide and fluticasone have less effect than BDP on HPA axis function.[78,82] In children no suppression of urinary cortisol is seen with doses of BDP of 800 μg or less.[83–85] In studies where plasma cortisol has been measured at frequent intervals there was a significant reduction in cortisol peaks with doses of inhaled BDP as low as 400 μg daily,[86] although this does not appear to be dose related in the range 400–1000 μg.[87,88] However, the clinical significance of these effects is not certain.

Overall, the studies that are not confounded by concomitant treatment with oral steroids have consistently shown that there are no significant suppressive effects on HPA axis function at doses of ≤ 1500 μg in adults and ≤ 400 μg in children.

Effects on Bone Metabolism

Steroids lead to a reduction in bone mass by direct effects on bone formation and resorption and indirectly by suppression of the pituitary–gonadal and HPA axes, effects on intestinal calcium absorption, renal tubular calcium reabsorption and secondary hyperparathyroidism (Fig. 15.5).[89] The effects of oral steroids on osteoporosis and increased risk of vertebral and rib fractures are well known, but there are no reports suggesting that long-term treatment with inhaled steroids is associated with an increased risk of fractures. Bone densitometry has been used to assess the effect of inhaled steroids on bone mass. Although there is evidence that bone density is less in patients taking high-dose inhaled steroids, interpretation is confounded by the fact that these patients are also taking intermittent courses of oral steroids.[90] A longitudinal study in adults found no evidence for a reduction in bone density in patients taking 400–1000 μg inhaled BDP over a 2-year period.[91]

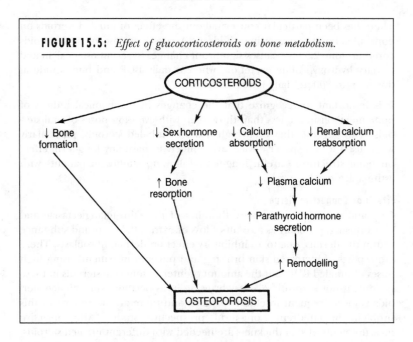

FIGURE 15.5: *Effect of glucocorticosteroids on bone metabolism.*

Changes in bone mass occur very slowly and several biochemical indices have been used to assess the short-term effects of inhaled steroids on bone metabolism. Bone formation has been measured by plasma concentrations of bone-specific alkaline phosphatase or serum osteocalcin, a non-collagenous 49-amino acid peptide secreted by osteoblasts. Bone resorption may be assessed by urinary hydroxyproline after a 12-hour fast, urinary calcium excretion and pyridinium cross-link excretion. It is important to consider the age, diet, time of day and physical activity of the patient in interpreting any abnormalities. It is also necessary to choose appropriate control groups as asthma itself may have an effect on some of the measurements, such as osteocalcin.[92] Inhaled steroids, even at doses up to 2000 μg daily, have no significant effect on calcium excretion, but acute and reversible dose-related suppression of serum osteocalcin has been reported with BDP and budesonide when given by conventional MDI.[93–97] Budesonide consistently has less effect than BDP at equivalent doses and only BDP increases urinary hydroxyproline at high doses.[98] However, with a large volume spacer even doses of 2000 μg daily of either BDP or budesonide are without effect on plasma osteocalcin concentrations.[79] Urinary pyridinium and deoxypyridinoline cross-links, which are a more accurate and stable measurement of bone and collagen degradation, are not increased with inhaled steroids (BDP > 1000 μg daily), even with intermittent courses of oral steroids.[90]

There has been particular concern about the effect of inhaled steroids on bone metabolism in growing children. A very low dose of oral steroids (prednisolone 2.5 mg) causes significant changes in serum osteocalcin and urinary hydroxyproline excretion, whereas daily BDP and budesonide at doses up to 800 μg daily have no effect.[92,99]

It is important to recognize that the changes in biochemical indices of bone metabolism are less than those seen with even low doses of oral steroids. This suggests that even high doses of inhaled steroids, particularly when used with a spacer device, are unlikely to have any long-term effect on bone structure. Careful long-term follow-up studies in patients with asthma are needed.

Effects on Connective Tissue
Oral and topical steroids cause thinning of the skin, telangiectasiae and easy bruising, probably as a result of loss of extracellular ground substance within the dermis, due to an inhibitory effect on dermal fibroblasts. There are reports of increased skin bruising and purpura in patients using high doses of inhaled BDP, but the amount of intermittent oral steroids in these patients is not known.[100,101] Easy bruising in association with inhaled steroids is more frequent in elderly patients and there are no reports of this problem in children. Long-term prospective studies with objective measurements of skin thickness are needed with different inhaled steroids.

Cataracts
Long-term treatment with oral steroids increases the risk of posterior subcapsular cataracts and there are several case reports describing cataracts in individual patients taking inhaled steroids.[20] In a study of 48 patients who were exposed to oral and/or high-dose inhaled steroids the prevalence of posterior subcapsular cataracts (27%) correlated with the daily dose and duration of oral steroids, but not with the dose and duration of inhaled steroids.[102] In a recent cross-sectional study in patients aged 5–25 years taking either inhaled BDP or budesonide no cataracts were found on slit-lamp examination, even in patients taking 2000 μg daily for over 10 years.[103]

Growth
There has been particular concern that inhaled steroids may cause stunting of growth and several studies have addressed this issue. Asthma itself (as with other chronic diseases) may have an effect on the growth pattern and has been associated with delayed onset of puberty and deceleration of growth velocity that is more pronounced with more severe disease.[104] However, asthmatic children appear to grow for longer, so that their final height is normal. The effect of asthma on growth makes it difficult to assess the effects of inhaled steroids on growth in cross-sectional studies, particularly as courses of oral steroids is a confounding factor. Longitudinal studies have demonstrated that there is no significant effect of inhaled steroids on statural growth in doses of up to 800 μg daily and for up to 5

years of treatment.[20,38,70,105,106] A prospective study of inhaled BDP (400 μg daily) versus theophylline in children with mild to moderate asthma showed no effect on height, although there was some reduction in growth velocity compared with children treated with theophylline.[107] However it is not possible to relate changes in growth velocity to final height as other studies have demonstrated that there is a "catch-up" period. In a longitudinal study in children aged 2–7 years with severe asthma, budesonide 200 μg daily had no effect on growth over 3–5 years.[85] A meta-analysis of 21 studies, including over 800 children, showed no effect of inhaled BDP on statural height, even with higher doses and long durations of therapy.[108]

Short-term growth measurements (knemometry) have demonstrated that even a low dose of an oral steroid (prednisolone 2.5 mg) is sufficient to give complete suppression of lower leg growth. However, inhaled budesonide up to 400 μg is without effect, although some suppression is seen with 800 μg and with 400 μg BDP.[109,110] The relationship between knemometry measurements and final height are uncertain since low doses of oral steroids that have no effect on final height cause profound suppression.

Metabolic Effects

Several metabolic effects have been reported after inhaled steroids, but there is no evidence that these are clinically relevant at therapeutic doses. In adults, fasting glucose and insulin are unchanged after doses of BDP up to 2000 μg daily[50] and in children with inhaled budesonide up to 800 μg daily.[111] In normal individuals high-dose inhaled BDP may slightly increase resistance to insulin.[112] However, in patients with poorly controlled asthma a high-dose BDP and budesonide paradoxically decrease insulin resistance and improve glucose tolerance, suggesting that the disease itself may lead to abnormalities in carbohydrate metabolism.[113] Neither BDP 2000 μg daily in adults nor budesonide 800 μg daily in children have any effect on plasma cholesterol or triglycerides.[50,111]

Haematological Effects

Inhaled steroids may reduce the numbers of circulating eosinophils in asthmatic patients,[10] possibly due to an effect on local cytokine generation in the airways. Inhaled steroids may cause a small increase in circulating neutrophil counts.[79,114]

Central Nervous System Effects

There are various reports of psychiatric disturbance, including emotional lability, euphoria, depression, aggressiveness and insomnia, after inhaled steroids. Only eight such patients have so far been reported, suggesting that this is very infrequent and a causal link with inhaled steroids has usually not been established.[20]

Safety in Pregnancy

Based on extensive clinical experience inhaled steroids appear to be safe in pregnancy, although no controlled studies have been performed. There is no evidence for any adverse effects of inhaled steroids on the pregnancy, the delivery or on the fetus.[20] It is important to recognize that poorly controlled asthma may increase the incidence of perinatal mortality and retard intrauterine growth, so that more effective control of asthma with inhaled steroids may reduce these problems.

COMPARISONS WITH OTHER THERAPIES

No other anti-asthma therapy is as effective in controlling asthma as corticosteroids, but other treatments may reduce the requirement for inhaled steroids and thus reduce the need for high doses. Cromones (sodium cromoglycate and nedocromil sodium) are less effective in controlling asthma than inhaled steroids, although they may sometimes be useful in patients with mild asthma.[115] It is recommended that sodium cromoglycate should be given prior to starting inhaled steroids in children, although it is important to recognize that the doses of inhaled steroid giving equivalent asthma control to cromones (100–400 μg daily) have no appreciable side-effects and have the additional advantages of twice daily administration and lower cost. Cromones may be useful in reducing the requirements for inhaled steroids in patients who have problems with local side-effects,[116] although others have not shown any steroid-sparing effect.[117]

Conventional β_2-agonists do not control asthma as effectively as inhaled steroids in either adults or children.[27,38] The long-acting inhaled β_2-agonist, salmeterol, appears to give equivalent, if not better, control of asthma when added to 400 μg BDP than increasing the dose of BDP to 1000 μg daily.[118]

Theophylline when used alone does not control asthma as effectively as inhaled steroids and is associated with more frequent side-effects.[107] However, theophylline may be useful in controlling asthma in patients with more severe disease and controlled studies designed to compare the effect of adding theophylline to low-dose inhaled steroid compared with increasing the dose of inhaled steroid are now needed.

CLINICAL USE OF INHALED STEROIDS

Inhaled steroids are now recommended as first-line therapy for all but the mildest of asthmatic patients.[23,27] Several inhaled steroids are now available for use, although their availability varies between countries (Table 15.2). Inhaled steroids should be started in any patient who needs to use a β-agonist inhaler for symptom control more than once daily (or possibly three times weekly). It is conventional to start with a low dose of inhaled

TABLE 15.2: *Inhaled steroids*

Drug	Trade name	Dose (μg/puff)
Beclomethasone dipropionate	Becotide/Beclovent/ Vanceril	MDI: 50, 100
	Becotide	Rotacaps: 100, 200, 400
	Becloforte	MDI: 250
	Becodisks	100, 200, 400
Budesonide	Pulmicort	MDI: 50, 200 Turbohaler: 200, 400
Betamethasone valerate	Bextosol	MDI: 100
Triamcinolone acetonide	Azmacort	MDI: 100
Flunisolide	Aerobid/Bronalide	MDI: 250
Fluticasone propionate	Flixotide	MDI: 50, 125 Disks: 50, 100, 250

steroid and to increase the dose until asthma control is achieved. However, this may take time and a preferable approach is to start with a dose of steroids in the middle of the dose range (400 μg twice daily) to establish control of asthma more rapidly. Once control is achieved (defined as normal or best possible lung function and infrequent need to use an inhaled β_2 agonist) the dose of inhaled steroid should be reduced in a step-wise manner to the lowest dose needed for optimal control. It may take as long as 3 months to reach a plateau in response and any changes in dose should be made at intervals of 3 months or more. When doses of ≤ 800 μg daily are needed a large volume spacer device should be used with an MDI and mouth-washing with a dry powder inhaler in order to reduce local and systemic side-effects. Inhaled steroids are usually given as a twice daily dose in order to increase compliance. When asthma is more unstable four times daily dosage is preferable.[60,119] For patients who require ≤ 400 μg daily once daily dosing appears to be as effective as twice daily dosing, at least for budesonide.[61]

The dose of inhaled steroid should be increased to 2000 μg daily if necessary, but higher doses may result in systemic effects and it may be preferable to add an oral steroid, since higher doses of inhaled steroids are expensive and have a high incidence of local side-effects. Nebulized budesonide has been advocated in order to give an increased dose of inhaled steroid and to reduce the requirement for oral steroids,[120] but this treatment is expensive and may achieve its effects largely via systemic absorption.

Most of the guidelines for asthma treatment suggest that additional bronchodilators (slow-release theophylline preparations, inhaled and oral long-acting β_2 agonists and inhaled anticholinergics) should be introduced after increasing the dose of inhaled steroid to 1600–2000 μg daily. However, an alternative approach is to introduce these treatments when patients are taking 800–1000 μg inhaled steroid daily. Carefully designed clinical trials of long duration are needed to determine the optimal approach.

SYSTEMIC STEROIDS

Oral or intravenous steroids may be indicated in several situations. Prednisolone, rather than prednisone, is the preferred oral steroid as prednisone has to be converted in the liver to the active prednisolone. In pregnant patients prednisone may be preferable as it is not converted to prednisolone in the fetal liver, thus diminishing the exposure of the fetus to glucocorticosteroids. Enteric-coated preparations of prednisolone are used to reduce side-effects (particularly gastric side-effects) and give delayed and reduced peak plasma concentrations, although the bioavailability and therapeutic efficacy of these preparations is similar to uncoated tablets. Prednisolone and prednisone are preferable to dexamethasone, betamethasone or triamcinolone, which have longer plasma half-lives and therefore an increased frequency of adverse effects.

Short courses of oral steroids (30–40 mg prednisolone daily for 1–2 weeks or until the peak flow values return to best attainable) are indicated for exacerbations of asthma, and the dose may be tailed off over 1 week once the exacerbation is resolved. The tail-off period is not strictly necessary,[121] but some patients find it reassuring.

Maintenance oral steroids are only needed in a small proportion of asthmatic patients with the most severe asthma that cannot be controlled with maximal doses of inhaled steroids (2000 μg daily) and additional bronchodilators. The minimal dose of oral steroid needed for control should be used and reductions in the dose should be made slowly in patients who have been on oral steroids for long periods (e.g. by 2.5 mg per month for doses down to 10 mg daily and thereafter by 1 mg per month). Oral steroids are usually given as a single morning dose as this reduces the risk of adverse effects since it coincides with the peak diurnal concentrations. There is some evidence that administration in the afternoon may be optimal for some patients who have severe nocturnal asthma.[122] Alternate day administration may also reduce adverse effects, but control of asthma may not be as good on the day when the oral dose is omitted in some patients.

Intramuscular triamcinolone acetonide (80 mg monthly) has been advocated in patients with severe asthma as an alternative to oral steroids.[123,124] This may be considered in patients in whom compliance is a particular problem, but the major concern is the high frequency of proximal myopathy associated with this fluorinated steroid. Some patients who do not respond well to prednisolone are reported to respond to oral betamethasone, presumably because of pharmacokinetic handling problems with prednisolone.[125]

STEROID-SPARING THERAPY

In patients who have serious side-effects with maintenance steroid therapy there are several treatments that have been shown to reduce the requirement for oral steroids. These treatments are commonly termed steroid sparing, although this is a misleading description that could be applied to any additional asthma therapy (including bronchodilators). The amount of steroid sparing with these therapies is not impressive.

Several immunosuppressive agents have been shown to have steroid effects, including methotrexate,[126–128] oral gold[129,130] and cyclosporin A.[131,132] These therapies all have side-effects that may be more troublesome than those of oral steroids and are therefore only indicated as an additional therapy to reduce the requirement of oral steroids. None of these treatments is very effective, but there are occasional patients who appear to show a particularly good response. Because of side-effects these treatments cannot be considered as a way to reduce the requirement for inhaled steroids. Side-effects are a problem with these immunosuppressive drugs and include nausea, vomiting, hepatic dysfunction, hepatic fibrosis, pulmonary fibrosis and increased infections for methotrexate and renal dysfunction for cyclosporin and oral gold. Several other therapies, including azathioprine, dapsone and hydroxychloroquine have not been found to be beneficial. The macrolide antibiotic troleandomycin is also reported to have steroid-sparing effects, but this is only seen with methylprednisolone and is due to reduced metabolism of this steroid, so that there is little therapeutic gain.[133]

ACUTE SEVERE ASTHMA

Intravenous hydrocortisone is given in acute severe asthma; the recommended dose is 200 mg.[26] While the value of corticosteroids in acute severe asthma has been questioned, others have found that they speed the resolution of attacks.[134] There is no apparent advantage in giving very high doses of intravenous steroids (such as methylprednisolone 1 g). Indeed, intravenous steroids in ventilated patients have occasionally been associated with an acute severe myopathy.[135] In a recent study no difference in recovery from acute severe asthma was seen whether intravenous hydrocortisone in doses of 50, 200 or 500 mg 6-hourly was used.[136] Intravenous steroids are indicated in patients with acute asthma if lung function is < 30% predicted and in whom there is no significant improvement with nebulized β_2 agonist. Intravenous therapy is usually given until a satisfactory response is obtained and then oral prednisolone may be substituted.

Oral prednisolone (40–60 mg) has a similar effect to intravenous hydrocortisone and is easier to administer.[134,137] Oral prednisolone is the preferred treatment for acute severe asthma, providing there are no contraindications to oral therapy.[26]

STEROID-RESISTANT ASTHMA (see also Chapter 37)

Although most patients with asthma respond to steroids, there is a small minority of patients who appear to be resistant to steroid therapy. Steroid resistance is defined by a lack of response to oral steroids (usually 40 mg prednisolone daily for 2 weeks).[138,139] Other patients require very high doses of oral steroids for control and these patients should be considered as part of the steroid-resistant asthma spectrum.[140] It is important before diagnosing steroid-resistant asthma to ensure that the patient has asthma, that there are no problems with compliance and that absorption of the oral steroid is normal.[140] There are no epidemiological surveys of true steroid-resistant asthma, but as strictly defined above this may only occur in 1 : 1000 to 1 : 10 000 asthmatic subjects. There is a tendency for these patients to have more severe asthma of a longer duration and nocturnal exacerbations. There is often a family history of asthma. Steroid resistance does not appear to be explained by pharmacokinetic problems, such as impaired absorption or rapid elimination of oral steroids.[141–143] The inhibitory effect of steroids on phytohaemagglutinin-stimulated growth of cultured blood monocytes is reduced in steroid-resistant patients compared with steroid-sensitive controls,[143,144] suggesting that there is a cellular defect in steroid responsiveness. Steroids also fail to suppress the release of cytokines from monocytes of resistant patients.[145] This defect is not confined to monocytes but is also seen in peripheral T lymphocytes,[141] and a defect in the skin blanching response to topical steroids has also been described in such patients.[146]

However, the precise mechanism of steroid resistance is not certain. There is no significant defect in binding of steroids to GR in monocytes or lymphocytes from these patients and no defect in nuclear transcription of GR.[141,142] This is in contrast to the rare patients with familial cortisol resistance who may have marked abnormalities in steroid receptor-binding parameters.[147,148] There is no evidence for lipocortin-1 autoantibodies in patients with steroid-resistant asthma,[149,150] as has been described in patients with steroid-resistant arthritis.[151,152] A recent study has suggested that there is impaired binding of GR to GRE and also a defect in the inhibitory effect of AP-1 activation on GRE binding in resistant compared with sensitive patients.[153] This would explain why resistance to the anti-inflammatory effects of steroids is seen in these patients, yet circulating cortisol levels, adrenal suppression in response to steroids and metabolic actions of steroids are apparently normal.

Resistance to steroids is not confined to asthma, but is also described in other conditions where steroids are required for disease control, including rheumatoid arthritis, leukaemias and transplant rejection.[138] Although patients with resistance to steroids may be an extreme, there may be a spectrum of steroid responsiveness. Down-regulation of steroid receptors after exposure to steroids *in vitro* is well described,[154,155] and there is some evidence that this can occur in circulating lymphocytes *in vivo* after oral steroid treatment. Reduction in GR mRNA has been described in human lung *in vitro* after exposure to high-dose steroids,[3] but whether this is important in asthmatic patients exposed to high-dose inhaled steroids is not known. Another possibility is that inflammation itself may counteract the anti-inflammatory effects of steroids through the direct interaction between GR and AP-1 (activated by exposure to pro-inflammatory cytokines)[1,156] or with the transcription factor CREB (cyclic AMP response element binding protein) activated by exposure to high dose β agonists.[157]

FUTURE DEVELOPMENTS

Because inhaled steroids are the most effective therapy currently available for asthma, perhaps the most useful advances in asthma therapy in the future may be the improvement of inhaled steroids so that systemic and local adverse effects are less likely. The use of new delivery devices has partly achieved the desired reduction in local and systemic effects, but novel types of steroid for inhalation or the development of non-steroidal drugs that mimic the essential anti-asthma effects of steroids are also a possibility. It is clear that there is a single type of GR[4] and therefore it is not possible to develop novel steroids that have a greater selectivity. Improvements in inhaled steroids must therefore be based on pharmacokinetic differences. Inhaled steroids exert their anti-asthmatic effects topically in the airways rather than via a systemic effect. This is demonstrated by a recent study in which a systemic dose of budesonide given to mimic the small systemic effect of inhaled budesonide (400 μg daily) was without anti-asthma effect.[158] New inhaled steroids may be developed by increasing the inactivation of the systemic component of the inhaled steroid and/or by potentiating the topical anti-inflammatory action of steroids in the airways.[159]

Several other anti-asthma drugs are now in development and will eventually have to be compared with inhaled steroids as a "gold standard".[160] It is unlikely that any of these treatments will replace inhaled steroids, although they may reduce the need for high doses. Inhaled steroids are here to stay and it is important to use them as effectively as possible.

INCREASED METABOLISM

The fraction of inhaled steroids deposited in the oropharynx and swallowed is available for absorption from the gastrointestinal tract. First-pass metabolism in the liver is therefore important in limiting the systemic effect of inhaled steroids. Budesonide has a very efficient first-pass metabolism (90%). The swallowed fraction of inhaled steroids is also markedly reduced by the use of a large volume spacer device or by mouth-washing. However, the major component of inhaled steroid that reaches the systemic circulation is derived from the respiratory tract. It can be calculated that for a steroid with 90% first-pass hepatic metabolism approximately 75% of the total systemic availability originates from the lung-absorbed fraction, and that mouth-rinsing after inhalation can enhance this figure to approximately 90%.[159] This calculation has recently been supported by *in vivo* experiments in human volunteers, where the oral absorption was completely blocked by administration of charcoal by mouth.[74] The large lung-absorbed fraction could be reduced by the development of inhaled steroids that are inactivated in the lung or in the circulation by esterases. Examples of such steroids are fluocortinbutyl ester (hydrolysed in tissue and blood) and tixocortol pivalate (inactivated in blood by *S*-methyltransferases).[159] However the same properties reduce the topical potency of these steroids, resulting in local metabolism in the airways, and neither of these drugs has useful anti-asthma effects. It is possible that steroids with a higher receptor affinity could be developed to exert a topical action before metabolism occurs.

INCREASED BINDING

Currently effective inhaled steroids derived from lipophilic substitution in the 17α, 17β positions of the glucocorticoid structure have a high affinity for GR and also have a high mucosal uptake and retention in airways and lung.[159,161,162] However increasing the local tissue retention time carries the risk of more troublesome local effect in the oropharynx. More selective targeting of the inhaled steroid to the key target cells may be another approach in the future, although it is likely that several target cells are involved in asthma. One possibility is to target airway macrophages by the use of liposomes coated with surface receptors that trigger phagocytosis.[159]

GENOMIC SELECTIVITY

Steroids exert their anti-inflammatory and immunomodulatory effect by regulating gene transcription via several different mechanisms, as discussed above. By the use of site-directed mutagenesis of GR it is possible to differentiate some of these mechanisms so that some receptor mutants may more selectively mediate a particular type of genomic mechanism. It is possible that different types of steroid might be developed in the future that may cause conformational changes in the receptor to lead to more selective genomic effects.

CONCLUSIONS

Glucocorticosteroids are by far the most effective anti-asthma therapy currently available. The problem of side-effects encountered with oral steroids has largely been avoided by the development of potent inhaled steroids. Inhaled steroids are very effective in controlling asthma symptoms and in reducing asthma exacerbations. There is also preliminary evidence that they may prevent irreversible airway changes and may reduce asthma mortality. An important consideration is their risk–benefit ratio and inhaled steroids have now been studied more extensively than any other drug in both adults and children. These studies, conducted in normal volunteers and asthmatic patients of varying severity, have demonstrated that, irrespective of the inhaled steroid, there are minimal systemic effects, even using the most sensitive indicators, at doses of ≤ 400 µg in children or ≤ 800 µg in adults. At higher doses there is some evidence for systemic effects, although this is less noticeable with budesonide and fluticasone than with BDP. Even at high doses (up to 2000 µg daily) there is little evidence of any adverse effects, although occasional patients may have idiosyncratic responses. The small risk of adverse effects at high doses of inhaled steroids has to be offset against the risks of not adequately controlling severe asthma. The risk of systemic absorption is markedly reduced by the use of spacer devices with MDIs and by mouth-washing with dry powder inhalers and these should be used whenever doses of ≥ 800 µg daily are needed for asthma control. More detailed dose–response curves for beneficial and adverse effects of different inhaled steroids are needed. Additional long-term studies of the effects of inhaled steroids in adults and children are needed, taking into account long-term benefits, adverse effects and costs. It is also important that other anti-asthma treatments, including new therapies, such as leukotriene antagonists and selective phosphodiesterase inhibitors, are compared with inhaled steroids in long-term studies.

REFERENCES

1 Barnes PJ, Adcock IM. Anti-inflammatory actions of steroids: molecular mechanisms. *Trends Pharmacol Sci* 1993; 14: 436–41.

2 Taylor IK, Shaw RJ. The mechanism of action of corticosteroids in asthma. *Respir Med* 1993; 4: 261–78.

3 Adcock IM, Bronnegard M, Barnes PJ. Glucocorticoid receptor mRNA localization and expression in human lung. *Am Rev Respir Dis* 1991; 143: A628.

4 Muller M, Renkawitz R. The glucocorticoid receptor. *Biochim Biophys Acta* 1991; 1088: 171–82.

5 Beato M. Gene regulation by steroid hormones. *Cell* 1989; 56: 335–44.

6 Schleimer RP. Effects of glucocorticoids on inflammatory cells relevant to their therapeutic application in asthma. *Am Rev Respir Dis* 1990; 141: S59–S69.

7 Lamas AM, Leon OG, Schleimer RP. Glucocorticoids inhibit eosinophil responses to granulocyte-macrophage colony-stimulating factor. *J Immunol* 1991; 147: 254–9.

8 Laitinen LA, Laitinen A, Haahtela T. A comparative study of the effects of an inhaled corticosteroid, budesonide, and of a β_2-agonist, terbutaline, on airway inflammation in newly diagnosed asthma. *J Allergy Clin Immunol* 1992; 90: 32–42.

9 Djukanovic R, Wilson JW, Britten YM *et al.* Effect of an inhaled corticosteroid on airway inflammation and symptoms of asthma. *Am Rev Respir Dis* 1992; 145: 669–74.

10 Evans PM, O'Connor BJ, Fuller RW, Barnes PJ, Chung KF. Effect of inhaled corticosteroids on peripheral eosinophil counts and density profiles in asthma. *J Allergy Clin Immunol* 1992; 91: 643–9.

11 Robinson DS, Hamid Q, Ying S *et al.* Prednisolone treatment in asthma is associated with modulation of bronchoalveolar lavage cell IL-4, IL-5 and IFN-γ cytokine gene expression. *Am Rev Respir Dis* 1993; 148: 401–6.

12 Sousa AR, Poston RN, Lane SJ, Narhosteen JA, Lee TH. Detection of GM-CSF in asthmatic bronchial epithelium and decrease by inhaled corticosteroids. *Am Rev Respir Dis* 1993; 147: 1557–61.

13 Boschetto P, Rogers DF, Fabbri LM, Barnes PJ. Corticosteroid inhibition of airway microvascular leakage. *Am Rev Respir Dis* 1991; 143: 605–9.

14 Shimura S, Sasaki T, Ikeda K, Yamauchi K, Sasaki H, Takishima T. Direct inhibitory action of glucocorticoid on glycoconjugate secretion from airway submucosal glands. *Am Rev Respir Dis* 1990; 141: 1044–9.

15 Jeffery PK, Godfrey RW, Ädelroth E, Nelson F, Rogers A, Johansson S-A. Effects of treatment on airway inflammation and thickening of basement membrane reticular collagen in asthma. *Am Rev Respir Dis* 1992; 145: 890–9.

16 Burke C, Power CK, Norris A, Condez A, Schmekel B, Poulter LW. Lung function and immunopathological changes after inhaled corticosteroid therapy in asthma. *Eur Respir J* 1992; 5: 73–9.

17 Barnes PJ. Effect of corticosteroids on airway hyperresponsiveness. *Am Rev Respir Dis* 1990; 141: S70–S76.

18　Bel EH, Timers MC, Zwinderman AH, Dijkman JH, Sterk PJ. The effect of inhaled corticosteroids on the maximal degree of airway narrowing to methacholine. *Am Rev Respir Dis* 1991; 143: 109–13.

19　Barnes PJ. Antiinflammatory therapy in asthma. *Ann Rev Med* 1993; 44: 229–49.

20　Barnes PJ, Pedersen S. Efficacy and safety of inhaled steroids in asthma. *Am Rev Respir Dis* 1993; 148: S1–S26.

21　König P. Inhaled corticosteroids – their present and future role in the management of asthma. *J Allergy Clin Immunol* 1988; 82: 297–306.

22　Reed CE. Aerosol glucocorticoid treatment of asthma: adults. *Am Rev Respir Dis* 1990; 140: S82–S88.

23　Barnes PJ. A new approach to asthma therapy. *N Engl J Med* 1989; 321: 1517–27.

24　National Heart, Lung and Blood Institute – National Asthma Education Programme Expert Panel Report. Guidelines for the diagnosis and management of asthma. *J Allergy Clin Immunol* 1991; 88: 425–534.

25　International Consensus Report on Diagnosis and Management of Asthma. *Clin Exp Allergy* 1992; 22 (suppl 1): 1–72.

26　British Thoracic Society. Guidelines on the management of asthma. *Thorax* 1993; 48 (suppl): S1–S24.

27　Haahtela T, Jarvinen M, Kava T *et al.* Comparison of a β_2-agonist terbutaline with an inhaled steroid in newly detected asthma. *N Engl J Med* 1991; 325: 388–92.

28　Juniper EF, Kline PA, Vanzieleghem MA, Ramsdale EH, O'Byrne PM, Hargreave FE. Effect of long-term treatment with an inhaled corticosteroid (budesonide) on airway hyperresponsiveness and clinical asthma in non-steroid-dependent asthmatics. *Am Rev Respir Dis* 1990; 142: 832–6.

29　Kerrebijn KF, van Essen-Zandvliet EEM, Neijens HJ. Effect of long-term treatment with inhaled corticosteroids and beta-agonists on bronchial responsiveness in asthmatic children. *J Allergy Clin Immunol* 1987; 79: 653–9.

30　Vathenen AS, Knox AJ, Wisniewski A, Tattersfield AE. Time course of change in bronchial reactivity with an inhaled corticosteroid in asthma. *Am Rev Respir Dis* 1991; 143: 1317–21.

31　Toogood JH. High dose inhaled steroid therapy for asthma. *J Allergy Clin Immunol* 1989; 83: 528–36.

32　Salmeron S, Guerin J-C, Godard P *et al.* High doses of inhaled corticosteroids in unstable chronic asthma. *Am Rev Respir Dis* 1989; 140: 167–71.

33　Lacronique J, Renon D, Georges D, Henry-Amar M, Marsac J. High-dose beclomethasone: oral steroid-sparing effect in severe asthmatic patients. *Eur Respir J* 1991; 4: 807–12.

34　Barnes PJ. Inflammatory mechanisms and nocturnal asthma. *Am J Med* 1988; 85(suppl 1B): 64–70.

35 Dahl R, Pedersen B, Hägglöf B. Nocturnal asthma: effect of treatment with oral sustained-release terbutaline, inhaled budesonide and the two in combination. *J Allergy Clin Immunol* 1989; 83: 811–5.

36 Wempe JB, Tammeling EP, Postma DS, Auffarth B, Teengs JP, Koëter GH. Effects of budesonide and bambuterol on circadian variation of airway responsiveness and nocturnal asthma symptoms of asthma. *J Allergy Clin Immunol* 1992; 90: 349–57.

37 Juniper EF, Kline PA, Vanzieleghem MA, Hargreave FE. Reduction of budesonide after a year of increased use: a randomized controlled trial to evaluate whether improvements in airway responsiveness and clinical asthma are maintained. *J Allergy Clin Immunol* 1991; 87: 483–9.

38 van Essen-Zandvliet EE, Hughes MD, Waalkens HJ, Duiverman EJ, Pocock SJ, Kerrebijn KF. Effects of 22 months of treatment with inhaled corticosteroids and/or beta$_2$-agonists on lung function, airway responsiveness and symptoms in children with asthma. *Am Rev Respir Dis* 1992; 146: 547–54.

39 Waalkens HJ, van Essen-Zandvliet EE, Hughes MD *et al.* Cessation of long-term treatment with inhaled corticosteroids (budesonide) in children with asthma results in deterioration. *Am Rev Respir Dis* 1993; 148: 1252–7.

40 Ilangovan P, Pedersen S, Godfrey S, Nikander K, Novisky N, Warner JO. Nebulised budesonide suspension in severe steroid-dependent preschool asthma. *Arch Dis Child* 1993; 68: 356–9.

41 Gleeson JGA, Price JF. Controlled trial of budesonide given by Nebuhaler in preschool children with asthma. *BMJ* 1988; 297: 163–6.

42 Bisgard H, Munck SL, Nielsen JP, Peterson W, Ohlsson SV. Inhaled budesonide for treatment of recurrent wheezing in early childhood. *Lancet* 1990; 336: 649–51.

43 Dompeling E, van Schayck CP, Molema J, Folgering H, van Grusven PM, van Weel C. Inhaled beclomethasone improves the course of asthma and COPD. *Eur Respir J* 1992; 5: 945–52.

44 Haahtela T, Järvinen M, Kava T *et al.* First-line treatment of newly detected asthma: an inhaled steroid? One year's follow-up after two years treatment. *Eur Respir J* 1992; 5 (suppl 15): 13S.

45 Pedersen S, Agertoft L. Effect of long term budesonide treatment on growth, weight and lung function in children with asthma. *Am Rev Respir Dis* 1993; 147: A265.

46 Ernst P, Spitzer WD, Suissa S *et al.* Risk of fatal and near fatal asthma in relation to inhaled corticosteroid use. *JAMA* 1992; 268: 3462–4.

47 Watson A, Lim TK, Joyce H, Pride NB. Failure of inhaled corticosteroids to modify bronchoconstrictor or bronchodilator responses in middle-aged smokers with mild airflow obstruction. *Chest* 1992; 101: 350–5.

48 Kertjens HAM, Brand PLP, Hughes MD *et al.* A comparison of bronchodilator therapy with or without inhaled corticosteroid therapy for obstructive airways disease. *N Engl J Med* 1992; 327: 1413–9.

49 Pauwels RA, Löfdahl C-G, Pride NB, Postma DS, Laitinen LA, Ohlsson SV. European Respiratory Society study on chronic obstructive pulmonary disease (EUROSCOP): hypothesis and design. *Eur Respir J* 1992; 5: 1254–61.

50 Ebden P, Jenkins A, Houston G, Davies BH. Comparison of two high-dose corticosteroid aerosol treatments, beclomethasone dipropionate (1500 mcg/day) and budesonide (1660 mcg/day) for chronic asthma. *Thorax* 1986; 41: 869–74.

51 Baran D. A comparison of inhaled budesonide and beclomethasone dipropionate in childhood asthma. *Br J Dis Chest* 1987; 81: 170–5.

52 Szefler S. Glucocorticoid therapy for asthma: clinical pharmacology. *J Allergy Clin Immunol* 1991; 88: 147–65.

53 Wurthwein G, Rohdewald P. Activation of beclomethasone dipropionate by hydrolysis to beclomethasone-17-monophosphate. *Biopharm Drug Dispos* 1990; 11: 381–94.

54 Chaplin MD, Rooks W, Svenson EW, Couper WC, Nerenberg C, Chu NI. Flunisolide metabolism and dynamics of a metabolite. *Clin Pharmacol Ther* 1980; 27: 402–13.

55 Ryrfeldt A, Andersson P, Edsbacker S, Tonnesson M, Davies D, Pauwels R. Pharmacokinetics and metabolism of budesonide, a selective glucocorticoid. *Eur J Respir Dis* 1982; 63 (suppl 122): 86–95.

56 Mollman H, Rohdewald P, Schmidt EW, Salomon V, Derendorf H. Pharmacokinetics of triamcinolone acetonide and its phosphate ester. *Eur J Clin Pharmacol* 1985; 29: 85–9.

57 Harding SM. The human pharmacology of fluticasone propionate. *Respir Med* 1990; 84 (suppl A): 25–9.

58 Toogood JH, Baskerville JC, Jennings B, Lefcoe NM, Johansson SA. Influence of dosing frequency and schedule on the response of chronic asthmatics to the aerosol steroid budesonide. *J Allergy Clin Immunol* 1982; 70: 288–98.

59 Meltzer EO, Kemp JP, Welch MJ, Orgel HA. Effect of dosing schedule on efficacy of beclomethasone dipropionate aerosol in chronic asthma. *Am Rev Respir Dis* 1985; 131: 732–6.

60 Malo J-L, Cartier A, Merland N *et al.* Four-times-a-day dosing frequency is better than twice-a-day regimen in subjects requiring a high-dose inhaled steroid, budesonide, to control moderate to severe asthma. *Am Rev Respir Dis* 1989;140: 624–8.

61 Jones AH, Langdon CG, Lee PS. Pulmicort Turbohaler once daily as initial prophylactic therapy for asthma. *Respir Med* 1994; 88: 293–300.

62 Toogood JH, Jennings B, Greenway RW, Chung L. Candidiasis and dysphonia complicating beclomethasone treatment of asthma. *J Allergy Clin Immunol* 1980; 65: 145–53.

63 Williams AJ, Baghat MS, Stableforth DE, Cryton RM, Shenos PM, Skinner C. Dysphonia caused by inhaled steroids: recognition of a characteristic laryngeal abnormality. *Thorax* 1983; 38: 813–21.

64 Brogden RN, Heel RC, Speight TM, Avery GS. Beclomethasone dipropionate. A reappraisal of its pharmacodynamic properties and therapeutic efficacy after a decade of use in asthma and rhinitis. *Drugs* 1984; 28: 99–126.

65 Brogden RN, McTavish D. Budesonide. An updated review of its pharmacological properties and therapeutic efficacy in asthma and rhinitis. *Drugs* 1992; 44: 375–407.

66 Lungren R, Soderberg M, Horstedt P, Stenling R. Morphological studies on bronchial mucosal biopsies from asthmatics before and after ten years treatment with inhaled steroids. *Eur Respir J* 1988; 1: 883–9.

67 Engel T, Heinig JH, Malling H-J, Scharing B, Nikander K, Masden F. Clinical comparison of inhaled budesonide delivered either by pressurized metered dose inhaler or Turbuhaler. *Allergy* 1989; 44: 220–5.

68 Geddes DM. Inhaled corticosteroids: benefits and risks. *Thorax* 1992; 47: 404–7.

69 Monson JP. Systemic effects of inhaled steroids. *Thorax* 1993; 48: 955–6.

70 Boner AL, Piacentini G. Inhaled corticosteroids in children. Is there a "safe" dosage? *Drug Safety* 1993; 9: 9–20.

71 Brown PH, Blundell G, Greening AP, Crompton GK. Do large volume spacer devices reduce the systemic effects of high dose inhaled corticosteroids? *Thorax* 1990; 45: 736–9.

72 Brown PH, Greening AP, Crompton GK. Large volume spacer devices and the influence of high dose beclomethasone dipropionate on hypothalamo–pituitary–adrenal axis function. *Thorax* 1993; 48: 233–8.

73 Selroos O, Halme M. Effect of a Volumatic spacer and mouth rinsing on systemic absorption of inhaled corticosteroids from a metered-dose inhaler and dry powder inhaler. *Thorax* 1991; 46: 891–4.

74 Thorsson L, Edsbäcker S. Lung deposition of budesonide from Turbuhaler is twice that from a pressurized metered dose inhaler (abstract). *Thorax* 1993; 48: 434.

75 Brown PH, Blundell G, Greening AP, Crompton GK. High dose inhaled corticosteroids and the cortisol induced response to acute severe asthma. *Respir Med* 1992; 86: 495–7.

76 Holt PR, Lowndes DW, Smithies E, Dixon GT. The effect of an inhaled steroid on the hypothalamic–pituitary–adrenal axis: which tests should be used? *Clin Exp Allergy* 1990; 20: 145–9.

77 Löfdahl CG, Mellstrand T, Svedmyr N. Glucocorticosteroids and asthma – studies of resistance and systemic effects of glucocorticosteroids. *Eur J Respir Dis* 1989; 65 (suppl 130): 69–79.

78 Pedersen S, Fuglsang G. Urine cortisol excretion in children treated with high doses of inhaled corticosteroids; a comparison of budesonide and beclomethasone. *Eur Respir J* 1988; 1: 433–5.

79 Brown PH, Matusiewicz SP, Shearing C, Tibi L, Greening AP, Crompton GK. Systemic effects of high dose inhaled steroids: comparison of beclomethasone dipropionate and budesonide in healthy subjects. *Thorax* 1993; 48: 967–73.

80 Sly RM, Imseis M, Frazer M *et al.* Treatment of asthma in children with triamcinolone acetonide aerosol. *J Allergy Clin Immunol* 1978; 62: 76–82.

81 Placcentini G, Sette L, Peroni DG, Bonizatto C, Bonetti S, Boner AL. Double blind evaluation of effectiveness and safety of flunisolide aerosol for treatment of bronchial asthma in children. *Allergy* 1990; 45: 612–6.

82 Fabbri L, Burge PS, Croonenburgh L *et al.* Comparison of fluticasone propionate with beclomethasone dipropionate in moderate to severe asthma treated for one year. *Thorax* 1993; 48: 817–23.

83 Prahl P. Adrenocortical suppression following treatment with beclomethasone and budesonide. *Clin Exp Allergy* 1991; 21: 145–6.

84 Bisgaard H, Damkjaer Nielsen M, Andersen B *et al.* Adrenal function in children with bronchial asthma treated with beclomethasone dipropionate or budesonide. *J Allergy Clin Immunol* 1988; 81: 1088–95.

85 Volovitz B, Amir J, Malik H, Kauschansky A, Varsano I. Growth and pituitary–adrenal function in children with severe asthma treated with inhaled budesonide. *N Engl J Med* 1993; 329: 1703–8.

86 Law CM, Honour JW, Marchant JL, Preece MA, Warner JO. Nocturnal adrenal suppression in asthmatic children taking inhaled beclomethasone dipropionate. *Lancet* 1986; i: 942–4.

87 Tabacknik E, Zadik Z. Diurnal cortisol secretion during therapy with inhaled beclomethasone dipropionate in children with asthma. *J Pediatr* 1991; 118: 294–7.

88 Philip M, Aviram M, Lieberman E *et al.* Integrated plasma cortisol concentration in children with asthma receiving long-term inhaled corticosteroids. *Pediatr Pulmonol* 1992; 12: 84–9.

89 Hosking DJ. Effect of corticosteroids on bone turnover. *Respir Med* 1993; 87 (suppl A): 15–21.

90 Packe GE, Douglas JG, MacDonald AF, Robins SP, Reid DM. Bone density in asthmatic patients taking high dose inhaled beclomethasone dipropionate and intermittent systemic steroids. *Thorax* 1992; 47: 414–7.

91 Luengo M, Del Rio L, Guanabens N, Picado C. Long-term effect of oral and inhaled glucocorticoids on bone mass in chronic asthma. A two year follow-up study. *Eur Respir J* 1991; 4(suppl 14): 342S.

92 König P, Hillman L, Cervantes CI. Bone metabolism in children with asthma treated with inhaled beclomethasone dipropionate. *J Pediatr* 1993; 122: 219-26.

93 Pouw GM, Prummel MF, Oustang H, Roos CM, Endert C. Beclomethasone inhalation decreases serum osteocalcin concentrations. *BMJ* 1991; 302: 627-8.

94 Teelucksingh S, Padfield PL, Tibi L. Inhaled corticosteroids, bone formation and osteocalcin. *Lancet* 1991; 338: 60-1.

95 Toogood JH, Jennings B, Hudsman AB, Baskerville J, Fraher LJ. Effects of dose and dosing schedule of inhaled budesonide on bone tumour. *J Allergy Clin Immunol* 1991; 88: 572-80.

96 Toogood JH, Crilly RG, Jones G, Nadeau J, Wells GA. Effect of high dose inhaled budesonide on calcium and phosphate metabolism and the risk of osteoporosis. *Am Rev Respir Dis* 1988; 138: 57-61.

97 Jennings B, Andersson K, Johannsson S. Assessment of systemic effects of inhaled glucocorticosteroids; comparison of the effects of inhaled budesonide and oral prednisolone on adrenal function and markers of bone tumour. *Eur J Clin Pharmacol* 1991; 40: 77-82.

98 Ali NJ, Capewell S, Ward MJ. Bone turnover during high dose inhaled corticosteroid treatment. *Thorax* 1991; 46: 160-4.

99 Wolthers OD, Pedersen S. Bone turnover in asthmatic children treated with oral prednisolone or inhaled budesonide. *Pediatr Pulmonol* 1993; 16: 341-7.

100 Capewell S, Reynolds S, Shuttleworth D, Edwards C, Finlay AY. Purpura and dermal thinning associated with high dose inhaled corticosteroids. *BMJ* 1990; 300: 1548-51.

101 Mak VHF, Melchor R, Spiro S. Easy bruising as a side-effect of inhaled corticosteroids. *Eur Respir J* 1992; 5: 1068-74.

102 Toogood JH, Markov AE, Baskerville J, Dyson C. Association of ocular cataracts with inhaled and oral steroid therapy during long term treatment for asthma. *J Allergy Clin Immunol* 1993; 91: 571-9.

103 Simons FER, Persaud MP, Gillespie CA, Cheang M, Shuckett EP. Absence of posterior subcapsular cataracts in young patients treated with inhaled glucocorticoids. *Lancet* 1993; 342: 736-8.

104 Russell G. Asthma and growth. *Arch Dis Child* 1993; 69: 695-8.

105 Balfour-Lynn L. Growth and childhood asthma. *Arch Dis Child* 1986; 61: 1049-55.

106 Ninan T, Russell G. Asthma, inhaled corticosteroid treatment and growth. *Arch Dis Child* 1992; 67: 703–5.

107 Tinkelman DG, Reed CE, Nelson HS, Offord KP. Aerosol beclomethasone dipropionate compared with theophylline as primary treatment of chronic, mild to moderately severe asthma in children. *Pediatrics* 1993; 92: 64–77.

108 Allen DB, Mullen M, Mullen B. A meta-analysis of the effects of oral and inhaled corticosteroids on growth. *J Allergy Clin Immunol* 1994; 93: 967–76.

109 Wolthers OD, Pedersen S. Growth in asthmatic children treated with budesonide. *Pediatrics* 1993; 90: 517–8.

110 Wolthers O, Pedersen S. Short term growth during treatment with inhaled fluticasone dipropionate and beclomethasone dipropionate. *Arch Dis Child* 1993; 68: 673–6.

111 Turpeinen M, Sorva R, Juntungen-Backman K. Changes in carbohydrate and lipid metabolism in children with asthma inhaling budesonide. *J Allergy Clin Immunol* 1991; 88: 384–9.

112 Kruszynska YT, Greenstone M, Home PD. Effect of high dose inhaled beclomethasone dipropionate on carbohydrate and lipid metabolism in normal subjects. *Thorax* 1987; 42: 881–4.

113 Kiviranta K, Turpeinen M. Effect of eight months of inhaled beclomethasone dipropionate and budesonide on carbohydrate metabolism in adults with asthma. *Thorax* 1993; 48: 974–8.

114 Toogood JH, Baskerville J, Jennings B. Use of spacers to facilitate inhaled corticosteroid treatment of asthma. *Am Rev Respir Dis* 1984; 129: 723–9.

115 Thomson NC. Nedocromil sodium: an overview. *Respir Med* 1989; 83: 269–76.

116 Svendsen UG, Jorgensen H. Inhaled nedocromil sodium as additional treatment to high dose inhaled corticosteroids in the management of bronchial asthma. *Eur Respir J* 1991; 4: 992–9.

117 Goldin JG, Bateman ED. Does nedocromil sodium have a steroid sparing effect in adult asthmatic patients requiring maintenance oral corticosteroids? *Thorax* 1988; 43: 982–6.

118 Greening AP, Ind PW, Northfield M, Shaw G. Added salmeterol versus higher-dose corticosteroids in asthma patients with symptoms on existing corticosteroids. *Lancet* 1994; 344; 219–24.

119 Toogood JH, Jennings B, Baskerville J, Andersson J, Johansson S-Å. Dosing regimen of budesonide and occurrence of oropharyngeal complications. *Eur J Respir Dis* 1984; 65: 35–44.

120 Otulana BA, Varma N, Bullock A, Higenbottam T. High dose nebulized steroid in the treatment of chronic steroid-dependent asthma. *Respir Med* 1992; 86: 105–8.

121 O'Driscoll BR, Kalra S, Wilson M, Pickering CAC, Caroll KB, Woodcock AA. Double blind trial of steroid tapering in acute asthma. *Lancet* 1993; 341: 324-7.

122 Beam WR, Ballard RD, Martin RJ. Spectrum of corticosteroid sensitivity in nocturnal asthma. *Am Rev Respir Dis* 1992; 145: 1082-6.

123 McLeod DT, Capewell SJ, Law J, MacLaren W, Seaton A. Intramuscular triamcinolone acetamide in chronic severe asthma. *Thorax* 1985; 40: 840-5.

124 Ogirala RG, Aldrich TK, Prezant DJ, Sinnett MJ, Enden JB, Williams MH. High dose intramuscular triamcinolone in severe life-threatening asthma. *N Engl J Med* 1991; 329: 585-9.

125 Grandordy B, Belmatoug N, Morelle A, De Lauture D, Marsac J. Effect of betamethasone on airway obstruction and bronchial response to salbutamol in prednisolone resistant asthma. *Thorax* 1987; 42: 65-71.

126 Mullarkey MF, Blumenstein BA, Mandrade WP, Bailey GA, Olason I, Wetzel CE. Methotrexate in the treatment of corticosteroid-dependent asthma. *N Engl J Med* 1988; 318: 603-7.

127 Mullarkey MF, Lammert JK, Blumenstein BA. Long-term methotrexate treatment in corticosteroid-dependent asthma. *Ann Intern Med* 1990; 112: 577-81.

128 Shiner RJ, Nunn AJ, Chung KF, Geddes DM. Randomized, double-blind, placebo-controlled trial of methotrexate in steroid-dependent asthma. *Lancet* 1990; 336: 137-40.

129 Klaustermeyer WB, Noritake DT, Kwong FK. Chrysotherapy in the treatment of corticosteroid-dependent asthma. *J Allergy Clin Immunol* 1987; 79: 720-5.

130 Nierop G, Gijzel WP, Bel EH, Zwinderman AH, Dijkman JH. Auranofin in the treatment of steroid dependent asthma: a double blind study. *Thorax* 1992; 47: 349-54.

131 Alexander AG, Barnes NC, Kay AB. Trial of cyclosporin in corticosteroid-dependent chronic severe asthma. *Lancet* 1992; 339: 324-8.

132 Szczeklik A, Nizankoska E, Dworski R, Domagala B, Pinis G. Cyclosporin for steroid-dependent asthma. *Allergy* 1991; 46: 312-5.

133 Nelson HS, Hamilos DL, Corsello PR, Levesque NV, Buchameier AD, Bucher BL. A double-blind study of troleandamycin and methylprednisolone in asthmatic patients who require daily corticoteroids. *Am Rev Respir Dis* 1993; 147: 398-404.

134 Engel T, Heinig JH. Glucocorticoid therapy in acute severe asthma – a critical review. *Eur Respir J* 1991; 4: 881-9.

135 Griffin D, Fairman N, Courson MD, Rawsthormne L, Grossman JE. Acute myopathy during treatment of status asthmaticus with corticosteroids and steroid muscle relaxants. *Chest* 1992; 102: 510-4.

136 Bowler SD, Mitchell CA, Armstrong JG. Corticosteroids in acute severe asthma: effectiveness of low doses. *Thorax* 1992; 47: 584–7.

137 Harrison BDN, Stokes TC, Hart GJ, Vaughan DA, Ali NJ, Robinson AA. Need for intravenous hydrocortisone in addition to oral prednisolone in patients admitted to hospital with severe asthma without ventilatory failure. *Lancet* 1986; i: 181–4.

138 Cypcar D, Busse WW. Steroid-resistant asthma. *J Allergy Clin Immunol* 1993; 92: 362–72.

139 Carmichael J, Paterson IC, Diaz P, Crompton GK, Kay AB, Grant IWB. Corticosteroid resistance in chronic asthma. *BMJ* 1981; 282: 1419–22.

140 Woolcock AJ. Steroid resistant asthma: what is the clinical definition? *Eur Respir J* 1993; 6: 743–7.

141 Corrigan C, Brown PH, Barnes NC *et al.* Glucocorticoid resistance in chronic asthma. *Am Rev Respir Dis* 1991; 144: 1016–25.

142 Lane SJ, Lee TH. Glucocorticoid receptor characteristics in monocytes of patients with corticosteroid-resistant bronchial asthma. *Am Rev Respir Dis* 1991; 143: 1020–4.

143 Alvarez J, Surs W, Leung DY, Ikle D, Gelfand EW, Szefler SJ. Steroid-resistant asthma: immunologic and pharmacologic features. *J Allergy Clin Immunol* 1992; 89: 714–21.

144 Poznansky MC, Gordon ACH, Douglas JG, Krajewski AS, Wyllie AH, Grant IWB. Resistance to methylprednisolone in cultures of blood mononuclear cells from glucocorticoid-resistant asthmatic patients. *Clin Sci* 1984; 67: 639–45.

145 Wilkinson JRW, Crea AEG, Clark TJH, Lee TH. Identification and characterization of a monocyte-derived neutrophil-activating factor in corticosteroid-resistant bronchial asthma. *J Clin Invest* 1989; 84: 1930–41.

146 Brown PH, Teelucksingh S, Matusiewicz SP, Greening AP, Crompton GK, Edwards CRW. Cutaneous vasoconstrictor responses to glucocorticoids in asthma. *Lancet* 1991; 337: 576–80.

147 Lamberts SWJ, Kioper JW, de Jong FH. Familial and iatrogenic cortisol receptor resistance. *J Steroid Biochem Molec Biol* 1992; 43: 385–8.

148 Malchoff DM, Brufsky A, McDermott P *et al.* A mutation of the glucocorticoid receptor in primary cortisol resistance. *J Clin Invest* 1993; 91: 1918–25.

149 Chung KF, Podgorski MR, Goulding NJ *et al.* Circulating autoantibodies to recombinant lipocortin-1 in asthma. *Respir Med* 1991; 95: 121–4.

150 Wilkinson JR, Podgorski MR, Godolphin JL, Goulding NJ, Lee TH. Bronchial asthma is not associated with auto-antibodies to lipocortin-1. *Clin Exp Allergy* 1990; 20: 189–92.

151 Hirata F, del Carmine R, Nelson CA *et al.* Presence of autoantibody for phospholipase inhibitory protein, lipomodulin, in patients with rheumatic diseases. *Proc Natl Acad Sci USA* 1981; 78: 3190–4.

152 Goulding NJ, Podgorski MR, Hall ND *et al.* Autoantibodies to recombinant lipocortin-1 in rheumatoid arthritis and systemic lupus erythematosus. *Ann Rheum Dis* 1989; 48: 843–50.

153 Adcock IM, Brown CR, Virdee H *et al.* DNA binding of glucocorticoid receptor from peripheral blood monocytes of steroid sensitive and resistant patients. *Am Rev Respir Dis* 1993; 147: A244.

154 Rosewicz S, McDonald AR, Maddux BA, Godfine ID, Miesfeld RL, Logsden CD. Mechanism of glucocorticoid receptor down-regulation by glucocorticoids. *J Biol Chem* 1988; 263: 2581–4.

155 Okret S, Dong Y, Brönnegård M, Gustafsson JÅ. Regulation of glucocorticoid receptor expression. *Biochimie* 1991; 73: 51–9.

156 Schüle R, Evans RM. Cross-coupling of signal transduction pathways: zinc finger meets leucine zipper. *Trends Genet* 1991; 7: 377–81.

157 Peters MJ, Adcock IM, Brown CR, Barnes PJ. β-Agonist inhibition of steroid-receptor DNA binding activity in human lung. *Am Rev Respir Dis* 1993; 147: A772.

158 Toogood JH, Frankism CW. A study of the antiasthma action of inhaled budesonide. *J Allergy Clin Immunol* 1990; 85: 872–80.

159 Brattsand R, Axelsson B. New inhaled glucocorticosteroids. In: Barnes PJ (ed.) *New Drugs for Asthma*, vol 2. London: IBC Technical Services Ltd, 1992: 192–207.

160 Barnes PJ. New drugs for asthma. *Eur Respir J* 1992; 5: 1126–36.

161 Miller-Larsson A, Lundin P, Brattsand R. Affinity for airway tissue of topical corticosteroid budesonide, but not hydrocortisone – study in a rat tracheal model *in situ. Eur Respir J* 1992; 5 (suppl 15): 364S.

162 Ryrfeldt Å, Persson G, Nilsson E. Pulmonary deposition of the potent glucocorticoid budesonide evaluated in an isolated perfused rat lung model. *Biochem Pharmacol* 1989; 38: 17–22.

KEY POINTS

1 Corticosteroids are by far the most effective anti-asthma therapy currently available.

2 Inhaled steroids are very effective in controlling asthma symptoms and in reducing asthma exacerbations.

3 Irrespective of the inhaled steroid, there are minimal systemic effects, even using the most sensitive indicators, at doses of $\leqslant 400$ µg in children or $\leqslant 800$ µg in adults.

4 Preliminary evidence suggests that inhaled steroids may prevent irreversible airway changes and may reduce asthma mortality.

16

ANTI-ALLERGIC DRUGS

André Cartier

Drugs with so-called anti-allergic properties were first developed to control the allergic reaction in asthma but these same drugs are often useful in the management of non-allergic individuals as the inflammatory process seen in the allergic reaction is common to both intrinsic and extrinsic asthma. The aim of this chapter is to describe both old and new so-called anti-allergic agents that are currently used in asthma.

Although corticosteroids have several anti-allergic properties, the term "anti-allergic agents" is reserved here for drugs with anti-inflammatory activity such as cromoglycate and nedocromil or for specific antagonists to mediators of inflammation such as antihistamines, including ketotifen (see also Chapter 18).

SODIUM CROMOGLYCATE

First synthesized in 1967, sodium cromoglycate, a derivative of chromone-2-carboxylic acid, was shown to be of value in 1976 by Howell and Altounyan.[1] Since then, several studies have shown its efficacy in the treatment of asthmatic subjects and in the prevention of exercise- and allergen-induced asthma.

Despite its prolonged use in the treatment of childhood and adult asthma,[2] the precise mode of action of sodium cromoglycate is not understood. Traditionally believed to prevent mast cell degranulation, sodium cromoglycate has a wide variety of other suppressive actions on inflammatory cells; in addition, there is some evidence that it may block neural reflex bronchoconstriction. Sodium cromoglycate is particularly effective in preventing the asthmatic reactions associated with inhaled allergen and the associated increase in airway responsiveness. This is the basis for its important role as a prophylactic anti-inflammatory drug in asthma. However, its effect on airway responsiveness is limited to atopic subjects currently exposed to relevant allergens, e.g. house-dust mites. Exerting no bronchodilator activity, sodium cromoglycate is used both on a chronic and on an as-needed basis in the management of asthma in children and adults.

Sodium cromoglycate is a very safe drug being virtually free of systemic side-effects. Occasionally, the potentially irritant nature of the relatively large amount of drug powder or of the aerosol may cause transient bronchoconstriction or cough, easily prevented by the prior administration of an inhaled β_2 agonist; it is rarely associated with nausea and headaches.

For the treatment of asthma, sodium cromoglycate is available for inhalation as a powder (20 mg per capsule), as a metered dose inhaler (MDI; 1 or 5 mg per puff, although the latter dosage is not available in all countries) or as a nebulizer solution (10 mg ml^{-1}).

In children, sodium cromoglycate has proved to be highly effective in controlling mild asthma symptoms, improving spirometry and airway responsiveness. It is at least as effective as theophylline in controlling symptoms of asthma but with fewer side-effects. Studies are lacking to show that it has any corticosparing effects in children with severe asthma, or that its combined use with inhaled corticosteroids has any advantage. When given to a child, although symptoms may be controlled within days, its full effect may take several weeks to be achieved, during which symptoms may still not be adequately controlled. It is then suggested to combine the use of sodium cromoglycate with inhaled corticosteroids for about 1 month and then try to taper the inhaled corticosteroids; if asthma is not adequately controlled by sodium cromoglycate alone, it should be stopped and replaced by inhaled corticosteroids. The usual dosage is either 20 mg (as a powder) or 2 mg (as an MDI) four times per day but this should be tapered to the lowest effective dosage once symptoms are under control; some authors recommend higher dosages of the MDI formulation, i.e. 10 mg three times daily. It should be given for at least 4 weeks before it is decided that it is clinically ineffective. Sodium cromoglycate is probably the best available first-line prophylactic anti-asthma drug in paediatric medicine.[3–5]

In adults, although studies have shown that sodium cromoglycate does improve control of symptoms in mild to moderate asthmatics,[6,7] it is generally replaced by inhaled corticosteroids, which are more effective. Sodium cromoglycate has no place in the treatment of acute asthma in either children or adults.

Used on an as-needed basis, sodium cromoglycate is very effective in preventing the bronchoconstriction induced by exercise or cold air; effective within only a few minutes, it does afford an effective protection for up to 6 hours[8] in the majority of subjects. This protective effect is dose related.[9] In some subjects, this blocking action is potentiated by inhaled β_2 agonists.[10] Sodium cromoglycate is also particularly effective in preventing the early and late asthmatic reactions following allergen exposure in sensitized individuals; it also prevents the increase in airway responsiveness seen after the late asthmatic reaction.[11] To be effective, it needs to be given just before the allergen exposure and should be repeated every 2 or 3 hours until end of exposure; if symptoms occur earlier, an inhaled β_2 agonist should be given to relieve symptoms and sodium cromoglycate should be repeated at a more frequent interval.

NEDOCROMIL SODIUM

Nedocromil is a pyrano-quinoline dicarboxylic acid derivative that shares similar pharmacological properties with sodium cromoglycate, although *in vitro* experiments and some clinical studies have shown a broader spectrum of activity. As with sodium cromoglycate, it has no place in the treatment of acute asthma.

Only available for inhalation as an MDI (2 mg per puff), it has also a very safe profile with virtually no systemic adverse effects; however, many patients feel that it has an unusual or bad taste (in up to nearly 30% of patients) that is sometimes associated with nausea. This is in fact, in my experience, a frequent cause of cessation of the drug or of poor compliance. Finally, nedocromil is sometimes associated with throat irritation and/or cough, which may be reduced by the use of a spacer, or with headaches.

Few long-term studies have directly compared nedocromil to sodium cromoglycate although several acute studies have shown that it affords similar or better bronchoprotection against exercise, cold air, irritants such as sodium metabisulphite, or exposure to allergens (preventing the early and late asthmatic reaction as well as the associated increase in airway responsiveness).[12,13] However, compared with sodium cromoglycate, the bronchoprotection against exercise or cold air produced by nedocromil, does not appear to exhibit a dose–response relationship, and its duration of action seems to be shorter;[14] 4 mg of nedocromil seems to be equivalent to 8–10 mg of sodium cromoglycate (MDI).

Long-term studies in adults, both atopic and non-atopic, have shown that nedocromil can improve the control of asthma.[12,13] The optimal dosage is 4 mg (two puffs) four times per day until maximal improvement has been achieved, when it should be tapered slowly in order to keep control of symptoms. Most clinical long-term studies have shown that it improves symptoms in subjects with mild asthma as well as in subjects with moderate to severe asthma already taking inhaled corticosteroids (low and high doses).[15,16] Although controversial, some studies show that it has also some corticosparing effect, allowing reduction of oral or inhaled corticosteroids in severe asthmatics.[17,18] However, the drug is not effective in all subjects and should be stopped after 4–6 weeks if no improvement is shown at that time.

When compared to inhaled corticosteroids given as beclomethasone dipropionate (BDP) 100 µg four times daily, nedocromil 4 mg four times daily allows a similar improvement in symptoms and airway responsiveness, but less improvement in spirometry;[19] this has been confirmed by others. Although nedocromil can be given as a first-line anti-inflammatory treatment in asthma, it is the view of most authors and guidelines that inhaled corticosteroids at low doses are still the first choice. Indeed, when considering that nedocromil affords a similar protection as low-dose inhaled corticosteroids at doses equivalent to one puff twice daily of the concentrated formulations (e.g. BDP 250 µg per puff or budesonide 200 µg per inhalation), but with a lower rate of success, a lesser improvement in forced expiratory volume in 1 s (FEV_1) and more compliance problems (requiring a four times daily regimen and associated with more local side-effects and no reduction in systemic side-effects), it is easy to choose low-dose inhaled corticosteroids as first-line prophylactic treatment of asthma. In long-term studies in adults, nedocromil was shown to be either superior[20] or similar[21] to sodium cromoglycate.

The clinical use of nedocromil in children is less well studied but it appears to improve control of symptoms and the need for rescue β_2 agonists in mild to severe asthmatics.[22]

KETOTIFEN

Ketotifen is a non-bronchodilating oral anti-asthmatic drug that has some clinical efficacy in the management of asthma.[23] Although *in vitro* studies have shown that it exerts some anti-inflammatory activity, no clinical human studies have confirmed these findings. It is mainly considered as an effective antihistamine. Despite its limited efficacy in the treatment of asthma, ketotifen is widely used around the world.

Ketotifen is a safe drug although frequently associated with drowsiness, particularly in the first 1–2 weeks of treatment, and occasionally with weight gain. Clinical studies with ketotifen are often poorly designed, rendering their interpretation difficult and several studies have shown conflicting results. Most studies have been done in children and have shown only marginal improvement in asthma control. The usual dosage is 1 mg twice a day.

Recently, a 12-month placebo-controlled study in infants with atopic dermatitis but not yet asthma[24] has shown that ketotifen effectively prevented the onset of asthma. If these data are confirmed by others, it will open a new avenue in the prevention of asthma and the clinical use of ketotifen.

SUMMARY

Among the anti-allergic drugs now available, sodium cromoglycate and nedocromil are the most useful in the treatment of asthma. While they share similar pharmacological activities, nedocromil has a broader spectrum of efficacy both in adults and children, atopic or not, whereas sodium cromoglycate is particularly useful in children, being considered a first-line prophylactic anti-inflammatory treatment in children. They are particularly effective in the prevention of exercise- or cold air-induced bronchoconstriction and allergen-induced early and late asthmatic reactions. However, for the chronic treatment of asthma, they are less potent than inhaled corticosteroids both in children and adults. Some studies on the new second-generation antihistamines and ketotifen show that these drugs may have a place in the treatment of asthma but further well-controlled and well-designed studies are required to clarify their position in the treatment of asthma.

REFERENCES

1 Howell JBL, Altounyan REC. A double-blind trial of disodium cromoglycate in the treatment of allergic bronchial asthma. Lancet 1976, ii: 539–42.

2 Thomson NC. Asthma. Anti-inflammatory therapies. Br Med Bull 1992; 48: 205–20.

3 Guidelines on the management of asthma. Statement by the British Thoracic Society, the British Paediatric Association, the Research Unit of the Royal College of Physicians of London, the King's Fund Centre, the National Asthma Campaign, the Royal College of General Practitioners, the General Practitioners in Asthma Group, the British Association of Accident and Emergency Medicine, and the British Paediatric Respiratory Group. Thorax 1993; 48: S1–S24.

4 Rachelefsky GS, Warner JO. International consensus on the management of pediatric asthma: a summary statement. Pediatr Pulmonol 1993; 15: 125–7.

5 International consensus report on diagnosis and treatment of asthma. Clin Exp Allergy 1992; 22 (suppl 1): 1–72.

6 Petty TL, Rollins DR, Christopher K, Good JT, Oakley R. Cromolyn sodium is effective in adult chronic asthmatics. Am Rev Respir Dis 1989; 139: 694–701.

7 Eigen H, Reid JJ, Dahl R et al. Evaluation of the addition of cromolyn sodium to bronchodilator maintenance therapy in the long-term management of asthma. J Allergy Clin Immunol 1987; 80: 612–21.

8　Bar-Yishay E, Gur I, Levy M, Volozni D, Godfrey S. Duration of action of sodium cromoglycate on exercise induced asthma: comparison of 2 formulations. Arch Dis Child 1983; 58: 624–7.

9　Tullett WM, Tan KM, Wall RT, Patel KP. Dose–response effect of sodium cromoglycate pressurised aerosol in exercise induced asthma. Thorax 1985; 40: 41–4.

10　Latimer KM, O'Byrne PM, Morris MM, Robert R, Hargreave FE. Bronchoconstriction stimulated by airway cooling. Better protection with combined inhalation of terbutaline sulphate and cromolyn sodium than with either alone. Am Rev Respir Dis 1983; 128: 440–3.

11　Cockcroft DW, Murdock KY. Comparative effects of inhaled salbutamol, sodium cromoglycate, and beclomethasone dipropionate on allergen-induced early asthmatic responses, late asthmatic responses, and increased bronchial responsiveness to histamine. J Allergy Clin Immunol 1987; 79: 734–40.

12　Brogden RN, Sorkin EM. Nedocromil sodium. An updated review of its pharmacological properties and therapeutic efficacy in asthma. Drugs 1993; 45: 693–715.

13　Parish RC, Miller LJ. Nedocromil sodium. DICP Ann Pharmacother 1993; 27: 599–606.

14　Konig P, Hordvik NL, Kreutz C. The preventive effect and duration of action of nedocromil sodium and cromolyn sodium on exercise-induced asthma (EIA) in adults. J Allergy Clin Immunol 1987; 79: 64–8.

15　A double-blind multicenter group comparative study of the efficacy and safety of nedocromil sodium in the management of asthma. North American Tilade Study Group. Chest 1990; 97: 1299–306.

16　Rebuck AS, Kesten S, Boulet LP et al. A 3-month evaluation of the efficacy of nedocromil sodium in asthma: a randomized, double-blind, placebo-controlled trial of nedocromil sodium conducted by a Canadian multicenter study group. J Allergy Clin Immunol 1990; 85: 612–7.

17　Boulet LP, Cartier A, Cockcroft DW et al. Tolerance to reduction of oral steroid dosage in severely asthmatic patients receiving nedocromil sodium. Respir Med 1990; 84: 317–23.

18　Bone MF, Kubik MM, Keaney NP et al. Nedocromil sodium in adults with asthma dependent on inhaled corticosteroids: a double blind, placebo controlled study. Thorax 1989; 44: 654–9.

19　Bel EH, Timmers MC, Hermans J, Dijkman JH, Sterk PJ. The long-term effects of nedocromil sodium and beclomethasone dipropionate on bronchial responsiveness to methacholine in nonatopic asthmatic subjects. Am Rev Respir Dis 1990; 141: 21–8.

20　Lal S, Dorow PD, Venho KK, Chatterjee SS. Nedocromil sodium is more effective than cromolyn sodium for the treatment of chronic reversible obstructive airway disease. Chest 1993; 104: 438–47.

21 Boldy DA, Ayres JG. Nedocromil sodium and sodium cromoglycate in patients aged over 50 years with asthma. *Respir Med* 1993; 87: 517–23.

22 Armenio L, Baldini G, Bardare M *et al.* Double blind, placebo controlled study of nedocromil sodium in asthma. *Arch Dis Child* 1993; 68: 193–7.

23 Grant SM, Goa KL, Fitton A, Sorkin EM. Ketotifen. A review of its pharmacodynamic and pharmacokinetic properties, and therapeutic use in asthma and allergic disorderes. *Drugs* 1990; 40: 412–48.

24 Iikura Y, Naspitz CK, Mikawa H *et al.* Prevention of asthma by ketotifen in infants with atopic dermatitis. *Ann Allergy* 1992; 68: 233–6.

KEY POINTS

1 The precise mode of action of sodium cromoglycate or nedocromil sodium is not understood.

2 Sodium cromoglycate and nedocromil sodium are safe drugs being virtually free of systemic side-effects.

3 Sodium cromoglycate is used particularly in children.

4 Both sodium cromoglycate and nedocromil sodium are effective in the prevention of exercise and allergen-induced asthma.

17

IMMUNOSUPPRESSIVE AGENTS

Paul S. Thomas and Duncan M. Geddes

INTRODUCTION

After the use of corticosteroids, immunosuppressive agents are a logical next step in asthma therapy, since oral corticosteroids are efficacious in controlling the symptoms and disease but have significant side-effects. Furthermore, corticosteroid response itself is variable, being incomplete in some patients and negligible in a minority. It has been difficult to show a clear benefit from adding immunosuppressive agents in a disease that is very variable, and only small numbers of patients require oral therapy. Therefore, only severe cases, poorly controlled by oral corticosteroids, have been studied. Most studies have used patients who are already on large doses of oral corticosteroids and have measured benefit by dose reduction, with the premise that this will reduce the incidence and prevalence of side-effects. A few studies have also kept corticosteroid dose constant and looked for improved control of asthma. There remain, however, the problems of polypharmacy and the introduction of drugs which themselves have well-recognized adverse effects. This brief review will consider the evidence for the efficacy and toxicity of these drugs (see also Chapter 41).

METHOTREXATE

MODE OF ACTION (Fig. 17.1)
Methotrexate is a di-folate reductase inhibitor that decreases intracellular folate, essential for the biosynthesis of thymidylate and purines. This results in decreased DNA and RNA synthesis, affecting replication and function of any active cell, including T lymphocytes. There is also some evidence that basophil histamine release may be inhibited, that interleukin (IL)-1 activity can be reduced and that neutrophil chemotaxis is inhibited. Methotrexate has been used for cancer chemotherapy, but in lower doses it has

FIGURE 17.1: *Schematic view of the points at which immunosuppressive agents can work in the inflammatory asthmatic response. The mechanism of the activity of gold is not clear and therefore not included.*

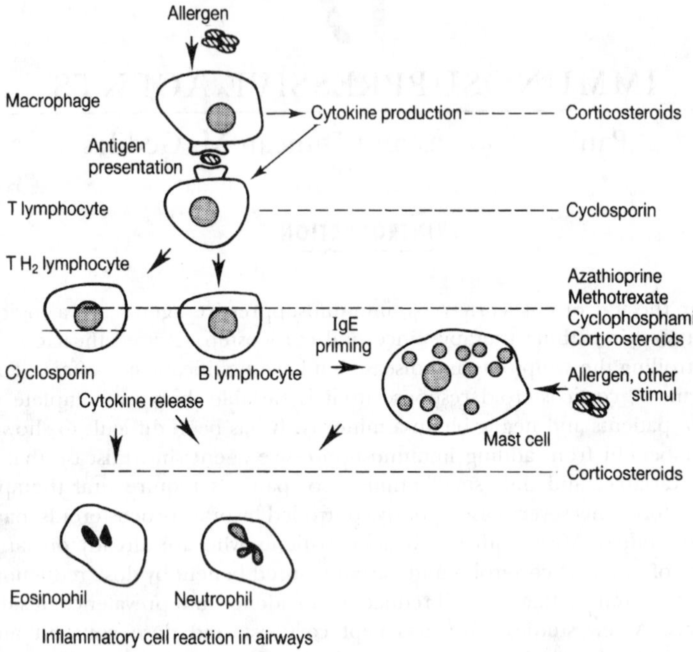

Inflammatory cell reaction in airways

also been used with some success in the treatment of rheumatoid arthritis and psoriasis. As these doses are smaller, there is debate whether the drug is acting as an immunosuppressive or as an anti-inflammatory. The two descriptors may be simply different ends of the same spectrum, related to the dose of drug given, and at the lower dose a predominantly anti-inflammatory effect is seen.

CLINICAL TRIALS

There have been several trials of methotrexate therapy in asthma. Mullarkey *et al.* initially observed ability to reduce corticosteroid dose in a case report and subsequently in an open trial[1] and therefore studied 22 patients in a double-blind cross-over trial.[2] Of the 14 patients who completed the trial, 13 were able to take a lower dose of prednisolone while on methotrexate, but details of the severity of asthma and the outcome of the treatment failures are not given. Furthermore, other anti-inflammatory treatment, such as inhaled corticosteroid was not optimized. A further open study on 31 patients from the same group suggests similar findings and proposes that the intramuscular route is more efficacious and better tolerated.[3] Shiner *et al.*[4] used a parallel, double-blind, 24-week study of 60 patients and were able to show ability to reduce prednisolone in the methotrexate group without loss of asthma control, but not in the placebo group. Similar results were seen in a small study of similar design,[5] but a parallel study of 19 patients taking either intramuscular methotrexate or placebo over 12 weeks was not able to demonstrate an improvement, nor was the airway reactivity altered.[6] A further double-blind cross-over trial lasting 24 weeks was unable to show a reduction in steroid dose or significant change in forced expiratory volume in 1 s (FEV_1), although the maximal mid-expiratory flow rate improved.[7] It must be pointed that many of the placebo-controlled studies show a significant reduction in corticosteroid requirement in the placebo group, which emphasizes that there is a large over-treatment tendency or placebo effect in this disease, and that treatment on enrolment may be suboptimal. Therefore the case reports, and uncontrolled, unblinded studies cannot be used as justification for this treatment.

DOSE

The methotrexate dose used in the studies varies – generally 15–30 mg weekly were used – but there is little evidence of a difference between intramuscular and oral routes.

SIDE-EFFECTS

Side-effects are usually mild and include elevation of liver enzyme values, which require close monitoring along with renal function. Disturbance of haemopoiesis is common with the higher doses given for neoplasia but rare with low doses, but these indices also require observation. Other side-effects include macrocytosis, hypogammaglobulinaemia, stomatitis, renal toxicity, teratogenesis and osteoporosis. Pulmonary reactions occur, including interstitial pneumonitis, which is probably an idiosyncratic alveolar reaction, reversible on cessation of methotrexate and already described in one asthmatic patient.[8] Also an insidious irreversible lower zone fibrosis can occur. The combination of methotrexate and prednisolone has been associated with *Pneumocystis* pneumonia in at least four asthmatic patients, fatal in one of these cases.[6,9,10] Methotrexate has been reported to induce asthma in one case.[11] Methotrexate should be avoided in those who abuse alcohol, and in both males and females who do not use effective contraception, since it is a teratogen. Sulphonamides, non-steroidal anti-inflammatory drugs and diuretics are contraindicated with concurrent methotrexate use, and there is probably competition for clearance with theophylline.[12]

Most of these side-effects occur quite rapidly and are likely to be reversed if methotrexate is stopped. Liver damage and pulmonary fibrosis may, in contrast, be insidious and irreversible. This has led to the recommendation of monthly liver enzyme testing, although significant liver fibrosis can occur in the absence of enzyme dysfunction, and a routine liver biopsy after each sequential 1.5 g in order to minimize the risks.[13,14] While this monitors liver dysfunction, similar guidelines have yet to be developed to ensure early detection of pulmonary fibrosis. Regular lung function testing and radiology would seem prudent, presumably at monthly intervals. Probably transbronchial biopsy to monitor pulmonary fibrosis would be too hazardous. It should be remembered that the clinical effect of methotrexate in rheumatoid arthritis is known to decline after a few years of treatment and no trial of this drug in asthma has addressed this question. The study by Shiner et al.[4] showed that there was no carry-over effect or long-term disease modification by methotrexate, as all benefit had disappeared by 10 weeks after treatment cessation.

PLACE IN THERAPY

While methotrexate offers the possibility of corticosteroid dose reduction, the risk of additional and potentially fatal side-effects mean that there are, as yet, no clear indications for methotrexate in asthma.

CYCLOSPORIN

MODE OF ACTION (see Fig. 17.1)

Cyclosporin A (or cyclosporine) is a cyclic peptide derived from a fungus that appears to have an ability to inhibit the activity of T lymphocytes (and other cells), preventing their activation. It may work by inhibition of the autocrine effects of lymphokines, with some selectivity for helper (CD4) cells.

CLINICAL TRIALS

A case report in the literature suggested benefit from using this agent,[15] and an uncontrolled trial on 12 patients attempted to reduce corticosteroid dosage over 9 months with concomitant administration of cyclosporin; six patients were able to reduce their corticosteroids, six were not.[16] Another study, which was a placebo-controlled cross-over trial,[17] was carried out in 33 oral corticosteroid-dependent patients, which led to improvements in airflow measurements and reduced the number of exacerbations. No systematic attempt was made to reduce the dose of oral corticosteroids, but this is the subject of current research.

DOSE

Alexander et al.[17] used an initial dose of 5 mg kg^{-1} daily and adjusted the dose thereafter to maintain whole-blood trough levels at 100–250 µg l^{-1}. Other studies have used an initial dose of 3 mg kg^{-1} daily.

SIDE-EFFECTS

Side-effects included elevated systolic blood pressure, and decline in renal function as evidenced by glomerular filtration rate and rise in serum urea.

These side-effects and those of hypertrichosis, tremor and headache appeared to be reversible after completion of the study. When used with other immunosuppressive agents, cyclosporin is known to be associated with lymphomas and the long-term safety of this drug in asthma has yet to be evaluated, but concerns regarding long-term use have been expressed.[18]

PLACE IN THERAPY

Use of cyclosporin has had a major impact upon transplantation,[19] and while its place in asthma therapy is likely to be less impressive, the results of trials will be of interest. To use this drug, physicians will have to monitor blood pressure, cyclosporin levels and indices of renal function. The results of trials in progress are awaited; trials on the feasibility of using the inhaled route of administration and upon the newer, related drugs for transplant immunosuppression will be of considerable interest.

GOLD

MODE OF ACTION

The intracellular mechanism of gold activity is not known, but it inhibits neutrophil generation of superoxide and lysosomal enzyme release, antibody-dependent cellular toxicity, IgE-mediated mediator release and reduces eicosanoid formation.

CLINICAL TRIALS

As yet there are only a few reports in the literature of gold therapy in the treatment of asthma. Parenteral gold salts have been used in Japanese studies[20,21] suggesting that corticosteroids could be reduced and that bronchial responsiveness was decreased. Two, small, unblinded American studies using parenteral and oral gold have suggested that there may be a steroid-sparing effect[22,23] and perhaps a reduction in anti-IgE leucocyte histamine release, but changes in bronchial responsiveness were not significant. A further double-blind placebo-controlled parallel study of 32 patients suggested that a mean reduction of about 4 mg of prednisolone could be achieved over 26 weeks in the group taking oral gold associated with a modest increase in FEV_1.[24] Four of the 15 patients taking gold developed eczema or dermatitis; two of these had to be withdrawn. The authors have suggested that oral gold is more easily tolerated than parenteral gold, but it is not clear that the bioavailability and drug levels are comparable.

DOSE

Most studies have used 25–50 mg per week in either divided daily oral doses or a weekly injection.

SIDE-EFFECTS

Proteinuria, skin disorders and gastrointestinal disturbances are common and blood dyscrasias, including aplastic anaemia, neurotoxic effects, hepatitis, pulmonary infiltrates and fibrosis can occur.

PLACE IN THERAPY

The literature suggests that the drug holds some promise in the treatment of severe asthma, but that more trials are needed and that the incidence of side-effects requiring treatment cessation is high. Clinical studies show that of those taking gold for rheumatoid arthritis, over 50% had stopped by 3–6 years due to toxicity or treatment failure.

AZATHIOPRINE

MODE OF ACTION (see Fig. 17.1)

Glutathione cleaves azathioprine into mercaptopurine, which is incorporated into, and interferes with, the synthesis of RNA and DNA. It is considered to be an immunosuppressive drug.

CLINICAL TRIALS

Two short-term studies have been reported.[25] One showed a small decrease in SG_{aw}, but 1 of 10 patients was withdrawn due to breathlessness. The other showed no difference between placebo and azathioprine and 3 of 13 patients had to be withdrawn due to an exacerbation of their asthma while on the drug. Unfortunately these studies were small, brief and with limited power, so a clinically useful steroid-sparing effect could have been missed. An appropriate dose cannot be suggested from the data available on asthmatic subjects.

SIDE-EFFECTS

Side-effects include leucocytopenia and thrombocytopenia, gastrointestinal disturbances, joint pains, rashes, fever, liver damage and pancreatitis. The dose should be reduced with concurrent allopurinol administration.

PLACE IN THERAPY

There is little in the current literature to substantiate its use in the treatment of asthma, but the drug has not been adequately assessed and no firm conclusions can be drawn. This is disappointing in view of the drug's relative lack of toxicity and established role as a steroid-sparing agent in other disorders.

OTHER AGENTS

TROLEANDOMYCIN

Troleandomycin has been studied by a number of investigators.[26–30] While it showed promise for steroid reduction in small, often uncontrolled trials, this has not been borne out in larger, long-term studies.[31] It also appears to increase the risk of long-term steroid-like side-effects[28,32] and its action may be by simply reducing the clearance of corticosteroids.[26,31] Some clinical benefit has also been noted in small studies on colchicine[33] and dapsone.[34]

INTRAVENOUS IMMUNOGLOBULIN

Intravenous immunoglobulin has also been considered for severe asthmatic patients (in the absence of immunodeficiency), on the basis of it having an immunomodulatory effect in diseases such as juvenile rheumatoid arthritis, Kawasaki disease and myasthenia gravis. Eight children were studied by Mazer *et al.*[35] in an uncontrolled study and showed steroid dose reduction and a fall in skin allergen reactivity and serum IgE. Further trials are awaited.

ROLE OF IMMUNOSUPPRESSIVE DRUGS IN ROUTINE ASTHMA MANAGEMENT

There is now some evidence that administration of methotrexate, cyclosporin and gold can usefully reduce the dose of oral corticosteroids in asthma. Gold and methotrexate can induce lung disease themselves and the combination of methotrexate and corticosteroids would appear to increase the risk of *Pneumocystis* pneumonia. The larger number of trials of methotrexate would currently favour this drug as a corticosteroid-sparing agent, but of the published trials only three have been adequately controlled, and one of these has shown no benefit. It would seem that the trials have generally used too few patients for too short a study period. At least one controlled study has suggested improved asthma control with cyclosporin, but immunosuppressive drugs have in general been assessed as corticosteroid-sparing drugs. Cyclosporin administration calls for regular blood sampling to ensure that non-toxic, therapeutic levels are achieved; therefore regular haematological, hepatic and renal surveillance is required for cyclosporin, and the other drugs mentioned above, to ensure that toxicity does not occur. There is little information on the long-term risk of oncogenesis.

There is no place for use of these drugs in patients who do not require long-term corticosteroids. Immunosuppressive therapy should be limited to those patients who are already on such doses of oral corticosteroids that are inducing important side-effects. These drugs should only be considered when the dose of prednisolone is always greater than 10 mg (0.14 mg kg^{-1}) or more per day and has been at this level for 12 months and there are related side-effects. The aim of treatment would then be to reduce steroid side-effects, without introducing a greater risk of side-effects from the immunosuppressive drug. In this context the uncertain long-term risks need to be borne in mind.

The need for use of high-dose oral corticosteroids should be critically appraised, since some patients who do not respond to this treatment can be managed without oral corticosteroids and some will be found not to have asthma. Treatment needs to be optimized before a label of cortico-steroid resistance is applied to the patient, and the patient referred to an asthma specialist for evaluation, such as outlined by Woolcock.[36]

The marked improvement in asthma control during placebo drug treat-ment (Fig. 17.2) emphasizes the need for optimizing inhaled corticosteroid treatment and for close monitoring with patient education. Currently, these drugs should be given either in the context of an organized clinical trial or at least as an individual, double-blinded, within-subject, placebo-controlled cross-over study (Fig. 17.3). Only by performing such closely monitored studies will unnecessary complications be avoided, and the exact place of these drugs in asthma management become clear. The role of immunosuppressive agents for improvement of asthma control and their topical use in milder forms of asthma remain important areas for future investigation. These drugs offer hope of treating those who are inherently resistant to oral corticosteroids or whose disease has become refractory to a dose of steroids that has acceptable levels of side-effects, and the trials need to continue.

FIGURE 17.2: *Effect of methotrexate upon mean daily dose of prednisolone. There is a significant fall in the treatment group, but the placebo group also shows some response up to 12 weeks. ●, Methotrexate; ○, placebo. *, P < 0.05; **, P < 0.005. (From Ref. 4 with permission.)*

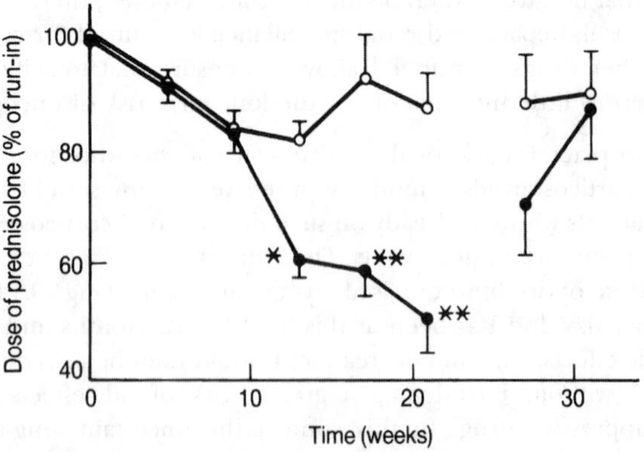

FIGURE 17.3: *Suggested algorithm for assessment and treatment of asthmatic patients who do not respond adequately to corticosteroids (PC_{20}), provocative concentration of histamine or methacholine causing a 20% fall in forced expiratory volume in 1 second; ATS, American Thoracic Society).*

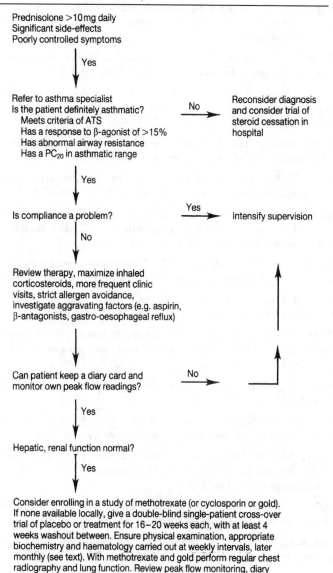

Prednisolone >10 mg daily
Significant side-effects
Poorly controlled symptoms

↓ Yes

Refer to asthma specialist
Is the patient definitely asthmatic?   No →   Reconsider diagnosis
  Meets criteria of ATS   and consider trial of
  Has a response to β-agonist of >15%   steroid cessation in
  Has abnormal airway resistance   hospital
  Has a PC_{20} in asthmatic range

↓ Yes

Is compliance a problem?   Yes →   Intensify supervision

↓ No

Review therapy, maximize inhaled
corticosteroids, more frequent clinic
visits, strict allergen avoidance,
investigate aggravating factors (e.g. aspirin,
β-antagonists, gastro-oesophageal reflux)

↓

Can patient keep a diary card and   No →
monitor own peak flow readings?

↓ Yes

Hepatic, renal function normal?

↓ Yes

Consider enrolling in a study of methotrexate (or cyclosporin or gold).
If none available locally, give a double-blind single-patient cross-over
trial of placebo or treatment for 16–20 weeks each, with at least 4
weeks washout between. Ensure physical examination, appropriate
biochemistry and haematology carried out at weekly intervals, later
monthly (see text). With methotrexate and gold perform regular chest
radiography and lung function. Review peak flow monitoring, diary
card and spirometry at end of trial. Always consider stopping the drug.

REFERENCES

1. Mullarkey MF, Webb DR, Pardee NE. Methotrexate in the treatment of steroid dependent asthma. *Ann Allergy* 1986; 56: 347–50.

2. Mullarkey MF, Blumenstein BA, Andrade WP, Bailey GA, Olason I, Wetzel CE. Methotrexate in the treatment of corticosteroid dependent asthma. *N Engl J Med* 1988; 318: 603–7.

3. Mullarkey MF, Lammert JK, Blumenstein BA. Long-term methotrexate in corticosteroid dependent asthma. *Ann Intern Med* 1990; 112: 577–81.

4. Shiner RJ, Nunn AJ, Chung KF, Geddes DM. Randomised double blind placebo controlled trial of methotrexate in steroid dependent asthma. *Lancet* 1990; ii: 137–40.

5. Dyer PD, Vaughan TR, Weber RW. Methotrexate in the treatment of steroid-dependent asthma. *J Allergy Clin Immunol* 1991; 88: 208–12.

6. Erzurum SC, Leff JA, Cochran JE *et al.* Lack of benefit of methotrexate in severe, steroid-dependent asthma. *Ann Intern Med* 1991; 114: 353–60.

7. Trigg CJ, Davies RJ. Comparison of methotrexate 30 mg per week with placebo in chronic steroid-dependent asthma: a 12-week double blind, cross-over study. *Respir Med* 1993; 87: 211–6.

8. Tsai JJ, Shin JF, Chen CH, Wang SR. Methotrexate pneumonitis in bronchial asthma. *Int Arch Allergy Appl Immunol* 1993; 100: 287–90.

9. Kuitert LM, Harrison AC. *Pneumocystis carinii* pneumonia as a complication of methotrexate treatment of asthma. *Thorax* 1991; 46: 936–7.

10. Vallerand H, Cossart C, Milosevic D, Lavaud F, Leone J. Fatal *Pneumocystis* pneumonia in asthmatic patient treated with methotrexate. *Lancet* 1992; 339: 1551.

11. Jones G, Mierins E, Karsh J. Methotrexate-induced asthma. *Am Rev Respir Dis* 1991; 143: 179–81.

12. Glynn-Barnhart AM, Erzurum SC, Leff JA *et al.* Pharmacokinetics of low-dose methotrexate in adult asthmatics. *Pharmacotherapy* 1992; 12: 383–90.

13. Lewis JH, Schiff E. Methotrexate-induced chronic liver injury: guidelines for detection and prevention. The ACG Committee on FDA-related matters. *Am J Gastroenterol* 1988; 83: 1337–45.

14. Health and Public Policy Committee, American College of Physicians. Methotrexate in rheumatoid arthritis. *Ann Intern Med* 1987; 107: 418–9.

15. Nizankowska E, Dworski R, Szczeklik A. Cyclosporin for a severe case of aspirin-induced asthma. *Eur Respir J* 1991; 4: 380.

16   Szczeklik A, Nizankowska E, Dworski R, Domagala B, Pinis G. Cyclosporin for steroid-dependent asthma. *Allergy* 1991; 46: 312–5.

17   Alexander AG, Barnes NC, Kay AB. Trial of cyclosporin in corticosteroid-dependent chronic severe asthma. *Lancet* 1992; 339: 324–8.

18   Myers BD, Newton L, Dyer P. The case against the indefinite use of cyclosporine. *Transplant Proc* 1991; 23: 41–2.

19   Margreiter R. Impact of cyclosporine on organ transplantation. *Transplant Proc* 1991; 23: 2180–2.

20   Muranaka M, Miyamoto T, Shida T *et al.* Gold salt in the treatment of bronchial asthma – a double blind study. *Ann Allergy* 1978; 40: 132–7.

21   Muranaka M, Nakajima K, Suzuki S. Bronchial responsiveness to acetylcholine in patients with bronchial asthma after long-term treatment with gold salt. *J Allergy Clin Immunol* 1981; 67: 350–6.

22   Klaustermeyer WB, Noritake DT, Kwong FK. Chrysotherapy in the treatment of corticosteroid-dependent asthma. *J Allergy Clin Immunol* 1987; 79: 720–5.

23   Bernstein DI, Bernstein IL, Bodenheimer SS, Pietrusko RG. An open study of Auranofin in the treatment of steroid-dependent asthma. *J Allergy Clin Immunol* 1988; 81: 6–16.

24   Nierop G, Gizjel WP, Bel EH, Zwinderman AH, Dijkman JH. Auranofin in the treatment of steroid dependent asthma: a double blind study. *Thorax* 1992; 47: 349–54.

25   Hodges NG, Brewis RAL, Howell JBL. An evaluation of azathioprine in severe chronic asthma. *Thorax* 1971; 26: 734–9.

26   Ball BD, Hill MR, Brenner M, Sanks R, Szefler SJ. Effect of low-dose troleandomycin on glucocorticoid pharmacokinetics and airway hyperresponsiveness in severely asthmatic children. *Ann Allergy* 1990; 65: 37–45.

27   Menz G, Rothe T, Schmitt M *et al.* Experiences with a combination therapy of methylprednisolone and troleandomycin in severe bronchial asthma requiring high-dose corticoids. *Pneumologie* 1990; 44 (suppl): 238–40.

28   Flotte TR, Loughlin GM. Benefits and complications of troleandomycin (TAO) in young children with steroid-dependent asthma. *Pediatr Pulmonol* 1991; 10: 178–82.

29   Schivaram U, Cash M. Use of troleandomycin as a steroid-sparing agent in both asthma and chronic obstructive pulmonary disease. *J Assoc Academic Minority Physicians* 1991; 2: 131–3.

30   Kamada AK, Hill MR, Ikle DN, Brenner AM, Szefler SJ. Efficacy and safety of low-dose troleandomycin therapy in children with severe, steroid-requiring asthma. *J Allergy Clin Immunol* 1993; 91: 873–82.

31 Nelson HS, Hamilos DL, Corsello PR, Levesque NV, Buchmeier AD, Bucher BL. A double-blind study of troleandomycin and methylprednisolone in asthmatic patients who require daily corticosteroids. Am Rev Respir Dis 1993; 147: 398–404.

32 Harris R, German D. The incidence of corticosteroid side effects in chronic steroid-dependent asthmatics on TAO (troleandomycin) and methylprednisolone. Ann Allergy 1989; 63: 110–1.

33 Schwarz YA, Kivity S, Ilfield DN et al. A clinical and immunologic study of colchicine in asthma. J Allergy Clin Immunol 1990; 85: 578–82.

34 Berlow BA, Liebhaber MI, Dyer Z, Spiegel TM. The effect of dapsone in steroid-dependent asthma. J Allergy Clin Immunol 1991; 87: 710–5.

35 Mazer BD, Giclas PC, Gelfand EW. Immunomodulatory effects of intravenous immunoglobulins in severe steroid-dependent asthma. Clin Immunol Immunopathol 1989; 53: S156–S163.

36 Woolcock AJ. Steroid resistant asthma: what is the clinical definition? Eur Respir J 1993; 6: 743–7.

KEY POINTS

1   Asthma is an inflammatory disease, and should be amenable to immunomodulatory therapy.

2   Methotrexate appears to have a steroid-sparing effect but it has significant side-effects, which can be as severe as the steroids themselves. Its effect may also decline with time.

3   Gold and azathioprine are as yet of unproved value in the treatment of asthma.

4   Cyclosporin appears to enable a reduction in steroid dose, but has marked side-effects.

5   All the immunomodulatory drugs mentioned have to be considered experimental. They should be given after careful review of the patient and treatment has been carried out and in the context of a clinical trial.

6   When prescribing immunomodulatory drugs, the clinician must always ask whether the new therapy is as safe as the current treatment.

18

MEDIATOR ANTAGONISTS AND OTHER NEW AGENTS

Elliot Israel and Jeffrey M. Drazen

This chapter focuses on the utility of agents whose mechanism of action is to inhibit the synthesis or action of specific chemical mediators in the management of asthma. We address the utility of antihistamines, platelet activating factor antagonists and agents active on the 5-lipoxygenase pathway. Even though inhaled diuretics do not act by inhibiting the synthesis or action of an inflammatory mediator, their use in asthma is reviewed in this chapter.

HISTAMINE ANTAGONISTS

Histamine has been implicated as a mediator of asthmatic bronchoconstriction since the demonstration that inhaled histamine produced bronchoconstriction in humans. The antihistamines that became available in the 1950s did not permit adequate evaluation of the therapeutic role of histamine antagonism in the treatment of asthma due to their anticholinergic and sedative side-effects. The development of H_1-receptor antagonists with markedly reduced side-effects has permitted a re-exploration of the effects of histamine antagonism in asthma. However, it is important to bear in mind that these new H_1 antagonists frequently possess anti-allergic properties besides their antihistaminic effects. Various compounds have been shown to inhibit eosinophil migration,[1] histamine release,[2] mast cell degranulation[3,4] and leukotriene release.[5]

INDUCED ASTHMA

Allergen

Histamine can be detected in biological fluids during allergen-induced early asthmatic responses[6] and antihistamines increase the amount of allergen required to produce an early asthmatic response.[7-10] An inconsistent effect has been noted on the allergen-induced late response. In one study, azelastine was shown to diminish the late response[11] while no such effect was seen in a subsequent examination of the effects of this drug.[12] Cetirizine had been shown to produce a statistically significant reduction in the late response without an effect on the early response.[13]

Exercise and Hyperventilation

Treatment with antihistamines has been shown to attenuate the response to exercise and isocapnic hyperventilation.[14–17] In the case of cetirizine, this effect was only seen when the drug was administered by inhalation rather than by the oral route.[18]

CLINICAL ASTHMA

Antihistamines have been shown to have effects on resting asthmatic airway tone as evidenced by an improvement in baseline forced expiratory volume in 1 s (FEV_1).[19–21] While studies with chronic use of antihistamines have not demonstrated a significant change in airway responsiveness[22] they have been able to show a reduction in both symptoms and a need for β agonists.[22–25]

SUMMARY

Histamine appears to play a role in mediating part of the bronchospastic response to allergen, as well as some of the response to exercise and hyperventilation; antihistamines may be used to attenuate a degree of the response to these asthmogenic stimuli. In mild asthmatics, the third-generation H_1-receptor antagonists improve symptoms as well, but it is not clear that they offer any incremental therapeutic value over currently available treatments. Studies have not yet defined whether there is a role for antihistamines in the treatment of more chronic and severe asthma.

PLATELET ACTIVATING FACTOR

Platelet activating factor (PAF), 1-O-alkyl-2-acetyl-sn-glycero-e-phosphocholine, is an inflammatory mediator produced by alveolar macrophages, eosinophils, platelets, mast cells and neutrophils.[26,27] It transduces its effects via specific PAF receptors (Fig. 18.1). A number of agents have been developed with the capacity to inhibit signal transduction by PAF at its receptor. PAF has been implicated in the pathogenesis of asthma because administration of exogenous PAF to humans causes acute bronchoconstriction,[28–30] mucosal oedema,[31] inflammatory cell recruitment,[32] increased mucous production[33] and a possible increase in airway hyperresponsiveness.[28–30] In addition, PAF has been recovered from bronchoalveolar lavage fluid of asthmatics[34] and from the plasma of asthmatic children.[35]

FIGURE 18.1: *Schematic diagram of the various metabolic pathways leading to the availability of chemical mediators derived from membrane phospholipid. The agents that have been used in clinical trials are indicated at their site of proposed action. Details about the trials with each agent are given in the appropriate section of the text.*

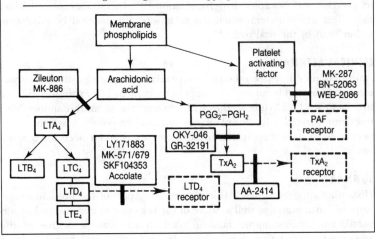

PAF ANTAGONISTS IN INDUCED ASTHMA

Allergen

UK-74,505, a potent and selective PAF antagonist that inhibits PAF-induced bronchoconstriction, failed to inhibit allergen-induced early and late asthmatic responses.[36] However, daily administration of BN 52063, another PAF antagonist, for 3 days, partially attenuated the acute bronchoconstriction induced by the inhalation of allergen.[37] BN 52021, a similar compound, produced some inhibition of the early response to allergen but had no effect on methacholine responsiveness.[38] Another PAF antagonist, WEB-2086, a hetrazepine with proven *in vivo* activity, failed to inhibit the early and late bronchospastic responses to allergen or the hyperresponsiveness to methacholine or histamine that follows antigen exposure.[39,40] MK-287, another antagonist of the *in vivo* effects of PAF, failed to inhibit the response to house-dust mite inhalation.[41]

Exercise and Hyperventilation

PAF antagonists have not shown effectiveness in blocking the asthmatic airway response to exercise or the hyperventilation of cold, dry air. BN 52063 failed to inhibit the acute bronchoconstriction following exercise.[42] SCH-37370, a dual PAF and histamine antagonist, did not appear to inhibit the response to cold, dry air isocapnic hyperventilation to any greater degree than would have been expected due to its antihistaminic properties alone.[43]

SUMMARY

Although exogenously administered PAF can mimic the physiological events that occur in asthma, the currently available PAF antagonists have not proved effective in preventing induced asthmatic bronchoconstriction or airway hyperresponsiveness. Since several molecular species of PAF exist,[44] several receptors have been identified[45] and PAF may act as an intracellular messenger,[46] it may be necessary to develop antagonists with greater avidity for specific receptor subtypes or greater intracellular activity than those currently available.

AGENTS MODIFYING THE METABOLISM OF ARACHIDONIC ACID

Arachidonic acid is cleaved from cell membrane phospholipids as a result of the action of phospholipases. The free arachidonic acid so liberated serves as a substrate for a number of enzyme systems;[47,48] the cyclooxygenase and 5-lipoxygenase systems are those of greatest relevance to the lung. A number of agents have been discovered or developed whose action is to alter either the metabolism of arachidonic acid or the action of the metabolic products formed from arachidonic acid at specific receptors. Some of the agents that have been studied in asthma in humans are detailed in Fig. 18.1 and are considered in detail below.

THROMBOXANE SYNTHESIS INHIBITORS AND RECEPTOR ANTAGONISTS

Recovery of Thromboxane A_2 Metabolites in Asthma

Thromboxane $(Tx)A_2$ is derived from the PGG_2–PGH_2 complex by the action of thromboxane synthase. Increased amounts of thromboxane metabolites, including TxB_2, 2,3 dinor-TxB_2 and 11-dehydro-TxB_2, have been recovered in the urine from patients during acute severe asthma.[49] However there is not agreement about whether allergen challenge results in increased urinary recovery of TxA_2 metabolites.[49,50]

Thromboxane Synthesis Inhibitors and Receptor Antagonists in Induced Asthma

OKY-046, a thromboxane inhibitor, inhibited exercise-induced asthma in 7 out of 11 patients.[51] In contrast GR32191, a structurally distinct thromboxane synthase inhibitor, had no salutary effect on exercise-induced asthma.[52] CGS 13080, another thromboxane synthase inhibitor, had a small but significant effect on allergen-induced early asthmatic responses, but not late asthmatic responses or airway hyperresponsiveness.[53]

Thromboxane Synthesis Inhibitors and Receptor Antagonists in Spontaneous Asthma

GR32191, when given at a dose of 40 mg four times a day failed to exhibit a positive effect on airway physiology, asthma symptoms or asthma medication use in patients with moderate to severe asthma.[54]

Thromboxane Synthesis Inhibitors and Receptor Antagonists on Airway Responsiveness

OKY-046, a thromboxane synthesis inhibitor, decreases airway responsiveness by about a single doubling dilution.[55,56] AA-2414, an antagonist at the TxA_2 receptor, inhibits the response to aerosol methacholine such that the inhaled concentration required to decrease the FEV_1 by 20% is approximately doubled.[57]

Summary

These data indicate a minimal role for thromboxanes in induced or spontaneous asthma. Thromboxanes may, in part, mediate the airway hyperresponsiveness of asthma, but this has yet to be clearly established.

FISH OILS

Fish oils contain eicosapentaenoic acid (EPA) and docosahexaenoic acid (DCHA). EPA can substitute for arachidonic acid as a substrate for the lipoxygenase and cyclooxygenase pathways, diminishes the capacity of neutrophils to respond to chemotactic stimuli and to adhere to endothelial cells, and some of the products derived from the enzymatic processing of EPA and DCHA by lipoxygenase and cyclooxygenase are diminished in biopotency compared with the homologous products derived from arachidonic acid. This spectrum of effects has led to trials in which fish oils, rich in EPA and DCHA, were used in the treatment of asthma and allergic rhinitis.

Treatment with fish oil of patients showing allergen-induced asthmatic responses attenuated the allergen-induced late response, but did not alter their overall asthma severity.[58] The lack of effect of fish oils in chronic stable asthma has been confirmed by another group in a 10-week crossover study,[59] while Dry and Vincent[60] showed a salutary effect on airflow obstruction in a group of 12 asthmatic subjects treated using a double-blind protocol with fish oil for 1 year.

A placebo-controlled parallel trial in which 25 subjects with pollen sensitivity were treated for 6 months with fish oil failed to show a salutary effect on asthma severity or hay fever symptoms over the 6 months encompassing the pollen seaon.[61] Taken together these data suggest that fish oil treatment has little to offer in the treatment of asthma or allergic rhinitis.

LEUKOTRIENE SYNTHESIS INHIBITORS AND RECEPTOR ANTAGONISTS

Trials with a number of different agents active on the 5-lipoxygenase pathway have appeared in the literature (Table 18.1). LY171883, MK571

TABLE 18.1: *Antagonists at the LTD_4 receptor used in clinical asthma trials*

Agent	Route of administration[a]			Approximate fold shift in LTD_4 response (systemic dose)	Reference
	Oral	i.v.	Aerosol		
LY171883	Yes	No	No	8	62
MK571(691)	Yes	Yes	No	40	63
SKF104353	No	No	Yes	?	
Accolate (ICI204219)	Yes	No	Yes	120	64

[a] Route of administration used in published clinical trial; does not indicate pharmaceutical availability.

(MK691), SKF104353 and accolate (ICI204219) are inhibitors of the action of leukotriene (LT)D_4 and LTE_4 at their receptor, and have been used in multiple clinical trials.[65–81] In addition, results of clinical trials with zileuton (A64077), an inhibitor of the 5-lipoxygenase enzyme, and MK886, an inhibitor of the 5-lipoxygenase activating protein (FLAP), have also been published.[82–85]

Studies in Induced Asthma

There have been three general types of trials in induced asthma; trials with cold air- or exercise-induced asthma, studies in allergen-induced asthma and studies in aspirin-induced asthma.

Exercise-induced asthma Over six separate trials have been conducted with various agents active on the 5-lipoxygenase pathway in exercise- or cold air-induced asthma.[65,69,74,80,83] Each of the compounds studied inhibited the induced asthmatic response. It is important to note that even though the LTD_4 receptor antagonists used in these trials differ in their capacity to inhibit the action of LTD_4 by approximately a factor of 10, their effectiveness in this form of induced asthma was quite similar. The failure of agents with increasing potency as LTD_4 receptor antagonists to have a graded effect on the asthmatic response suggests that there is a component of exercise- and cold air-induced asthma that is not leukotriene mediated. Furthermore, these data suggest that agents which are capable of inhibiting the 5-lipoxygenase pathway by a factor of about 10 are adequate for full inhibition of this response.

Allergen-induced asthma Each of the LTD$_4$ receptor antagonists studied in the allergen-induced asthma model inhibits the early phase of allergen-induced bronchoconstriction; the more potent LTD$_4$ receptor antagonists also inhibit the allergen-induced late response.[70-73,77-79] Clinical trials in the same model with inhibitors of the 5-lipoxygenase enzyme or the FLAP antagonist have had varied results. In one trial, zileuton had a small and statistically insignificant effect on the allergen-induced early response and no effect on the late response.[75] A trial with MK886,[82] a FLAP inhibitor, showed a significant inhibitory effect on the allergen-induced early response. Although the exact reason for the failure of zileuton to inhibit allergen-induced asthma is not known, it may be related to the timing of the dosing of the 5-lipoxygenase inhibitor and the allergen inhalation. When one examines the effects of the various LTD$_4$ receptor antagonists in allergen-induced asthma, there appears to be a direct relationship between the potency of the receptor antagonists and their capacity to inhibit the allergen response. The more potent the receptor antagonist, the greater the inhibition.

Aspirin-induced asthma This syndrome is covered in detail in Chapter 32. It is important to note that the bronchospastic, as well as the systemic, reactions to aspirin are probably mediated by products of the 5-lipoxygenase pathway. Although trials of the chronic treatment of individuals with aspirin sensitivity have not been completed, it seems likely that agents active on the 5-lipoxygenase pathway will become the treatment of choice for this condition.

Inhibition of Asthmatic Bronchoconstriction

If patients with mild to moderate asthma are not given bronchodilator medications they develop spontaneous reversible bronchoconstriction over a course of 6–12 hours. This so-called "asthmatic bronchoconstriction" can be reversed by agents active on the 5-lipoxygenase pathway. Oral administration of accolate (ICI204219) or intravenous administration of MK-571/679 results in an 8–20% improvement in FEV$_1$.[71,73,76] β-Agonist aerosols in the same patients increase the FEV$_1$ by 20–30%, an effect approximately twice as great as that resulting from the LTD$_4$ receptor antagonist. Importantly, the effects of the β-adrenergic agonist are *additive* with the effects of the LTD$_4$ receptor antagonists, suggesting that distinct contractile mechanisms are involved in each response. Administration of zileuton, an inhibitor of 5-lipoxygenase, to subjects with asthmatic bronchoconstriction[85] results in a similar degree of bronchodilation, i.e. a 10–15% increase in FEV$_1$. These data indicate that a significant component of "asthmatic bronchoconstriction" is directly due to the action of leukotrienes at their receptors and that the stimuli which result in leukotriene synthesis are continuously activated. Importantly, similar studies done in normal subjects or in very mild asthmatic patients have not shown reversal of airway tone; thus the effect of agents active on the 5-lipoxygenase pathway appears to be a unique aspect of moderate asthma.

Studies in Chronic Stable Asthma

Two trials with agents active on the 5-lipoxygenase pathway in chronic stable asthma have been published. In the first, LY171883, an antagonist at the LTD_4 receptor capable of shifting the LTD_4 dose–response curve about 5–8 fold in normal subjects,[62] was given to patients with mild asthma in a 6-week parallel placebo-controlled trial.[66] In this trial the patients receiving the LTD_4 receptor antagonist had a significant increase in FEV_1, approximately 250 ml, over the 6 weeks of the trial. There was also a decrease in asthma symptoms as well as a decrease in medication use in those asthma patients who were using their inhalers more frequently.

In a recently completed trial,[85] the effects of zileuton at two doses were compared with placebo in a double-blind parallel trial of 4 weeks duration. Zileuton's efficacy was demonstrated by a 30% decrease in urinary LTE_4 excretion. In this trial patients receiving high-dose zileuton had a significant increase in their FEV_1 compared with patients taking placebo, while patients receiving the lower dose of zileuton had an effect whose magnitude was between these two groups. In the group receiving high-dose zileuton, there was a decrease in asthma medication use, a decrease in asthma symptoms and an increase in the morning peak flow.

Summary

An increasing body of data suggests that agents active on the 5-lipoxygenase pathway are safe and effective treatment for asthma. Their role in the day-to-day treatment of asthma will probably only be established once they are available for general use.

DIURETICS

Since Bianco and colleagues first reported that inhaled furosemide inhibits the airway narrowing induced by exercise in asthmatic subjects,[86] there have been many studies that have attempted to further define the effect of diuretics in asthma and to investigate their mechanism of action. Aside from the obvious possible effects on the local fluid and electrolyte milieu and resultant alteration of airway liquid, several additional possible mechanisms have been advanced to account for the effects of inhaled diuretics. These include inhibition of mediator release from inflammatory cells,[87,88] stimulation of prostaglandin E_2 production[89] and inhibition of respiratory tract neural responses.[90] While the precise mechanism of the observed effect is unclear, the studies do suggest that the effect is independent of the renal diuretic potency of the drug. In addition, efficacy is dependent on the inhalational route of administration, suggesting that very high local concentrations are required and/or that the target cell is located in the airway epithelium.

DIURETICS IN INDUCED ASTHMA

The effects of diuretics have been studied extensively in laboratory-induced asthma models in humans. While some of these studies have produced contradictory results several patterns have emerged. For the most part, diuretics appear to be effective against "indirect" challenges (those that produce their effects via release of bronchoactive mediators) rather than against those that produce direct smooth muscle contraction. Inhaled diuretics have been shown to blunt the early response to inhaled allergen,[91–93] and the reaction to exercise,[86,94] hyperventilation,[95–98] sodium metabisulphite,[99–101] adenosine monophosphate,[100,102,103] hypertonic saline,[104] lysine aspirin[105] and distilled water.[88,106–108] Diuretics have been shown to be less effective in preventing the airway response to methacholine, histamine or prostaglandin $F_{2\alpha}$.[95,97,99,102]

SUMMARY

Clinical studies of the effects of diuretics in spontaneous asthma are currently underway. However, preliminary data suggest that furosemide is not effective in the treatment of bronchospasm of patients presenting to the emergency room.[109] The studies in induced asthma suggest that the inhaled diuretics may have a prophylactic role in the treatment of asthma similar to that of cromolyn and related compounds. However, in the case of furosemide, such a role may be limited due to the apparent short duration of its effect.[96,103]

REFERENCES

1. Fadel R, Herpin-Richard N, Rihoux JP, Henocq E. Inhibitory effect of cetirizine 2HCl on eosinophil migration *in vivo*. Clin Allergy 1987; 17: 373–9.

2. Naclerio RM, Kagey-Sobotka A, Lichtenstein LM, Freidhoff L, Proud D. Terfenadine, an H_1 antihistamine, inhibits histamine release *in vivo* in the human. Am Rev Respir Dis 1990; 142: 167–71.

3. Chand N, Pillar J, Diamantis W, Perhach JL Jr, Sofia RD. Inhibition of calcium ionophore (A23187)-stimulated histamine release from rat peritoneal mast cells by azelastine: implications for its mode of action. Eur J Pharmacol 1983; 96: 227–33.

4. Fields DA, Pillar J, Diamantis W, Perhach JL Jr, Sofia RD, Chand N. Inhibition by azelastine of nonallergic histamine release from rat peritoneal mast cells. J Allergy Clin Immunol 1984; 73: 400–3.

5. Temple DM, McCluskey M. Loratadine, an antihistamine, blocks antigen- and ionophore-induced leukotriene release from human lung *in vitro*. Prostaglandins 1988; 35: 549–54.

6   Busse WW, Swenson CA. The relationship between plasma histamine concentrations and bronchial obstruction to antigen challenge in allergic rhinitis. *J Allergy Clin Immunol* 1989; 84: 658–66.

7   Phillips MJ, Ollier S, Gould C, Davies RJ. Effect of antihistamines and antiallergic drugs on responses to allergen and histamine provocation tests in asthma. *Thorax* 1984; 39: 345–51.

8   Gong H Jr, Tashkin DP, Dauphinee B, Djahed D, Wu TC. Effects of oral cetirizine, a selective H_1 antagonist, on allergen- and exercise-induced bronchoconstriction in subjects with asthma. *J Allergy Clin Immunol* 1990; 85: 632–41.

9   Chan TB, Shelton DM, Eiser NM. Effect of an oral H_1-receptor antagonist, terfenadine, on antigen-induced asthma. *Br J Dis Chest* 1986; 80: 375–84.

10   Curzen N, Rafferty P, Holgate ST. Effects of a cyclo-oxygenase inhibitor, flurbiprofen, and an H_1 histamine receptor antagonist, terfenadine, alone and in combination on allergen induced immediate bronchoconstriction in man. *Thorax* 1987; 42: 946–52.

11   Rafferty P, Ng WH, Phillips G *et al*. The inhibitory actions of azelastine hydrochloride on the early and late bronchoconstrictor responses to inhaled allergen in atopic asthma. *J Allergy Clin Immunol* 1989; 84: 649–57.

12   Twentyman OP, Ollier S, Holgate ST. The effect of H_1-receptor blockade on the development of early- and late-phase bronchoconstriction and increased bronchial responsiveness in allergen-induced asthma. *J Allergy Clin Immunol* 1993; 91: 1169–78.

13   Wasserfallen JB, Leuenberger P, Pecoud A. Effect of cetirizine, a new H_1 antihistamine, on the early and late allergic reactions in a bronchial provocation test with allergen. *J Allergy Clin Immunol* 1993; 91: 1189–97.

14   Hartley JP, Nogrady SG. Effect of an inhaled antihistamine on exercise-induced asthma. *Thorax* 1980; 35: 675–9.

15   Patel, KR. Terfenadine in exercise induced asthma. *BMJ* 1984; 288: 1496–7.

16   Finnerty JP, Holgate ST. Evidence for the roles of histamine and prostaglandins as mediators in exercise-induced asthma: the inhibitory effect of terfenadine and flurbiprofen alone and in combination. *Eur Respir J* 1990; 3: 540–7.

17   Thompson AB, Huerta G, Robbins RA *et al*. The bronchitis index. A semiquantitative visual scale for the assessment of airways inflammation. *Chest* 1993; 103: 1482–8.

18   Ghosh SK, De Vos C, McIlroy I, Patel KR. Effect of cetirizine on exercise induced asthma. *Thorax* 1991; 46: 242–4.

19   Kemp JP, Meltzer EO, Orgel HA *et al*. A dose–response study of the bronchodilator action of azelastine in asthma. *J Allergy Clin Immunol* 1987; 79: 893–9.

20 Rafferty P, Holgate ST. Terfenadine (Seldane) is a potent and selective histamine H_1 receptor antagonist in asthmatic airways. Am Rev Respir Dis 1987; 135: 181–4.

21 Hopp RJ, Townley RG, Agrawal DK, Bewtra AK. Terfenadine effect on the bronchoconstriction, dermal response, and leukopenia induced by platelet-activating factor. Chest 1991; 100: 994–8.

22 Rafferty P, Jackson L, Smith R, Holgate ST. Terfenadine, a potent histamine H_1-receptor antagonist in the treatment of grass pollen sensitive asthma. Br J Clin Pharmacol 1990; 30: 229–35.

23 Taytard A, Beaumont D, Pujet JC, Sapene M, Lewis PJ. Treatment of bronchial asthma with terfenadine; a randomized controlled trial. Br J Clin Pharmacol 1987; 24: 743–6.

24 Bruttmann G, Pedrali P, Arendt C, Rihoux JP. Protective effect of cetirizine in patients suffering from pollen asthma. Ann Allergy 1990; 64: 224–8.

25 Kemp JP, Bernstein IL, Bierman CW et al. Pemirolast, a new oral nonbronchodilator drug for chronic asthma. Ann Allergy 1992; 68: 488–91.

26 Barnes PJ, Chung KF, Page CP. Platelet-activating factor as a mediator of allergic disease. J Allergy Clin Immunol 1988; 81: 919–34.

27 Page CP. The role of platelet-activating factor in asthma. J Allergy Clin Immunol 1988; 81: 144–52.

28 Cuss FM, Dixon CMS, Barnes PJ. Effects of inhaled platelet activating factor on pulmonary function and bronchial responsiveness in man. Lancet 1986; ii: 189–92.

29 Kaye MG, Smith LJ. Effects of inhaled leukotriene D_4 and platelet-activating factor on airway reactivity in normal subjects. Am Rev Respir Dis 1990; 141: 993–7.

30 Rubin AH, Smith LJ, Patterson R. The bronchoconstrictor properties of platelet-activating factor in humans. Am Rev Respir Dis 1987; 136: 1145–51.

31 Hamasaki Y, Mojarad M, Saga T, Tai HH, Said SI. Platelet-activating factor raises airway and vascular pressures and induces edema in lungs perfused with platelet-free solution. Am Rev Respir Dis 1984; 129: 742–6.

32 Archer CB, Page CP, Morley J, Macdonald DM. Accumulation of inflammatory cells in response to intracutaneous platelet activating factor (Paf-acether) in man. Br J Dermatol 1985; 112: 285–90.

33 Steiger J, Bray MA, Subramanian N. Platelet activating factor (PAF) is a potent stimulator of porcine tracheal fluid secretion in vitro. Eur J Pharmacol 1987; 142: 367–72.

34 Stenton SC, Court EN, Kingston WP et al. Platelet-activating factor in bronchoalveolar lavage fluid from asthmatic subjects. Eur Respir J 1990; 3: 408–13.

35 Hsieh, KH, Ng CK. Increased plasma platelet-activating factor in children with acute asthmatic attacks and decreased in vivo and in vitro production

of platelet-activating factor after immunotherapy. *J Allergy Clin Immunol* 1993; 91: 650–7.

36 Kuitert LM, Hui KP, Uthayarkumar S *et al.* Effect of the platelet-activating factor antagonist UK-74,505 on the early and late response to allergen. *Am Rev Respir Dis* 1993; 147: 82–6.

37 Guinot P, Brambilla C, Duchier J, Braquet P, Bonvoisin B, Cournot A. Effect of BN 52063, a specific PAF-acether antagonist, on bronchial provocation test to allergens in asthmatic patients. A preliminary study. *Prostaglandins* 1987; 34: 723–31.

38 Hsieh KH. Effects of PAF antagonist, BN52021, on the PAF-, methacholine-, and allergen-induced bronchoconstriction in asthmatic children. *Chest* 1991; 99: 877–82.

39 Wilkens H, Wilkens JH, Bosse S *et al.* Effects of an inhaled paf-antagonist (web 2086 bs) on allergen-induced early and late asthmatic responses and increased bronchial responsiveness to methacholine. *Am Rev Respir Dis* 1991; 143 (suppl): A812.

40 Freitag A, Watson RM, Matsos G, Eastwood C, O'Byrne PM. Effect of a platelet activating factor antagonist, WEB-2086, on allergen induced asthmatic responses. *Thorax* 1993; 48: 594–8.

41 Bel EH, Desmet M, Rossing TH, Timmers MC, Dijkman JH, Sterk PJ. The effect of a specific oral PAF-antagonist, MK-287, on antigen-induced early and late asthmatic reactions in man (abstract). *Am Rev Respir Dis* 1991; 143 (suppl): A811.

42 Wilkens JH, Wilkens H, Uffmann J, Bovers J, Fabel H, Frolich JC. Effects of a PAF-antagonist (BN 52063) on bronchoconstriction and platelet activation during exercise induced asthma. *Br J Clin Pharmacol* 1990; 29: 85–91.

43 Dermarkarian RM, Israel E, Rosenberg MA *et al.* The effect of SCH-37370, a dual platelet activating factor (PAF) and histamine antagonist, on the bronchoconstriction induced in asthmatics by cold, dry air isocapnic hyperventilation (ISH) (abstract). *Am Rev Respir Dis* 1991; 143 (suppl): A812.

44 Pinckard RN, Ludwig JC, McManus LM. Platelet activating factors. In: Gallin JI, Goldstein IM, Snyderman R (eds) *Inflammation: Basic Principles and Clinical Correlates.* New York: Raven Press, 1988: 139–67.

45 Stewart AG, Dusting GJ. Characterization of receptors for platelet-activating factor on platelets, polymorphonuclear leukocytes and macrophages. *Br J Pharmacol* 1988; 94: 1225–33.

46 Stewart AG, Phillips WA. Intracellular platelet-activating factor regulates eicosanoid generation in guinea-pig resident peritoneal macrophages. *Br J Pharmacol* 1989; 98: 141–8.

47 Samuelsson B, Dahlen SE, Lindgren JA, Rouzer CA, Serhan CN. Leukotrienes and lipoxins: structures, biosynthesis, and biological effects. *Science* 1987; 237: 1171–6.

48 Piper PJ. Formation and actions of leukotrienes. *Physiol Rev* 1984; 64: 744–61.

49 Taylor IK, Ward PS, O'Shaughnessy KM *et al.* Thromboxane A_2 biosynthesis in acute asthma and after antigen challenge. *Am Rev Respir Dis* 1991; 143: 119–25.

50 Sladek K, Dworski R, Fitzgerald GA *et al.* Allergen-stimulated release of thromboxane A_2 and leukotriene E_4 in humans. Effect of indomethacin. *Am Rev Respir Dis* 1990; 141: 1441–5.

51 Hoshino M, Fukushima Y. Effect of OKY-046 (thromboxane A_2 synthetase inhibitor) on exercise-induced asthma. *J Asthma* 1991; 28: 19–29.

52 Finnerty JP, Twentyman OP, Harris A, Palmer JB, Holgate ST. Effect of GR32191, a potent thromboxane receptor antagonist, on exercise induced bronchoconstriction in asthma. *Thorax* 1991; 46: 190–2.

53 Manning PJ, Stevens WH, Cockcroft DW, O'Byrne PM. The role of thromboxane in allergen-induced asthmatic responses. *Eur Respir J* 1991; 4: 667–72.

54 Coleman RA. GR32191 and the role of thromboxane A_2 in asthma – preclinical and clinical findings. *Agents Actions Suppl* 1991; 34: 211–20.

55 Fujimura M, Sakamoto S, Matsuda T. Attenuating effect of a thromboxane synthetase inhibitor (OKY-046) on bronchial responsiveness to methacholine is specific to bronchial asthma. *Chest* 1990; 98: 656–60.

56 Fujimura M, Nishioka S, Kumabashiri I, Matsuda T. Mifune J. Effects of aerosol administration of a thromboxane synthetase inhibitor (OKY-046) on bronchial responsiveness to acetylcholine in asthmatic subjects. *Chest* 1990; 98: 276–9.

57 Fujimura M, Sakamoto S, Saito M, Miyake Y, Matsuda T. Effect of a thromboxane A_2 receptor antagonist (AA-2414) on bronchial hyperresponsiveness to methacholine in subjects with asthma. *J Allergy Clin Immunol* 1991; 87: 23–7.

58 Arm JP, Horton CE, Spur BW, Mencia-Huerta JM, Lee TH. The effects of dietary supplementation with fish oil lipids on the airways response to inhaled allergen in bronchial asthma. *Am Rev Respir Dis* 1989; 139: 1395–400.

59 Stenius-Aarniala B, Aro A, Hakulinen A, Ahola I, Seppala E, Vapaatalo H. Evening primrose oil and fish oil are ineffective as supplementary treatment of bronchial asthma. *Ann Allergy* 1989; 62: 534–7.

60 Dry J, Vincent D. Effect of a fish oil diet on asthma: results of a 1-year double-blind study. *Int Arch Allergy Appl Immunol* 1991; 95: 156–7.

61 Thien FCK, Menciahuerta JM, Lee TK. Dietary fish oil effects on seasonal hay fever and asthma in pollen-sensitive subjects. *Am Rev Respir Dis* 1993; 147: 1138–43.

62 Phillips GD, Rafferty P, Robinson C, Holgate ST. Dose-related antagonism of leukotriene D_4-induced bronchoconstriction by p.o. administration of LY-171883 in nonasthmatic subjects. *J Pharmacol Exp Ther* 1988; 246: 732–8.

63 Kips JC, Joos GF, Delepeleire I *et al*. MK-571, a potent antagonist of leuko-triene D_4-induced bronchoconstriction in the human. *Am Rev Respir Dis* 1991; 144: 617–21.

64 Smith LJ, Geller S, Ebright L, Glass M, Thyrum PT. Inhibition of leukotri-ene D_4-induced bronchoconstriction in normal subjects by the oral LTD_4 receptor antagonist ICI 204,219. *Am Rev Respir Dis* 1990; 141: 988–92.

65 Israel E, Juniper EF, Callaghan JT *et al*. Effect of a leukotriene antagonist, LY171883, on cold air-induced bronchoconstriction in asthmatics. *Am Rev Respir Dis* 1989; 140: 1348–53.

66 Cloud ML, Enas GC, Kemp J *et al*. A specific LTD_4/LTE_4-receptor antagon-ist improves pulmonary function in patients with mild, chronic asthma. *Am Rev Respir Dis* 1989; 140: 1336–9.

67 Fuller RW, Black PN, Dollery CT. Effect of the oral leukotriene D_4 antagon-ist LY171883 on inhaled and intradermal challenge with antigen and leu-kotriene D_4 in atopic subjects. *J Allergy Clin Immunol* 1989; 83: 939–44.

68 Christie L, Lee TH. The effects of SKF104353 on aspirin induced asthma. *Am Rev Respir Dis* 1991; 144: 957–8.

69 Manning PJ, Watson RM, Margolskee DJ, Williams VC, Schwartz JI, O'Byrne PM. Inhibition of exercise-induced bronchoconstriction by MK-571, a potent leukotriene D_4-receptor antagonist. *N Engl J Med* 1990; 323: 1736–9.

70 Rasmussen, JB, Margolskee DJ, Eriksson LO, Williams VC, Andersson KE. Leukotriene (LT) D_4 is involved in antigen-induced asthma: a study with the LTD_4 receptor antagonist, MK-571. *Ann NY Acad Sci* 1991; 629: 436.

71 Gaddy JN, Margolskee DJ, Bush RK, Williams VC, Busse WW. Bronchodil-ation with a potent and selective leukotriene D_4 (LTD_4) antagonist (MK-571) in patients with asthma. *Am Rev Respir Dis* 1992; 146: 358–63.

72 O'Shaughnessy KM, Taylor IK, O'Connor B, O'Connell F, Thomson H, Dollery CT. Potent Leukotriene-D(4) receptor antagonist ICI-204,219 given by the inhaled route inhibits the early but not the late phase of allergen-induced bronchoconstriction. *Am Rev Respir Dis* 1993; 147: 1431–5.

73 Impens N, Reiss TF, Teahan JA *et al*. Acute bronchodilation with an intra-venously administered leukotriene-D(4) antagonist, MK-679. *Am Rev Respir Dis* 1993; 147: 1442–6.

74 Makker HK, Lau LC, Thomson HW, Binks SM, Holgate ST. The protective effect of inhaled leukotriene-D(4) receptor antagonist ICI-204,219 against exercise-induced asthma. *Am Rev Respir Dis* 1993; 147: 1413–8.

75 Hui KP, Taylor IK, Taylor GW *et al*. Effect of a 5-lipoxygenase inhibitor on leukotriene generation and airway responses after allergen challenge in asthmatic patients. *Thorax* 1991; 46: 184–9.

76 Hui KP, Barnes NC. Lung function improvement in asthma with a cysteinyl-leukotriene receptor antagonist. *Lancet* 1991; 337: 1062–3.

77 Dahlen SE, Dahlen B, Eliasson E *et al.* Inhibition of allergic bronchocon-
striction in asthmatics by the leukotriene-antagonist ICI-204,219. *Adv Prostaglandin Thromboxane Leukotriene Res* 1991; 21A: 461–4.

78 Findlay SR, Barden JM, Easley CB, Glass M. Effect of the oral leukotriene
antagonist, ICI 204,219, on antigen-induced bronchoconstriction in subjects with asthma. *J Allergy Clin Immunol* 1992; 89: 1040–5.

79 Taylor IK, O'Shaughnessy KM, Fuller RW, Dollery CT. Effect of cysteinyl-
leukotriene receptor antagonist ICI 204.219 on allergen-induced bronchoconstriction and airway hyperreactivity in atopic subjects. *Lancet* 1991; 337: 690–4.

80 Finnerty JP, Wood-Baker R, Thomson H, Holgate ST. Role of leukotrienes
in exercise-induced asthma: inhibitory effect of ICI 204219, a potent LTD_4
receptor antagonist. *Am Rev Respir Dis* 1992; 145: 746–9.

81 Smith LJ, Glass M, Minkwitz MC. Inhibition of leukotriene D(4)-induced
bronchoconstriction in subjects with asthma – a concentration–effect study
of ICI-204,219. *Clin Pharmacol Ther* 1993; 54: 430–6.

82 Friedman BS, Bel EH, Buntinx A *et al.* Oral leukotriene inhibitor (MK-
886) blocks allergen-induced airway responses. *Am Rev Respir Dis* 1993; 147: 839–44.

83 Israel E, Dermarkarian R, Rosenberg M *et al.* The effects of a 5-lipoxygen-
ase inhibitor on asthma induced by cold, dry air. *N Engl J Med* 1990; 323: 1740–4.

84 Israel E, Fischer AR, Rosenberg MA *et al.* The pivotal role of 5-lipoxygenase
products in the reaction of aspirin-sensitive asthmatics to aspirin. *Am Rev Respir Dis* (in press).

85 Israel E, Rubin P, Kemp JP *et al.* The effect of inhibition of 5-lipoxygenase
by zileuton in mild to moderate asthma. *Ann Intern Med* 1993; 119: 1059–66.

86 Bianco S, Vaghi A, Robuschi M, Pasargiklian M. Prevention of exercise-
induced bronchoconstriction by inhaled frusemide. *Lancet* 1988; ii: 252–5.

87 Anderson SD, He W, Temple DM. Inhibition by furosemide of inflammatory mediators from lung fragments (letter). *N Engl J Med* 1991; 324: 131.

88 Moscato G, Dellabianca A, Falagiani P, Mistrello G, Rossi G, Rampulla C.
Inhaled furosemide prevents both the bronchoconstriction and the
increase in neutrophil chemotactic activity induced by ultrasonic "fog" of
distilled water in asthmatics. *Am Rev Respir Dis* 1991; 143: 561–6.

89 Miyanoshita A, Terada M, Endou H. Furosemide directly stimulates prosta-
glandin E_2 production in the thick ascending limb of Henle's loop. *J Pharmacol Exp Ther* 1989; 251: 1155–9.

90 Elwood W, Lotvall JO, Barnes PJ, Chung KF. Loop diuretics inhibit cholinergic and noncholinergic nerves in guinea pig airways. *Am Rev Respir Dis* 1991;
143: 1340–4.

91 Bianco S, Pieroni MG, Refini RM, Rottoli L, Sestini P. Protective effect of
inhaled furosemide on allergen-induced early and late asthmatic reactions.
N Engl J Med 1989; 321: 1069–73.

92 Robuschi M, Pieroni M, Refini M *et al.* Prevention of antigen-induced early obstructive reaction by inhaled furosemide in (atopic) subjects with asthma and (actively sensitised) guinea pigs. *J Allergy Clin Immunol* 1990; 85: 10–6.

93 Verdiani P, Di Carlo S, Baronti A, Bianco S. Effect of inhaled frusemide on the early response to antigen and subsequent change in airway reactivity in atopic patients. *Thorax* 1990; 45: 377–81.

94 Pavord ID, Wisniewski A, Tattersfield AE. Inhaled frusemide and exercise induced asthma: evidence of a role for inhibitory prostanoids. *Thorax* 1992; 47: 797–800.

95 Grubbe RE, Hopp R, Dave NK, Brennan B, Bewtra A, Townley R. Effect of inhaled furosemide on the bronchial response to methacholine and cold-air hyperventilation challenges. *J Allergy Clin Immunol* 1990; 85: 881–4.

96 O'Donnell, WJ, Rosenberg M, Niven RW, Drazen JM, Israel E. Acetazolamide and furosemide attenuate asthma induced by hyperventilation of cold, dry air. *Am Rev Respir Dis* 1992; 146: 1518–24.

97 Netzel M, Hopp RJ, Buzzas R, Dowling P, Palmeiro E, Bewtra AK. Effect of inhaled amiloride on the bronchial response to methacholine and cold air hyperventilation challenges. *Chest* 1993; 103: 484–7.

98 Seidenberg J, Dehning J, von der Hardt H. Inhaled frusemide against cold air induced bronchoconstriction in asthmatic children. *Arch Dis Child* 1992; 67: 214–7.

99 Nichol GM, Alton EW, Nix A, Geddes DM, Chung KF, Barnes PJ. Effect of inhaled furosemide on metabisulfite- and methacholine-induced bronchoconstriction and nasal potential difference in asthmatic subjects. *Am Rev Respir Dis* 1990; 142: 576–80.

100 O'Connor BJ, Chung KF, Chen-Worsdell YM, Fuller RW, Barnes PJ. Effect of inhaled furosemide and bumetanide on adenosine 5'-monophosphate- and sodium metabisulfite-induced bronchoconstriction in asthmatic subjects. *Am Rev Respir Dis* 1991; 143: 1329–33.

101 Yeo CT, O'Connor BJ, Chen-Worsdell M, Barnes PJ, Chung KF. Protective effect of loop diuretics, piretanide and frusemide, against sodium metabisulphite-induced bronchoconstriction in asthma. *Eur Respir J* 1992; 5: 1184–8.

102 Polosa R, Lau LC, Holgate ST. Inhibition of adenosine 5'-monophosphate- and methacholine-induced bronchoconstriction in asthma by inhaled frusemide. *Eur Respir J* 1990; 3: 665–72.

103 Polosa R, Rajakulasingam K, Prosperini G, Church MK, Holgate ST. Relative potencies and time course of changes in adenosine 5'-monophosphate airway responsiveness with inhaled furosemide and bumetanide in asthma. *J Allergy Clin Immunol* 1993; 92: 288–97.

104 Rodwell LT, Anderson SD, du Toit JI, Seale JP. The effect of inhaled frusemide on airway sensitivity to inhaled 4.5% sodium chloride aerosol in asthmatic subjects. *Thorax* 1993; 48: 208–13.

105 Vargas FS, Croce M, Teixeira LR, Terra-filho M, Cukier A, Light RW. Effect of inhaled furosemide on the bronchial response to lysine-aspirin inhalation in asthmatic subjects. *Chest* 1992; 102: 408–11.

106 Bianco S, Robuschi M, Vaghi A, Pieroni MG, Sestini P. Protective effect of inhaled piretanide on the bronchial obstructive response to ultrasonically nebulized H_2O. A dose–response study. *Chest* 1993; 104: 185–8.

107 Robuschi M, Gambaro G, Spagnotto S, Vaghi A, Bianco S. Inhaled frusemide is highly effective in preventing ultrasonically nebulised water bronchoconstriction. *Pulmon Pharmacol* 1989; 187–91.

108 Foresi A, Pelucchi A, Mastropasqua B, Cavigioli G, Carlesi RM, Marazzini L. Effect of inhaled furosemide and torasemide on bronchial response to ultrasonically nebulized distilled water in asthmatic subjects. *Am Rev Respir Dis* 1992; 146: 364–9.

109 Dworkin F, Hager D, Shapiro D, Posner L, Luks D. Karpel J. Inhaled furosemide is not effective in acute asthma (abstract). *Am Rev Respir Dis* 1993; 147: A298.

KEY POINTS

Agents active on the 5-lipoxygenase pathway:

1 Aspirin-induced asthma will respond dramatically to this treatment.

2 Expect maximal effects after 3–4 weeks of chronic treatment.

19

BRONCHODILATORS

John W. Jenne

INTRODUCTION

While controversy swirls around them, β_2 agonists are still the core of bronchodilator therapy today, and they are no less appreciated by the patient. While their use has been considerably lessened by concomitant inhaled corticosteroid therapy, they are still necessary for symptomatic treatment. The introduction of new, long-acting agents has brought excitement to this field with respect to their remarkably prolonged anti-spasmolytic activity. Use of anti-muscarinic agents is gradually expanding and there is real hope for developing compounds with more receptor subtype specificity. While the use of theophylline has declined and become more selective, increased knowledge of phosphodiesterase isozyme families is pushing a search for more selective and organ-specific inhibitors, aimed at both spasmolytic and anti-inflammatory actions. There is promise that drugs activating potassium channels may become practical, with both spasmolytic and anti-neural reflex actions. An appreciation for the role of cyclic GMP in muscle relaxation may result in compounds directed towards its synthesis. Indeed, with today's advances in muscle and receptor pharmacology there is as much excitement in their mechanisms as in their clinical application.

β-ADRENERGIC DRUGS

EVOLUTION OF β_2-AGONIST BRONCHODILATORS (Fig. 19.1)

Only the highlights can be presented, but the reader is referred to an engaging account of this history for more detail.[1] *Adrenaline* (epinephrine in the USA) was extracted and shortly thereafter synthesized in the early 1900s. While extremely valuable in acute asthma, it had unwanted pressor and cardiovascular effects. However, when its bronchodilator activity was increased by replacing the terminal methyl group with an isopropyl group

FIGURE 19.1: *β-Adrenergic agonists in use, and their evolution toward more β₂-selective compounds, with alterations to the N-terminal group of isoproterenol (non-selective) and changes in the catechol ring structure producing more prolonged activity. Only fenoterol is not available in the USA. In some cases, the two names shown represent nomenclature in the USA and Europe. Bitolterol is hydrolysed to colterol. (From Jenne JW. Pharmacology in the respiratory patient. In: Hodgkin JE (ed) Pulmonary Rehabilitation: Guidelines to Success. New York: JB Lippincott, 1992: 135–99, with permission.)*

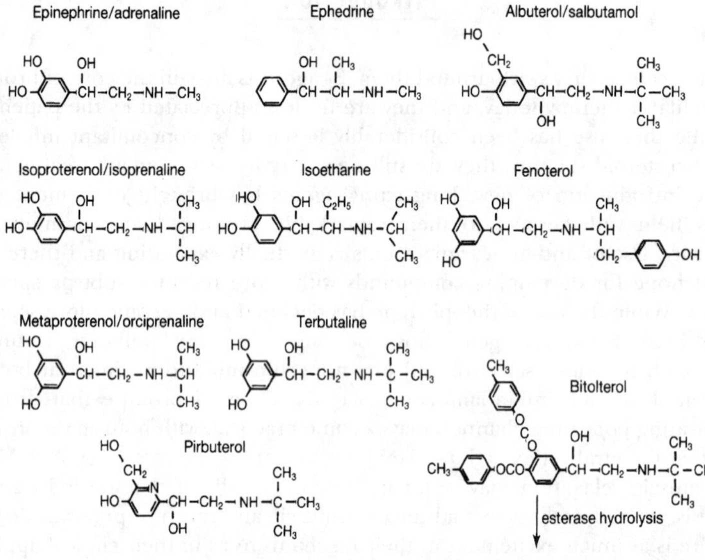

to produce isoprenaline (isoproterenol in the USA), with a loss of pressor effect and, in fact, vasodilatation, the concept of dual α and β adrenergic receptors was established.[2] *Ephedrine* was introduced in the 1930s, and then combined with theophylline and a barbiturate in fixed combinations, the latter to counteract CNS stimulation. This formulation was surprisingly effective, but was strongly and, perhaps, unfairly criticized in the 1970s for its fixed combination as clinicians began to individualize dosing, particularly theophylline.

In 1967, Lands proposed distinct β₁ and β₂ receptor subtypes, the former present in heart, adipose tissue and small intestine, and the latter in bronchi, vasculature and uterus.[3] (It is believed that a third subtype, β₃, causes lipolysis of fat and may exist in myocardium.) Many compounds were synthesized in an attempt to increase the β_2 activity, but with their catechol nucleus they had the disadvantage of rapid inactivation by catechol-*O*-methyltransferase (COMT). One of these was *isoetharine*, popular in the 1960s and 1970s for use by inhalation. A considerable advance was made when the catechol group of isoproterenol was replaced by a 3,5-OH resorcinol group with a resulting prolongation of action. The compound metaproterenol (orciprenaline) achieved wide use despite its weak or non-existent β_2 selectivity.

β_2 Selectivity was achieved with three compounds. *Salbutamol* (albuterol in the USA) was created by adding a *t*-butyl group on the side-chain and a hydroxymethyl group to replace an OH group in the catechol ring to create a saligenin. *Terbutaline* was created by adding the *t*-butyl group to the resorcinol compound and *fenoterol* was created by adding a hydroxyphenyl group to the side-chain of metaproterenol, creating a highly potent β_2 agonist, but one also active on β_1 receptors. A number of other compounds were created but never competed successfully, except perhaps pirbuterol, with an N inserted in the ring. It is equally potent at 200 μg per puff as salbutamol and, incidentally, its canister contains 300 puffs.

A significant theoretical development has been the recognition that β_2 receptors constitute an appreciable proportion of β receptors in the right atrium, and particularly the rate-determining tissues.[4] Thus, β_2-selective compounds in sufficient doses still cause cardioacceleration, something traditionally attributed to β_1 activity.

A new era has begun with the advent of slow-acting β_2 agonists. Two prodrugs have been introduced that hydrolyse slowly to active compounds. *Bitolterol* and its metabolites are hydrolysed to colterol, and *bambuterol* hydrolyses to terbutaline. Tulobuterol has even more active metabolites. Another approach has been to create highly lipophilic compounds (Fig. 19.2). *Salmeterol* has a long lipophilic tail that adheres tightly to regions in the receptor or adjacent to it while its head engages the active site. Even when displaced by soterol, activity resumes after the antagonist is washed free.[5] *Formoterol* is even more potent, but less adherent. Its high lipophilicity retains it in the receptor region. Lessons learned during the evolution of β_2 agonists have been discussed by David Jack in the 1990 Lilly Prize Lecture.[6]

These long-acting compounds hold great promise for their twice-daily convenience and 24-hour effectiveness, thus sparing the asthmatic patient from the feast–famine cycle of the previous agents (see below). Only an asthmatic patient can fully appreciate this feature. Current concerns over these agents centre around the questions of tachyphylaxis (or some related detrimental action) consequent to their "regular use" and whether their sustained relief of bronchospasm will undercut the need for some anti-inflammatory agents.

FIGURE 19.2: *Structure of new long-acting β_2 agonists, formoterol and salmeterol, compared with salbutamol. Note the addition of lipophilic groupings.*

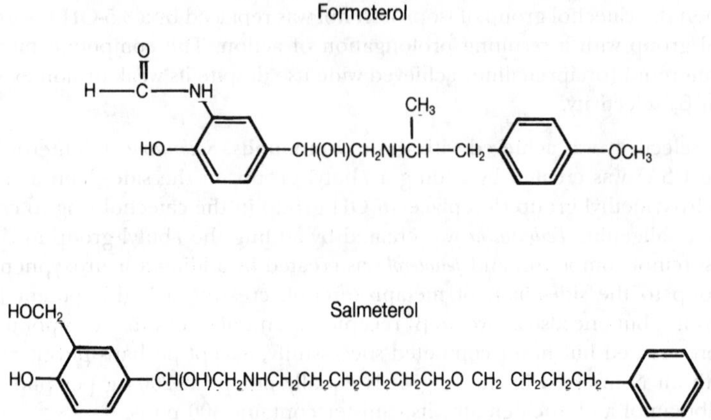

PHYSIOLOGICAL ACTIONS OF β AGONISTS

Large doses of β_2 agonist carry with them some risk of adverse metabolic and cardiac events, despite their beneficial effects on the airways.[7–10] These effects are summarized in Table 19.1.

Hypokalaemia during intensive therapy is a matter of concern as it might favour arrhythmias, especially in patients with heart disease. It should be anticipated, with potassium infusion, in high doses. For example, 10.0 mg salbutamol by nebulization causes a drop in K^+ of 0.62 mEq l^{-1} (0.62 mmoles l^{-1}).[11] Arterial Po_2 can drop transiently, but significantly due to worsened $\dot{V}/\dot{Q}$ relationships. Supplemental O_2 is recommended. Skeletal muscle tremor,[12] while not serious, is distressing, highly variable, proportionate to baseline tremor and shows some tachyphylaxis, while bronchodilation is relatively resistant. Therefore, responses studied in normal subjects may be more marked than those on therapy.

Effect of β Agonists on the β-Receptor Subtypes of the Heart

Administration of a β_2 agonist systemically produces a rise in heart rate by two mechanisms: (1) response to a fall in systemic vascular resistance, and (2) stimulation of β_2 receptors in the sinoatrial (SA) node and right atrium. Much is known now about cardiac β-receptor subtypes and the effects of specific bronchodilators. β_2 Receptors coexist with β_1 in the hearts of most species, but are in the overall minority.[13,14] They constitute a higher proportion in humans than other mammals and are most numerous, proportionately, in the order SA node > right atrium > ventricle.[4]

TABLE 19.1: *Actions of β_2 agonists*

Heart
Tachycardia: SA node, right atrium
Increased cardiac output: peripheral vasodilatation
Inotropism: left ventricle (β_1 and β_2)
ECG: increased QT_c, decreased $Q-S_2I$, T wave
Myocardial necrosis: proportionately β_1, animals; ? humans
Arrhythmias: most asymptomatic, concern when heart disease

Lung
Bronchodilation: large, small airways
Mucociliary: ciliary beat frequency; mucous and serous cells;
   Cl^-, H_2O, epithelium; surfactant secretion
Pulmonary vasodilatation: decreased Po_2 ($\dot{V}/\dot{Q}$)
Anti-inflammatory: mast cells, PMN, decreased capillary
   permeability

Systemic
Hypokalaemia: insulin release, muscle Na^+/K^+-ATPase
Hyperglycaemia: glycogenolysis, gluconeogenesis
Increased free fatty acids: lipolysis ($\beta_2 > \beta_1$,?β_3)
Hypomagnesaemia
Thermogenesis: increased O_2, CO_2, RQ $= k$
Increased pulse pressure: decreased peripheral resistance
Tremor: increased force, fast twitch fibres; decreased force,
   slow twitch fibres
Increased lactate
Increased cAMP: various tissues ($\beta_2 > \beta_1$)
Increased renin
Uterine relaxation
Detrusor relaxation

The effect of either subtype (rate vs. force) depends upon its *location*, and the effects of a drug depend upon its *efficacy* for that subtype. In the right atrium, both subtypes increase rate.[4] Salbutamol, terbutaline and salmeterol are partial agonists while fenoterol, metaproterenol and isoproterenol are full agonists (with greater E_{max}).[15,16] Thus, in guinea-pig right atrium, Brittain showed that isoproterenol and metaproterenol were full agonists for rate, with parallel log-dose–response curves, but salbutamol and trimetoquinol were partial agonists, with flattened curves that did not reach the same response at any concentration.[15] The same relationships apply to the left atrial effects on force.[15]

In the human left ventricle, β_2 receptors are outnumbered by β_1, but both subtypes produce force.[17] Salbutamol and fenoterol have affinity for both β_1 and β_2 subtypes, but while fenoterol has efficacy for both, salbutamol has efficacy for only β_2, and is a partial agonist at that. Fenoterol's intrinsic activity (or E_{max}) far exceeds that of salbutamol on force (130% increase vs. 11%).[18,19] Thus, this explains, on a pharmacological level, the greater effects of fenoterol on both rate and force.

When salbutamol and metaproterenol are given intravenously to dogs in equal doses, metaproterenol greatly exceeds salbutamol in its effect on force production, oxygen uptake and reduction of energy stores of the myocardium.[20] Metaproterenol cannot be recommended for high-intensity nebulized therapy for this reason. In humans, the effects of salbutamol or terbutaline on rate are not affected at lower doses by β_1 blockers,[21] but at higher doses β_1 blockers cause some reduction and they lose some β_2 selectivity.

Anti-inflammatory Effects

The extent to which β_2 agonists, particularly salmeterol and formoterol, exert anti-inflammatory effects in the airways is receiving much attention. In a sufficient dose, salbutamol,[22] salmeterol,[23] and formoterol[24] completely obliterate the allergen-induced late phase response, but the question has been whether this is merely functional antagonism or whether there is some true anti-inflammatory action. Salbutamol by metered dose inhaler (MDI) inhibits the appearance of histamine and neutrophil chemotactic factor in blood,[25] consistent with its ability to inhibit mast cell discharge from sensitized lung fragments at low concentrations.[26] Both formoterol[27] and salmeterol[28] inhibit release of histamine, leukotriene (LT)C_4 and prostaglandin (PG)D_2 at considerably lower concentrations. However, β_2 agonists also inhibit release of heparin from sensitized mast cells, and since heparin has anti-inflammatory actions it has been argued that this could be a detrimental action.[29]

Anti-permeability effects of β_2 agonists in post-capillary venules have been studied for some time in experimental animal preparations[30] and are seen with both salbutamol and salmeterol.[31] In the guinea-pig, formoterol and salbutamol inhibit bradykinin- and histamine-induced airway microvascular leakage.[32] They also inhibit H_2O_2 release from sensitized eosinophils, the latter action blocked but not shared by salmeterol.[33] Formoterol inhibits the appearance of eosinophils and macrophages in the bronchoalveolar lavage fluids of the allergen-induced late response in guinea-pig airways, and decreases bronchial reactivity following challenge.[34] But while β_2 agonists inhibit the respiratory burst of human peripheral neutrophils quite readily,[35] the ability of salmeterol and formoterol to inhibit release of LTB$_4$, PGE$_2$ and interleukin (IL)-1β from human peripheral mononuclear cells in culture occurs only at relatively high concentrations and not through a β_2-mediated process.[36] Clearly, much more needs to be learned about the mechanisms whereby β_2 agonists may exert anti-inflammatory actions. At least it seems likely that they are able to inhibit discharge of mediators from sensitized mast cells and to inhibit an inflammatory increase in microvascular permeability. Their actions will likely supplement but not replace actions of inhaled corticosteroids.

PHARMACODYNAMICS OF INHALED β AGONISTS

Dose-Response in Stable Asthma

In stable asthma, a complex, unknown mix of factors regulating airway tone is added to more permanent structural changes in the airways. Certainly, during acute allergenic challenge, something is known of the mediators discharged, but what is involved during the stable state? Can the net response be considered consistent with functional antagonism?

Barnes and Pride performed full cumulative dose–response curves to salbutamol by MDI in eight stable asthmatic subjects with mild to severe airway obstruction (Fig. 19.3).[37] In four, repeat studies were done with isoproterenol. There was a log-dose relationship with decreasing FEV_1. Those patients with an initial FEV_1 above 1.5 l achieved their plateau of maximum response (E_{max}) at 100–200 μg of salbutamol, while those whose FEV_1 was below 1.5 l required much more, about 1000 μg to reach their E_{max}, and this was at a lower level. The results are consistent with the concept of overall functional antagonism, but the decreased plateau of FEV_1 in the most severe cases also indicates an element of irreversible obstruction, perhaps much of it permanent. Once the peak bronchodilator effect is reached, additional drug only prolongs the response.[38] The study illustrates the need for sometimes considerably increasing the dose and perhaps combining bronchodilators in the severe cases shown, assuming that anti-inflammatory agents are being used appropriately as well.

Dose-Response in Nocturnal Asthma

Recent studies have brought out new information regarding the dysfunction in nocturnal asthma. In a preliminary presentation, dose–response studies with salbutamol by MDI were described in 12 mild to moderate asthmatic subjects with nocturnal bronchospasm.[39] During the day (mean FEV_1 72% predicted) only one puff was usually necessary to normalize pulmonary function. During nocturnal bronchospasm (mean FEV_1 47% predicted), an average of eight puffs was required, although in some patients even 16 puffs did not reach a plateau, with a suggestion moreover that the plateau would be lower when finally reached. This study has implications of strong antagonistic forces and/or β-adrenergic dysfunction in nocturnal asthma. It is reminiscent of studies by Joad et al. demonstrating the limited response to β agonists for night-time symptom control.[40]

A recent study of allergic asthmatic subjects with and without nocturnal asthma and normal subjects may provide some clues.[41] Surprisingly, there were no day–night differences in plasma adrenaline, cyclic AMP or cortisol

FIGURE 19.3: *Cumulative dose–response curves for salbutamol (●) and isoprenaline (○) by MDI in eight stable asthmatic subjects with varying degrees of impaired FEV₁. Dosing was continued until a plateau was reached. The figure illustrates that the principle of functional antagonism applies in actual asthma. (From Ref. 37 with permission.)*

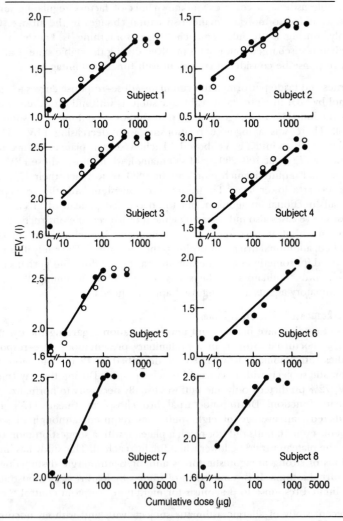

in any group. However, all groups had a doubling of their plasma histamine at night. In those with nocturnal asthma, β-adrenergic receptor density was decreased in peripheral mononuclear cells and neutrophils harvested during nocturnal attacks, and the ability of the latter to generate cyclic AMP *in vitro* was profoundly depressed at night compared with daytime. It is not known, of course, whether this dysfunction applies to asthmatic airways, but if it does it could profoundly affect their ability to resist the elevated plasma or tissue histamine levels to which asthmatic subjects are peculiarly sensitive.

Long-acting β_2 Agonists

The advent of long-acting β_2 agonists administered twice daily are milestones in improved bronchodilator therapy. Corresponding to its slightly greater potency *in vitro*, dose–response curves for formoterol *in vivo* suggest an optimal dose for the mild to moderate asthmatic subject to be 24 μg b.i.d. (Fig. 19.4)[42] and, for salmeterol, 50 μg b.i.d.[43]

The onset of action of formoterol at 24 μg is nearly as rapid as salbutamol. One minute after inhalation, salbutamol (200 μg) had reached 63% of its maximum response, but formoterol was close behind at 47%.[44] A 12-μg dose has a slower onset (Fig. 19.4). At 24 μg formoterol is satisfactory for both rescue and maintenance therapy.

With salmeterol at 50 μg there is some delay. Beach *et al.* studied the difference between salbutamol and salmeterol in recovery rate from a methacholine challenge.[45] Recovery with 200 μg salbutamol was 90% complete at 4.8 min compared with 9.6 min with 50 μg salmeterol. Since the bronchoconstriction from methacholine was wearing off simultaneously, the true rates may be slower. They conclude that "salmeterol is likely to be less effective as rescue medication than salbutamol for rapid relief of symptoms". A study in children showed a 5-min delay in onset of response to 50 μg salmeterol.[46] However, a 100-μg dose may still be quite effective as rescue medication. This needs to be studied in detail.

Compared with salbutamol, both drugs are spectacularly successful in maintaining pulmonary function around the clock. Figure 19.5 illustrates this using 50 μg salmeterol every 12 hours vs. salbutamol 200 μg every 6 hours in mild to moderate asthmatic subjects.[47] Night awakenings lessened compared with salbutamol. While 50 μg b.i.d. did not eliminate nocturnal variation in peak flow, sleep quality and quantity were significantly better with either 50 or 100 μg salmeterol compared with placebo.[48] Against methacholine-induced responsiveness, 50 μg salmeterol also provides 12-hour protection,[49] although protection against methacholine challenge by 50 μg salmeterol b.i.d. led to some tolerance by the fourth week.[50] For 283 patients with moderate to severe disease studied over 12 weeks, salmeterol 100 μg b.i.d. provided superior results to 50 μg b.i.d. in peak flow and general control of the disease, although the incidence of mild side-effects

FIGURE 19.4: *Ratio of post- to pre-treatment FEV₁ following inhalation of placebo (●), salbutamol (▲) and formoterol 12 μg (□) and 24 μg (■) in 16 children with asthma. Values represent means ± 1 SEM. Asterisks denote significant differences from placebo: *, P < 0.05; **, P < 0.01; ***, P < 0.001. Daggers indicate significant differences between formoterol and salbutamol: †, P < 0.01; ‡, P < 0.01. (From Ref. 42 with permission.)*

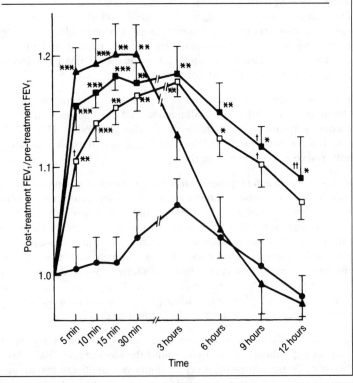

was greater. Improvement was distinctly better on the larger dose and maximized sooner.[51]

Bronchodilation vs. Protection against Constriction

There is pharmacodynamic evidence that these actions are quite different and more complex than meets the eye. The ability of metaproterenol[52] and fenoterol[53] to protect against methacholine or histamine challenge subsides more rapidly than the bronchodilator response in stable asthma

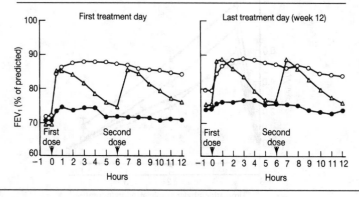

FIGURE 19.5: *Mean FEV₁ in the treatment groups (salbutamol 200 μg every 6 hours and salmeterol 50 μg every 12 hours) as a percentage of the predicted value on the first and last days of treatment. For the second dose, placebo was given to the salmeterol and placebo groups and salbutamol to the salbutamol group. ○, Salmeterol (n = 75 first treatment day; n = 68 last treatment day); △, salbutamol (n = 73 first treatment day; n = 66 last treatment day); ●, placebo (n = 77 first treatment day; n = 63 last treatment day). (From Ref. 47 with permission.)*

(Fig. 19.6), and against exercise metaproterenol has completely lost its effect by 2 hours.[54]

Dose-Response in Acute Asthma

The response to a given dose of inhaled β agonist is unpredictable. When 20 adults were given nebulized fenoterol in successive doses to a total of 3.0 mg, the response varied greatly,[55] but the response to the initial 0.5 mg was predictive of the final response and bore no relationship to the initial FEV_1. However, the longer the duration of the episode, the more sluggish was the response. If less than 24 hours the response was rapid, while those episodes lasting 14 days or more responded very sluggishly. In such cases, corticosteroids are essential to treat the obstructing inflammatory component.

Despite individual variability, there is a correlation between total dose of β_2 agonist administered and the response for the group as a whole. After an initial dose of 0.15 mg kg^{-1} salbutamol by nebulization, Schuh showed that a group of asthmatic children responded more rapidly to 0.15 mg kg^{-1} (every 20 min for 6 doses) than 0.05 mg kg^{-1} per dose.[56] Plasma levels averaged 19.8 ng ml^{-1} (range 0.9–46.3) on the high dose, and 12.4 ng ml^{-1} (range

FIGURE 19.6: *(a) Activity ratio at several times after one (△) and two (▲) puffs of salbutamol, two (□) and four (■) puffs of metaproterenol, and placebo aerosol (●). The "activity ratios" represent the PC_{20} for histamine after drug divided by PC_{20} before drug. (b) The effect on FEV_1 of the same doses. Note that the maximum bronchodilator effect is sustained for at least 2 hours, while the activity ratio is falling. (From Ref. 52 with permission.)*

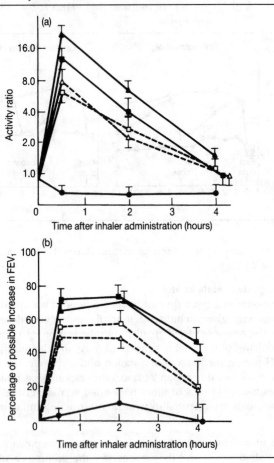

6.6–34) on the low dose. The considerable variability of levels is worth noting, probably reflecting mainly differences in absorption and hence drug delivered to the lung. This will have a bearing on response and side-effects.

The question of dosing frequency is a fascinating problem, first raised by Robertson et al. who showed that after an initial dose of 0.15 mg kg^{-1} by nebulization, patients responded better to dosing every 20 min than every 60 min using the same total dose.[57] After each 60-min dose, there was a peak response followed by a decline, suggesting that under these conditions of severe bronchospasm rapid dissipation of drug from the site resulted in more spasm and less access to the next dose (Fig. 19.7).

APPROACHES TO THE LIFE-THREATENING ATTACK OF ASTHMA

Continuous Nebulization for Poor Responders

Dosing every 20 min is essentially continuous nebulization. Kelly et al. reported success with continuous nebulization of terbutaline (0.4 mg kg^{-1} hour^{-1}) in seven children in whom repeated single applications by nebulization had failed.[58] They later described similar results in 22 children with salbutamol. Doses of salbutamol ranged from 6 to 30 mg hour^{-1} with a mean dose of 0.67 mg kg^{-1} hour^{-1} and a mean duration of 37 hours (range 1–96 hours).[59] Moler described superior results with continuously nebulized terbutaline in 19 children when the same dose of 4 mg hour^{-1} given intermittently had failed.[60] The average total time of nebulization was 15.4 hours (3–37 hours). The six patients with a P_aCO$_2$ over 45 mmHg (6 kPa) would, in the past, have been treated with intravenous isoproterenol.

The above studies were not controlled and some of the success may have simply been due to the time lapse during which corticosteroids were having some effect. However, a recent publication compares continuous nebulization of 0.3 mg kg^{-1} hour^{-1} salbutamol in children to the same total dose given over 20 min every hour through the same apparatus. On the continuous regimen, there was a superior resolution of the asthma score despite greater severity initially (Fig. 19.8).[61]

A question is when to commence such therapy, assuming that the hospital has acquired experience with the set-up. Certainly, after several nebulizations or applications by MDI have failed, one would be justified in commencing continuous nebulization in children and probably adults. Of course, it must be accompanied by continuous monitoring (ECG, oxygen, serum electrolytes determination, potassium administration if nebulization is prolonged and corticosteroids).

It should be emphasized that plasma levels of drug will vary considerably between patients and that toxic and therapeutic levels are higher for salbutamol than terbutaline. Terbutaline becomes quite toxic, with headache, tremor and tachycardia when mean levels reach 6.8 ng ml^{-1}.[62] When

FIGURE 19.7: *Change in FEV_1 from baseline at 20-min intervals in two groups of children with severe asthma. Group 1 (●) received salbutamol 0.15 mg kg^{-1} (▲) initially and at hourly intervals; Group 2 (○) received salbutamol 0.15 mg kg^{-1} (▲) initially and salbutamol 0.05 mg kg^{-1} every 20 min (△) thereafter. Values represent mean changes in FEV_1 from baseline, expressed as the percentage predicted (± 1 SEM). Note that both groups had a similar response to the initial dose of salbutamol. Thereafter, Group 1 continued to improve during the first hour but Group 2 showed deterioration, on the average, prior to the next dose. At 60 min, the mean change in FEV_1 was significantly less in Group 2 than in Group 1 ($P < 0.05$). (From Ref. 57 with permission.)*

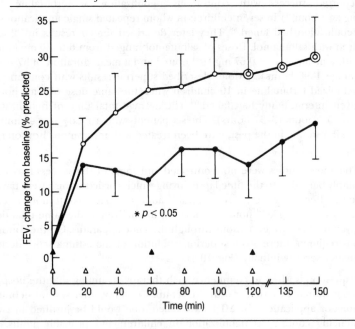

salbutamol (0.4 mg kg^{-1} hour^{-1}) was continuously nebulized to adults for 4 hours to a mean total dose of 96 mg, plasma levels varied from 11.0 to 61.5 ng ml^{-1} (mean 37.7). One of seven patients developed supraventricular tachycardia by 3 hours, which abated after 30 min when nebulization was stopped. Serum K$^+$ dropped an average of 0.8 mEq l^{-1}.[63]

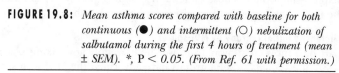

FIGURE 19.8: *Mean asthma scores compared with baseline for both continuous (●) and intermittent (○) nebulization of salbutamol during the first 4 hours of treatment (mean ± SEM). *, P < 0.05. (From Ref. 61 with permission.)*

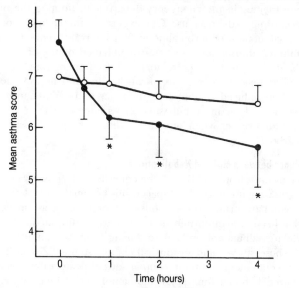

This dose of salbutamol is about four times as large and twice as long as the Medical Letter guidelines for treatment of severe asthma, 2.5 mg every 20 min times six.[64] The latter can be calculated to deliver about 0.1 mg kg^{-1} hour^{-1} for only 2 hours. The dosing schedule of Kelly *et al.*[59] with salbutamol in children delivers a mean of 0.67 mg kg^{-1} hour^{-1} for a mean of 37 hours; Schuh's children dosed at 0.15 mg kg^{-1} per 20 min for 2 hours, some of whom had levels in the 40 ng ml^{-1} range.[56] Apparently children are more robust in their ability to withstand β_2 agonists. It would seem prudent to limit the dose rate of salbutamol in adults to 0.1–0.2 mg kg^{-1} hour^{-1} and to proceed with great care beyond 4 hours.

Subcutaneous Dosing for Non-responders?

Appel *et al.* randomized asthmatic subjects between a regimen of 15 mg metaproterenol every 30 min times three and 0.3 mg adrenaline subcutaneously times three.[65] At 90 min, patients were crossed over to the other regimen. The results clearly showed that a significant fraction (18 of 46) did not respond to the nebulized route but, in most cases, responded to the injected route. The reverse was not true. Those who finally required adrenaline were patients in whom the attack was of longer duration. The principle is important. Those patients responding poorly to nebulization in the first few hours should be given a parenteral (subcutaneous) trial.

High-intensity Initial Therapy by MDI-spacer

As part of a movement away from wet nebulization now taking place in the USA and Canada, several groups have advocated the MDI with spacer as prime therapy in the emergency department, titrating the number of puffs according to the response. One expert committee has advocated four puffs of salbutamol or terbutaline at 30-s intervals followed by one puff each minute until either a response is obtained or the patient develops disturbing side-effects (e.g. tremor).[66] The dose of four puffs can be repeated as needed at intervals of 20–30 min until improvement is sustained, then reduced in dose and frequency to a maintenance schedule. There is a need for more published experience with these regimens, as well as studies of behaviour of serum levels of the β_2 agonist and fluorohydrocarbons.

Equivalence between MDI and Nebulization?

How many puffs from an MDI are the equivalent of a dose by nebulization? With increasing use of the MDI-spacer, this becomes very relevant. Despite several comparisons of dose–response curves in stable asthmatic subjects, there has been little uniformity of opinion, with ratios varying from 1 : 12.5 (i.e. 200 μg salbutamol by MDI to 2.5 mg by nebulization[67]) to 1 : 1 or 1 : 2.[68] These studies and various others are summarized in Table 19.2. In two recent emergency-room comparisons of acute asthma with patients randomized between four puffs salbutamol and 2.5 mg by nebulization every 30 min, rates of improvement were the same.[69,70] Thus, four puffs seems a minimal figure, and it may be more.

Intravenous β_2 Agonists for Life-threatening Asthma

Most experience has been gained in children. Salbutamol or terbutaline may be given intravenously over 10 min, but the peak concentrations reached are only transient unless followed by a maintenance dose. Thus, 250 μg terbutaline given to adults[71] gave peak concentrations of 7.7 ± 1.5 ng ml^{-1} and 5 μg kg^{-1} salbutamol produced a mean peak of about 14 ng ml^{-1}. In children, Dietrich *et al.* used a 10 μg kg^{-1} load, given over 30 min, and repeated 30 min later by a second loading dose, then maintained at 0.5 μg kg^{-1} min^{-1} for an average of 44 hours.[72] There were no elevations of the creatine phosphokinase (CPK)-MB band. An aggressive approach with terbutaline has been outlined by Uden with nomograms for loading, and maintenance of 0.1–0.5 μg kg^{-1} min^{-1}.[73] With salbutamol, a 10 μg kg^{-1} loading dose over 10 min followed by step-wise increases of maintenance dose up to an average of 1.7 μg kg^{-1} min^{-1} for 36 hours was used successfully in children who otherwise would have required mechanical ventilation.[74] One can assume that these maintenance doses provide very high drug levels, since only 0.133 μg kg^{-1} min^{-1} salbutamol infused into adults for 5 hours plateaued at levels that averaged 20 ng ml^{-1}.[75] Based

TABLE 19.2: *Ratios of equivalent dose (MDI/nebulizer) in various studies using dose–response curves*

Study	Ratio MDI : nebulizer	Drug	Spacer	Nebulizer
Cushley *et al.* (1983)	1 : 1	Terbutaline	With and without	Dose leaving face mask
Mestitz *et al.* (1989)	1 : 2	Terbutaline	No	2.0 ml, face mask
Blake *et al.* (1991)	1 : 2.5	Salbutamol	Yes	2.0 ml, mouthpiece PC_{20} endpoint
Madsen *et al.* (1982)	1 : 4	Terbutaline	Yes	2.0 ml, face mask
Weber *et al.* (1979)	1 : 7	Terbutaline	No	1.0 ml, IPPB, Y tube
Harrison *et al.* (1983)	1 : 12.5	Salbutamol	No	2.0 ml

From Jenne JW, Tashkin DP. Beta adrenergic agonists. In: Weiss EB, Stain M (eds) *Bronchial Asthma. Mechanisms and Therapeutics.* Boston: Little, Brown and Co., 1993: 700–48.

on this, a loading dose of 10 μg kg^{-1} over 10 min followed by a maintenance dose of 0.1–0.2 μg kg^{-1} min^{-1} administered by syringe pump should provide high therapeutic levels but heart rate, blood pressure and serum potassium must be monitored closely. One would hesitate to use such a regimen in the older adult but, if faced with any patient who has intractable asthma and is being mechanically ventilated, an intravenous infusion is certainly worth trying.

Dosing in Mechanically Ventilated Patients

The use of aerosolized β_2 agonists in these patients has been reviewed in detail.[76] There is a paucity of published experimental data to recommend a particular approach. It is clear that the percentage of the dose deposited in the lung, even with the use of a holding chamber, is considerably less than in the non-ventilated patient. Fuller *et al.* calculated that 5.6% (mean) of fenoterol was deposited using an MDI and holding chamber, compared with 1.2% by nebulization.[77] Others have found about 2.9%[78] and 2.2% for nebulization.[79] A shocking ineffectiveness of one adaptor for the MDI was recently published showing that 100 puffs of salbutamol administered over 60 min produced no effect on peak airway measurements as recorded by the ventilator, in contrast to even 2.5 mg salbutamol by nebulization.[80] However, using a Monaghan Aerovent holding chamber, Dhand *et al.* found that 10 puffs at 30-s intervals produced significant improvement in pressures and inspiratory resistance as measured by a pulmonary mechanics computer.[81] Fink *et al.* individualized MDI dosing by using up to 40 puffs of salbutamol applied to 85 patients. In those 50 patients responding by ventilator measurements, responses commenced at mean doses of 10 puffs and became maximum at 22 puffs.[82] Gay *et al.* have demonstrated responses in peak pressure and expiratory flow using as little as 1.8 mg of nebulized metaproterenol applied directly to the endotracheal inlet by special adaptor.[83] Bernasconi nebulized 1.2 mg of fenoterol and produced a significant response, but this was gone by 3 hours.[84] There is a great need to evaluate the individual equipment and routines and technique used for delivery.

TOXICITY OF INHALED β_2 AGONISTS

Adverse Effects on the Heart

The current emphasis on high-dose therapy with inhaled β_2 agonists in the emergency-department treatment of acute asthma has prompted careful study of the toxic response to these drugs and, particularly, comparisons of fenoterol and salbutamol. In this situation, it is not known how much drug is reaching the peripheral airways to be absorbed. The intense treatment used in the life-threatening attack, added to the amounts taken by the patient during the preceding 24 hours and the effects of hypoxaemia, produce a highly uncertain situation from the standpoint of toxicity, and the need for careful monitoring.

In cumulative dosing in normal subjects, fenoterol has produced greater effects on heart rate and the QT_c interval than salbutamol, similar in degree to isoproterenol.[85,86] But both "β_1-like" (my term) and β_2 effects are more strongly stimulated. There are also greater effects on the drop in K^+ and the increase in plasma cAMP, both β_2 responses.[87] When fenoterol, salbutamol and formoterol were administered by MDI in doses of 400 μg every 30 min times five, the responses of heart rate, QT_c interval, QS_2I (inotropic effect) and K^+ were all more abrupt and more pronounced for fenoterol[88] than salbutamol (Fig. 19.9).

Studies in stable asthmatic subjects already using these drugs have also been done. When 400 μg of drug was applied at 0, 30, 40 and 45 min, and responses followed to 60 min, peak responses after the 400 μg (low dose) and 1600 μg (high dose) were recorded. The authors concluded that "both

FIGURE 19.9: *The effects of treatment by MDI on heart rate (HR), electromechanical systole (QS_2I), potassium (K^+) and QT_c interval. Drug was administered at 400-µg doses at 0, 30, 60, 90 and 120 min. □, Placebo; ●, fenoterol; ■, salbutamol; ○, formoterol. (From Ref. 88 with permission.)*

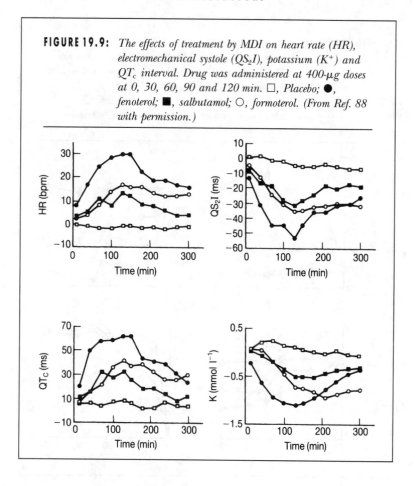

fenoterol and isoproterenol resulted in greater positive inotropic stimulation than did salbutamol, and fenoterol caused the greater fall in potassium levels".

A few studies have also been conducted with nebulized drug in stable asthmatic subjects. Figure 19.10 shows responses to 5.0 mg of salbutamol and fenoterol, each dose repeated at 60 min for those four of eleven subjects able to tolerate it.[90] The response to 0.5 mg ipratropium bromide is also included. Bremner et al.[90] contend that while the maximum bronchodilator effects of salbutamol and fenoterol are similar, the cardiovascular effect of fenoterol is greater as is the effect on K^+. They state, "The observed difference between fenoterol and salbutamol provides a plausible mechanism which may explain the increased risk of death associated with fenoterol in severe asthma". Added to this is the fact that each puff of

FIGURE 19.10: *The effects of treatment (mean ± SEM) with nebulized drugs on heart rate (HR), electromechanical systole (QS₂I), plasma K⁺ and FEV₁ in the four subjects who received two consecutive doses of drug.* ◇, *Ipratropium bromide 0.5 mg;* ■, *fenoterol;* □, *salbutamol, each at 5.0 mg. (From Ref. 90 with permission.)*

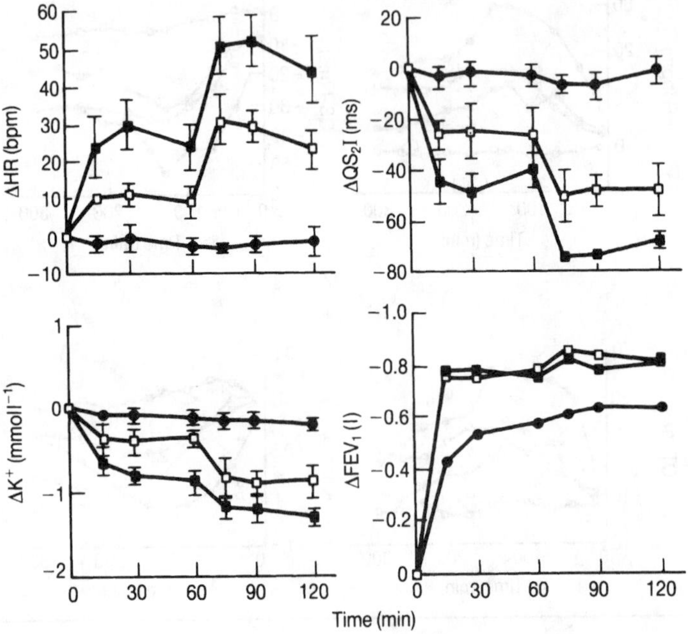

fenoterol had (until recently) twice the dose by weight contained in a puff of salbutamol.

Myocardial Necrosis

Myocardial toxicity during intensive β-agonist therapy has been a concern, especially since Food and Drug Administration (USA) specialists have experimentally produced a characteristic necrosis of the papillary muscle and apical subendocardium, and fatal arrhythmias, during isoproterenol administration to fat rats, dogs and rabbits.[91,92] At much larger doses, this also occurred with intravenous terbutaline, and, ironically, was potentiated by corticosteroids and aminophylline, the very drugs used in treating acute asthma and therefore candidates for asthma mortality. Animals surviving these lesions were subsequently more resistant. While myocardial fractions of the CPK have been strongly elevated during intravenous isoproterenol therapy,[93] lack of elevation during intravenous terbutaline therapy has been reassuring. The cardiac damage is a function of the β_1 component. β_2-Selective agents are highly preferred for intravenous administration.

Toxicity in the Elderly

One is always concerned about toxicity, but I am convinced that more patients suffer because of under-treatment than over-treatment. The various regimens published have been used, for the most part, in children or otherwise healthy adult asthmatic subjects. In the acute attack, patients with known myocardial disease require continuous monitoring and supplemental O_2 as needed to maintain oxygenation when receiving the least dose (e.g. 2.5 mg) that provides relief; older patients without known heart disease nevertheless require heightened surveillance for induced arrhythmias. When 5.0 mg of nebulized salbutamol was administered to elderly patients, two of twenty developed increased runs of atrial fibrillation and two developed increased ventricular ectopy, one with a short burst of ventricular tachycardia, although all were asymptomatic.[94] Case reports of angina or myocardial infarction occurring during nebulization of 5-mg doses of salbutamol are convincing enough to warrant caution in the older age group.[95]

Adverse Effects on the Airways?

Increasing knowledge of the mechanisms of β_2-adrenergic tachyphylaxis and desensitization gained from shorter-term *in vitro* studies with cells and tissues contrasts with lack of knowledge of these processes in patients, who are exposed to much lower concentrations over long periods. What is more, asthmatic subjects may differ from normal subjects. As reviewed in 1982, it appeared that normal subjects on 1600 µg per 24 hours of salbutamol by MDI were capable of developing tachyphylaxis of the bronchodilator response to inhaled salbutamol, which was reversible with intravenous corticosteroids, while the airways of atopic normal and asthmatic subjects seemed to be relatively resistant,[96] although subsensitivity was still produced in systemic responses.[9] Some authors have been able to demonstrate a degree of airway tachyphylaxis in the bronchodilator response of asthmatic subjects with ordinary use of inhaled[97] or oral[98] β_2 agonists, most convincing when examining the area under the curve.[99] Others, using dose–response curves, have not[96] and it has been generally concluded that tachyphylaxis of a "clinically significant" degree does not develop in the airways of the stable asthmatic subject.

New findings are beginning to emerge suggesting that the airways of asthmatic subjects may indeed develop a degree of tolerance or tachyphylaxis to inhaled β_2 agonists. This is manifested as a loss of the airways' protective ability against various challenges, as well as a reduction in their ability to withstand challenge, perhaps due to tolerance induced in endogenous β_2-agonist functions.[100] Evidence is also accumulating that the β_2-mediated relaxation of airway smooth muscle has become impaired in patients dying during an acute attack. The New Zealand and Saskatchewan studies, at first focusing on fenoterol, have prompted a deeper look into the issue of inhaled β_2 agonists.

Upon withdrawal of several weeks' regular inhalation of β_2 agonists, including salmeterol, a small but temporary (24–56 hour) increase in responsiveness to methacholine or histamine challenge occurs[101,102] and even some loss of forced expiratory flow.[103] Perhaps related, there is also greater rate of decline in peak flow or FEV_1 in patients while taking regular as opposed to "as needed" inhaled β_2 agonists over longer periods, up to 48 weeks;[104,105] this is possibly related to induced subsensitivity of mechanisms maintaining airway patency and, what is more feared perhaps, a structural phenomenon. Control of asthma has been said to be worsened[105] and bronchial hyperresponsiveness to methacholine increased,[105] although this had not been observed previously with histamine challenge over 4 weeks.[106]

Others, failing to find increased responsiveness to methacholine, or a decrease in bronchodilator effectiveness, nevertheless have found that patients regularly using β_2 agonists develop impaired protection by their MDI against methacholine challenge[107,108] and even greater impairment against an inflammatory challenge, using AMP[108] or allergen,[107] both consistent with development of some drug tolerance.[100]

These distinctions are subtle, complex and poorly understood. In general, but not always,[105] these studies have been carried out with mild asthmatic subjects who were not on inhaled corticosteroids, or on regular β_2 agonist use before the trial. A study of patients on salmeterol for only 8 weeks, who were also on inhaled corticosteroids, found no differences in methacholine responsiveness and no rebound 60 hours after stopping.[109] If, indeed, inhaled corticosteroids are able to prevent such adverse changes, this becomes another reason for their use in patients on continual β_2-agonist treatment.

Desensitization During Acute Severe Asthma

Asthmatic airways studied after death following fatal asthma show impaired bronchodilator responses to β agonists, but not theophylline, as studied by two groups.[110,111] This intriguing area is beyond the scope and space of this discussion, but suffice it to say that, despite an increase in β_2 receptor density, both groups conclude that the evidence of a marked (up to 17-fold) decrease in relaxant potency suggests a defect distal to the receptor, perhaps in its coupling to adenylyl cyclase. It is known that an allergic challenge impairs β_2-adrenergic responses of peripheral lymphocytes[112] and also that inflammatory events and mediators of diverse kinds affect β_2-adrenergic function.[113] Is it possible that the impaired muscle receptor function found after death arises from the inflammatory events during the fatal attack, perhaps augmented by tachyphylaxis from extensive, but necessary, treatment? Corticosteroids could be critical in minimizing these possibilities.

EPIDEMIOLOGICAL STUDIES ON SAFETY OF β_2 AGONISTS AND THE QUESTIONS THEY RAISE

The questions surrounding the use of β_2 agonists have been summarized.[114] Most clinicians are aware of the temporary increase in asthma deaths in the mid-1960s that was generally attributed to the introduction and withdrawal of a "Forte" strength of isoproterenol (0.4 mg per puff compared with 0.08 mg per puff previously used). Countries not sharing this rise in death rates had no access to the Forte preparation.

Next to receive critical scrutiny was the β_2-selective drug fenoterol. In the New Zealand asthma epidemic of the late 1970s and early 1980s, an excess mortality was found in those patients who had been using fenoterol, in contrast to those using salbutamol[115] with some properties similar to isoproterenol. Since the dose/puff of fenoterol was twice that of salbutamol and, microgram per microgram, it was even more potent systemically, a case was made that fenoterol quantitatively and qualitatively was dangerous to patients. These investigators believe that fenoterol *per se* is at fault. A behaviouristic alternative explanation was that perhaps patients with such an effective agent waited too long before seeking medical help.

Now, interesting and provocative further questions have arisen from a retrospective case-control analysis of 8 years of experience in Saskatchewan, documenting a relationship between fatal and near-fatal episodes of asthma and their regular use of inhaled β_2 agents.[116] While that initial publication especially singled out fenoterol, the criticism became a class indictment when doses of fenoterol and salbutamol were expressed in terms of micrograms of drug used instead of number of puffs or canisters. The odds ratio then became equal. In the original study, 129 patients were matched with 665 control subjects, adjusting for the number of hospitalizations for asthma and other demographic variables. While the thrust of the study was to indict the heavy use of β_2 agonists, the authors recognized the alternative possibility that those using more drug might have inherently more severe disease. Their recommendation in any case was to employ anti-inflammatory agents on a larger scale, in an attempt to decrease the regular use of inhaled β_2 agonists.

Such general condemnation of β_2 agonists has been countered by authorities with years of favourable experience with salbutamol[117] and terbutaline.[118] Criticism has been directed towards the Saskatchewan study, questioning the validity of the control group. The authors have now published their further attempts to answer this criticism, adjusting for severity factors after further examining each hospital admission and after interviewing the physicians caring for the patients for the 2 years prior to the event.[119] Their conclusions remain the same, and are again directed towards β_2 agonists as a class. The risk-ratio is only slightly higher for fenoterol than salbutamol (2.5 vs. 2.0). Despite this prodigious effort, the uncertainty must remain. If one uses death or near death to select the cases, can one ever be sure that the control group is matched when selected retrospectively?

MUSCARINIC ANTAGONISTS

The formulae of muscarinic antagonists in use are shown in Fig. 19.11. Note the presence of a positive charge on the quaternary ammonium compounds that prevents their absorption.

Most studies have shown that, in the recommended doses, muscarinic antagonists are more effective in chronic obstructive pulmonary disease

FIGURE 19.11: *Formulae of five "non-absorbable" anti-cholinergic anti-muscarinic compounds and the parent and absorbable compound, atropine. Ipratropium bromide and glycopyrrolate bromide are available both by MDI and in solution and may be nebulized. (From Gross NJ, Skorodin MS. Anticholinergic agents. In: Jenne JW, Murphy S (eds)* Drug Therapy in Asthma. Research and Clinical Practice. Vol 31 of Lung Biology in Health and Disease Series. *New York: Marcel Dekker, 1987: 615 with permission.)*

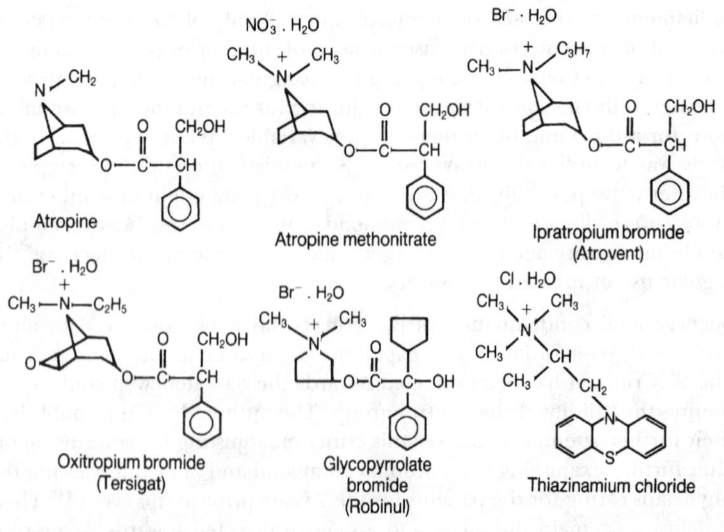

(COPD), i.e. chronic bronchitis, emphysema, than in asthma. Full dose–response curves for fenoterol and ipratropium bromide over a range of 1–16 puffs showed the superiority of ipratropium bromide in the bronchitic patients, while in asthma the action of the β_2 agonist far exceeded that of the anti-muscarinic. Yet both curves rose in parallel, indicating that anti-muscarinics indeed have an action in asthma.[120] Similar conclusions have been reached with nebulized ipratropium bromide and salbutamol, along with a demonstration of the relative ineffectiveness of ipratropium against histamine-induced bronchospasm in either condition.[121] Most recently, these agents have been compared in a large series of asthmatic and bronchitic patients, with the conclusion that, in general, chronic bronchitic patients respond better to 80 μg ipratropium bromide by MDI than to 400 μg salbutamol, whereas the reverse is true for asthmatic patients.[122] A significant proportion of each category responded equally to both, however. Significantly, measurements were taken 60 min after the dose to obtain the full benefit of ipratropium bromide.

In chronic stable asthma, ipratropium bromide on average produces a smaller and more delayed response than salbutamol, whether delivered by MDI,[123] or in large doses by nebulization (Fig. 19.10).[90] van Schayck makes the point, however, that non-allergic and older patients may respond as well to the anti-muscarinic.[122] Obviously, the β_2 agonist is the treatment of choice for rapid relief of bronchospasm, but the delayed action of the anti-muscarinic is useful during multiple dosing.

COMBINED THERAPY IN ACUTE ASTHMA AND EXACERBATIONS OF COPD
What is the relative benefit of adding anti-muscarinic agents to intensive β_2-agonist therapy in these acute conditions? The results of two studies involving significant numbers of patients are rather unexpected. Thus, 0.5 mg nebulized ipratropium bromide added to 1.25 mg nebulized fenoterol produced an additive effect on FEV_1 *in only the asthma group*.[124] In another study involving 56 asthmatic subjects and 47 patients with COPD, when 0.5 mg ipratropium bromide was added to 10 mg salbutamol by nebulization, the result was similar.[125] Clearly, there is parasympathetic tone in acute asthma that is being addressed by the anti-muscarinic agent. However, it is not at all clear why the same should not apply to COPD. It may be that the anti-muscarinic agent in asthma is adding effectiveness by inhibiting mediator release.

THEOPHYLLINE AND OTHER PHOSPHODIESTERASE INHIBITORS

INDICATIONS FOR THEOPHYLLINE
In the 1970s and early 1980s, theophylline (1,3-dimethylxanthine) was the mainstay of bronchodilator therapy in the USA. Information on its pharmacokinetics, the development of sustained-release preparations and serum

level monitoring all facilitated its use. However, the new emphasis on anti-inflammatory therapy, combined with the simplicity and safety of inhaled β_2 agonists, led to a decline in theophylline use except for certain select circumstances where its properties still offer certain advantages that justify its use (Table 19.3); when long-acting β_2 agonists are found to meet certain of these select needs, the use of theophylline will diminish.

ACTIONS OF THEOPHYLLINE

Figure 19.12 shows the theophylline molecule along with enprofylline (3-propylxanthine), which lacks the 1-methyl group but is a more potent bronchodilator. Bronchodilating and anti-inflammatory actions reside in the 3-position, while adenosine antagonism resides in the 1-methyl group. Thus, whether an action of theophylline is due to adenosine antagonism can be determined by comparing the action of the two compounds. Table 19.4 lists the actions of theophylline and whether adenosine antagonism is involved.

Bronchodilation

Through its inhibition of phosphodiesterase $(PDE)_{III}$ and PDE_{IV} (see below), as well as other postulated mechanisms,[126] theophylline relaxes smooth muscle and inhibits PDE_{III} at similar concentrations (40–100 μM). *In vivo* its bronchodilating action depends entirely on the position of its serum levels on the dose–response curve for that patient (Fig. 19.13). In some cases, levels between 5 and 10 $\mu g\,ml^{-1}$ may suffice but, for most patients, a level in the 10–15 $\mu g\,ml^{-1}$ range is an optimal compromise between efficacy and safety from minor toxic effects (nausea, vomiting,

---

TABLE 19.3: *Indications for theophylline*

Nocturnal bronchospasm that persists despite full use of other agents

Asthma so poorly controlled that systemic corticosteroids are needed, intermittently or continuously

Asthma severe enough to warrant hospitalization and in whom mechanical ventilation may be needed

COPD severe enough to produce significant blood gas abnormalities, and/or limiting dyspnoea

Hypoventilatory entities, namely neonatal apnoea and sleep apnoea or hypopnoea in which other measures are rejected or unsatisfactory

Miscellaneous socio-economic entities: oral drug preferences, economy, convenience or practicality. Some asthmatic children fall in the latter category

FIGURE 19.12: *Theophylline (1,3-dimethylxanthine) and enprofylline (3-propylxanthine). Smooth muscle relaxation resides in the 3-position, while adenosine antagonism resides in the 1-methyl group, accounting for actions not shared by enprofylline.*

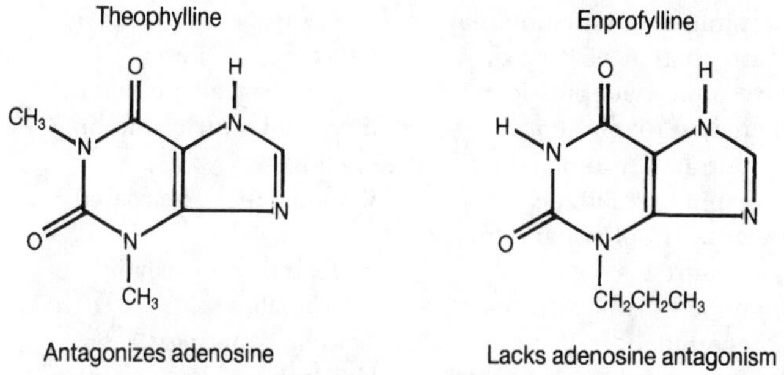

Theophylline — Antagonizes adenosine

Enprofylline — Lacks adenosine antagonism

headache, nervousness, tachycardia), which may commence at 20 μg ml^{-1} or a little higher. Racineux *et al.*[127] compared the dose–response curves for theophylline and salbutamol in stable asthma, using doses of 20 μg ml^{-1} or up to four puffs, respectively (Fig. 19.13). A level of 15 μg ml^{-1} theophylline was equivalent to two puffs of salbutamol on the FEV_1 response, and somewhat less on airway conductance. Levels between 10 and 15 μg ml^{-1} were equal to at least one puff of salbutamol at its peak effect. Hence, in the proper range, theophylline is not a "weak" bronchodilator as often claimed.

Theophylline produces at least additive bronchodilation with other drugs[128] and elevates both pre- and post-bronchodilator response to an MDI;[129] some studies suggest its action is actually over-additive with β agonists, even increasing their E_{max} (maximum relaxation).[130] Additivity is perhaps best exemplified by studies in COPD, a number of which have been done recently to compare the actions of agents alone and in combination. In the asthmatic patient, any over-additivity has been ascribed to the action of a systemic bronchodilator facilitating airway distribution of an inhaled bronchodilator.[131]

EFFECT OF THEOPHYLLINE ON RESPIRATORY MUSCLE FORCE

In 1981, Aubier *et al.* showed that intravenous aminophylline increased maximum transdiaphragmatic pressure (P_{di}) produced by unilateral single twitch supramaximal electrode stimulation of phrenic nerves in normal males.[132] At serum level of 13 μg ml^{-1}, theophylline increased the ratio of P_{di} to E_{di} (diaphragm electrical activity) an average of 16% during resistive breathing at all frequencies of stimulation and markedly delayed the onset

TABLE 19.4: *Actions of theophylline in humans.*

Useful action	Adverse action
Bronchodilation	CNS stimulation including seizures[a]
Respiratory stimulation and attenuation of hypoxic respiratory depression[a]	Relaxation of lower oesophageal sphincter
Increased diaphragm contractility and reduced diaphragm fatigue[a]	Increased gastric volume, acidity[a]
Decreased pulmonary artery pressure	Vasodilatation, increased heart rate
Increased cardiac output (combination of inotropism, increased rate, decreased peripheral resistance)	Increased myocardial irritability
	Nausea, vomiting
	Headache
Anti-inflammatory effect (including inhibition late phase response, anti-PAF, anti-permeability)	Cerebral vasconstriction[a]
	Decreased red cell mass due to decreased interferon[a]
Relief of syndrome "X" (angina with negative angiogram)[a]	Increased catecholamines, cyclic AMP, lipolysis, glucose, metabolic acidosis
Excretion of salt and water[a]	
Restoration of sinus rhythm in asystolic cardiac arrest[a]	

[a] Mediated by adenosine receptor antagonism.
PAF, platelet activating factor.
From Jenne JW. Pharmacology in the respiratory patient. In: Hodgkin JE (ed) *Pulmonary Rehabilitation. Guidelines to Success.* New York: J.B. Lippincott, 1992: 135–99.

of fatigue. If applied following induction of fatigue, recovery of normal strength was accelerated. While much controversy has been generated over this issue, I believe the evidence that supports an effect on respiratory muscles is more rigorous. Since enprofylline does not share this effect,[133] the effect depends on adenosine antagonism and would not likely be matched by any new phosphodiesterase inhibitor. Studies in normal subjects suggest that the effect is not simply the result of an improved diaphragmatic position in a hyperinflated lung.[134] While theophylline increases respiratory drive in the dog at higher concentrations[135] (and

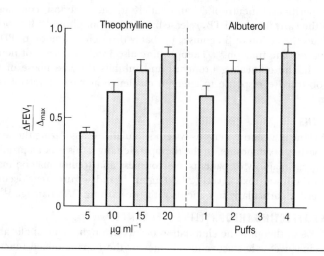

FIGURE 19.13: *Dose–response to theophylline and albuterol (salbutamol) in asthma, using mean values from 13 subjects. Aminophylline was given intravenously to approximately 5, 10, 15 and 20 μg ml⁻¹ theophylline levels, and albuterol was given to the same subjects as one, two, three and four puffs. The response is calculated in terms of the maximum change in FEV₁ achieved by either means. (Adapted from Ref. 127.)*

likely does so in neonatal apnoea), the effect in humans at usual concentrations is an improvement in P_{di}/E_{di}.[136] There is as yet no evidence that theophylline improves central fatigue or neuromuscular transmission.

HEART AND CIRCULATION

As theophylline levels are increased from 5 to 20 μg ml⁻¹, there is an inotropic effect as indicated by a shortening of the QS_2 interval. Combination with 2.5 mg nebulized salbutamol is synergistic.[137] At 15 μg ml⁻¹, the rate also begins to increase and there is acceleration of intra-cardiac conduction. Supraventricular arrhythmias occur at toxic levels, enhanced by adenosine antagonism. Multifocal atrial tachycardia is particularly characteristic.[138] Theophylline causes a decrease in venous and arterial tone, producing a decrease in pulmonary and peripheral vascular resistance. There is increased right and left ventricular ejection fraction but a decrease in stroke work.[139] In COPD, a 20–30% reduction in mean pulmonary artery pressure persists even with chronic therapy.[139] In the mid-therapeutic range, these actions are useful in the COPD patient, but with acute theophylline poisoning serious hypotension and various arrhythmias may develop.

With aminophylline loading, there is an approximately 25% reduction in cerebral blood flow, probably due to antagonism of adenosine, a vasodilator. However, this subsides with chronic use.[140] There is also a drop in jugular venous P_{O_2}.

Effect on Inflammation

Theophylline is synergistic with β agonists in inhibiting release of mediators from sensitized lung.[141] It inhibits the respiratory burst of human peripheral neutrophils and, at $18 \, \mu g \, ml^{-1}$, almost completely inhibits the early phase of LTB_4 release by calcium ionophore.[142] It strongly potentiates the action of β agonists, probably through inhibition of PDE_{IV} in the particulate fraction.[143] Theophylline also inhibits release of neuropeptides in the guinea-pig bronchus and inhibits the late phase of the airway obstructive response to allergen challenge at mean levels of only $9.7 \, \mu g \, ml^{-1}$.[144]

Effect on CNS

Theophylline is a central nervous system stimulant, antagonizing the sedating properties of adenosine. In the therapeutic range, this is not a problem for the great majority of patients. Nervousness and tremor may be manifested in the lower toxic levels $(20-30 \, \mu g \, ml^{-1})$ and seizures may occur at higher levels, particularly in patients with pre-existing CNS damage.[145]

FACTORS AFFECTING THEOPHYLLINE CLEARANCE

About 90% of theophylline elimination occurs through its metabolic alteration to inactive or less active metabolites by the hepatic mixed function oxidases utilizing the cytochrome P450 system. The normal activities of this system vary appreciably, and are induced or inhibited by host variables such as liver disease or congestive heart failure, and by various drugs.[146] Those factors having a significant effect (over 25%) are listed in Table 19.5.

THEOPHYLLINE DOSING

The reader is referred to a recent review for dosing of theophylline in children and infants, as well as further discussion of theophylline as a bronchodilator.[147]

Tips on Oral Theophylline Dosing in Adults (Table 19.6)

(1) The physician should first consider whether the patient

    (a) is a smoker, elderly, thin or fat;

    (b) has liver disease, recurring left heart failure, a history of arrhythmias or seizures (all of which are relative contraindications);

    (c) is on drugs that reduce or increase elimination rate.

TABLE 19.5: *Effect of host factors and interfering drugs on theophylline clearance and half-life*

Age	$t_{\frac{1}{2}}$ (hours) mean (range)	Clearance increased (shorter $t_{\frac{1}{2}}$)		Clearance decreased (longer $t_{\frac{1}{2}}$)		
		25–50%	50–75%	25–50%	50–90%	($t_{\frac{1}{2}}$ highly variable)
Adults (NS)[a]	8.7 (6.1–12.8)	Barbiturates	Tobacco[b], marijuana	Cimetidine		
Adults (NS)[a]	7.7 (5.3–11.3)	Sulfinpyrazone	Phenytoin	Ciprofloxacin	Unstable patient	
Premature infants	30.2 (14.4–57.7)	High-protein diet	Carbamazepine	Erythromycin	Heart failure	
Newborns	24.0		Rifampicin	Sustained fever	Severe liver disease	
Children (1–9 years)	3.7 (2.0–10.0)			Oral contraceptives	Sepsis	
Elderly	10.2 (7.1–13.3)			Troleandomycin		
				Propranolol		
				Allopurinol		
				Cor pulmonale		

[a] Mean clearance in non-smoking (NS) adults is about 40 ml kg^{-1} hour^{-1}.
[b] Low-tar cigarettes may have small effect.
From Gross NJ, Jenne JW, Hess D. In: Tobin MJ (ed) *Principles and Practices of Mechanical Ventilation*. New York: McGraw-Hill, 1993: 1077–123.

TABLE 19.6: *Theophylline dosing recommendations for adults*

Intravenous aminophylline

Patient off theophylline

Loading: 6 mg kg^{-1} ideal body weight over 20 min to produce
average level of 10 μg ml^{-1} (range 7–17)[a]

Maintenance

 Non-smokers, elderly, critically ill in ICU: 0.5 mg kg^{-1} hour^{-1}
 Current smokers: 0.7 mg kg^{-1} hour^{-1}
 Unstable patient: 0.2 mg kg^{-1} hour^{-1} (or none)

Patient on theophylline (or not sure)

Draw level, begin maintenance, then load as needed

Monitor

Loading: 30–60 min after load, adjust up as needed
Maintenance: re-measure *12–24 hours and daily thereafter,*
 adjusting infusion rate to maintain levels of 10–15 μg ml^{-1}.
 Limit to acute phase

Oral theophylline

Adaptation phase (optional): half full dose, then full dose
Initial full dose, then adjust[b]: 500–600 mg daily
Monitor: after 48 hours, or next appointment, adjust to
 10–15 μg ml^{-1} using small increments. Yearly thereafter

[a] Some authors advocate larger loading doses, aiming at 15 μg ml^{-1}.
[b] Typically non-smokers will require 10 mg kg^{-1} daily (500–800 mg) and
smokers 13 mg kg^{-1} daily (700–1200 mg).
Modified from Jenne JW. Pharmacology in the respiratory patient. In:
Hodgkin JE (ed) *Pulmonary Rehabilitation: Guidelines to Success.* New
York: J.B. Lippincott Co., 1992: 135–99.

(2) Dosing is a two-step process:

 (a) an initial, conservative dose up to 600 mg per 24 hours, followed by a serum level; and

 (b) dose-adjustment to bring levels into the 10–15 μg ml^{-1}
 range, using small, incremental increases.

 Levels are best measured after 48 hours of no missed doses,
 but this may await an early next appointment provided the
 patient is instructed regarding side-effects.

(3) A twice-daily slow-release preparation is used initially. If nocturnal symptoms persist, the dosing may be staggered to increase nocturnal levels, or a once-daily preparation taken in the evening.

(4) The patient is thoroughly instructed. Mild symptoms may only be transient. Nausea, vomiting, headache or jitteriness call for stopping the drug. Patients should never increase the dose on their own (more of the "breathing pill"). They should understand the concept of a narrow therapeutic range. They should keep the bottle secured from other family members.

THEOPHYLLINE TOXICITY

Monitoring of levels is clearly the way to reduce these problems. It is difficult to assess the true incidence of toxicity from theophylline, due to referral bias or the practical problems of developing prospective data in meaningful numbers. Under the most favourable clinical circumstances, with routine monitoring of levels in outpatients, a large Seattle home maintenance organization reported only 7.8 hospitalizations for toxicity per 10 000 person-years of therapy, from a total of 220 000 prescriptions.[148]

However, when 5557 levels were analysed from an emergency department of a university hospital–VA complex, 55% were under 10 μg ml^{-1}, 10% over 20 μg ml^{-1} and 2.8%, or 116 cases, over 30 μg ml^{-1} (167 μM).[149] From these, four grades of toxicity were developed (Table 19.7): 50% of cases fell in Grade 1, 38% in Grade 2, or moderate, and 7% in grades 3 or 4, severe and life-threatening; 12% of cases were due to acute overdose (suicidal). Figure 19.14 shows the acute and chronic categories and the serum levels. This figure is representative of conclusions first drawn by Olson et al.,[150] namely that the spectrum of toxicity and its prognosis differs between the acute overdose and those with chronic over-medication. In the acute cases, it is possible to predict major toxicity from the serum levels and hence the prophylactic need for charcoal haemoperfusion, namely a level in the 80–100 μg ml^{-1} range. The three cases dying with fulminant toxicity in the Sessler series[149] had status epilepticus, shock, ventricular fibrillation or refractory atrial flutter, and all had levels over 100 μg ml^{-1}. The four deaths in chronic cases had much lower levels, and three had serious underlying disease that could have been contributory. Of the seven with chronic seizures one died, and all had levels under 42 μg ml^{-1}. Thus, chronically elevated levels over 30 μg ml^{-1} have the potential for moderate to severe toxicity.

Management of Theophylline Toxicity

The approach used so successfully by Parr et al.[151] is reproduced here (Table 19.8), the great majority being cases of acute suicidal overdose.

TABLE 19.7: *Manifestations of toxicity and grades of severity*[a]

Grade 1
Vomiting
Abdominal pain
Diarrhoea
Nervousness
Tremor
Tachycardia ($>$ 120 beats/minute)
Mild hypokalaemia (2.5–3.5 mEq l^{-1})

Grade 2
Haematemesis
Lethargy or disorientation
Supraventricular tachyarrhythmia[b]
Frequent ventricular premature beats
Hypotension (mean blood pressure $<$ 60 mmHg, improves with
   standard therapy)
Severe hypokalaemia ($<$ 2.5 mEq l^{-1})
Acid–base disturbance (arterial pH $<$ 7.20 or $>$ 7.60)
Rhabdomyolysis

Grade 3
Seizure, non-repetitive
Sustained ventricular tachycardia
Shock (mean blood pressure $<$ 60 mmHg that is refractory to
   standard)

Grade 4
Status epilepticus
Ventricular fibrillation
Cardiac arrest

[a] The grades of toxicity were defined as follows: Grade 1, self-limited
toxicity that typically has no major impact; Grade 2, toxicity that
typically requires close observation, electrocardiographic monitoring, or
specific medical intervention; Grade 3, toxicity that typically requires
immediate intervention and/or often progresses to Grade 4 toxicity;
and Grade 4, toxicity that is often fatal.
[b] Includes atrial fibrillation or flutter, multifocal atrial tachycardia and
paroxysmal supraventricular tachycardia.
From Ref. 149.

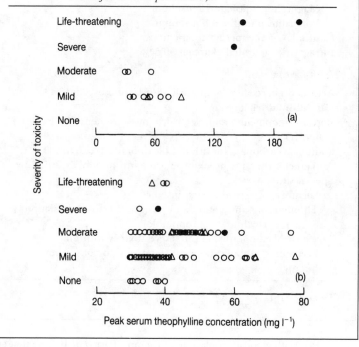

FIGURE 19.14: *Correlation between peak serum theophylline concentrations (STC) (mg l⁻¹) and severity of toxicity for 14 acute overdose (a) and 102 chronic over-medication (b) cases. Severity of toxicity is displayed as none, mild, moderate, severe and life-threatening according to categories in Table 19.7. Individual cases are adults (○) or children (△). Solid symbols denote fatal cases. There was a significant correlation (P < 0.01) between STC and severity for acute overdoses but not chronic over-medication. (From Ref. 149 with permission.)*

Further Points on Managing Toxicity

(1) Make every effort to distinguish acute from chronic toxicity. Treatment and prognosis differ.

(2) Include theophylline in any toxic screen of attempted suicide by overdose.

(3) With rising levels or increasing symptoms, admit the patient to an intensive care unit for monitoring and full press of conservative therapy.

TABLE 19.8: *Management schedule for theophylline poisoning*

Emergency department

History and examination, ECG monitoring commenced
Establish i.v. access, 0.9% sodium chloride infusion
Blood for laboratory investigation: theophylline level, sodium,
potassium, urea, glucose, creatinine, full blood count, arterial
blood gases
Electrolyte therapy commenced:
Potassium chloride 20 mM hour^{-1}
Magnesium sulphate 10 mM hour^{-1}
Potassium phosphate 5 mM hour^{-1}
Gastric lavage or ipecacuanha emesis
Intragastric, activated charcoal 50 g

Intensive care unit

Activated charcoal 20 g 2-hourly with lactulose 20 ml
Careful fluid balance
Repeat theophylline and electrolyte measurements (at least 4-
hourly)
Sodium bicarbonate for arterial bicarbonate (< 16 mmol l^{-1})
Anti-emetic therapy: prochlorperazine, droperidol ± ranitidine
Special situations:
Seizures: diazepam in first instance
Thiopentone, intubation and positive pressure ventilation
Serious arrhythmias: ? propranolol
Charcoal haemoperfusion for severe toxicity with life-
threatening complications, unresponsive to conservative
therapy

From Ref. 151.

(4) With vigorous replacement therapy, Parr *et al.* believe that charcoal haemoperfusion can be reserved for those few instances
where toxic events fail to respond to specific therapy.[151]

(5) In animal models of theophylline-induced seizures, phenobarbital is superior to phenytoin. Following diazepam and intubation, phenobarbital is the drug of choice in a dose of
10 mg kg^{-1} i.v. over 30 min, repeated if needed.

(6) Intravenous phenobarbital is also valuable in decreasing the
seizure threshold of those showing CNS excitation. This could
be life-saving. It controls vomiting as well.

THE CONTINUING SEARCH FOR AN IMPROVED PHOSPHODIESTERASE INHIBITOR

Recent years have seen a growing interest in developing phosphodiesterase inhibitors that would retain the spasmolytic and anti-inflammatory qualities of theophylline, but through greater organ selectivity would minimize the side-effects. Enprofylline is a possible improvement. It avoids the life-threatening toxicity of seizures and is cleared by the kidneys. However, it produces at least as much nausea and headache as theophylline and may be no more acceptable to the patient.

The history and potential of this field have been comprehensively reviewed.[152] Bronchial (and pulmonary artery) smooth muscle contains five PDE "families", each with several subtypes. While all five hydrolyse both cAMP and cGMP, PDE_{IV} and PDE_V are much more selective for cAMP and cGMP, respectively.

The relaxant efficacy of inhibiting each family is $PDE_{III} > PDE_{IV} > PDE_V$. Inhibition of PDE_{III} and PDE_{IV} together produces at least additive relaxation,[152] or is even synergistic when using the specific inhibitors SK&F 94120 and rolipram. PDE_{III} but not PDE_{IV} inhibition potentiates isoproterenol relaxation of LTD_4-contracted bronchi, while PDE_V inhibition potentiates relaxation by nitroprusside, presumably operating through the cGMP mechanism of relaxation.

In addition, PDE_{IV} inhibition exerts an anti-inflammatory effect on polymorphonuclear leucocyte mediator release[143] and combination $PDE_{III/IV}$ inhibition would be expected to do the same. In fact, theophylline has shown such activity and synergizes strongly with isoproterenol in inhibiting the release of mediators from activated polymorphonuclear leucocytes.[142] It is ironic that theophylline, which combines many of these inhibitory actions, is handicapped by a narrow therapeutic range and such variable metabolism. Despite the theoretical promise of more potent and selective PDE inhibitors, it may be some time before any of them reach the drug market.

CONCLUDING COMMENT

With the increased emphasis on anti-inflammatory therapy of asthma, bronchodilators are assuming a subsidiary role as a "mop-up" operation. However, there is no substitute for their vigorous use in the acute attack, nor in managing the residual bronchospasm that still plagues the asthmatic patient. Constricted airways still kill patients. The receptor pharmacology of the airways will still demand the present classes of agents, very likely in their present forms, with occasional new compounds such as the long-acting β_2 agonists. What will develop, however, is the mode of delivering them, the philosophy of their use and their combinations, and an increased understanding of their adverse effects. Nothing will replace clinical judgement.

REFERENCES

1 O'Donnell SR. The development of beta receptor agonist drugs. In: Beasley R, Pearce NE (eds) *The Role of Beta Receptor Agonist Therapy in Asthma Mortality.* Boca Raton: CRC Press, 1993: 4–26.

2 Ahlquist RP. A study of adrenotropic receptors. Am J Physiol 1948; 153: 586–600.

3 Lands AM, Arnold A, McAuliff JP *et al.* Differentiation of receptor systems activated by sympathomimetic amines. Nature 1967; 214: 597–8.

4 Kaumann AJ. Is there a third heart beta-adrenoceptor? Trends Pharmacol Sci 1989; 10: 316–20.

5 Nials AT, Sumner MT, Johnson M, Coleman RA. Investigation into factors determining the duration of action of the β_2-adrenoceptor agonist, salmeterol. Br J Pharmacol 1993; 108: 507–15.

6 Jack D. A way of looking at agonism and antagonism: Lessons from albuterol, salmeterol, and other β-adrenoceptor agonists. Br J Clin Pharmacol 1991; 31: 501–14.

7 Kendall MJ, Haffner C. The acute unwanted effects of beta$_2$ receptor agonist therapy. In: Beasley R, Pearce NE (eds) *The Role of Beta Receptor Agonist Therapy in Asthma Mortality.* Boca Raton: CRC Press, 1993: 163–99.

8 Lipworth BJ, McDevitt DG, Struthers AD. Systemic β-adrenoceptor responses to salbutamol given by metered-dose inhaler alone and with pear shaped spacer attachment: comparison of electrocardiographic hypokalaemic and haemodynamic effects. Br J Clin Pharmacol 1989; 27: 837–42.

9 Lipworth BJ, Struthers AD, McDevitt DG. Tachyphylaxis to systemic but not to airway responses during prolonged therapy with high dose inhaled salbutamol in asthmatics. Am Rev Respir Dis 1989; 140: 586–92.

10 Lipworth BJ, Tregaskis BF, McDevitt DG. β-Adrenoceptor responses to inhaled salbutamol in the elderly. Br J Clin Pharmacol 1989; 28: 725–9.

11 Allon M, Dunlay R, Copkney C. Nebulized albuterol for acute hyperkalemia in patients on dialysis. Ann Intern Med 1989; 110: 426–9.

12 Jenne JW, Ridley DF, Marcucci R, Druz WS, Rook JC. Objective and subjective tremor responses to oral beta-2 agents on first exposure. Am Rev Respir Dis 1982; 126: 607–10.

13 Buxton BF, Jones CR, Molenaar P, Summers RJ. Characterization and auto-radiographic localization of beta adrenoceptor subtypes in human cardiac tissues. *Br J Pharmacol* 1987; 92: 299–310.

14 Brodde OE, Daul A, Wellstrein A, Palm D, Michael MC, Backerugh JJ. Differentiation of $beta_1$ and $beta_2$ adrenoceptor mediated effects in humans. *Am J Physiol* 1988; 251: H119–206.

15 Brittain RT. A comparison of the pharmacology profile of salbutamol with that of isoproterenol, orciprenaline (metaproterenol) and trimetoquinol. *Postgrad Med J* 1971; 47: 11–6.

16 Ball DI, Brittain RT, Coleman RA *et al.* Salmeterol, a novel, long-acting $β_2$-adrenoceptor agonist: characterization of pharmacological activity *in vitro* and *in vivo*. *Br J Pharmacol* 1991; 104: 665–71.

17 Kaumann AJ, Hall JA, Murray KJ, Walls FC, Brown MJ. A comparison of the effects of adrenaline and noradrenaline in human heart. The role of $beta_1$ and $beta_2$ adrenoceptors in the stimulation of adenylate cyclase and contractile force. *Eur Heart J* 1989; 10 (suppl B): 29–37.

18 Mugge A, Posselt D, Reimer U, Schmitz W, Scholz H. Effects of the $beta_2$ adrenoceptor agonists fenoterol and salbutamol on force of contraction in isolated human ventricular myocardium. *Klin Wochenschr* 1985; 63: 26–31.

19 Burgess CD. An overview of experimental methods. In: Beasley R, Pierce NE (eds) *The Role of Beta Receptor Agonist Therapy in Asthma Mortality.* Boca Raton: CRC Press, 1993: 128–48.

20 Naylor WG, McInnes I. Salbutamol and orciprenaline-induced changes in myocardial function. *Cardiovasc Res* 1972; 6: 725–33.

21 Hall JA, Petch MC, Brown MJ. Intracoronary injections of salbutamol demonstrate the presence of functional $beta_2$ adrenoceptors in the human heart. *Circ Res* 1989; 65: 546–53.

22 Twentyman OP, Finnerty JP, Holgate ST. The inhibitory effect of nebulized albuterol on the early and late asthmatic reactions and increase in airway responsiveness provoked by inhaled allergen in asthma. *Am Rev Respir Dis* 1991; 14: 782–7.

23 Twentyman OP, Finnerty JP, Harris A, Palmer J, Holgate ST. Protection against allergen-induced asthma by salmeterol. *Lancet* 1990; 336: 1338–42.

24 Palmqvist M, Balder B, Lowhagen D, Melander B, Svedmyr N, Wahlander L. Late asthmatic reaction decreased after treatment with salbutamol and formoterol, a new long-acting beta-2 agonist. *J Allergy Clin Immunol* 1992; 89: 844–9.

25 Howarth PH, Durham SR, Lee TH, Kay AB, Church MK, Holgate ST. Influence of albuterol, cromolyn sodium and ipratropium bromide on the airway circulating mediator response to allergen bronchial provocation in asthma. *Am Rev Respir Dis* 1985; 132: 986–92.

26 Church MK, Hiroi J. Inhibition of IgE-dependent histamine release from human dispersed lung mast cells by anti-allergic drugs and salbutamol. Br J Pharmacol 1987; 90: 421–9.

27 Tomioka K, Yamada T, Tachikawa S. Effects of formoterol (BD40A), a β-adrenoceptor stimulant on isolated guinea-pig lung parenchymal strips and antigen-induced SRS-A release in rats. Arch Int Pharmacodyn 1984; 267: 91–102.

28 Butchers PR, Vardey CJ, Johnson M. Salmeterol: a potent and long-acting inhibitor of inflammatory mediator release from human lung. Br J Pharmacol 1991; 104: 672–6.

29 Page CP. One explanation of the asthma paradox: inhibition of natural anti-inflammatory mechanisms by beta-2 agonists. Lancet 1991; 337: 717–20.

30 Erjefalt I, Persson CGA. Pharmacological control of plasma exudation in the tracheobronchial airways. Am Rev Respir Dis 1991; 143: 1008–14.

31 Wheland CJ, Johnson M. Inhibition by salmeterol of increased vascular permeability and granulocyte accumulation in guinea pig lung and skin. Br J Pharmacol 1992; 105: 831–8.

32 Advenier C, Qian Y, Koune JD, Molimard M, Candenas ML, Naline E. Formoterol and salbutamol inhibit bradykinin- and histamine-induced airway microvascular leakage in guinea pig. Br J Pharmacol 1992; 105: 792–8.

33 Rabe KF, Giembycz MA, Dent G, Perkins RS, Evans P, Barnes PJ. Salmeterol is a competitive antagonist at beta-adrenoceptors mediating inhibition of respiratory burst in guinea pig eosinophils. Eur J Pharmacol 1993; 231: 305–8.

34 Sugiyama H, Okada C, Bewtra AK, Hope RJ, Townley RG. The effect of formoterol on the late asthmatic phenomenon in guinea pigs. J Allergy Clin Immunol 1992; 89: 858–66.

35 Nielson CP. β-Adrenergic modulation of the polymorphonuclear leukocyte respiratory burst is dependent upon the mechanism of cell activation. J Immunol 1987; 139: 2392–7.

36 Linden M. The effect of beta 2-adrenoceptor agonists and a corticosteroid, budesonide, on the secretion of inflammatory mediators from monocytes. Br J Pharmacol 1992; 107: 156–60.

37 Barnes PJ, Pride NB. Dose–response curves to inhaled beta-adrenoceptor agonists in normal and asthmatic subjects. Br J Pharmacol 1983; 15: 677–82.

38 Ruffin RE, Obminski G, Newhouse MT. Aerosol salbutamol administration of IPPB: lowest effectiveness. Thorax 1978; 33: 689–93.

39 Beaty R, Harman E, Molino L, Hendeles L. The dose–response of albuterol during acute attacks of nocturnal asthma. Am Rev Respir Dis 1992; 145: A66.

40 Joad JP, Ahrens RC, Lindgren SC, Weinberger MW. Relative efficacy of maintenance therapy with theophylline, inhaled albuterol and the combination for chronic asthma. J Allergy Clin Immunol 1987; 79: 78–85.

41 Szefler S, Ando R, Cicutto LC, Surs W, Hill MW, Martin RJ. Plasma hista-
    mine, epinephrine, cortisol, and leukocyte β-adrenergic receptors in noc-
    turnal asthma. *Clin Pharmacol Ther* 1991; 49: 59–68.

42 Becker AB, Simons FER, McMillan JL, Faridy T. Formoterol, a new long-
    acting selective β_2 adrenergic receptor agonist. Double-blind comparison
    with salbutamol and placebo in children with asthma. *J Allergy Clin Immunol* 1989;
    84: 891–5.

43 Kemp JP, Bierman CW, Cocchetto DM. Dose–response study of inhaled
    salmeterol in asthmatic patients with 24-hour spirometry and Holter moni-
    toring. *Ann Allergy* 1993; 70: 316–22.

44 Derom EY, Pauwels R. Time course of bronchodilating effect of inhaled
    formoterol, a potent and long-acting sympathomimetic. *Thorax* 1992; 47: 30–3.

45 Beach JR, Young CL, Stenton SC, Avery AJ, Walters EH, Hendrick DJ. A
    comparison of the speeds of action of salmeterol and salbutamol in revers-
    ing methacholine-induced bronchoconstriction. *Pulm Pharmacol* 1992; 5: 133–5.

46 Simon SE, Soni NR, Watson WTA, Becker AB. Bronchodilator and
    bronchoprotective effects of salmeterol in young patients with asthma. *J
    Allergy Clin Immunol* 1992; 90: 840–6.

47 Pearlman DS, Chervinsky P, LaForce C *et al.* A comparison of salmeterol
    with albuterol in the treatment of mild to moderate asthma. *N Engl J Med* 1992;
    327: 1420–5.

48 Fitzpatrick MF, Mackay T, Driver H, Douglas NJ. Salmeterol in nocturnal
    asthma: a double blind, placebo controlled trial of a long-acting inhaled
    β_2 agonist. *BMJ* 1990; 301: 1365–8.

49 Derom EY, Pauwels R, van der Straeten ME. The effect of inhaled salmet-
    erol on methacholine responsiveness in subjects with asthma up to 12
    hours. *J Allergy Clin Immunol* 1992; 89: 811–5.

50 Cheung D, Timmers MD, Zwinderman AH, Bel EH, Dijkman JH, Sterk PJ.
    Long-term effects of a long-acting beta-2 adrenoceptor agonist, salmeterol,
    on airway hyperresponsiveness in patients with mild asthma. *N Engl J Med* 1992;
    327: 1198–203.

51 Palmer JR, Stuart AM, Shepherd G, Viskum K. Inhaled salmeterol in the
    treatment of patients with moderate to severe reversible obstructive airways
    disease – a 3 month comparison of the efficacy and safety of twice-daily
    salmeterol (100 micrograms) with salmeterol (50 micrograms). *Respir Med*
    1992; 86: 409–17.

52 Ahrens RC, Harris JB, Milavetz G, Annis L, Ries R. Use of bronchial provo-
    cation with histamine to compare the pharmacodynamics of inhaled albut-
    erol and metaproterenol in patients with asthma. *J Allergy Clin Immunol* 1987; 79:
    876–82.

53 Salome CM, Schoeffel RE, Woolcock AJ. Effect of aerosol and oral fenoterol on histamine and methacholine challenge in asthmatic subjects. *Thorax* 1981; 36: 580–4.

54 Konig P, Eggleston A, Serby CW. Comparison of oral and inhaled metaproterenol for prevention of exercise-induced asthma. *Clin Allergy* 1981; 11: 597–604.

55 Mitchell CA, Armstrong JG, Bartholomew MA, Scicchitano R. Nebulized fenoterol in severe asthma: determinants of the dose response. *Eur J Respir Dis* 1983; 64: 340–6.

56 Schuh S. High versus low-dose frequently administered nebulized albuterol in children with severe, acute asthma. *Pediatrics* 1989; 83: 513–8.

57 Robertson CF, Smith F, Beck R, Levison H. Response to frequent low doses of nebulized salbutamol in acute asthma. *J Pediatr* 1985; 106: 672–4.

58 Kelly HW, McWilliams B, Katz R, Crowley M, Murphy S. Safety of frequent high dose nebulized terbutaline in children with acute asthma. *Ann Allergy* 1990; 64: 229–33.

59 Katz RW, Kelly HW, Crowley M. Safety of continuous nebulized albuterol for bronchospasm in infants and children. *Pediatrics* 1993; 92: 666–9.

60 Moler FW, Hurwitz ME, Custer JR. Improvement in clinical asthma score and P_aCO_2 in children with severe asthma treated with continuously nebulized terbutaline. *J Allergy Clin Immunol* 1988; 81: 1101–9.

61 Papo MC, Frank JA, Thompson AE. A prospective randomized study of continuous versus intermittent nebulized albuterol for severe status asthmaticus in children. *Crit Care Med* 1993; 21: 1479–86.

62 Fuglsang G, Pedersen S, Borgstrom L. Dose–response relationships of intravenously administered terbutaline in children with asthma. *J Pediatr* 1989; 114: 315–20.

63 Lin RY, Smith AJ, Hergenroeder P. High serum albuterol levels and tachycardia in adult asthmatics treated with high-dose continuously aerosolized albuterol. *Chest* 1993; 103: 221–5.

64 Anonymous. Drugs for asthma. *Medical Letter* 1987; 29: 13.

65 Appel DW, Karpel JP, Sherman M. Epinephrine improves expiratory flow rates in patients with asthma who do not respond to inhaled metaproterenol sulfate. *J Allergy Clin Immunol* 1989; 84: 90–8.

66 Hargreave FE, Dolovich J, Newhouse MT. The assessment and treatment of asthma. A conference report. *J Allergy Clin Immunol* 1990; 85: 1098–111.

67 Harrison BA, Pierce RJ. Comparison of wet and dry aerosol salbutamol. *Aust N Z J Med* 1983; 13: 29–33.

68 Mestitz H, Copeland JM, McDonald CF. Comparison of outpatient nebulized vs metered dose inhaled terbutaline in chronic air flow obstruction. *Chest* 1989; 96: 1237–40.

69 Colacone MA, Wokove N, Kreisman H. Dose response to inhaled salbutamol administered by metered dose inhaler or wet nebulizer in the treatment of acute asthma. *Am Rev Respir Dis* 1991; 143: A650.

70 Idros AH, McDermott MF, Raucci JC, Morrabel A, McGorray S, Hendeles L. Emergency department treatment of severe asthma. *Chest* 1993; 103: 665–72.

71 Leferink JG, Van den Berg W, Wagemaker-Engels J *et al.* Pharmacokinetics of terbutaline, a β_2-sympathomimetic, in healthy volunteers and asthmatic patients. *Arzneim Forsch* 1982; 32: 159–64.

72 Dietrich KA, Conrad SA, Romero MD. Creatine kinase (CK) isoenzymes in pediatric status asthmaticus treated with intravenous terbutaline. *Crit Care Med* 1991; 19: 539.

73 Uden DL. Guidelines for intravenous terbutaline use in status asthmaticus. In: Weiss EB, Stein M (eds) *Bronchial Asthma. Mechanisms and Therapeutics.* Boston: Little, Brown & Co., 1993: 1226.

74 Bohn D, Kalloghian A, Jenkins J, Edmonds J, Barker G. Intravenous salbutamol in the treatment of status asthmaticus in children. *Crit Care Med* 1984; 12: 892–6.

75 Fairfax AJ, McNabb WR, Davis HJ, Spiro SG. Slow-release oral salbutamol and aminophylline in nocturnal asthma: relation of overnight changes in lung function and plasma drug levels. *Thorax* 1980; 35: 526–30.

76 Gross NJ, Jenne JW, Hess D. Bronchodilator therapy. In: Tobin MJ (ed) *Principles and Practice of Mechanical Ventilation.* New York: McGraw-Hill, 1994: 1077–123.

77 Fuller HD, Dolovich MB, Posmituck G, Wong Pak W, Newhouse MT. Pressurized aerosol versus jet aerosol delivery to mechanically ventilated patients. Comparison of dose to the lungs. *Am Rev Respir Dis* 1990; 141: 440–4.

78 MacIntyre NR, Silver RM, Miller CW, Schuler F, Coleman RE. Aerosol delivery in intubated, mechanically ventilated patients. *Crit Care Med* 1985; 13: 81–4.

79 Thomas SHL, O'Doherty MJ, Fidler HM, Page CJ, Treacher DF, Nunan TO. Pulmonary deposition of a nebulized aerosol during mechanical ventilation. *Thorax* 1993; 48; 154–9.

80 Manthous CA, Hall JB, Schmidt GA, Wood LDH. Metered dose inhaler versus nebulized albuterol in mechanically ventilated patients. *Am Rev Respir Dis* 1993; 148: 1567–70.

81 Dhand R, Jubran A, Tobin MJ. Response to bronchodilator administration by metered dose inhaler in mechanically ventilated patients with COPD (abstract). *Am Rev Respir Dis* 1993; 147: A895.

82 Fink JB, Cohen NH, Covington J, Mahlmeister MJ. Titration for optimal dose response to bronchodilators using MDI and spacer in ventilated adults (abstract). *Respir Care* 1991; 36: 1321.

83 Gay PC, Rodarte JR, Tayyab M, Hubmayer RD. Evaluation of bronchodilator responsiveness in mechanically ventilated patients. Am Rev Respir Dis 1987; 136: 880–5.

84 Bernasconi M, Brandolese R, Poggi R, Manzino E, Rossa A. Dose–response effects and time course of effects of inhaled fenoterol on respiratory mechanics and arterial oxygen in mechanically ventilated patients with chronic airflow obstruction. Intensive Care Med 1990; 16: 108–14.

85 Crane J, Burgess C, Beasley R. Cardiovascular and hypokalemic effects of inhaled salbutamol, fenoterol and isoprenaline. Thorax 1989; 44: 136–40.

86 Wong CS, Pavord ID, Williams J, Britton JE, Tattersfield AE. Bronchodilator cardiovascular and hypokalemic effects of fenoterol, salbutamol, and terbutaline in asthma. Lancet 1990; 336: 1396–9.

87 Scheinin M, Kaulus MM, Laurikainen E, Allonen H. Hypokalemia and other non-bronchial effects of inhaled fenoterol and salbutamol. A placebo controlled dose–response study in healthy volunteers. Br J Clin Pharmacol 1987; 24: 645–53.

88 Bremner P, Woodman K, Burgess C et al. A comparison of the cardiovascular and metabolic effects of formoterol, salbutamol and fenoterol. Eur Respir J 1993; 6: 204–10.

89 Windom HH, Burgess CD, Siebers RWL et al. The pulmonary and extrapulmonary effects of inhaled β-agonists in patients with asthma. Clin Pharmacol Ther 1990; 48: 296–301.

90 Bremner P, Burgess C, Beasley R et al. Nebulized fenoterol causes greater cardiovascular and hypokalemic effects than equivalent bronchodilator doses of salbutamol in asthmatics. Respir Med 1992; 86: 419–23.

91 Joseph X, Whitehurst VE, Bloom S, Balazs T. Enhancement of cardiotoxic effects of beta-adrenergic bronchodilators by aminophylline in experimental animals. Fundam Appl Toxicol 1981; 1: 443–7.

92 Sly RM, Jenne JW, Cohn J. Toxicity of beta-adrenergic drugs. In: Jenne JW, Murphy S (eds) Drug Therapy for Asthma. Research and Clinical Practice. Vol. 31, Lung Biology in Health and Disease. New York: Marcel Dekker, 1987: 953–96.

93 Maguire JF, Geha RS, Umetsu DJ. Myocardial specific creatinine phosphokinase isozyme elevation in children with asthma treated with intravenous isoproterenol. J Allergy Clin Immunol 1986; 78: 631–6.

94 Higgins RM, Cookson WOCM, Lane DJ, John SM, McCarthy GL, McCarthy ST. Cardiac arrhythmias caused by nebulized beta-agonist therapy. Lancet 1987; ii: 863–4.

95 Shovlin CL, Tam FWK. Salbutamol nebulizer and precipitation of critical cardiac ischemia. Lancet 1990; 335: 258.

96 Svedmyr NLV, Larson SA, Thiringer G. Development of resistance in beta adrenergic receptors of asthmatic patients. Chest 1976; 69: 479–83.

97 Weber RW, Smith KA, Nelson HS. Aerosolized terbutaline in asthmatics: Development of subsensitivity with long-term administration. *J Allergy Clin Immunol* 1982; 70: 417–22.

98 Jenne JW, Chick TW, Strickland RD, Wall FJ. Subsensitivity of beta responses during therapy with long-acting beta-2 preparation. *J Allergy Clin Immunol* 1977; 59: 383–90.

99 Repsher LH, Anderson JA, Bush RK *et al.* Assessment of tachyphylaxis following prolonged therapy of asthma with inhaled albuterol aerosol. *Chest* 1984; 85: 34–8.

100 Britton J. Tolerance to beta-agonists in asthma. *Lancet* 1993; 342: 818–9.

101 Vathenen AS, Knox AJ, Higgens BG, Britton JR, Tattersfield AE. Rebound increase in bronchial responsiveness after treatment with inhaled terbutaline. *Lancet* 1988; i: 554–8.

102 Kraan J, Koeter GH, Mark VD, Sluiter HJ, de Vries K. Changes in bronchial hyperreactivity induced by 4 weeks of treatment with anti-asthmatic drugs in patients with allergic asthma: A comparison between budesonide and terbutaline. *J Allergy Clin Immunol* 1985; 76: 628–36.

103 Wahedna I, Wong CS, Wisniewski AFZ, Pavord ID, Tattersfield AE. Asthma control during and after cessation of regular beta$_2$ agonist treatment. *Am Rev Respir Dis* 1993; 148: 707–12.

104 Kerrebijn KG, van Essen-Zandvliet EM, Neijens HJ. Effect of long-term treatment with inhaled corticosteroids and beta-agonists on the bronchial responsiveness in children with asthma. *J Allergy Clin Immunol* 1987; 79: 653–9.

105 Sears MR, Taylor DR, Print CG *et al.* Regular inhaled beta-agonist treatment in bronchial asthma. *Lancet* 1990; 336: 1391–6.

106 Ramsdell JW, Nachtweg JF, Moser KM. Bronchial hyperreactivity in chronic obstructive bronchitis. *Am Rev Respir Dis* 1982; 126: 829–32.

107 Cockcroft DW, McParland CP, Britto SA, Swyztun VA, Rutherford BC. Regular induced salbutamol and airways responsiveness to allergen. *Lancet* 1993; 342: 833–6.

108 O'Connor BJ, Aikman SL, Barnes PJ. Tolerance to the nonbronchodilator effects of inhaled β$_2$-agonists in asthma. *N Engl J Med* 1992; 327: 1204–8.

109 Booth H, Fishwick K, Harkawat R, Devereux G, Hendrick DJ, Walters EH. Changes in methacholine induced bronchoconstriction with the long acting β$_2$-agonist salmeterol in mild to moderate asthmatic patients. *Thorax* 1993; 48: 1121–4.

110 Spina D, Rigby PJ, Paterson JW, Goldie RG. Autoradiographic localization of β-adrenoceptors in asthmatic human lung. *Am Rev Respir Dis* 1989; 140: 1410–5.

111 Bai TR, Prasad FW. Abnormalities in airway smooth muscle in fatal asthma. *Am Rev Respir Dis* 1990; 141: 552–7.

112 Dooper MWSM, Timmerman A, Aalbers R, DeMonchy JGR, Kauffman HF. Desensitization of the adenylyl cyclase system in peripheral blood mononuclear cells from patients with asthma three hours after allergen challenge. J Allergy Clin Immunol 1993; 92: 559–66.

113 Nijkamp FP, Henricks PAJ. Receptors in airway disease. Beta-adrenoceptors in lung inflammation. Am Rev Respir Dis 1990; 141: 5145–50.

114 Barnes PJ, Chung KF. Questions about inhaled β_2-adrenoceptor agonists in asthma. Trends Pharmacol Sci 1992; 13: 20–3.

115 Pearce N, Grainger M, Crane J et al. Case-control study of prescribed fenoterol and death from asthma in New Zealand, 1977–1981. Thorax 1990; 45: 170–5.

116 Spitzer WO, Suisa S, Ernst P et al. The use of beta-agonists and the risk of death and near-death from asthma. N Engl J Med 1992; 326: 501–6.

117 Nelson HS, Szefler SJ, Martin RJ. Regular inhaled beta-adrenergic agonists in the treatment of bronchial asthma: Beneficial or detrimental? Am Rev Respir Dis 1991; 144: 249–50.

118 Lofdahl C-G, Svedmyr N. Beta-agonists – friends or foes? Eur Respir J 1991; 4: 1161–5.

119 Ernst P, Habbick B, Suisa S et al. Is the association between inhaled beta-agonists and life-threatening asthma because of confounding by severity? Am Rev Respir Dis 1992; 148: 75–9.

120 Marlin GE, Bush DE, Berend N. Comparison of ipratropium bromide and fenoterol in asthma and chronic bronchitis. Br J Clin Pharmacol 1976; 6: 647–9.

121 Higgens BG, Powell RM, Cooper S, Tattersfield AE. Effect of salbutamol and ipratropium bromide on the airway calibre and bronchial reactivity in asthma and chronic bronchitis. Eur Respir J 1991; 4: 415–20.

122 van Schayck CP, Folgering H, Harbers H, Maas KL, van Weel C. Effect of allergy and age on responses to salbutamol and ipratropium bromide in moderate asthma and chronic bronchitis. Thorax 1991; 46: 355–9.

123 Ruffin RE, Fitzgerald JD, Rebuck AS. A comparison of the bronchodilator activity of Sch 1000 and salbutamol. J Allergy Clin Immunol 1977; 59: 136–41.

124 Rebuck AS, Read J. Assessment and management of severe asthma. Am J Med 1971; 51: 788–98.

125 O'Driscoll BR, Taylor RJ, Horsley MG, Chambers DK, Bernstein A. Nebulized salbutamol with and without ipratropium bromide in acute airflow obstruction. Lancet 1989; 1: 1489.

126 Jenne JW. Physiology and pharmacodynamics of theophylline. In Jenne JW, Murphy S (eds) Drug Therapy for Asthma. Research and Clinical Practice. Vol. 31 Lung Biology in Health and Disease. New York: Marcel Dekker, 1987: 297–334.

127 Racineux JL, Troussier J, Tureant A. Comparison of bronchodilator effects of salbutamol and theophylline. Bull Eur Physiopathol Respir 1981; 17: 799–806.

128 Wolfe JD, Tashkin DP, Calvarese B, Simmons M. Bronchodilator effects of terbutaline and aminophylline alone and in combination in asthmatic patients. *N Engl J Med* 1978; 298: 363–7.

129 Appel DW. Effect of aminophylline when added to metaproterenol sulfate and beclomethasone diproprionate aerosol. *J Allergy Clin Immunol* 1984; 73: 291–7.

130 Billing B, Dahlquist R, Gal M. Separate and combined use of terbutaline and theophylline in asthmatics. *Eur J Respir Dis* 1982; 63: 399–402.

131 Svedmyr K, Svedmyr N. Does theophylline potentiate inhaled β_2-agonists? *Allergy* 1982; 37: 101–10.

132 Aubier M, De Troyer A, Sampson M, Macklem PT, Roussos C. Aminophylline improves diaphragmatic contractility. *N Engl J Med* 1981; 305: 249–52.

133 Murciano D, Aubier M, Viires N, Mal H, Pariente R. Effects of theophylline and enprofylline on diaphragmatic contractility. *J Appl Physiol* 1983; 54: 460–4.

134 Okubo S, Konno K, Ishizaki T, Kubo M, Suganuma T, Takizawa T. Effect of theophylline on respiratory neuromuscular drive. *Eur J Clin Pharmacol* 1987; 33: 85–8.

135 Aubier MA, Murciano D, Viires N, Lecocguig Y, Palacios S, Pariente R. Increased ventilation caused by improved diaphragmatic efficiency during aminophylline infusion. *Am Rev Respir Dis* 1983; 127: 148–54.

136 Murciano D, Aubier MA, Lecocquic Y, Pariente R. Effect of theophylline on diaphragmatic strength and fatigue in patients with chronic obstructive pulmonary disease. *N Engl J Med* 1984; 311: 349–53.

137 Burgess CD, Crane J, Graham AN, Maling TJB. The hemodynamic effects of aminophylline and salbutamol alone and in combination. *Clin Pharmacol Ther* 1986; 40: 550–3.

138 Bitter G, Friedman HS. The arrhythmogenicity of theophylline. A multivariate analysis of clinical determinants. *Chest* 1992; 99: 1415–20.

139 Matthay RA, Berger SA, Davies R *et al.* Improvement in cardiac performance by oral long-term theophylline in chronic obstructive pulmonary disease. *Am Heart J* 1982; 104: 1022–6.

140 Bowton DL, Alford PT, Prough DS, Stump DA, Motsinger S. The effect of chronic theophylline therapy on brain blood flow and function. *Chest* 1990; 98: 215.

141 Orange RP, Austin WG, Austen KF. Immunologic release of histamine and slow-reactive substances of anaphylaxis from human lung. I. Modulation by agents influencing cellular levels of cyclic 3', 5'-adenosine monophosphate. *J Exp Med* 1971; suppl 134: 136.

142 Nielson CP, Crowley JJ, Cusack BJ, Vestal RE. Therapeutic concentrations of theophylline and enprophylline potentiate catecholamine effects and inhibit leukocyte activation. *J Allergy Clin Immunol* 1986; 78: 660–7.

143 Nielson CP, Vestal RE, Sturm RJ, Heaslip R. Effects of selective phosphodi-esterase inhibitors in the polymorphonuclear leukocyte respiratory burst. *J Allergy Clin Immunol* 1990; 86: 801–8.

144 Ward AJM, McKenniff M, Evans JM, Page CP, Costello JF. Theophylline – an immunomodulatory role in asthma? *Am Rev Respir Dis* 1993; 147: 518–23.

145 Covelli HD, Knodel AR, Keppner BT. Predisposing factors to apparent theophylline-induced seizures. *Ann Allergy* 1985; 54: 411–5.

146 Jusko WJ, Gardner MJ, Mangione A, Schentag JJ, Koup JR, Vance JW. Factors affecting theophylline clearance: age, tobacco, marijuana, cirrhosis, congestive heart failure, obesity, oral contraceptives, benzodiazepines, barbiturate and ethanol. *J Pharm Sci* 1979; 68: 1358–66.

147 Hendeles L, Weinberger M, Szefler SJ. Safety and efficacy of theophylline in children with asthma. *J Pediatr* 1992; 120: 177–83.

148 Derby LE, Jick SS, Langbis JC, Johnson LE, Jick H. Hospital admission for xanthine toxicity. *Pharmacotherapy* 1990; 10: 112–4.

149 Sessler CN. Theophylline toxicity: clinical features of 116 consecutive cases. *Am J Med* 1990; 88: 567–72.

150 Olson KR, Benowitz NL, Woo OF, Pond SM. Theophylline overdose: acute single ingestion versus chronic repeated overmedication. *Am J Emerg Med* 1985; 3: 386–94.

151 Parr MJ, Anaes FC, Day AC, Kletchko SL, Crone PD, Rankin APN. Theophylline poisoning – a review of 64 cases. *Intensive Care Med* 1990; 16: 394–8.

152 Torphy TJ, Undem BJ. Phosphodiesterase inhibitors: new opportunities for the treatment of asthma. *Thorax* 1991; 46: 512–23.

KEY POINTS

1 β₂-Adrenergic drugs relax bronchial smooth muscle through several direct mechanisms and indirectly by suppressing cholinergic traffic. In experimental preparations, they also inhibit mediator release from sensitized lung and inhibit microvascular leakage.

2 The principle of "functional antagonism" applies grossly to β₂ agonists as bronchodilators. The greater the contractile forces, the more β agonist is required to overcome it, providing a rationale for adjusting dose to the severity of bronchospasm.

3   The route of choice is aerosolization. Increasing emphasis is being placed on the metered dose inhaler (MDI), often with a holding chamber, rather than wet nebulization, for reasons of flexibility and economy. Provided anti-inflammatory therapy is in place, titration of dose by MDI is advocated for acute and chronic situations; 400–600 μg by MDI is the equivalent of 2.5 mg by wet nebulization.

4   The ultra-long-acting β_2 agonists, salmeterol and formoterol, usually dosed at 50 and 12–24 μg every 12 hours, respectively, provide 24-hour coverage. The dose can be doubled for more severe asthma. They owe their prolonged action to high lipophilicity and enhanced receptor binding. Salmeterol has a slower onset of action and requires a rapidly acting compound for "rescue" purposes, while formoterol is its own rescue system. Anti-inflammatory therapy must be continued.

5   Anticholinergic drugs such as ipratropium or oxitropium bromide antagonize acetylcholine at the M_3 muscarinic receptor on the muscle membrane and at the M_2 receptor inhibiting adenylyl cyclase activity. While less potent in asthma than β_2 agonists, they still prolong their overall "envelope" of bronchodilation, and are able to add bronchodilation when nebulized in the severe, poorly responsive, acute attack.

6   Theophylline is a non-specific phosphodiesterase inhibitor and adenosine antagonist. Both its useful and toxic actions have steep dose–response curves. Besides adding bronchodilation, it increases respiratory centre output, resists diaphragmatic fatigue and possibly force, and possibly has anti-inflammatory effects.

7   Despite its narrow therapeutic range and variable clearance requiring careful dose adjustment and monitoring, theophylline retains popularity. It finds use in nocturnal asthma and more severe asthmatic patients. While its use is controversial in acute, severe asthma, it may be useful against the fatiguing respiratory muscles in the most severe cases.

8 β_2 Agonists have received recent bad press, largely derived from retrospective epidemiological studies in heavy users and historical controls. Whatever the validity of this approach, anti-inflammatory therapy is the acknowledged cornerstone of asthma treatment. Bronchodilators are nevertheless necessary to treat residual bronchospasm and acute attacks. Prospective studies indicate that chronic β_2-agonist treatment does indeed cause some increase in underlying airway responsiveness to non-specific and inflammatory challenges, and probably a degree of tachyphylaxis. Bronchi removed after fatal asthma attacks show reduced β-adrenergic bronchodilatory response, perhaps due to a combination of inflammatory and drug-induced desensitization. At present, corticosteroids are the best hope for combating these effects as well.

20

DELIVERY SYSTEMS

Graham K. Crompton

Inhaled remedies have been used for many centuries in the treatment of respiratory disorders[1] and bronchodilator aerosols have been used in the treatment of asthma at least since 1935.[2] Various types of inhaler device were used in the early days, many being driven by air generated from a hand-squeezed rubber bulb. The introduction of the pressurized metered dose inhaler (PMDI) in 1956 was a major advance and its popularity with patients and clinicians is reflected by the sales of this device in the decade after its introduction.[3] When corticosteroid therapy became available in the PMDI this allowed topical therapy to replace oral treatment in the majority of adult asthmatic patients – a revolution in the management of asthma in adults. Spacer devices or holding chambers made PMDI therapy available to all but very young children. Dry powder inhalers (DPIs) have provided alternative drug delivery systems and the available choice of PMDI, PMDI plus spacer system or a DPI now makes it possible for the vast majority of patients with reversible airflow limitation to be treated with bronchodilator and anti-inflammatory drugs with inhalation systems they can use efficiently. Nebulizers are less convenient than PMDIs and DPIs, but have an important role in the long-term treatment of some young children, and in the treatment of severe acute asthma.

THE PRESSURIZED METERED DOSE INHALER

The PMDI has been used widely in clinical practice since the early 1960s. It consists of a canister and a plastic actuator. When the canister is depressed into the actuator a measured amount of aerosol is released, which is determined by a valve in the actuator into which the canister nozzle is seated. Within the canister is drug either as a suspension or as a solution with fluorocarbon propellants at a pressure of approximately 3 atm (303 kPa). The canister also contains a dispersant or lubricant to ensure accurate functioning of the valve during the multiple actuations of the inhaler. The aerosol released from the PMDI consists of large droplets of propellant within which the drug is enclosed either as a solid crystal or as a liquid.[4] The propellants evaporate rapidly as soon as they leave the canister and this "flashing" breaks up the liquid stream into droplets that continue to evaporate as they move away from the canister at an initial velocity exceeding 30 m s^{-1}.[5] Because of the high velocity of drug particles, the effects of evaporating propellants and the hygroscopicity of the drug, together with the anatomy of the respiratory tract, the majority of drug impacts in the oropharynx even when a PMDI is used efficiently. Less than 25% of the drug dose reaches the lungs,[6,7] but because all drugs do not possess similar characteristics with regard to hygroscopicity and electrostatic charge the same device will deliver a reproducible amount of the same drug, but it cannot be assumed that a similar proportion of a different drug will reach the intrapulmonary airways. This is also true of dry powder delivery systems.

The most efficient way of using a PMDI is as follows.[8]

(1) Shake the canister thoroughly.

(2) Place the mouthpiece of the actuator between the lips.

(3) Breathe out steadily.

(4) Release the dose while taking a slow, deep breath in.

(5) Hold breath in while counting to 10.

These instructions appear to be simple but many if not the majority of adults cannot use a PMDI efficiently when the only instruction they receive is the manufacturer's package insert.[9-14] Also, more than 10% of patients develop an inefficient inhalation technique simply with continued use of this device,[9,13] the majority of these being those who had difficulty in learning how to use the PMDI initially. The main problem experienced is difficulty in coordinating dose release during an inspiratory manoeuvre,[13] but a significant proportion of patients cannot continue to inhale through the mouth when the propellants are released into the oropharynx ("cold Freon effect"), and it is rarely possible for these patients to overcome this problem. Children and the elderly have the greatest difficulties using the unmodified PMDI efficiently, and attempts to make this device easier to use have been made; the most successful is the development of holding chambers or "spacers" and a modification of the inhaler to make it breath actuated.

SPACERS OR HOLDING CHAMBERS

The droplet size of aerosols released from pressurized inhalers is dependent on the distance from the actuator orifice, a greater distance allowing more evaporation of propellants. It was found that by attaching tubes to the actuator that the total amount of drug lost in the actuator, tube and mouth was reduced.[15] This and subsequent experiments led to the design and development of spacer devices of different sizes. Such devices were found to increase drug availability to the lung and at the same time decrease unwanted drug deposition in the oropharynx,[16,17] although there was considerable initial scepticism about their clinical value.[18] A small-volume extension tube spacer has been shown to improve the efficiency of the PMDI by partially compensating for poor inhalation technique,[19] but large-volume spacers or holding chambers have proved to be of much more clinical value.[16,20-22] A one-way valve at the mouthpiece of large-volume spacer devices enables them to contain the aerosol before inhalation, and although more particles are lost within the spacer more of the aerosol leaving the device is able to penetrate the lungs. This has been shown to be the case with a 750-ml spacer (Nebuhaler) and a smaller device (Aerochamber),[22] but not all large-volume spacers have been shown to increase pulmonary deposition compared with the PMDI.[7] The efficiency of spacer devices in terms of increasing pulmonary deposition of drug is dependent upon a number of factors including their size, the characteristics of the one-way valve, the electrostatic charge of the plastics used to manufacture the device and the drug being discharged from a PMDI into the spacer.

Large-volume spacer devices decrease oropharyngeal deposition of drug and their use is recommended for inhaled steroids,[23,24] to decrease systemic effects and oropharyngeal candidiasis.[25-30] Use of spacers for inhaled corticosteroid treatment does not cause much inconvenience since most patients take these drugs twice daily and do not, therefore, have to carry the spacer with them during the day. However, bulky spacers for as-required bronchodilator therapy are much less convenient and are now rarely used for such treatment unless the patient is unable to use any of the alternative drug delivery systems. Large-volume spacers are now most often used in young children since many are unable to use the conventional PMDI, the breath-actuated PMDI (p. 345) and the dry powder delivery systems (p. 346). In adults their main use is when PMDI corticosteroid therapy has to be used in high dose.[23] They can be used as alternatives to nebulizers in chronic[31] and severe acute asthma.[32] Spacers do not decrease drug available for deposition in the area of the vocal cords and do not therefore protect against inhaled steroid-related dysphonia.[33]

Some Indications for the Use of Large-Volume Spacers

(1) High-dose steroid therapy to decrease oropharyngeal drug deposition and thereby lessen the risk of candidiasis and systemic activity from drug swallowed.

(2) Inability to synchronize dose release from a PMDI with inspiration.

(3) For the administration of high doses of a β-agonist instead of using a nebulizer.

THE BREATH-ACTUATED METERED DOSE INHALER

Attempts have been made to make the conventional PMDI easier to use by making it breath actuated, since the most common problem patients have using this device is coordination of dose release with inspiration.[13] Early models were somewhat clumsy and made a loud click when actuated, and were not successful. The most recently introduced breath-actuated PMDI (Autohaler) has design features that have, in the main, overcome the problems of its predecessors. The canister is completely enclosed within the body of the actuator; there is a latching lever at the top of the inhaler and when this is used to "prime" the device prior to inhalation a blocking system prevents valve actuation. This consists of a vane and a three-component triggering mechanism that is housed between the inhaler valve and the inhaler mouthpiece orifice. When "primed" the valve is actuated by an inspiratory flow of about $30 \, \mathrm{l \, min^{-1}}$.[34] The Autohaler is easier to use than the conventional PMDI[35,36] and can be triggered by patients with severe airflow obstruction.[37]

DISADVANTAGES OF METERED DOSE INHALERS

Problems of coordination of dose release with inspiration can be overcome by the breath-actuated PMDI or a spacer system, and the "cold Freon" effect is not a problem when large-volume spacers are used. However, problems inherent in the basic design of the PMDI have not yet been solved completely. These problems concern the propellants and surfactants/lubricants, which are, of course, essential to allow the device to function. The propellants provide the vehicle in which the drug particles are carried at high velocity from the valve and the surfactant/lubricants are necessary to lubricate the valve and to prevent aggregation of drug particles. The propellants are chlorofluorocarbons (CFCs) and mixtures of two or three of these substances are used to achieve the desired vapour pressure and spray characteristics. There is a numbering system for CFCs that indicates the number of carbon, hydrogen, chlorine and fluorine atoms. The CFCs used in medicinal aerosols are CFC 11, 12 and 114. For many years these were considered to be inert, but in the 1960s their safety was questioned,[38–40] but the majority decision now is that they are safe in the quantities necessary to allow the inhalation of therapeutic doses of drugs.[41–44] However CFCs are now under threat because of their effect on the environment. In the 1980s the ozone "hole" over Antarctica was discovered and in 1987 27 nations agreed in Montreal to reduce hard CFC consumption by 50% by 1999. Subsequently this was seen to be inadequate and in 1989 representatives of over 80 nations agreed, in principle, to eliminate hard CFCs by the end of the century.[45] In certain Western countries this ban has been brought forward to 1995 and in some the ban is already in force, although medical aerosols are exempt. This has stimulated the pharmaceutical industry to find alternative non-CFC propellants for medicinal aerosols and tetrafluoroethane is such a compound undergoing clinical trial. The other clinically important disadvantage of many PMDIs is the irritant effects of some of the presently used lubricants or surfactants. Cough and decrease in ventilatory function have been shown to be produced by these compounds in up to one-third of patients using PMDIs.[46–48] This is an underestimated clinical problem that should be addressed at the same time as CFC replacement.

DRY POWDER INHALERS

Dry powder inhalation systems depend entirely upon the patient's inspiratory effort and are generally easier to use than PMDIs. The first successful dry powder inhaler (Spinhaler) was introduced in 1969 and it was shown subsequently that the majority of patients unable to use the PMDI were able to cope with the Spinhaler.[9] However, this device was available only for the inhalation of sodium cromoglycate, but in the late 1970s the Rotahaler[49] became available for use with salbutamol and beclomethasone dipropionate. Equipotency of the Rotahaler and the PMDI was demonstrated for salbutamol[50–52] and beclomethasone dipropionate[53–55] and a dry powder inhaler for use with fenoterol (Italseber) was also shown to be at least as effective as the PMDI in asthmatic children.[56] The availability of dry powder inhalers for bronchodilator and steroid therapy made inhaled treatment available to a larger population of patients and was generally welcomed.[57,58] However, the first dry powder inhalers were single-dose devices and had to be reloaded with a cartridge/capsule containing micronized drug and a lactose or glucose carrier/vehicle each time they were used. However, they are more convenient than large-volume spacers for bronchodilator therapy since they are small and easy to carry.

The second generation of dry powder inhalers contain many doses and are preferred to single-dose devices by most patients. The Diskhaler/Rotadisk blister system was designed to be equivalent to the Rotahaler/Rotacaps cartridge system in terms of drug delivery both *in vitro* and in clinical practice.[59] The Diskhaler has been found to be equivalent to the Rotahaler with regard to efficacy and safety for both salbutamol and beclomethasone dipropionate.[59] The numbered blisters, arranged within a circular disc, each contain a unit dose of salbutamol, salmeterol, beclomethasone dipropionate or fluticasone propionate. A needle mechanism in the Diskhaler pierces individual blisters making the powder available for inhalation through the mouthpiece. The device is breath actuated and claimed to be efficient at low inspiratory flow rates.[59] When required the next dose is made available as lifting the lid rotates the circular blister pack and allows the needle to pierce another blister. The number of doses remaining in the device is visible through a window on its external surface. When all four or eight blisters have been punctured the device has to be opened so that another Rotadisk can be loaded. The aluminium foil blister packs protect the drug and lactose vehicle against adverse effects of moisture. In a

Glaxo handling study, 70% of patients preferred the Diskhaler to single-dose dry powder devices and 53% of a large number of patients already using a PMDI expressed a preference for the eight-dose Diskhaler.[59]

The Turbuhaler is a 50, 100 or 200 dose dry powder inhaler that has been designed to deliver micronized drug alone.[60] It is loaded in the upright position (45° or more from the horizontal) by rotating the turning grip at the bottom of the device. This action fills a cluster of machined conical holes in a rotating dosing disc, scrapers removing surplus drug as the disc revolves beneath them. The numbers and sizes of holes are tailored for dose and different drugs. The Turbuhaler is breath actuated by the patient breathing in as quickly and as deeply as is comfortable through the mouthpiece after the device is loaded. The inhaler has an in-built resistance to airflow since it has been designed with spiral-shaped channels in the mouthpiece. These create turbulent flow in order to deaggregate drug particles. A dose-indicator window shows when there are 20 or fewer doses remaining in the device. A desiccant is stored in the base of the Turbuhaler to ensure that the interior of the device and the drug powder remain dry. When not being used the inhaler must have its watertight cover screwed back in place to protect it against moisture. The spiral channels in the mouthpiece cause inspiratory flow resistance and an inspiratory flow in excess of $30 \, l \, min^{-1}$ is required for the device to function efficiently.[61] The vast majority of adult patients can generate inspiratory flows of $30 \, l \, min^{-1}$ or more[62] during an episode of acute asthma, and the Turbuhaler has been reported to be as effective as the PMDI used with a large-volume spacer for the administration of terbutaline in the treatment of patients with acute airways obstruction.[63]

Dry powder inhalers are easier to use than the conventional PMDI since they overcome the PMD's main problem of synchronizing dose release with inspiration. In general, dry powder inhalers are preferable to the conventional PMDI[64] because of their ease of use and lack of propellants and additives, except for carriers (vehicles) such as lactose. Carrier powders have large particles that are much in excess of the respirable range and are, therefore, deposited in the upper respiratory tract and only rarely cause any adverse effects such as cough.[50,53,54,65] The dry powder devices are less bulky than spacers and are as easy to use as the breath-actuated PMDI (Autohaler), although some dry powder devices are less convenient because of the need to reload cartridges/capsules or discs frequently. Clinical comparisons of different dry powder devices indicate that patients prefer multidose devices to single-dose inhalers.[66,67] and a meta-analysis of all available studies showed that 58% of 530 patients preferred a multidose dry powder inhaler to the PMDI.[68] The major drawback of dry powder inhalers is that their efficient use depends upon the patient being able to generate sufficient inspiratory flow to allow drug to reach the bronchi in therapeutic amounts. The various dry powder inhalers have different inspiratory resistances but comparisons of intra-pulmonary drug deposition and clinical efficacy of the devices used at different inspiratory flow rates have not been made. Children under the age of 6 years may not be able to generate an inspiratory flow sufficient to use the Turbuhaler; the younger the child the more likely that this is the case.[61] It is known[61] that the Turbuhaler is less efficient when inspiratory flow is below $30 \, l \, min^{-1}$ compared with $60 \, l \, min^{-1}$, and the Rotahaler has only about 10% of its maximum bronchodilator effect at inspiratory flow rates of $40 \, l \, min^{-1}$.[69] Until direct comparisons of all the dry powder devices have been made and data about optimal inspiratory flow rates for the different devices are available it should be assumed that, unlike the PMDI, the most efficient way of using dry powder inhalers is to breathe in from residual volume as quickly and as deeply as possible. There is great need for much more research with dry powder devices,[70] since it cannot be assumed that all have similar characteristics in terms of the proportion of the nominal dose delivered to the target organ, and distribution of drug within the lungs. Compared with the PMDI the Diskhaler is almost 50% less efficient in delivering salbutamol to the lungs and has a pattern of intra-pulmonary deposition similar to that produced by the PMDI without a spacer.[7] According to the manufacturers the Diskhaler was designed to be equivalent to the Rotahaler in terms of drug delivery both *in vitro* and in clinical practice.[59] Distribution of drug and clinical effects of terbutaline sulphate delivered from a Turbuhaler were reported to be similar to those of the PMDI,[71] but more recent studies have found the Turbuhaler to produce a mean lung deposition in the order of twice that of the PMDI with terbutaline[72] and budesonide.[73] Greater efficacy of the Turbuhaler compared with the PMDI is supported by clinical studies of inhaled steroids.[74–76] When dry powder inhalers are used for steroid administration patients should be encouraged to gargle/mouth rinse to decrease systemic effects from drug deposited in the mouth and throat,[77] which can be swallowed and have a varying degree of systemic activity that is dependent on the drug being used.

It is clear that with the proliferation of new delivery systems the clinician has to be aware of major differences in efficacy between inhalers and must not assume that all drug delivery systems are the same in terms of the amount of the nominal dose that is delivered to the target organ and deposited in the oropharynx. This is of particular importance with inhaled steroid therapy since a change of inhaler could decrease or increase the amount of drug available to a patient and therefore lead to inadequate disease control, or on the other hand the systemic consequences of a dose increase.

NEBULIZERS

Nebulizers are of two types: jet and ultrasonic.

JET NEBULIZERS

There are many different makes of jet nebulizer and they have widely differing characteristics with regard to the generation of drug particles within the respirable range (1–10 μm) that can be inhaled and deposited in the lung.[78,79] The performance of individual nebulizers is influenced by many factors such as the flow rate of the driving gas (air or oxygen), the duration of nebulization, the nature of the solution or suspension being nebulized and the amount of liquid in the chamber of the nebulizer.[80–83] For clinical purposes it is essential to at least be aware of the driving gas flow rate at which a nebulizer functions most efficiently.

Jet nebulizers work by compressed air or oxygen entering a chamber in the nebulizer through a narrow tube. The opening of the gas inlet tube meets that of a liquid inlet tube, and a venturi effect produces a pressure drop that causes the liquid to flow and break up into droplets of various sizes. Large droplets impact on baffles and a fine aerosol follows the gas stream out of the nebulizer. An increase in gas pressure used to operate the nebulizer will actually decrease particle size.

ULTRASONIC NEBULIZERS

Ultrasonic nebulizers use high-frequency sound waves produced from a piezoelectric crystal. The vibrations are focused on the surface of the liquid in order to create a fountain from which large and small droplets are emitted. The particle size of the generated aerosol varies, depending on the frequency of the ultrasonic vibrations. In general, ultrasonic nebulizers are less efficient for drug delivery than jet nebulizers.

SOME INDICATIONS FOR THE USE OF NEBULIZERS

(1) Treatment of severe acute asthma with β-agonists and ipratropium bromide in hospital.

(2) Supervised treatment of severe acute asthma in the home by general practitioners.

(3) Treatment of severe acute asthma in ambulances.

(4) Domiciliary treatment of chronic asthma in young children and selected adults with "brittle" asthma.

(5) Domiciliary treatment of selected patients with chronic obstructive airways disease.

(6) Administration of antimicrobial drugs in diseases such as cystic fibrosis, bronchiectasis and AIDS.

(7) Inhalation of hypertonic saline to induce the production of sputum.

REFERENCES

1   Miller WF. Aerosol therapy in acute and chronic disease. *Arch Intern Med* 1973; 131: 148–55.

2   Greaser JB, Rowe AH. Inhalation of epinephrine for relief of asthmatic symptoms. *J Allergy* 1935; 6: 415.

3   Inman WHW, Adelstein AM. Rise and fall of asthma mortality in England and Wales in relation to use of pressurised aerosols. *Lancet* 1969; ii: 279–85.

4   Morén F. Pressurised aerosols for oral inhalation. *Int J Pharm* 1981; 8: 1–10.

5   Newman SP, Clarke SW. Therapeutic aerosols 1 – physical and practical considerations. *Thorax* 1983; 38: 881–6.

6   Newman SP, Morén F, Pavia D, Sheahan NF, Clarke SW. Deposition of pressurised aerosols in the human respiratory tract. *Thorax* 1981; 36: 52–5.

7   Melchor R, Biddiscome MF, Mak VHF, Short MD, Spiro SG. Lung deposition patterns of directly labelled salbutamol in normal subjects and in patients with reversible airflow obstruction. *Thorax* 1993; 48: 506–11.

8   Newman SP, Pavia D, Clarke SW. How should a pressurized β-adrenergic bronchodilator be inhaled? *Eur J Respir Dis* 1981; 62: 3–21.

9   Paterson IC, Crompton GK. Use of pressurised aerosols by asthmatic patients. *BMJ* 1976; 1: 76–7.

10 Orehek J, Gayrard P, Grimaud CH, Charpin J. Patient error in use of bronchodilator metered aerosols. *BMJ* 1976; 1: 76.

11 Epstein SW, Manning CPR, Ashley MJ, Corey PN. Survey of the clinical use of pressurized aerosol inhalers. *Can Med Assoc J* 1979; 120: 813–6.

12 Gayrard P, Orehek J. Inadequate use of pressurized aerosols by asthmatic patients. *Respiration* 1980; 40: 47–52.

13 Crompton GK. Problems patients have using pressurized aerosol inhalers. *Eur J Respir Dis* 1982; 63 (suppl 119): 101–4.

14 de Blaquiere P, Christensen DB, Carter WB, Martin TR. Use and misuse of metered-dose inhalers by patients with chronic lung disease. *Am Rev Respir Dis* 1989; 140: 910–6.

15 Morén F. Drug deposition of pressurized inhalation aerosols 1. Influence of actuator tube design. *Int J Pharm* 1978; 1: 205–12.

16 Lindgren SB, Formgren H, Morén F. Improved aerosol therapy of asthma: effect of actuator tube size on drug availability. *Eur J Respir Dis* 1980; 61: 56–61.

17 Newman SP, Morén F, Pavia D, Little F, Clarke SW. Deposition of pressurized suspension aerosols inhaled through extension devices. *Am Rev Respir Dis* 1981; 124: 317–20.

18 Konig P. Spacer devices used with metered-dose inhalers. Breakthrough or gimmick? *Chest* 1985; 88: 276–84.

19 Bloomfield P, Crompton GK, Winsey NJP. A tube spacer to improve inhalation of drugs from pressurized aerosols. *BMJ* 1979; 2: 1479.

20 Crompton GK. Inhalation devices. *Eur J Respir Dis* 1982; 63: 489–92.

21 Dorow P, Hidinger KG. Terbutaline aerosol from a metered dose inhaler via a 750 ml spacer. Effect on large and small airways. *Eur J Clin Pharmacol* 1982; 22: 511–4.

22 Newman SP, Millar AB, Lennard-Jones TR, Morén F, Clarke SW. Improvement of pressurised aerosol deposition with Nebuhaler spacer device. *Thorax* 1984; 39: 935–41.

23 British Thoracic Society, Research Unit of the Royal College of Physicians of London, King's Fund Centre, National Asthma Campaign. Guidelines on the management of asthma. *Thorax* 1993; 48 (suppl): S1–S24.

24 Sackner MA, Kim CS. Auxiliary MDI aerosol delivery systems. *Chest* 1985; 88 (suppl): 161s–170s.

25 Prahl P, Jensen T. Decreased adreno-cortical suppression utilising the Nebuhaler for inhalation of steroid aerosols. *Clin Allergy* 1987; 17: 393–8.

26 Brown PH, Blundell G, Greening AP, Crompton GK. Do large volume spacer devices reduce the systemic effects of high dose inhaled corticosteroids? *Thorax* 1990; 45: 740–2.

27 Farrer M, Francis AJ, Pearce SJ. Morning serum cortisol concentrations after 2 mg inhaled beclomethasone dipropionate in normal subjects: effect of a 750 ml spacing device. *Thorax* 1990; 45: 740–2.

28 Brown PH, Matusiewicz SP, Shearing C, Tibi L, Greening AP, Crompton GK. Systemic effects of high dose inhaled steroids: comparison of beclomethasone dipropionate and budesonide in healthy subjects. *Thorax* 1993; 48: 967–73.

29 Toogood JH, Jennings B, Baskerville J, Newhouse M. Assessment of a device for reducing oropharyngeal complications during beclomethasone treatment of asthma. *Am Rev Respir Dis* 1981; 123: 113.

30 Toogood JH, Baskerville J, Jennings B, Lefcoe NM, Johansson SA. Use of spacers to facilitate inhaled corticosteroid treatment of asthma. *Am Rev Respir Dis* 1984; 129: 723–9.

31 O'Reilly JF, Buchanan DR, Sudlow MF. Pressurised aerosol with conical spacer is an effective alternative to nebuliser in chronic stable asthma. *BMJ* 1983; 286: 1548.

32 Morgan MDL, Singh BV, Frame MH, Williams SJ. Terbutaline aerosol given through pear spacer in acute severe asthma. *BMJ* 1982; 285: 849–50.

33 Toogood JH, Jennings B, Baskerville J, Johansson SA. Clinical use of spacer systems for corticosteroid inhalation therapy: a preliminary analysis. *Eur J Respir Dis* 1982; 63 (suppl 62): 100–7.

34 Baum EA, Bryant AM. The development and laboratory testing of a novel breath-actuated pressurised inhaler. *J Aerosol Med* 1988; 1: 219–20.

35 Crompton G, Duncan J. Clinical assessment of a new breath-actuated inhaler. *Practitioner* 1989; 233: 268–9.

36 Newman SP, Weisz AWB, Talaee N, Clarke SW. Improvement of drug delivery with a breath actuated pressurised aerosol for patients with poor inhaler technique. *Thorax* 1991; 46: 712–6.

37 Fergusson RJ, Lenny J, McHardy GJR, Crompton GK. The use of a new breath-actuated inhaler by patients with severe airflow obstruction. *Eur Respir J* 1991; 4: 172–4.

38 Speizer FE, Doll R, Heaf P. Observations on recent increase in mortality from asthma. *BMJ* 1968; 1: 339–43.

39 Speizer FE, Wegman DH, Ramirez A. Palpitation rates associated with fluorocarbon exposure in a hospital setting. *N Engl J Med* 1975; 292: 624–6.

40 Bass M. Sudden sniffing death. *JAMA* 1970; 212: 2075–9.

41 Dollery CT, Williams FM, Draffan GH *et al.* Arterial blood levels of fluorocarbons in asthmatics following the use of pressurized aerosols. *Clin Pharmacol Ther* 1974; 15: 59–66.

42 Thompson PJ, Dhillon P, Cole P. Addiction to aerosol treatment: the asthmatic alternative to glue sniffing. *BMJ* 1983; 287: 1515.

43 Brennan PO. Addiction to aerosol treatment. *BMJ* 1983; 287: 1877.

44 O'Callaghan C, Milner AD. Aerosol treatment abuse. *Arch Dis Child* 1988; 63: 70.

45 Newman SP. Metered dose pressurized aerosols and the ozone layer. *Eur Respir J* 1990; 3: 495–7.

46 Yarbrough J, Mansfield L, Ting S. Metered dose inhaler induced bronchospasm in asthmatic patients. *Ann Allergy* 1985; 55: 25–7.

47 Shim CS, Williams MH. Cough and wheezing from beclomethasone dipropionate aerosol are absent after triamcinalone acetonide. *Ann Intern Med* 1987; 106: 700–3.

48 Williamson I, Matusiewicz S, Brown P, Crompton G, Greening AP. Frequency of voice problems and cough in patients using aerosol steroid preparations. *Thorax* 1991; 46: 769P.

49 Hallworth GW. An improved design of powder inhaler. *Br J Clin Pharmacol* 1977; 4: 689–90.

50 Duncan D, Paterson IC, Harris D, Crompton GK. Comparison of the bronchodilator effects of salbutamol inhaled as a dry powder and by conventional pressurised aerosol. *Br J Clin Pharmacol* 1977; 4: 669–71.

51 Hetzel MR, Clark TJH. Comparison of salbutamol Rotahaler with conventional pressurized aerosol. *Clin Allergy* 1977; 7: 563–8.

52 Hartley JPR, Nogrady SG, Gibby OM, Seaton A. Bronchodilator effects of dry salbutamol powder administered by Rotahaler. *Br J Clin Pharmacol* 1977; 4: 673–5.

53 Carmichael J, Duncan D, Crompton GK. Beclomethasone dipropionate dry-powder inhalation compared with conventional aerosol in chronic asthma. *BMJ* 1978; 2: 657–8.

54 Morrison Smith J, Gwynn CM. A clinical comparison of aerosol and powder administration of beclomethasone dipropionate in asthma. *Clin Allergy* 1978; 8: 479–81.

55 Edmunds AT, McKenzie S, Tooley M, Godfrey S. A clinical comparison of beclomethasone dipropionate delivered by pressurised aerosol and as a powder from a Rotahaler. *Arch Dis Child* 1979; 54: 233–5.

56 Chambers S, Dunbar J, Taylor B. Inhaled powder compared with aerosol administration of fenoterol in asthmatic children. *Arch Dis Child* 1980; 55: 73–4.

57 Crompton GK. Inhalation devices. *Eur J Respir Dis* 1982; 63: 489–92.

58 Croner S, Hedenskog NI, Odelram H. Salbutamol by powder or spray inhalation in childhood asthma. *Allergy* 1980; 35: 589–92.

59 Meldrum L, Wheeler AWE, Huskisson SC, Palmer JBD. International Diskhaler Handling Study STC 406, Glaxo Group Research Ltd, Greenford, Middlesex, UK.

60 Wetterlin K. Turbuhaler: a new powder inhaler for administration of drugs to the airways. *Pharm Res* 1988; 5: 506–8.

61 Pedersen S, Hansen OR, Fugsland G. Influence of inspiratory flow rate upon the effect of a Turbuhaler. *Arch Dis Child* 1990; 65: 308–10.

62 Brown PH, Greening AP, Crompton GK. Peak inspiratory flow rates in acute asthma: are they adequate for efficient use of a Turbuhaler? *Thorax* 1992; 47: 239P.

63 Tonnesen F, Laursen LC, Ibsen T, Evald T, St Åhl E. Terbutaline powder in acute bronchial obstruction. *Lancet* 1991; 337: 1099–100.

64 Crompton GK. New inhalation devices. *Eur Respir J* 1988; 1: 679–80.

65 Brown PH, Lenney J, Armstrong S, Ning ACWS, Crompton G. Breath-actuated inhalers in chronic asthma: comparison of Diskhaler and Turbuhaler for delivery of beta-agonists. *Eur Respir J* 1992; 5: 1143–5.

66 Anani A, Higgins AJ, Crompton GK. Breath-actuated inhalers; comparison of terbutaline Turbuhaler with salbutamol Rotahaler. *Eur Respir J* 1989; 2: 640–2.

67 Stallaert RALM. The Bricanyl Turbuhaler, efficacy and acceptability compared to the Ventolin Rotahaler. Abstract, XIII International Congress of Allergy and Clinical Immunology, Montreux, October 1988.

68 Sinninghe Damsté HEJ. Turbuhaler – a clinical overview. In: *Turbuhaler – a non-CFC metered dose inhaler.* Report of a symposium held at the 8th Congress of the International Society for Aerosols in Medicine, Davos, Switzerland, April 1991. Amsterdam: Excerpta Medica, 1992: 12–3.

69 Pedersen S. How to use a Rotahaler. Arch Dis Child 1986; 61: 11–4.

70 Richards R, Saunders M. Need for a comparative performance standard for dry powder inhalers. Thorax 1993; 48: 1186–7.

71 Newman SP, Morén F, Trofast E, Talaee N, Clarke SW. Deposition and clinical efficacy of terbutaline sulphate from Turbuhaler, a new multi-dose powder inhaler. Eur Respir J 1989; 2: 247–52.

72 Pauwels R, Derom E. Deposition and pharmacodynamics of terbutaline inhaled via Turbuhaler. J Aerosol Med 1991; 4 (suppl 1): A187.

73 Thorsson L, Edsbäcker S. Lung deposition of budesonide from Turbuhaler is twice that from a pressurised metered dose inhaler (MDI). Thorax 1993; 4: 434.

74 Brambilla C, Braunstein G, Lacronique J, Allaert F, Godard P, Duroux P. Comparison between beclomethasone dipropionate by metered dose inhaler and budesonide by Turbuhaler in asthmatic adults. Am Rev Respir Dis 1992; 145: A737.

75 Engel T, Heinig JH, Malling H-J, Scharling B, Nikander K, Madsen F. Clinical comparison of inhaled budesonide delivered either via pressurized metered dose inhaler or Turbuhaler. Allergy 1989; 44: 220–5.

76 Sinninghe Damsté HEJ, Oostinga P, Heeringa A. Clinical comparison of inhaled budesonide administered via a pressurized metered dose inhaler or via Turbuhaler in patients with bronchial asthma. Eur Respir J 1989; 2: (suppl 8): 861s.

77 Selroos O, Halme M. Effect of a Volumatic spacer and mouth rinsing on systemic absorption of inhaled corticosteroids from a metered dose inhaler and dry powder inhaler. Thorax 1991; 46: 891–4.

78 Hardy JG, Newman SP, Knoch M. Lung deposition from four nebulisers. Respir Med 1993; 87: 461–5.

79 Thomas SHL, O'Doherty MJ, Graham A *et al.* Pulmonary deposition of nebulised amiloride in cystic fibrosis: comparison of two nebulisers. Thorax 1991; 46: 717–21.

80 Clay MM, Pavia D, Newman SP, Clarke SW. Factors influencing the size distribution of aerosols from jet nebulisers. Thorax 1983; 38: 755–9.

81 Clay MM, Pavia D, Newman SP, Lennard-Jones T, Clarke SW. Assessment of jet nebulisers for lung aerosol therapy. Lancet 1983; ii: 592–4.

82 Newman SP, Pellow PGD, Clarke SW. The flow–pressure characteristics of compressors used for inhalation therapy. Eur J Respir Dis 1987; 71: 122–6.

83 DHSS. Health Equipment Information. An evaluation of powdered nebulisers. Department of Health and Social Security. HEI No 180, February 1988.

KEY POINTS

1 The pressurized metered dose inhaler has been in clinical use for over 30 years. Only about 50% of adult patients can use it efficiently if the only tuition they have is reading the manufacturer's instruction pamphlet.

2 The main problem patients have using a pressurized metered dose inhaler is coordinating dose-release with inhalation. Some patients cannot continue to breathe in after the dose has been released into the mouth because of the sensation produced by the propellant (cold Freon effect).

3 The most important manoeuvre in the use of a pressurized metered dose inhaler is release of the dose during a slow inspiration.

4 Spacer devices (holding chambers) overcome the problem of coordinating dose-release with inhalation, decrease oropharyngeal deposition and increase pulmonary deposition of drug. Spacer devices can be used by the vast majority of patients except for very young children.

5 Dry powder inhaler devices are dependent upon the patient's inspiratory effort. The inspiratory flow required for the efficient use of each device is different. The best compromise instruction for the use of all dry powder devices is to breathe out fully and then breathe in through the inhaler as quickly as is possible for as long as possible.

6 In general dry powder devices are easier to use than the conventional metered dose inhaler.

7 Dry powder inhalers: an inspiratory flow of at least 30 l min^{-1} is required for the efficient use of dry powder inhalers such as the Turbuhaler and Rotahaler. Young children are unlikely to be able to achieve such an inspiratory flow.

8 Nebulizers: for most clinical purposes jet nebulizers are more efficient than ultrasonic.

9 The performance of jet nebulizers is affected by a number of factors. The clinician should at least be familiar with the optimal gas flow rates of nebulizers.

21

IMMUNOTHERAPY

S.R. Durham

Immunotherapy involves the subcutaneous injection of increasing concentrations of an allergen extract followed by "maintenance" injections for several years. The aim is to induce a state of immunological and clinical tolerance with a marked reduction (or absence) of clinical symptoms following subsequent natural allergen exposure. The approach is logical and complementary to allergen avoidance strategies. Thus both depend upon an accurate clinical and immunological diagnosis of the cause of symptoms (generally obtained from the clinical history and allergen skin-prick tests) and attempt to alleviate symptoms through either elimination of the cause or modification of the host response to that cause. However, in assessing the potential value of immunotherapy, efficacy must be balanced against side-effects.

Although widely practised in the USA and Europe, the use of immunotherapy in the UK has diminished markedly following a report in 1986 by the Committee on Safety of Medicines.[1] The report questioned the safety of this form of therapy in the UK. A recent position paper of the British Society of Allergy and Clinical Immunology[2] concluded that immunotherapy was indicated in patients with severe seasonal rhinitis unresponsive to pharmacological treatments but not indicated in patients with asthma because evidence for efficacy was less convincing and the risk of side-effects was greater in asthmatic subjects. The International Guidelines on Asthma Management[3] suggest that specific immunotherapy may be indicated in asthmatic subjects with clearly defined allergies when avoiding allergens is not possible and when medications fail to control symptoms. The position paper of the European Academy of Allergy and Immunology[4] similarly advocates cautious use of immunotherapy for rhinitis and asthma. In this chapter the role of allergen immunotherapy is considered for rhinitis and asthma separately and an attempt made to balance efficacy with side-effects. Possible mechanisms of immunotherapy are considered in the context of future improvements in this form of treatment.

IMMUNOTHERAPY FOR RHINITIS

Seasonal allergic rhinitis in the UK is most commonly due to allergy to grass pollen, although symptoms during the spring may be due to tree pollens whereas late summer and early autumn coincide with symptoms induced by weeds and mould spores.[5] Avoidance of pollen allergens is difficult, although simple advice such as wearing sunglasses and keeping windows tight shut in cars and buildings may be helpful. Recent advances in treatment include the availability of topical nasal corticosteroids and oral H_1-selective antihistamines with a low sedative profile.[6] Despite these measures a small proportion of patients may have persistent symptoms. It is this group of patients who may benefit from pollen immunotherapy. Double-blind placebo-controlled trials have shown that immunotherapy is effective in patients with seasonal pollinosis due to grass pollen.[7-10] In one study[10] 40 patients with severe symptoms uncontrolled by conventional anti-allergic drugs were treated with a biologically standardized alum-precipitated depot grass pollen extract (or matched placebo injections). There was a marked reduction in both seasonal symptoms and the use of rescue medication (Fig. 21.1). Systemic side-effects were infrequent (1 in 500 injections), occurred within 10 min of injection and responded promptly to adrenaline. Further controlled studies have shown that immunotherapy with birch pollen,[11] ragweed[12] and mould allergens[13] may also be effective for rhinitis in carefully selected patients. Perennial rhinitis due to house-dust mite allergy may require long-term use of topical and oral medications. Several studies of mite immunotherapy have shown efficacy.[14-16] One study that involved use of an aqueous extract was efficacious, although provoked frequent systemic reactions.[14] A standardized depot extract of *Dermatophagoides pteronyssinus* was efficacious (although less so) and did not result in systemic reactions.[15]

Only one study has compared the efficacy of immunotherapy for allergic rhinitis with pharmacotherapy.[17] Treatment with an aqueous topical corticosteroid nasal spray was more effective than treatment with a poorly standardized low-potency ragweed extract. With regard to long-term efficacy, an uncontrolled trial of immunotherapy for tree pollen allergy suggested clinical improvement was maintained for 6 years after discontinuation of treatment.[18] A previous controlled open study in children which employed crude extracts of allergens suggested that immunotherapy for rhinitis in this age group may reduce the frequency of development of asthma.[19] No firm conclusions can be drawn and clearly further studies employing modern biologically standardized extracts are required.

IMMUNOTHERAPY FOR ASTHMA

The role of immunotherapy for asthma is controversial. Asthma is frequently multifactorial and only occasionally due to sensitivity to a single

FIGURE 21.1: *Average weekly grass pollen counts (1989) (a), and symptom (b) and drug (c) scores for Alutard SQ (●) and placebo (○) groups. Arrows represent the beginning (15 May) and end (25 July) of pollen season. (From Varney VA et al. BMJ 1991; 302: 265–9, with permission.)*

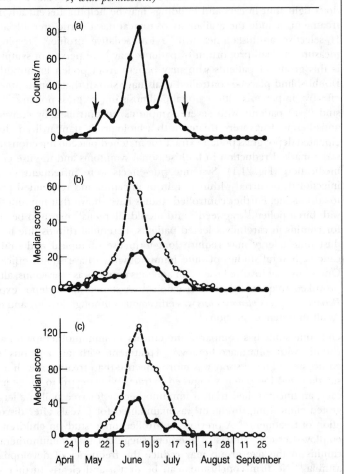

inhaled aeroallergen. The exception is grass pollen-induced asthma where several studies have confirmed that injection immunotherapy is effective in reducing asthma symptoms and treatment requirements.[8,9,20,21] Studies of immunotherapy in asthmatic patients with house-dust mite sensitivity have produced conflicting results.[22–27] Several studies did not show benefit[22,25,26] although, at least in one study,[25] the total dose of mite allergen administered was low. Mite immunotherapy appears to be more effective in children, where two double-blind trials[23,24] have shown an improvement in terms of reduced treatment requirements and inhibition of late asthmatic responses following bronchial provocation.

Immunotherapy in patients with cat-induced asthma have in general focused on the results of bronchial provocation tests,[28,29] which may or may not relate to clinical efficacy. The immediate asthmatic response after bronchial challenge has been reduced. One study demonstrated a decrease in asthma symptoms after exposure to cats.[30] A major problem in considering the role of immunotherapy for asthma is that no comparative studies of immunotherapy with pharmacotherapy have been performed.

IMMUNOTHERAPY IN CHILDREN

Immunotherapy appears to have a greater beneficial effect in children than adults. This is clearly demonstrated in asthmatic children with house-dust mite allergy. The arbitrary cut-off age below which immunotherapy is not recommended has been set at 5 years. The majority of trials of immunotherapy in children have focused on asthma and allergic rhinoconjunctivitis tends to be less prominent in this age group. However, there is a tendency for spontaneous improvement in childhood and further, more prolonged, controlled trials of immunotherapy are required.

SAFETY

Adverse reactions to allergen immunotherapy may occasionally occur. These range from large immediate or delayed skin responses to immediate life-threatening anaphylaxis. Delayed systemic reactions are far less common, in general taking the form of rhinitis, urticaria or lethargy. In patients with asthma delayed bronchospasm may occur. This is important and in all countries immunotherapy guidelines recommend a period of observation following allergen injections. Anaphylaxis, although relatively rare, almost always occurs within minutes, is easily identifiable and responds promptly to treatment with adrenaline. In contrast asthmatic patients, particularly those with unstable or poorly controlled asthma, are susceptible to the development of delayed bronchospasm, which may occur after the patient has left the clinic and in the absence of medical supervision and treatment. This represents the major objection to allergen immunotherapy for asthma. In 1986 the report by the British Committee on Safety of Medicines[1] identified 26 fatalities over the previous 30 years following allergen immunotherapy in the UK. In the 17 patients in whom the indication for injection immunotherapy was known, 16 of these patients received immunotherapy for treatment of asthma (i.e. not rhinitis). Similarly, recent reports from the USA[31,32] have revealed that between 1987 and 1991 there were 19 deaths associated with immunotherapy, of which at least 16 occurred in patients with asthma. Thus patients with asthma are at greater risk of developing life-threatening systemic reactions.

MECHANISM OF IMMUNOTHERAPY

The mechanism by which immunotherapy reduces symptoms on re-exposure to allergen are largely unknown. In patients with seasonal pollinosis, there is an initial increase in allergen-specific IgE concentrations. IgE concentrations subsequently return to baseline, although there is a blunting of the usual seasonal increases in IgE during natural pollen exposure.[33] The "blocking antibody theory" is based on the consistent finding of elevated IgG_4 concentrations.[34,35] However these changes in serum antibody concentrations do not appear to be related to the clinical response and may possibly represent a "bystander effect" following exposure to high concentrations of allergen during injection immunotherapy. Immunotherapy has also been shown to reduce effector cells including mast cells[36,37] and eosinophils[38,39] in the target organ. The mechanism of immunotherapy may relate to its ability to inhibit allergen-induced late responses.[10,40] For example, ragweed immunotherapy reduced eosinophils in nasal washings following allergen challenge in a dose-dependent manner according to the total dose of allergen given during immunotherapy.[38] More recent studies have focused on the role of the T lymphocyte in orchestrating local mast cell migration, tissue eosinophilia and local IgE regulation.[10] For example, successful grass pollen immunotherapy was associated with a decrease in the late cutaneous response and a decrease in infiltrating CD4+ T lymphocytes and activated eosinophils in late cutaneous biopsies following intradermal allergen. *In situ* hybridization studies of both cutaneous and nasal biopsies have suggested that there may be a change in the profile of cytokines produced by infiltrating T lymphocytes in favour of a "T_{H1} type" response with increase in local production of interferon-γ. This may reflect the development of T-lymphocyte tolerance as observed during *in vitro* studies of immunological tolerance induction.[41,42] The above work suggests alternative approaches to immunotherapy. For example, immunosuppressive therapy using cyclosporin A has recently been shown to be effective in patients with severe asthma.[43] An alternative strategy may be the use of anti-CD4 monoclonal antibodies, an approach that has been used in rheumatoid disease.[44] Antibodies or antagonists directed against specific cytokines, particularly interleukin (IL)-4, and IL-5 may possibly be effective.[45,46] An interesting possibility is the development of peptides that recognize sensitized T lymphocytes but do not bind IgE.[47] These so-called non-stimulatory peptides may have the potential to modify T-lymphocyte function without provoking IgE-mediated mast cell activation. The risk of anaphylaxis and other IgE-mediated side-effects might thereby be markedly reduced.

CONCLUSIONS

When considering allergen injection immunotherapy the benefits, side-effects, cost and duration of symptomatic treatment and patient preference must be balanced against those of immunotherapy. At present immunotherapy is recommended in the UK in patients with seasonal allergic rhinitis who fail to respond to treatment with topical corticosteroids and antihistamines.[2] In Europe, pollen immunotherapy is considered an adjunct to drug therapy and is introduced earlier.[4] Although immunotherapy for perennial rhinitis due to mite sensitivity is effective, further studies using standardized vaccines should be performed in order to monitor safety and identify safe protocols.

Allergen immunotherapy is a controversial treatment for asthma. It has been shown to be efficacious in pollen asthma and, particularly, mite asthma in children. The efficacy of immunotherapy has not been compared with pharmacological treatment. In view of the potential for serious side-effects, immunotherapy is not currently indicated for the treatment of asthma.

Immunotherapy should only be performed with standardized extracts of proven efficacy and in specialist centres with the availability of resuscitation measures.

REFERENCES

1   Committee on the Safety of Medicines. CSM update: Desensitizing vaccines. *BMJ* 1986; 293: 948.

2   Position Paper on Allergen Immunotherapy. Report of a BSACI Working Party. *Clin Exp Allergy* 1993; 23 (suppl 3): 1–44.

3   International Consensus Report on Diagnosis and Treatment of Asthma. National Heart, Lung, and Blood Institute, National Institutes of Health, Bethesda, Maryland 20892, USA, 1992; Publication No. 92-3091: 1–72.

4   Malling HV, Weeke B. Immunotherapy. European Academy of Allergy and Immunology position paper. *Allergy* 1993; 48 (suppl 14): 1–35.

5   Varney V. Hayfever in the United Kingdom. *Clin Exp Allergy* 1991; 21: 757–62.

6   Naclerio RM. Allergic rhinitis. *N Engl J Med* 1991; 325: 860–9.

7   Frankland AW, Augustin R. Prophylaxis of summer hayfever and asthma. A controlled trial comparing crude grass pollen extracts with the isolated main protein component. *Lancet* 1954; i: 1055–7.

8   Bousquet J, Maasch HJ, Hejjaoui A *et al.* Double blind placebo-controlled immunotherapy with mixed grass pollen allergoids. III. Efficacy and safety of unfractionated and high molecular weight preparations in rhinoconjunctivitis and asthma. *J Allergy Clin Immunol* 1989; 84: 546–56.

9   Bousquet J, Hejjaoui A, Soussana M, Michel FB. Double-blind placebo-controlled immunotherapy with mixed grass pollen allergoids. IV. Comparison of the safety of two dosages of a high molecular weight allergoid. *J Allergy Clin Immunol* 1990; 85: 490–7.

10   Varney VA, Hamid QA, Gaga M *et al.* Influence of grass pollen immunotherapy on cellular infiltration and cytokine mRNA expression during allergen-induced late-phase cutaneous responses. *J Clin Invest* 1993; 92: 644–51.

11   Viander M, Koivikko A. The seasonal symptoms of hyposensitized and untreated hayfever patients in relation to birch pollen counts: correlations with nasal sensitivity, prick tests and RAST. *Clin Allergy* 1978; 8: 387–96.

12   Lichtenstein LM, Norman PS, Winkenwerder WL. A single year of immunotherapy for ragweed hayfever: immunologic and clinical studies. *Ann Intern Med* 1971; 75: 663–71.

13   Malling HJ, Dreborg S, Weeke B. Diagnosis and immunotherapy of mould allergy. V. Clinical efficacy and side effects of immunotherapy with *Cladosporium herbarum*. *Allergy* 1986; 41: 507–19.

14   Ewan PW, Alexander MM, Snape C, Ind PW, Agrell B. Effective hyposensitization in allergic rhinitis using a potent partially purified extract of house dust mite. *Clin Allergy* 1988; 18: 501–8.

15   Corrado OJ, Pastorello E, Ollier S *et al.* A double-blind study of hyposensitization with an alginate conjugated extract of *D. pteronyssinus* "Conjuvac" in patients with perennial rhinitis. *Allergy* 1989; 44: 108–15.

16   McHugh SM, Lavelle B, Kemeny DM, Patel S, Ewan PW. A placebo-controlled trial of immunotherapy with two extracts of *D. pteronyssinus* in allergic rhinitis, comparing clinical outcome with changes in antigen-specific IgE, IgG and IgG subclasses. *J Allergy Clin Immunol* 1990; 86: 521–32.

17   Juniper EF, Kline PA, Ramsdale EH, Hargreave FE. Comparison of the efficacy and side effects of aqueous steroid nasal spray (budesonide) and allergen-injection immunotherapy (Pollinex-R) in the treatment of seasonal allergic rhinoconjunctivitis. *J Allergy Clin Immunol* 1990; 85: 606–11.

18   Mosbech H, Osterballe O. Does the effect of immunotherapy last after termination of treatment? Follow-up study in patients with grass pollen rhinitis. *Allergy* 1988; 43: 523–9.

19 Johnstone DE, Dutton A. The value of hyposensitization therapy for bronchial asthma in children. A 14 year study. *Pediatrics* 1968; 42: 793.

20 Bousquet J, Hejjaoui A, Michel FB. Specific immunotherapy in asthma. *J Allergy Clin Immunol* 1990; 86: 292–305.

21 Reid MJ, Moss RB, Yao-Pi Hsa MS, Kwasnicki JC, Commerford TM, Nelson BL. Seasonal asthma in northern California. Allergic causes and efficacy of immunotherapy. *J Allergy Clin Immunol* 1986; 78: 590–600.

22 Gaddie J, Skinner C, Palmer KNV. Hyposensitization with house dust mite vaccine in bronchial asthma. *BMJ* 1976; 2: 561–2.

23 Warner JO, Price JF, Soothill JF, Hey EN. Controlled trial of hyposensitization to *Dermatophagoides pteronyssinus* in children with asthma. *Lancet* 1978; ii: 912–5.

24 Price JF, Warner JO, Hey EN, Turner MW, Soothill JF. A controlled trial of hyposensitization with tyrosine-absorbed *Dermatophagoides pteronyssinus* antigen in childhood asthma. *In vivo* aspects. *Clin Allergy* 1984; 14: 209–19.

25 British Thoracic Association. A trial of house dust mite extract in bronchial asthma. *Br J Dis Chest* 1979; 73: 260–70.

26 Pauli G, Bessot JC, Bigot H *et al.* Clinical and immunologic evaluation of hyposensitization with tyrosine-absorbed *Dermatophagoides pteronyssinus* extract: a double-blind placebo-controlled trial. *Clin Allergy* 1984; 14: 209–19.

27 Bousquet J, Calvagvac P, Guérin B *et al.* Immunotherapy with standardized *Dermatophagoides pteronyssinus* extract: I. *In vivo* and *in vitro* parameters after a short course of immunotherapy. *J Allergy Clin Immunol* 1985; 76: 734–44.

28 Sundin B, Lilja G, Graff-Lonnevig V *et al.* Immunotherapy with partially purified and standardized animal dander extracts. 1. Clinical results from a double-blind study on patients with animal dander asthma. *J Allergy Clin Immunol* 1986; 77: 478–87.

29 van Metre TE, Marsh DG, Adkinson NF *et al.* Immunotherapy for cat asthma. *J Allergy Clin Immunol* 1988; 82: 1053–8.

30 Ohman JL, Findlay SR, Leitermann KM. Immunotherapy in cat-induced asthma. Double-blind trial with evaluation of *in vivo* and *in vitro* responses. *J Allergy Clin Immunol* 1984; 74: 230–9.

31 Reid MJ, Lockey RF, Turkeltaub PC, Platts-Mills TAE. Fatalities from immunotherapy and skin testing (abstract). *J Allergy Clin Immunol* 1990; 85: 180.

32 Reid MJ, Lockey RF, Turkeltaub PC, Platts-Mills TAE, Lehrer SB. Fatalities from immunotherapy 1990–91. *J Allergy Clin Immunol* 1992; 89: abstract no. 823.

33 Lichtenstein LM, Ishizaka K, Norman PS, Sobotka AK, Hill BM. IgE antibody measurements in ragweed hayfever. Relationship to clinical severity and the results of immunotherapy. *J Clin Invest* 1973; 52: 472–82.

34 Djurup R. The subclass nature and clinical significance of the IgG antibody response in patients undergoing allergen specific immunotherapy. *Allergy* 1985; 40: 469–86.

35 Creticos P, van Metre TE, Mardingley MR, Rosenberg GL, Adkinson NF. Dose–response of IgE and IgG antibodies during ragweed immunotherapy. *J Allergy Clin Immunol* 1984; 73: 94–104.

36 Creticos P, Adkinson NF, Kagey-Sobotka A *et al.* Nasal challenge with ragweed pollen in hayfever patients. Effect of immunotherapy. *J Clin Invest* 1985; 76: 2247–53.

37 Otsuka H, Mezawa A, Ohnishi M, Okubo K, Seki H, Okuda M. Changes in nasal metachromatic cells during allergen immunotherapy. *Clin Exp Allergy* 1991; 21: 115–9.

38 Furin MJ, Norman PS, Creticos PS *et al.* Immunotherapy decreases antigen-induced eosinophil migration into the nasal cavity. *J Allergy Clin Immunol* 1991; 88: 27–32.

39 Rak S, Lowhägen O, Venge P. The effect of immunotherapy on bronchial hyperresponsiveness and eosinophil cationic protein in pollen allergic patients. *J Allergy Clin Immunol* 1988; 82: 470–80.

40 Fling JA, Ruff ME, Parker WA *et al.* Suppression of the late cutaneous response by immunotherapy. *J Allergy Clin Immunol* 1989; 83: 101–9.

41 O'Hehir RE, Yssel H, Verma S, de Vries JE, Spits H, Lamb JR. Clonal analysis of differential lymphokine production in peptide and superantigen induced T cell anergy. *Int Immunol* 1991; 3: 819–26.

42 Lake RA, O'Hehir RE, Verhoef A, Lamb JR. CD28 mRNA rapidly decays when activated T cells are functionally energized with specific peptide. *Int Immunol* 1993; 5: 461–6.

43 Alexander A, Barnes NC, Kay AB. Trial of cyclosporin in corticosteroid-dependent chronic severe asthma. *Lancet* 1993; 339: 324–8.

44 Herzog C, Walker C, Müllert E *et al.* Anti-CD4 antibody treatment of patients with rheumatoid arthritis. I. Effect on clinical course and circulating T cells. *J Autoimmun* 1989; 2: 627–42.

45 Fanslow WC, Clifford KN, Rubin AS, Voice RF, Beckman MP, Widmer MB. Regulation of alloreactivity *in vivo* by IL-4 and the soluble IL-4 receptor. *J Immunol* 1991; 147: 535–40.

46 Chand N, Harrison JE, Rooney S *et al.* Anti-IL-5 monoclonal antibody inhibits allergic late phase bronchial eosinophilia in guinea pigs: a therapeutic approach. *Eur J Pharmacol* 1992; 211: 121–3.

47 O'Hehir RE, Busch R, Rothbard JB, Lamb JR. An *in vitro* model of peptide-mediated immunomodulation of the human T cell response to *Dermatophagoides* spp. (house dust mite). *J Allergy Clin Immunol* 1990; 87: 1120–7.

KEY POINTS

1   Allergen injection immunotherapy retains a place in treatment of seasonal allergic rhinitis unresponsive to anti-allergic drugs. The use of immunotherapy for asthma is controversial in view of attendant increased risks.

2   Patients with asthma are at greater risk of developing life-threatening systemic reactions to allergen injection immunotherapy.

3   Important issues for future research include the influence of immunotherapy in modifying disease progression, the evaluation of different immunotherapy protocols in terms of efficacy and safety, the optimum duration of immunotherapy and evaluation of factors contributing to adverse reactions.

22

OTHER FORMS OF TREATMENT

R. Bhagat and D.W. Cockcroft

INTRODUCTION

This chapter is a brief review of several treatment modalities (pharmacological, surgery and "alternative"; Table 22.1) that have limited, uncertain or unproven value in the specific management of asthma. Some of these (e.g. exercise, yoga) may improve general well-being.

TABLE 22.1: *Other forms of treatment*

Treatment	Efficacy
Pharmacological	
Calcium channel blockers	Slight (however "safe" vs. β blockers)
Diuretics (inhaled)	Slight
Magnesium	Slight
Mucolytics	Controversial (may cause bronchospasm)
α-Adrenergic agonists	Limited
Immunoglobulins	Uncertain
Surgery	Not recommended
Alternative	
Acupuncture	Limited
Homoeopathy	Probably nil
Yoga	Indirect benefit
Hypnosis	Selected cases
Ionizers	Nil

PHARMACOLOGICAL

CALCIUM CHANNEL BLOCKERS

Calcium is involved in excitation–contraction coupling of muscles and release of mediators/secretions from cells.[1-3] These processes are affected by intracellular, membrane-bound and extracellular calcium levels. The regulation of calcium levels is assisted by two types of cell membrane calcium channels, voltage-dependent and receptor-operated channels. The voltage-dependent channels, which open in response to a wave of rapid depolarization, are found predominantly in smooth muscles of arteries and are blocked by currently available calcium blockers.[4,5]

Several trials have used calcium channel blockers in asthmatic subjects.[6-25] Results have been variable and not encouraging after acute or chronic administration prior to histamine, methacholine and allergen challenges.[11-25] However, there has been some success in prevention of exercise-induced bronchospasm.[6-8,13,15] Although there is evidence for presence of voltage-dependent channels in the airway smooth muscles,[26] the relative inability of calcium blockers to prevent asthma[6-25] indicates that some other mechanism, probably receptor-operated channels, may play a significant role.[27,28] More specific calcium channel blockers are sought.[29]

The most important conclusion is that calcium channel blockers (unlike β-adrenergic blockers) can be safely used for other indications in asthmatic subjects.

DIURETICS

Inhaled furosemide inhibits bronchoconstriction induced by adenosine monophosphate,[30,31] cold air hyperventilation[32] and exercise;[33] however, methacholine PC_{20} is unaltered.[32,34] Further, inhaled furosemide has been shown to protect against allergen-induced early and late asthmatic responses.[34] These effects are not seen with oral or intravenous furosemide.[33] The absence of similar responses with bumetanide,[30,31] a stronger Na^+,K^+-ATPase inhibitor, suggests an alternative mechanism. Acetazolamide, a carbonic anhydrase inhibitor, has also been shown to reduce cold air hyperventilation-induced bronchoconstriction.[35] The clinical implications of these effects compared with other asthma medications requires further evaluation.

MAGNESIUM

During an episode of acute severe asthma, calcium is also involved in mediator release.[1-3] Intravenous magnesium, perhaps acting as a physiological antagonist to calcium,[36] has been shown to cause a rapid, short bronchodilating effect less than that of β$_2$ agonists.[37,38] Intravenous magnesium sulphate has been used for the management of acute severe asthma[37-40] and can shift the histamine PC_{20} by almost one doubling concentration.[41] However, two studies in acute severe asthma failed to demonstrate any benefits of this therapy.[42,43]

MUCOLYTICS

Mucous plugging the tracheobronchial tree in asthmatic subjects is well recognized; even mild asthmatic subjects have some amount of impaired mucociliary clearance.[44] Most studies and reviews on control of mucous hypersecretion have concentrated on pulmonary conditions other than asthma.[45-47] This perhaps is a reflection of the fact that most pharmacological methods for mucous management are already in use for therapy of asthma, i.e. corticosteroids, adrenergic drugs and methylxanthines.[46,48]

α-ADRENERGIC ANTAGONISTS

There is evidence to support the presence of α receptors in the airways;[49,50] however, they appear to play a limited role in asthma as demonstrated by studies on α-adrenergic antagonists in asthma.[51-54] Although some studies have shown partial prevention of exercise-induced bronchospasm by α blockers,[51,52] studies in histamine- or allergen-induced bronchospasm have not met with much success.[53,54] The situation is further complicated by a report of reduction of exercise-induced bronchospasm by inhaled α_1-adrenergic agonist, methoxamine,[55] and the bronchodilating effects of α_2 agonists.[56] Thus the role of α-adrenergic receptors in asthma remains unclear.

IMMUNOGLOBULINS

In the past immunoglobulins have been used for management of asthma, especially in children, but there is no rationale for their use except in hypoimmune states coexisting with asthma. However, a recent open-label study demonstrated that high-dose intravenous immunoglobulins may have a steroid-sparing effect.[57]

SURGERY

Carotid body resection (glomectomy), both unilateral and bilateral, was carried out in asthmatic subjects during the early 1960s for management of breathlessness. However, the procedures were stopped when unilateral glomectomy was shown to be no better than a sham surgery, while bilateral glomectomy reduced the sensitivity of the central nervous system to hypoxaemia and hypercarbia, thus further aggravating the clinical condition although the patient felt less dyspnoeic.[58] Surgery is used only for associated conditions like nasal polyps or chronic sinusitis. Although lungs from donors without asthma have been transplanted in asthmatic patients without subsequent development of asthma,[59] the role of lung transplant in asthma is more of scientific curiosity.

ALTERNATIVE MEDICINE

Alternative medicine is the practice of non-orthodox systems of therapy. Well-recognized alternative medical systems for asthma include acupuncture, homoeopathy, yoga, hypnosis and ionizer therapy.[60] The spectrum of therapies also includes speleotherapy (cave-dwelling), bracelets, chihuaua sniffing, element-containing syrups[61] and free medicine dispensed inside a live (expensive) fish.[62] Alternative medicine encompasses all folk remedies and therapeutic measures that are often scientifically inexplicable. Almost one-third of doctors in one study admitted to referring patients for alternative medical treatment,[63] while about 45% of asthmatic families either consulted or followed advice of alternative medicine practitioners.[64] Indeed, some modern asthma therapies are derived from herbal folk remedies, e.g. ephedrine from ma-huang, anti-cholinergic alkaloids from *Datura stramonium*, khellin (the basis of cromoglycate) from *Ammi visnaga* and theophylline from tea.[65]

The absence of double-blind, randomized, cross-over, placebo-controlled trials in carefully selected subjects is responsible for much scepticism of alternative therapy. This section provides an overview of some of the widely followed medical systems for asthma so that physicians can advise patients properly and help safeguard against quacks, who often infiltrate the ranks of practitioners of alternative medicine.

ACUPUNCTURE

Acupuncture is an ancient Chinese art of restoring the "balance of Ying and Yang energies" by stimulating specific nodal points on the body surface at specific depth without local anaesthesia with stainless steel needles that are either rotated or vibrated.[60,66,67] Acupuncture is efficacious in chronic osteoarticular pain by stimulating endogenous endorphin release.[68] However, results of acupuncture in asthma are variable.[69–72] Meta-analysis of 13 studies found that no study earned more than 72% on the quality scale; 8 of the 13 favoured acupunture.[67]

"Din Chuan" is the most widely accepted nodal point[60,72] and is located approximately 4 cm deep bilaterally on the back 3 cm lateral to midpoint of C7 and T1 spinous processes. Stimulation of Din Chuan may improve expiratory flow rates but does not improve airway hyperresponsiveness.[72] The limited efficacy of acupuncture in reversing acute bronchospasm[72] or exercise-induced bronchospasm[73,74] is less than β agonists. Thus, the benefit of acupuncture over conventional therapy in the management of asthma is controversial.

HOMOEOPATHY

The principles of homoeopathy include (1) "like cures like", and (2) use of exceedingly high dilutions of an active agent.[60] A substance that causes the symptoms is given in very high dilutions (isopathy). Serial 10- or 100-fold dilutions are repeated along with succussion (intensive shaking) to produce dilutions as weak as $1/100^{12}$ (referred to as C_{12}), which are unlikely to contain even a single molecule of the original agent.[75] Many homoeopathy trials[75] in chronic disorders show some success. A few studies involve dilute sublingual allergen extracts in hay fever and/or asthma pollinosis. The majority of the trials are designed suboptimally. The effect of the dilutions beyond molecular concentration is explained by the spatial reorientation of water molecules by succussion with the basic substance.[76] This has been the cause of conflict between sceptical scientists and proponents of homoeopathy.[76–80]

YOGA

Yoga is a system of complete health care, consisting of exercises that include asanas (postural exercises), pranayama (breathing exercises), kriyas (like neti and vaman dhouti, i.e. nasal and stomach wash) and meditation.[81–83] Several studies on yoga in asthma[82–85] have demonstrated objective improvement in peak flow symptom score and drug intake in addition to subjective improvement. One study[86] demonstrated a one-dose shift of histamine PC_{20} after practising pranayama for 2 weeks. There is a need for standardization of yogic techniques, and to understand physiopathological mechanisms.

HYPNOSIS

Psychological factors, especially emotions and stress, may contribute to asthma morbidity and mortality.[87,88] Hypnosis is a technique used for alleviating stress; several trials have shown that it benefits asthmatic subjects.[89–91] A multicentre trial of hypnosis in asthma demonstrated small benefits, although five of the six objective measurements showed no difference.[92] Hypnosis reduces exercise-induced bronchospasm but less so than cromoglycate.[93]

The efficacy of hypnosis depends upon the practitioner's experience and the susceptibility of the patient.[94] Further, the bronchoconstrictive response can be modified by suggestion.[95] Thus hypnosis can help a tense, anxious asthmatic subject and perhaps play a role in changing the neurotic attitude of the subject to the disease.

IONIZER THERAPY

Large numbers of negatively or positively charged molecules in the environment inhibit bacterial growth, affect influenza mortality in rats and affect the life expectancy of rats.[96] Negative ions deplete serotonin concentrations in mice and rabbit trachea.[96,97] Ions can be produced artificially by thermionic emission, charge separation, γ-radiation or high voltage discharge[98] and in nature by shearing of water as in waterfalls, movements of large masses of air or by cosmic rays.[96]

Some benefit was initially seen in asthmatic subjects using ionizers.[99,100] However, two well-controlled studies found no benefits with ionizers,[98,101] while one of them reported an increase in nocturnal dry cough in spite of a fall in airborne allergen.[101] Thus ionizers have no role in the management of asthma, but may aid environmental control; benefits need to be objectively documented.

ACKNOWLEDGEMENTS

The authors would like to thank Jacquie Bramley for assistance in preparing this manuscript. Dr R. Bhagat is a Fellow of the Saskatchewan Lung Association.

REFERENCES

1 Kirkpatrick CT. Excitation and contraction in bovine tracheal smooth muscle. *J Physiol* 1975; 244: 263-81.

2 Foreman JC, Hallett MB, Mongar JL. The relationship between histamine and $^{45}Ca^{++}$ uptake by mast cells. *J Physiol* 1977; 271: 193-214.

3 Holgate ST, Church MK. Control of mediator release from mast cells. *Ann Allergy* 1982; 12 (suppl): 5-13.

4 Triggle DJ, Swamy VC. Pharmacology of agents that affect calcium. Agonists and antagonists. *Chest* 1980; 78 (suppl): 174-9.

5 Braunwald E. Mechanisms of action of calcium-channel-blocking agents. *N Engl J Med* 1982; 307: 1618-27.

6 Patel KR. Calcium antagonists in exercise induced asthma. *BMJ* 1981; 282: 932-3.

7 Barnes PJ, Wilson NM, Brown MJ. A calcium antagonist, nifedipine, modifies exercise induced asthma. *Thorax* 1981; 36: 726-30.

8 Cerrina J, Denjean A, Alexandre G, Lockhart A, Duroux P. Inhibition of exercise induced asthma by a calcium antagonist, nifedipine. *Am Rev Respir Dis* 1981; 123: 156-60.

9 Williams DO, Barnes PJ, Vickers HP, Rudolf M. Effect of nifedipine on bronchomotor tone and histamine reactivity in asthma. *BMJ* 1981; 283: 348.

10 Malik S, O'Reilly J, Sudlow MF. Effects of sublingual nifedipine on inhaled histamine and methacholine-induced bronchoconstriction in atopic subjects. *Thorax* 1982; 37: 230.

11 So SY, Lam WK, Yu DYC. Effect of calcium antagonists on allergen induced asthma. *Clin Allergy* 1982; 12: 595-600.

12 Patel KR, Kerr JW. Calcium antagonists in experimental asthma. *Ann Allergy* 1982; 12 (suppl): 15–20.

13 Corris PA, Nariman S, Gibson GJ. Nifedipine in the prevention of asthma induced by exercise and histamine. *Am Rev Respir Dis* 1983; 128: 991–2.

14 Miadonna A, Tedeschi A, Leiggieri E, Cootini M, Restuccia M, Bianchini C. Effect of verapamil on allergen-induced asthma in patients with respiratory allergy. *Ann Allergy* 1983; 51: 201–4.

15 McIntyre E, Fitzgibbon B, Otto H, Minson R, Alpers J, Ruffin R. Inhaled verapamil in histamine induced bronchoconstriction. *J Allergy Clin Immunol* 1983; 71: 375–81.

16 Mathews JI, Richey HM III, Ewald FW Jr, Glending DL. Nifedipine does not alter methacholine induced bronchial reactivity. *Ann Allergy* 1984; 53: 462–7.

17 Popa VT, Somani P, Simon V. The effect of inhaled verapamil on resting bronchial tone and airway contractions induced by histmaine and acetylcholine in normal and asthmatic subjects. *Am Rev Respir Dis* 1984; 130: 1006–13.

18 Ozenne G, Moore ND, Leprevost A *et al.* Nifedipine in chronic bronchial asthma: a randomised, double blind, cross over trial against placebo. *Eur J Respir Dis* 1985; 67: 238–43.

19 Moscato G, Danna P, Dorigo N *et al.* Effect of nifedipine on hyperreactive bronchial responses to methacholine. *Ann Allergy* 1986; 56: 145–9.

20 Schwartzstein RH, Fanta CH. Orally administered nifedipine in chronic stable asthma: comparison with an orally administered sympathomimetic. *Am Rev Respir Dis* 1986; 134: 262–5.

21 Ballester E, Roca J, Rodriguez-Roisin R, Agusti-Vidal A. Effect of nifedipine on arterial hypoxaemia occurring after methacholine challenge in asthma. *Thorax* 1986; 41: 468–72.

22 Fish JE, Norman PS. Effect of calcium channel blocker, verapamil, on asthmatic airway responses to muscarinic, histaminergic and allergenic stimuli. *Am Rev Respir Dis* 1986; 133: 730–4.

23 Molho M, Gruzman C, Katz I, Lidgi M, Chaniac A. Nifedipine in asthma: dose related effect on bronchial tone. *Chest* 1987; 91: 667–70.

24 Ferrari M, Olivieri M, Gasperi MD, Lechi A. Differential effects of nifedipine and diltiazem on methacholine-induced bronchospasm in allergic asthma. *Ann Allergy* 1989; 63: 196–200.

25 Kivity S, Brayer M, Topilsky M. Combined effects of nifedipine and diltiazem on methacholine induced bronchoconstriction in asthmatic patients. *Ann Allergy* 1992; 68: 175–9.

26 Marthan R, Martin C, Amedee T, Mironneau J. Calcium channel currents in isolated smooth muscle cells from human bronchus. *J Appl Physiol* 1989; 66: 1706–14.

27   Murray RK, Kotlifoff MI. Receptor-activated calcium influx in human airway smooth muscle cells. *J Physiol* 1991; 435: 123–44.

28   Murray LE. Effects of a receptor operated channel blocker on intracellular calcium in human airway smooth muscle cells. *Am Rev Respir Dis* 1992; 145: A205.

29   Ritchie DM, Kirschner T, Moore JB *et al.* Experimental antiasthmatic activity of RWJ 22108: a bronchoselective calcium entry blocker. *Int Arch Allergy Immunol* 1993; 100: 274–82.

30   O'Connor BJ, Chung KF, Chen-Worsdell YM, Fuller RW, Barnes PJ. Effect of inhaled furosemide and bumetanide on adenosine 5'-monophosphate and sodium metabisulfite-induced bronchoconstriction in asthmatic subjects. *Am Rev Respir Dis* 1991; 143: 1329–33.

31   Polosa R, Holgate ST. Inhaled furosemide is more effective than inhaled bumetanide in reducing airway responsiveness to adenosine 5'-monophosphate (AMP) in asthma. *Am Rev Respir Dis* 1991; 143 (suppl): A549.

32   Grubbe RE, Hopp R, Dave NK, Brennan B, Bewtra A, Townley R. Effect of inhaled furosemide on the bronchial response to methacholine and cold air hyperventilation challenges. *J Allergy Clin Immunol* 1990; 85: 881–4.

33   Bianco S, Vaghi A, Robuschi M, Pasargiklian M. Prevention of exercise induced bronchoconstriction by inhaled furosemide. *Lancet* 1988; ii: 252–5.

34   Bianco S, Pieroni MG, Refini RM, Rottoli L, Sestini P. Protective effect of inhaled furosemide on allergen-induced early and late asthmatic reactions. *N Engl J Med* 1989; 321: 1069–71.

35   O'Donnell WJ, Rosenberg MA, Niven RW, Drazen JM, Israel E. Inhaled acetazolamide attenuates bronchoconstriction induced by cold-air hyperventilation. *Am Rev Respir Dis* 1991; 143 (suppl): A211.

36   Levine BS, Coburn JW. Magnesium the mimic/antagonist of calcium. *N Engl J Med* 1984; 310: 1253–5.

37   Okayama H, Aikawa T, Okayama M, Sasaki H, Mue S, Takishima T. Bronchodilating effect of intravenous magnesium sulfate in bronchial asthma. *JAMA* 1987; 257: 1076–8.

38   Rolla G, Bucca C, Caria E *et al.* Acute effect of intravenous magnesium sulfate on airway obstruction of asthmatic patients. *Ann Allergy* 1988; 61: 388–91.

39   Skobeloff EM, Spivey WH, McNamara RM, Greenspon L. Intravenous magnesium sulfate for the treatment of acute asthma in the emergency department. *JAMA* 1989; 262: 1210–3.

40   Noppen M, Vanmaele L, Impens N, Schandevyl W. Bronchodilating effect of intravenous magnesium sulfate in acute severe asthma. *Chest* 1990; 97: 373–6.

41   Rolla G, Bucca C, Bugrani M, Arossa W, Spinaci S. Reduction of histamine-induced bronchoconstriction by magnesium in asthmatic subjects. *Allergy* 1987; 42: 186–8.

42 Green SM, Rothrock SG. Intravenous magnesium for acute asthma: failure to decrease emergency treatment duration or need for hospitalisation. *Ann Emerg Med* 1992; 21: 260–5.

43 Tiffany BR, Berk WA, Todd IK, White SR. Magnesium bolus or infusion fails to improve expiratory flow in acute asthma exacerbations. *Chest* 1993; 104: 831–4.

44 Bateman JRM, Pavia D, Sheahan NF, Agnew JE, Clarke SW. Impaired tracheobronchial clearance in patients with mild stable asthma. *Thorax* 1983; 38: 463–7.

45 Sutton PP, Parker RA, Webber BA *et al.* Assessment of forced expiratory technique, postural drainage and directed coughing in chest physiotherapy. *Eur J Respir Dis* 1983; 64: 62–8.

46 Clarke SW. Management of mucous hypersecretion. *Eur J Respir Dis* 1987; 71 (suppl 153): 136–44.

47 Clarke SW. Rationale of airway clearance. *Eur Respir J* 1989; 2 (suppl 7): 599S–604S.

48 Ziment I. Theophylline and mucociliary clearance. *Chest* 1987; 92 (suppl): 38S–42S.

49 Fleisch JH, Maling HM, Brodie BB. Evidence for existence of alpha adrenergic receptors in mammalian trachea. *Am J Physiol* 1970; 218: 596–9.

50 Barnes PJ, Dollery CT, MacDermott J. Increased pulmonary α-adrenergic and reduced β-adrenergic receptors in experimental asthma. *Nature* 1980; 285: 569–71.

51 Barnes PJ, Wilson NM, Vickers H. Prazosin, an alpha$_1$-adrenoceptor antagonist partially inhibits exercise induced asthma. *J Allergy Clin Immunol* 1981; 68: 411–5.

52 Walden SM, Bleecker ER, Chahal K, Britt EJ, Mason P, Permutt S. Effect of alpha-adrenergic blockade on exercise-induced asthma and conditioned air. *Am Rev Respir Dis* 1984; 130: 357–62.

53 Barnes PJ, Ind PW, Dollery CT. Inhaled prazosin in asthma. *Thorax* 1981; 36: 378–81.

54 Jenkins C, Breslin ABX, Marlin GE. The role of alpha and beta-adrenoceptors in airway hyperresponsiveness to histamine. *J Allergy Clin Immunol* 1985; 75: 364–72.

55 Din Xuan AT, Chaussain M, Regnard J, Lockhart A. Pretreatment with an inhaled α_1-adrenergic agonist, methoxamine, reduces exercise induced asthma. *Eur Respir J* 1989; 2: 409–14.

56 Din Xuan AT, Lockhart A. Bronchial effects of α_2-adrenoceptor agonist and of other antihypertensive agents in asthma. *Am J Med* 1989; 87 (suppl 3C): 34S–37S.

57 Mazer BD, Gelfand EW. An open label study of high-dose intravenous immunoglobulin in severe childhood asthma. *J Allergy Clin Immunol* 1991; 87: 976–83.

58 Busey JF, Fenger EPK, Hepper NG *et al.* Current status of the surgical treatment of pulmonary emphysema and asthma. A statement by the committee. Am Rev Respir Dis 1968; 97: 486-9.

59 Corris PA, Dark JH. Aetiology of asthma: lessons from lung transplantation. Lancet 1993; 341: 1369-71.

60 Lane DJ, Lane TV. Alternative and complementary medicine for asthma. Thorax 1991; 46: 787-97.

61 Kalyonov AF, Selcuk ZT, Iskendarani A *et al.* Alternative and complementary medicine (letter). Thorax 1992; 47: 762.

62 *India Abroad,* Toronto edn, 1993, 6 August, p. 24.

63 Reilly DT. Young doctor's views on alternative medicine. BMJ 1983; 287: 337-9.

64 Donnelly WJ, Spykerboer JE, Thong YH. Are patients who use alternative medicine dissatisfied with orthodox medicine? Med J Aust 1985; 142: 539-41.

65 Ziment I, Stein M. Inappropriate and unusual remedies. In: Weiss EB, Stein M (eds) *Bronchial Asthma: Mechanisms and Therapeutics,* 3rd edn. Boston: Little Brown & Co., 1993: 1145.

66 Aldridge D, Pietroni PC. Clinical assessment of acupuncture in asthma therapy: discussion paper. J R Soc Med 1987; 80: 222-4.

67 Kleijnen J, Reit G, Knipschild P. Acupuncture and asthma: a review of controlled trials. Thorax 1993; 46: 798-801.

68 Clement-Jones V, McLoughlin L, Tomlin S, Besser GM, Rees LH, Wen HL. Increased β-endorphin but not met-enkephalin levels in human cerebrospinal fluid after acupuncture for recurrent pain. Lancet 1980; ii: 946-8.

69 Tashkin DP, Kroenig RJ, Bresler DE, Simmons M, Coulson AH, Kerschnav H. A controlled trial of real and simulated acupuncture in the management of chronic asthma. J Allergy Clin Immunol 1985; 76: 855-64.

70 Mitchell P, Wells JE. Acupuncture for chronic asthma: a controlled trial with six months follow-up. Am J Acupuncture 1989; 17: 5-13.

71 Takishima T, Mue S, Tamura G, Ishihara T, Watanabe K. The bronchodilating effect of acupuncture in patients with acute asthma. Ann Allergy 1982; 48: 44-9.

72 Yu DYC, Lee SP. Effect of acupuncture on bronchial asthma. Cli Sci Mol Med 1976; 51: 503-9.

73 Morton AR, Fazio SM, Miller D. Efficacy of laser–acupuncture in the prevention of exercise-induced asthma. Ann Allergy 1993; 70: 295-8.

74 Fung PK, Chow OKW, So SY. Attenuation of exercise-induced asthma by acupuncture. Lancet 1986; ii: 1419-21.

75 Kleijnen J, Knipschild P, ter Riet G. Clinical trials of homeopathy. BMJ 1991; 302: 316-23.

76 Davenas E, Beauvais F, Amara J *et al.* Human basophil degranulation triggered by very dilute antiserum against IgE. *Nature* 1988; 333: 816–8.

77 Maddox J, Randi J, Stewart WW. "High-dilution" experiments a delusion. *Nature* 1988; 334: 287–90.

78 Benveniste J. Dr Jacques Benveniste replies. *Nature* 1988; 334: 29.

79 Maddox J. Waves caused by extreme dilution. *Nature* 1988; 335: 760–3.

80 Benveniste J. Benveniste on Benveniste affair. *Nature* 1988; 335: 759.

81 Goyeche JRM, Abo Y, Ikemi Y. Asthma: the yoga perspective. Part II: yoga therapy in treatment of asthma. *J Asthma* 1982; 19: 189–201.

82 Nagendra HR, Nagarathna R. An integrated approach of yoga therapy for bronchial asthma: a 3–54 month prospective study. *J Asthma* 1986; 23: 123–37.

83 Tandon MK. Adjunct treatment with yoga in chronic severe airway obstruction. *Thorax* 1978; 33: 514–7.

84 Nagarathna R, Nagendra HR. Yoga for bronchial asthma: a controlled study. *BMJ* 1985; 291: 1077–9.

85 Jain SC, Rai L, Valecha A, Jha UK, Bhatnagar SOD, Ram K. Effect of yoga training on exercise tolerance in adolescents with childhood asthma. *J Asthma* 1991; 28: 437–42.

86 Singh V, Wisniewski A, Britton J, Tattersfield A. Effect of yoga breathing exercises (pranayama) on airway reactivity in subjects with asthma. *Lancet* 1990; 335: 1381–3.

87 Barnes PJ, Chung FK. Difficult asthma: cause for concern. *BMJ* 1989; 299: 695–8.

88 Strunk RC. Deaths due to asthma: new insights into sudden unexpected deaths, but the focus remains on prevention. *Am Rev Respir Dis* 1993; 148: 550–2.

89 White HC. Hypnosis in bronchial asthma. *J Psychosom Res* 1961; 5: 272–9.

90 Maher-loughnan GP, MacDonald N, Mason AA, Fry L. Controlled trial of hypnosis in the symptomatic treatment of asthma. *BMJ* 1962; ii: 371–6.

91 Morrison JB. Chronic asthma and improvement with relaxation induced by hypnotherapy. *J R Soc Med* 1988; 81: 701–4.

92 A report to the research committee of the British Tuberculosis Association. Hypnosis for asthma – a controlled trial. *BMJ* 1968; 4: 71–6.

93 Ben-Zvi Z, Spohn WA, Young SH, Kattan M. Hypnosis for exercise-induced asthma. *Am Rev Respir Dis* 1982; 125: 392–5.

94 Ewer TC, Stewart DE. Improvement in bronchial hyperresponsiveness in patients with moderate asthma after treatment with a hypnotic technique: a randomised control trial. *BMJ* 1986; 293: 1129–32.

95 Horton DJ, Suda WL, Kinsman RA, Souhrada J, Spector SL. Bronchoconstrictive suggestion in asthma: a role of airways hyperreactivity and emotions. *Am Rev Respir Dis* 1978; 117: 1029–38.

96 Kreuger AP, Reed EJ. Biological impact of small air ions. *Science* 1976; 193: 1203-13.

97 Kreuger AP, Smith RF. The biological mechanism of air ion action: negative ion effect on the concentration and metabolism of 5HT in the mammalian respiratory tract. *J Gen Physiol* 1960; 44: 269-72.

98 Nogardy SG, Furnass SB. Ionizers in the management of bronchial asthma. *Thorax* 1983; 38: 919-22.

99 Osterballe O, Weeke B, Albrechtsen O. Influence of small atmospheric ions on the airways in patients with bronchial asthma. *Allergy* 1979; 34: 187-94.

100 Ben-Dov I, Amirav I, Shochina M, Amitai I, Bar-Yishay E, Godfrey S. Effect of negative ionisation of inspired air on the response of asthmatic children to exercise and inhaled histamine. *Thorax* 1983; 38: 584-8.

101 Warner JA, Marchant JL, Warner JO. Double blind trial of ionisers in children with asthma sensitive to house-dust mite. *Thorax* 1993; 48: 330-3.

KEY POINTS

1 Treatments outlined here have limited, uncertain or unproven value.

2 Some treatments may indirectly improve the (or any) condition by improvement in general well-being.

23

PATIENT EDUCATION

Martyn R. Partridge

INTRODUCTION

To ensure that the good treatments that are available for asthma reach the patients, and are taken, requires:

- well-educated health professionals;

- well-organized health services;

- adequate personal and/or government finance;

- easy-to-take drugs with a good benefit/side-effect profile;

- attention being paid to clear communication and patient education.

It is of no value having excellent treatments available if they are not used.

Guidelines, whether national[1] or international,[2] may be useful in the education of health professionals and they provide a framework for local asthma task forces or planning teams to adapt and make locally relevant. Suggested members of a local asthma task force are shown in Table 23.1 and the sort of issues that they may tackle are shown in Table 23.2. From such national guidelines may thus be derived departmental or practice protocols and it is at this level that the benefit of guidelines is seen.[3,4] Such protocols are essential if a multidisciplinary approach to the care of those with asthma is adopted and guidelines provide us with a "common language" – nothing unsettles the patient with asthma more than to appear to be receiving conflicting messages from different members of the health professional team.

The evidence available suggests that in addition to under-diagnosis or delayed diagnosis (which may be a particular problem in the elderly[5,6]), many patients receive too little in the way of treatment and too little regular preventative therapy.[7,8] However even when the correct diagnosis is made and the correct treatment is given it is suggested that many patients,

TABLE 23.1: *Possible members of a local asthma task force set up to adapt national or international guidelines for local use*

Respiratory physician
Paediatrician
Primary care physician
Practice nurse
Respiratory nurse
Allergist
Pharmacist
Manager
Health planner
Patient support group
Health educationalist

TABLE 23.2: *Possible issues to be considered by a local asthma task force in each district*

What is the size of the problem of asthma?
Are mainly children or adults affected?
Who will provide care?
   Primary care – doctor or nurse
   Secondary care
   Other
What arrangements will be made for shared care?
Who will follow up those who have attended the accident and
   emergency department?
Will treatments/inhaler devices/peak flow rates be
   standardized?
Will there be a central educational resource centre?
What public education problems are there in this district (e.g.
   misconceptions about local environmental issues, need for
   training of schoolteachers, etc.)?

adults and children, may not take treatment as previously discussed with their health professionals.[9–12] A key factor in determining whether or not a patient complies with therapy relates to the quality of communication between patient and health professional.[13] All the national and international guidelines stress the importance of patient education. What is meant by the term and what does it involve?

COMMUNICATION AND EDUCATION

There are two key parts to the process of education:

(1) the passage of information and the acquisition by the patient of certain skills;

(2) a change in behaviour.

It is important to realize that knowledgeable patients do not automatically alter their behaviour or their attitude towards illness. A number of barriers to education may exist and this reinforces the cardinal role of clear communication in patient education. Some potential barriers to education are listed in Table 23.3. In any type of communication there is a sender, a message and a recipient and in an ideal world this is a circular model with the recipient also acting as a sender, and the sender as a recipient (Fig. 23.1).

THE SENDER

In the case of patient education the sender may be a person delivering verbal messages, or another transmitter such as the written word, audiovisual material, interactive computer, or poster. In one study patients expressed a preference to hear information about their condition from a doctor,[14] whilst in a recent poll of 1631 members of the UK National Asthma Campaign, when asked who they would prefer to see when seeking medical advice, 5% expressed a preference to see a nurse, 44% a doctor and 48% did not mind which (personal communication, National Asthma Campaign, London, 1993). In other situations the sender may be a trained educator or even a member of a support group.

TABLE 23.3: *Potential barriers to education*

Disbelief regarding diagnosis
Misconceptions about the nature of the condition
Belief that relieving drugs are best
Distrust of all medications
Belief that by altering environment, attacks can be avoided
Feeling of stigmatization
Drugs cause side-effects
"It won't happen to me"
Depression
"Steroid phobia"
Denial based on feeling of not being in control

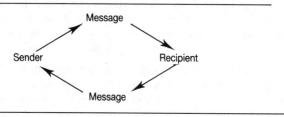

FIGURE 23.1: *Clear communication is an essential component of patient education, and involves consideration being paid to the message and to the recipient so that "wants" are matched with "needs".*

Patients rarely recall more than 50% of what they have heard for more than 5 min after the end of a consultation and some form of reinforcement of messages is therefore necessary. This may be done by the same sender on a subsequent occasion (and by the time the same message has been given more than three times retention approaches 100%), or a verbal message may be reinforced by different routes. Supplementing verbal advice with specific *written* information about a complicated series of proposed treatment changes has been shown to greatly enhance compliance.[15] In a survey of 699 UK health professionals (personal communication, National Asthma Campaign, London, 1993) asthma was the commonest condition for which they gave information booklets (asthma 92%, heart disease 84%, diabetes 80%, cancer 34%, epilepsy 17%) but clearly not all with the condition receive such materials. Indeed in the 1993 poll of 1631 members of the National Asthma Campaign only 39% had ever received booklets or leaflets and only 4% had ever seen a video on the subject. Two-thirds had received a demonstration of how to use their inhaler devices but only 27% reported receiving written instructions on how/when to take their medicines. Giving the written word alone may not alter patient behaviour[16] and nor does the use of audio tapes.[17] However such seemingly negative trials are not arguments against patient education as a whole. What they tell us is that materials must be of the highest quality (written for a reading age appropriate for the population) and they can only be expected to influence behaviour as part of a wider package. Sometimes materials act only as a source of satisfaction to the patient,[18,19] and sometimes as a means of giving the patient the information they need to enable them to ask more meaningful questions of the health professional – they are thus an important prerequisite of patient education, not an education in themselves.

As an alternative to written information, video tapes are particularly appropriate to those with poor literacy skills and are useful in teaching techniques such as use of a metered dose inhaler.[20] In one study[14] videos were the second most preferred source of information (after the doctor). However preference does not always equate with effectiveness, for in another study patients expressed a preference for written information rather than audio tapes, although a simple knowledge study showed that they actually learnt more from the audio tape.[17] What is important is to have available an array of materials so that the same messages may be given to those with asthma by several different routes (Table 23.4). All should contain the same core materials and clearly some are more suitable for personal use and others for giving information to groups.

Clinicians should not lose sight of the fact that individuals with asthma do not live in a vacuum. Their illness may impact upon others around them; 18% of parents say that their children's asthma had either a great deal or quite a lot of influence on their lives, and 20% of cohabitees consider that their own life was influenced to a considerable degree by the asthma of the person with whom they live.[21] Furthermore of 397 cohabitees, 12% always made sure that the person with whom they live were taking their medication, and a further 30% usually, or occasionally, did so. Materials should thus be suitable for sharing, and videos especially can be watched by the whole family together. For particular audiences, e.g. schoolchildren, the sender may be something innovative such as playacting or drama, whilst for other recipients, e.g. physical education teachers, a lecture and demonstration may be more appropriate.

THE MESSAGE - THE "NEEDS"
If these are the methods of "sending" information what of the message itself: what might those with asthma "need" to know. Likely needs are listed in Table 23.5 and these are probably non-controversial and require little explanation. However as a prerequisite for good compliance it is important that patients do know the diagnosis, understand their treatment and know that any risk applies to them and not just to the other person. No person with asthma (or parent of a child with asthma) should be left not knowing

TABLE 23.4: *Methods of giving information to those with asthma*

Verbal (by doctor, nurse or trained educator)
Written (leaflets, booklets, posters)
Audio tapes
Video tapes (for loan, or playing in waiting rooms, etc.)
Public lectures
Support group meetings
Newspaper/magazine articles
Drama

TABLE 23.5: *Summary of what patients "need" to know about their asthma*

The diagnosis and how it was made
How to use an inhaler
The difference between relievers and preventers
How to use a peak flow meter
Signs and symptoms that suggest worsening asthma and what to do if present
When and where they will be followed up

what to do in the event of deteriorating asthma, and yet the evidence suggests that too few are given explicit instructions about signs that suggest that their asthma is worsening and what to do under those circumstances. Whilst 47% of 1631 National Asthma Campaign members reported having received such advice, in a UK Primary Care Study[22] only 41% of those who had experienced an attack during the previous year had been given a self-management plan. It is not yet possible to define accurately who needs or benefits most from home peak flow monitoring. Many young children lack the physical skills necessary for their use and paediatricians remain uncertain as to which older children would benefit most. There is evidence that children have the same difficulty as adults in perceiving the severity of induced airway narrowing[23] and objective monitoring is therefore likely to be a useful adjunct to advice based upon subjective criteria. Parents have also been reported to find peak flow monitoring useful in the recognition of severe asthma attacks.[24] In adults, studies of induced airway narrowing have shown a poor correlation between subjective and objective parameters of severity[25] and, when this is extended to evaluation of perception of day-to-day variation in severity, the majority of asthmatic subjects in a community study were shown to be poor discriminators.[26] Table 23.6 outlines some of the current indications for home peak flow monitoring.

TABLE 23.6: *Possible uses of peak flow monitoring*

To aid in the diagnosis of asthma
To delineate possible environmental or occupational triggers
To assess efficacy of treatment
To give warning of impending attacks of asthma
To monitor the stepping down or tailing off of treatment
To get reassurance as to good control of asthma

THE RECIPIENT – THE "WANTS"

One of the potential barriers to effective patient education is a mis-matching of perception of what patients "need" to know and their list of what they "want" to know. If doctors believe that a patient needs to know the virtues and mode of action of inhaled steroids and spend valuable time on this subject, when what the patient actually *wanted* was to know what to avoid so that the asthma would go away, the result is likely to be dissatis-faction, poor compliance and a failure of the patient to alter behaviour in a manner that leads to improved asthma control. It is thus vital that patients are given adequate opportunity to express their "wants". These are likely to vary considerably in content from patient to patient. They can be elicited by open consultation where it is clear to patients that the time available is for them, and where they can declare their thoughts and con-cerns in an open unhurried manner, or they can be elicited by the judicious use of open-ended questions or prompts. Of patients' main wor-ries 76% may not be mentioned during a consultation[13] and so it is essen-tial that these are elicited. "How do you feel about having asthma?" or "What concerns you most about asthma?" may unleash concerns that would not otherwise have been elicited. The results from surveys in general prac-tice show that many people with asthma feel different to other people (26% of 210 interviewees), angry (38%), depressed (32%) and unable to enjoy a full life (39%).[27] Others express concern as to the unpredictable nature of the condition and a feeling of not being in control; by eliciting specific fears it may be possible to direct management more specifically, for example by giving a self-management plan, to enhance a feeling of being in control.

Possible "wants" may also be gleaned by studying those problems received by telephone helplines from asthma sufferers. Questions about side-effects of drugs are part of the reason for the calls in 42% of cases.[28] Knowledge of this means that clinicians can attempt to elicit such unspoken fears dur-ing routine consultations. Again, open-ended questions are to be pre-ferred. "How do you feel about your treatment?" or "Some people think steroids are dangerous, what do you think?" may elicit specific concerns that can then be tackled by the provision of both verbal and written infor-mation so that the patient may make more informed decisions about whether or not to take a certain treatment.

REINFORCEMENT AND REVISION

Those with asthma need to be reviewed at regular intervals for the follow-ing reasons.

(1) Asthma is usually a long-term condition.

(2) Asthma is a variable condition and advice and management may change.

(3) Much of the information given to the patient will be forgotten, or bad habits and techniques may arise with time.

(4) Giving control to patients does not equal abdication of health professional responsibility. Care should be provided within the context of a partnership. Self-management plans, where issued, should be regarded as plans for *guided* self-management and they require frequent review.

(5) Information needs to be given in a graded, easy to assimilate manner, with frequent revision and reinforcement of previously given messages, plus praise to the patient or parent when self-management has been optimal.

It is thus easy to realize that what is being discussed is good communication and the development of a partnership between patient and health professional, where wants and needs are continually matched and where education involves a series of consultations or sessions. The ground that would be covered in such an educational programme is shown in Table 23.7 and it is emphasized that this ground would be covered (and revised) using several adjunctive methods of giving information (verbal, written, videos, etc.).

INDIVIDUAL OR GROUP EDUCATION?

The theme so far has been one of good communication between patient and health professional, and individualized advice. The logic behind such an approach appears to be strong and it is now possible to select a number of published studies to demonstrate support for the approach that has been outlined. It is thus possible to show that intensive education and management programmes may reduce admissions for adult asthma in both American,[29] Australian[30] and German[31,32] studies and also in a recent British study where the educational intervention was by means of computer-assisted personalized booklets sent to patients.[33] It is also possible to show that such intervention can increase compliance,[34,35] understanding and inhaler technique,[36] and childrens' knowledge and self-management practices of parents.[37] However these studies suggest a certainty that is probably unjustified and there are numerous further areas requiring elucidation and research. In many of the interventions it was difficult to fully separate the effects of more regular supervision and optimized therapy from the educational intervention, and there is still no clear message as to whether it is preferable to communicate, educate and personalize advice on a one-to-one basis or whether there is a benefit for group education as an adjunct to individualized care. Thus an excellent study[38] of group vs. individual education vs. usual care appears to show a benefit for group education (perhaps by virtue of advanced support, reduction of feelings of stigmatization, etc.), but recruitment to such groups is not easy and others have highlighted differences in characteristics between those willing and suitable for group education and those who decline to participate.[39] It is also

TABLE 23.7: *Ground to be covered in an asthma education programme*

What is asthma?
What symptoms suggest a diagnosis of asthma?
What signs or symptoms suggest poorly controlled asthma or asthma that is slipping from control?
Recognizing triggers:
  Avoidable precipitating factors and what to do about them
  Non-avoidable factors such as colds, and what to do if they occur
Knowing the different types of medicines:
  Difference between relievers and preventers
  Other treatments for asthma
  Understanding "generics"
Selecting and using an inhaler device (and revision)
Training in the use of a peak flow meter
Using a peak flow meter as part of a guided self-management plan
How to review self-management plans
Specific issues:
  Asthma and pregnancy
  Going on holiday
  Aspirin and other medicines
  Smoking and asthma
  Occupational asthma
  Work and asthma
  Drug interaction
  Why follow-up is necessary
  Where to turn to for help

difficult to extrapolate from one health system and culture to another and programmes based upon 5-day educational courses as an inpatient[31,32] may be neither affordable nor practical in other countries.

It seems likely that the best outcome from patient education may result from the development of a partnership between patient (or parent) and health professional, in which communication is of the highest standard and where advice is individualized for that patient. The patient will be reviewed regularly and messages reinforced. Whilst care may be shared with others in the health professional team all will give the same message, and verbal advice will be supported by an array of written and audiovisual materials. All patients will be given advice about other sources of information and support associations, and for those who are keen further education will be offered within a group setting.

PUBLIC EDUCATION AND THE EDUCATION OF OTHERS IN CONTACT WITH THOSE WITH ASTHMA

SCHOOLTEACHERS

Children with asthma spend a significant time at school and asthma is the commonest reason for a child to need to take any medication during the school day. Despite this, care for those with asthma at school is often "disorganized"[40] and teachers often lack appropriate knowledge to provide safe care of those in their charge. However, 92% of teachers have been shown to want further information[41] and in several countries (e.g. USA, UK and Australia) specific materials or policies have been made available for schools.

OBSTETRICIAN AND MIDWIFE

Whilst most pregnant asthmatic subjects have uneventful pregnancies resulting in the delivery of healthy infants, 42% of patients need increased treatment for their asthma whilst pregnant and there is a higher incidence of pre-eclampsia and neonatal hypoglycaemia.[43] In addition, cessation of medication at the onset of pregnancy or fear about its use[28] is common and it is thus important to target antenatal clinics, obstetricians and midwives with appropriate advice and materials[43] so that they may reassure mothers of the safety of asthma therapies.

EMPLOYERS

Asthma caused by occupational exposure to a variety of sensitizing agents may account for up to 5% of all cases of the disease. Employers need to be aware of this possibility but health professionals need to be aware that new causes of occupational asthma may present at any time. A numerically larger problem may be that of asthma which is worsened by conditions at work, and in one survey of 420 working asthmatic subjects 9% had to change jobs because of their asthma, 41% felt restricted in the work they could do, 55% had problems with fumes or dust at work and 74% had problems with the smoking of others in the workplace (personal communication, Workers Poll 1992, National Asthma Campaign, London). Employers need to be aware of the importance of, for example, appropriate smoking policies.

THE WIDER PUBLIC

Increased awareness of asthma by the general public may be necessary to reduce feelings of stigmatization and to facilitate appropriate domestic and work environments for those with the condition. It is also necessary for the general public and politicians to be educated about the impact of pollution on those with established asthma but also to be aware of the need for research to highlight those indoor or outdoor factors in the environment that are responsible for the increasing prevalence of the condition.

REFERENCES

1. British Thoracic Society, British Paediatric Association, Royal College of Physicians of London, the Kings Fund Centre, the National Asthma Campaign *et al.* Guidelines on the management of asthma. *Thorax* 1993; 48: S1–S24. Summary charts. *BMJ* 1993; 306: 776–82.

2. National Heart Lung & Blood Institute, National Institutes of Health. International Consensus Report on Diagnosis and Management of Asthma. 1992; Pub. No. 92-3091.

3. Town L, Kwong T, Holst P, Beasley R. Use of a management plan for treating asthma in an emergency department. *Thorax* 1990; 45: 702–6.

4. Lim KL, Harrison BDW. A criteria based audit of inpatient asthma care. *J R Coll Physicians Lond* 1992; 26: 71–5.

5. Banerjee DC, Lee GS, Malik SR, Daly S. Underdiagnosis of asthma in the elderly. *Br J Dis Chest* 1987; 81: 23–9.

6. Holgate ST, Dow L. Airways disease in the elderly: an easy to miss diagnosis. *J Respir Dis* 1988; 9: 14–22.

7. Gellert AL, Gellert SL, Iliffe SR. Prevalence and management of asthma in a London inner city general practice. *Br J Gen Practice* 1990; 40: 197–201.

8. Blainey AD, Beale A, Lomas D, Partridge MR. The cost of acute asthma – how much is preventable? *Health Trends* 1991; 22: 151–3.

9. Horn CR, Essex E, Hill P *et al.* Does urinary salbutamol reflect compliance with inhaled drug regimens by asthmatics. *Respir Med* 1989; 84: 67–70.

10. Spector SL, Kingsman R, Mawhinny H *et al.* Compliance of patients with asthma with an experimental aerolised medication. Implications for controlled clinical trials. *J Allergy Clin Immunol* 1986; 77: 65–70.

11. Cramer JA, Mattson RH, Prevey ML, Scheyer RD, Ovellette G. How often is medication taken as prescribed? *JAMA* 1991; 261: 3273–7.

12. Coutts JA, Gibson NA, Paton JY. Measuring compliance with inhaled medication in asthma. *Arch Dis Child* 1992; 67: 332–3.

13. Korsch BM, Negrete VF. Doctor–patient communication. *Sci Am* 1972; 227: 66–72.

14 Partridge MR. Asthma education: more reading or more viewing? *J R Soc Med* 1986; 79: 326–8.

15 Pedersen S. Ensuring compliance in children. *Eur Respir J* 1992; 5: 143–5.

16 Hilton S, Sibbald B, Anderson HR, Freeling P. Controlled evaluation of the effects of patient education on asthma morbidity in general practice. *Lancet* 1986; i: 26–9.

17 Jenkinson D, Davison J, Jones S, Hawtin P. Comparison of effects of a self management booklet and audiocassette for patients with asthma. *BMJ* 1988; 297: 267–70.

18 George CF, Waters WE, Nicholas JA. Prescription information leaflets: a pilot study in general practice. *BMJ* 1983; 287: 1193–6.

19 Gibbs S, Waters WE, George CF. Communicating information to patients about medicines. *J R Soc Med* 1990; 83: 292–7.

20 Mulloy EMT, Albazzar MK, Warley ARH, Harvey JE. Video education for patients who use inhalers. *Thorax* 1987; 42: 719–20.

21 Applied Research & Communications Ltd. *The Life Quality of Asthmatics.* Uxbridge, Middlesex: Allen & Hanburys Ltd, 1990.

22 Neville RG, Clark RA, Hoskins G, Smith B. First national audit of acute asthma attacks in general practice. *BMJ* 1992; 306: 559–62.

23 Boner AL, DeStefan G, Piacentini GL *et al.* Perception of bronchoconstriction in chronic asthma. *J Asthma* 1992; 19: 323–30.

24 Lloyd BW, Ali MH. How useful do patients find home peak flow monitoring for children with asthma. *BMJ* 1992; 305: 1128–9.

25 Rubinfield AR, Pain MCF. The perception of asthma. *Lancet* 1976; i: 882–4.

26 Kendrick AH, Higgs CMB, Whitfield MJ, Laszlo G. Accuracy of perception of severity of asthma: patients treated in general practice. *BMJ* 1993; 307; 422–4.

27 Sibbald B. Patient self care in acute asthma. *Thorax* 1989; 44: 97–101.

28 Crone S, Partridge M, McLean F. Launching a national helpline. *Health Visitor* 1993; 66: 94–6.

29 Mayo PH, Richman J, Harris HW. Results of a program to reduce admissions for adult asthma. *Ann Intern Med* 1990; 112: 864–71.

30 Yoon R, McKenzie DK, Nauman A, Miles DA. Controlled trial evaluation of an asthma education programme for adults. *Thorax* 1993; 48: 1110–6.

31 Trautner C, Richter B, Berger M. Cost effectiveness of a structured treatment and teaching programme on asthma. *Eur Respir J* 1993; 6: 1485–91.

32 Worth H. Patient education in asthmatic adults. *Lung* 1990; (suppl): 463–8.

33 Osman L, Abdalla MI, Beattie JA *et al.* Reducing hospital admissions through computer supported education for asthma patients. *BMJ* 1994; 308: 568–71.

34. Bailey WC, Richards JM, Brooks M, Soong SJ, Windsor RA, Manzella BA. A randomized trial to improve self management practices of adults with asthma. *Arch Intern Med* 1990; 150: 1664–8.

35. Windsor RA, Bailey WC, Richards JM, Manzella B, Soong S-J, Brooks M. Evaluation of the efficacy and cost effectiveness of health education methods to increase medication adherence amongst adults with asthma. *Am J Public Health* 1990; 80: 1519–21.

36. Quigley C, Donaghy D, Mulloy E, McNicholas W. Evaluation of patient education in asthma management. *Eur Respir J* 1992; 5 (suppl): 95.

37. Taggart VS, Zuckerman AF, Sly RM *et al.* You can control asthma: evaluation of an asthma education program for hospitalized inner city children. *Patient Education and Counselling* 1991; 17: 35–47.

38. Wilson SR, Scamagai P, German DF *et al.* A controlled trial of two forms of self management education for adults with asthma. *Am J Med* 1993; 94: 564–76.

39. Yoon R, McKenzie DK, Miles DA, Barman A. Characteristics of attenders and non attenders at an asthma education programme. *Thorax* 1991; 46: 886–90.

40. Reynolds MA, Aylward P, Heaf DP. How much do school teachers know about asthma? *Pediatr Rev Commun* 1987; 2: 172–80.

41. Bevis M, Taylor B. What do school teachers know about asthma? *Arch Dis Child* 1990; 65: 622–5.

42. Stenius-Aarniala B, Piirila P, Teramo K. Asthma and pregnancy: a prospective study of 198 pregnancies. *Thorax* 1988; 43: 12–8.

43. National Institutes of Health. Report of the Working Group on Asthma and Pregnancy: Management of asthma during pregnancy. *US Department of Health, NIH Pub. No. 93-3279, 1993.*

SOURCE OF FURTHER MATERIALS FOR USE WITH THOSE WITH ASTHMA

Australia	National Asthma Campaign, 5th Floor, 615 St Kilda Road, Melbourne Victoria 3004, Australia.
France	"ASTHME", Programme National de Recherche et d'Education, 10 Rue du Commandant Schloesing, 75116 Paris France. Tel. 47 55 03 56; Fax 44 05 91 06.
Netherlands	Nederlands Astma fonds, Postbus 5 3830 AA Leusden, The Netherlands. Tel. 033 94 18 14; Fax 033 95 03 30.

New Zealand	The Asthma Foundation of New Zealand, PO Box 1459, 7th Floor, Rossmore House, 123 Molesworth Street, Wellington New Zealand. Tel. 011 64 4 499 4592 Fax 011 64 4 499 4594.
UK	National Asthma Campaign, Providence House, Providence Place, London N1 0NT. Tel. 44 171 226 2260; Fax 44 171 704 0740. (Materials in English, Welsh, Urdu, Bengali, Gujarati, Punjabi, Hindi). Telephone Helpline 9 a.m. to 9 p.m. Monday to Friday, 0345 010203.
USA	National Asthma Education Program, National Heart, Lung and Blood Institute, 9000 Rockville Pike, Building 31, Rm 4A-18, Bethesda MD 20892, USA.

AAFA/Asthma and Allergy Foundation of America, 1125 15th Street, NW
Suite 502, Washington DC 20005, USA. Tel. (202) 466-7643.

American Academy of Allergy and Immunology, 611 East Wells Street, Milwaukee WI 53202, USA. Tel. (414) 272-6071.

Allergy and Asthma Network/Mothers of Asthmatics, Inc., 3554 Chain Bridge Road, Suite 200, Fairfax VA 22030, USA. Tel. (703) 385-4403.

American Lung Association, 1740 Broadway, 14th Floor, New York, NY 10019-4374, USA. Tel. (212) 315 8700.

KEY POINTS

1 It is important to realize from the outset that the acquisition of knowledge does not automatically lead to an alteration in patient behaviour. Barriers to education that may be present should be sought and dismantled.

2 The same information should be offered to patients (or parents) on several occasions, and by several different routes. Video tapes are often underused and yet represent an excellent medium for demonstrating practical procedures, and they are particularly suitable for those with low literacy skills.

3   In one survey only one-quarter of patients with asthma had received written instructions on how and when to take their medicines.

4   Pregnant asthmatic patients need reassurance as to the safety and efficacy of their medication. Wherever possible this reassurance should be offered both verbally and by the use of printed booklets.

24

SELF-MANAGEMENT PLANS

Wendyl D'Souza, Julian Crane and Richard Beasley

INTRODUCTION

It is now acknowledged that most asthma attacks are managed by the individual asthmatic patient in the community without any consultation with the medical profession.[1] This suggests that appropriate self-management by the asthmatic patient could have a major influence on the significant morbidity and mortality associated with this common disease. One way in which this can be achieved is through the use of self-management plans whereby the health professional educates the asthmatic patient to successfully recognize deteriorating asthma and undertake the appropriate therapeutic response(s).

This approach is recommended in the recently published national and international guidelines, which state that asthma self-management plans are essential in the long-term treatment of adult asthma.[2–6] Although there are differences in the specific plans recommended, there is a general consensus regarding the basic principles on which the system of self-management should be based. These principles, which are summarised in the Key Points of this chapter, are also discussed in detail in many of the other chapters. In many respects, self-management plans simply represent one method whereby the patient and health professional can achieve these principles.

Asthma education programmes are sometimes considered synonymous with self-management plans,[7] however, this chapter focuses only on aspects associated with the standardized written self-management guidelines given to adult patients. Although the centrality of asthma education to self-management plans is undisputed and perhaps even impossible to separate, asthma education has been covered in the preceding chapter and will not be specifically discussed.

This chapter attempts, firstly, to outline the principal components of the self-management approach to the treatment of asthma. Secondly, clinical studies assessing the efficacy of management plans will be reviewed, with discussion of some of the practical features relating to their use. Finally, two international models will be presented to illustrate how theoretical considerations may be translated into practical examples of self-management plans.

ESSENTIAL COMPONENTS OF SELF-MANAGEMENT PLANS

The basic components of a self-management plan are discussed below.

THE RECOGNITION OF DETERIORATING ASTHMA (Table 24.1)

The recognition of unstable asthma requires the educated interpretation of both subjective and objective measures of asthma severity. The need for such an approach is illustrated by the descriptive asthma mortality surveys, undertaken during the last 20 years, which have reported the circumstances surrounding asthma deaths.[8-10] The most common and important factor associated with a fatal outcome has consistently been an inability of the patient to appreciate the severity of the attack, leading to an inevitable delay in seeking appropriate medical treatment and assistance.

The most likely explanation for these observations is that asthmatic patients base their assessment of the severity of an attack of asthma on their subjective perception of symptoms such as breathlessness, chest tightness and wheeze. However, this practice may be inadequate, as a significant proportion of chronic adult asthmatic patients may have minimal symptoms despite marked airflow obstruction.[11] Poor perception of asthma severity not only occurs in the situation of worsening asthma,[11] but also

---

TABLE 24.1: *Simple criteria for the patient to recognize asthma severity*

Unstable asthma
    Nocturnal symptoms
    Pre-bronchodilator PEFR < 70–80% of "best"

"Severe" asthma
    PEFR < 50–60% of "best"
    Requirements for frequent use of inhaled β_2 agonist

"Life-threatening" asthma
    PEFR < 30–40% of "best"
    Minimal to no response to frequent high doses of inhaled β_2 agonist

---

during recovery from a severe attack[12] and is most marked in patients with greatly increased airway hyperresponsiveness.[13] This suggests that those patients who are at the greatest risk of a severe attack of asthma are those most likely to underestimate the severity of such an attack.

These observations led to the identification of key symptoms to indicate to the patient significant worsening of their asthma. In particular the development of nocturnal asthma was recognized to be a good marker of unstable asthma, and the poor response to the increased use of inhaled β_2-agonist therapy an important marker of a severe attack requiring medical attention. Support for the use of the latter marker has come from a recent study in which the risk of death was reported to increase markedly with the use of more than two β_2-agonist metered dose inhalers (MDIs) per month, which is equivalent to more than 16 puffs per day.[14]

These findings have also led to the introduction and increasing use of peak flow meters to objectively measure the degree of airflow obstruction. While forced expiratory volume in 1 s (FEV_1) is considered the "gold standard" for the physician, the peak expiratory flow rate (PEFR) is an acceptable alternative for the patient as a portable, simple and practical test of lung function.[15] With education, the PEFR is a highly repeatable measurement[16] with predicted normal values calculated based on age, sex and height.[17] Because in many asthmatic patients the PEFR is consistently higher or lower than the mean predicted values, it is recommended that "personal best lung function" is determined, based on a period of preliminary lung function monitoring for 2–4 weeks. In patients with suboptimal lung function, it may be necessary to increase therapy, including a course of oral corticosteroids, to enable the best attainable PEFR to be determined. Although the determination of the "personal best" lung function as the ultimate therapeutic end-point can be time-consuming, it has the advantage of ensuring an objective baseline to gauge any subsequent deterioration in asthma control.

Subsequent asthma exacerbations are then most easily interpreted by patients when expressed as a percentage of this personal best value. The day-to-day variability of PEFR provides an index of asthma stability and/or severity for the physician but has limited use in self-management by the patient because of its complexity, requiring at least two readings and the use of a derived value from a formula.[18,19]

A morning pre-bronchodilator recording is probably the most sensitive method to identify inadequately controlled or deteriorating asthma. As the attack progresses, both pre- and post-bronchodilator recordings will be helpful to determine the response to therapy. In general patients should be encouraged to make recordings more often as their asthma becomes more severe.

Stable Asthma

Stable asthma may be defined as a combination of minimal symptoms (ideally none) day and night, no restriction to activities (including work and recreational exercise), infrequent need for inhaled β_2-agonist therapy (ideally none), optimal pulmonary function (a pre-bronchodilator PEFR > 80% of best), daily variation of PEFR < 20% (ideally < 10%) and no medication side-effects.[2,6,7]

"Unstable" Asthma (see Table 24.1)

The most reliable markers of unstable asthma are the development of nocturnal symptoms[20,21] and/or a pre-bronchodilator PEFR < 70–80% of best.[6] These markers are simple to determine and interpret, and should form the basis for the recognition of deteriorating asthma.

Other useful indicators of unstable asthma that are less specific include symptoms suggestive of a cold[22] and an increased need for bronchodilator use. The former recognizes that most exacerbations of asthma are associated with symptoms suggestive of a respiratory tract infection and, conversely, that such symptoms in an asthmatic patient frequently herald the onset of worsening asthma.[23] The latter is more difficult to define, as it depends on the baseline requirements for inhaled bronchodilator therapy. However, both an increased use of inhaled beta-agonist therapy and an absolute amount of more than three to four times daily have been suggested as an indication of deteriorating control.

"Severe" Asthma

Reductions in PEFR to < 50–60% predicted or personal best values[24] or the requirement for frequent inhaled β_2-agonist therapy[25] are considered to be the key markers of severe asthma. Both have been shown to be associated with sudden death or near fatal asthma. Once again, the exact amount of inhaled bronchodilator use is difficult to define; however self-administration by the patient more than every 2–4 hours, with the associated feature of reduced magnitude and duration of the bronchodilator effect, may be a useful guide.[5]

"Life-threatening" Asthma

The patient's perception that the attack has deteriorated further, a minimal or no response to bronchodilator medication, or a PEFR < 30–40% predicted or personal best values should suggest to the patient that their asthma is sufficiently severe to require emergency medical management. Other symptoms or signs, such as an inability to speak in short sentences, cyanosis or a pulse rate > 110–120 beats min^{-1} may also indicate a life-threatening attack;[6] however, these signs are likely to be too difficult for the patient to measure or interpret in this clinical situation.

THE SELF-MANAGEMENT OF DETERIORATING ASTHMA

Linking the assessment of asthma control with an appropriate therapeutic response represents one of the basic principles of patient self-management.

However, this approach may create problems for the patient, and the scientific validity of some of the treatment guidelines that have been recommended is uncertain. Because of these limitations, what is suggested in this section should be considered as guidelines only; specific treatments should be tailored by the physician to meet the requirements of individual patients. Whereas exacerbations in a particular patient often follow a specific pattern, patterns of exacerbations may vary markedly between patients.

Stable Asthma

The regular use of inhaled anti-inflammatory treatment represents the basis of the long-term treatment of adult self-management plans. For most adult patients, the anti-inflammatory therapy will be inhaled corticosteroids, delivered through an MDI or dry powder device, although inhaled sodium cromoglycate and nedocromil sodium represent useful alternatives in patients with mild disease. For stable asthma, the inhaled anti-inflammatory treatment can usually be taken according to a twice-daily regimen. This has been shown to be as effective as four times daily in stable asthma and has the advantage of improving compliance, especially when associated with a routine twice-daily activity, such as teeth-cleaning. Linked with mouth-rinsing, this also reduces systemic absorption and the likelihood of oral thrush with inhaled corticosteroids.

Inhaled bronchodilator therapy is recommended to be used for relief of symptoms, rather than regularly.[6] The use of bronchodilators in this way has stemmed from the concerns that regular inhaled β_2 agonists may make chronic asthma worse.[26] When incorporated in a self-management plan system, it has the advantage of allowing the frequency of use and the resulting response to be used as a guide of asthma severity.

Unstable Asthma

Although not rigorously tested, the introduction of or increase in the dose of inhaled anti-inflammatory therapy is considered to be one of the therapeutic responses to the recognition of unstable asthma. Thus, in the situation of unstable asthma, the patient is usually instructed to double the dose of inhaled corticosteroids or start this therapy, if not currently being used. The increased dose is then continued until stable asthma is achieved.

If patients remain unstable, frequently needing to double the dose of their inhaled corticosteroid therapy, then this higher dose becomes the new regular dose. Similarly, if patients have remained stable for a few (2–3) months, they can be instructed to halve the dose of their inhaled corticosteroid therapy while continuing to use their plan to monitor their response. As patients become more experienced, these dosage adjustments can be done with minimal medical assistance.

This method of varying the dose of inhaled anti-inflammatory therapy over long periods of time is consistent with the recommended guidelines for the long-term management of chronic persistent asthma in adults, in which

TABLE 24.2: *Adult asthma self-management plan studies*

Study	Design	Features of plan/programme	Reported improvements in markers of asthma severity
Beasley et al.[31]	Open, 6 month, hospital-based (n = 36)	Four-stage PEFR-based plan Specialist outpatient clinics	Nights woken, days lost from work, requirement for oral corticosteroids, % predicted FEV$_1$ and FVC
Charlton et al.[32]	Randomized, 12 month, community-based (n = 115)	Symptom vs. PEFR based plans Nurse-run general practice clinics Educational package	Requirements for oral steroids, nebulized medications, doctor consultations
Mayo et al.[37]	Randomized, 12 month, hospital-based (n = 104)	Non-standardized symptom and PEFR and self-management plan Shared patient care with nurse practitioner Open-door clinic policy and education programme	Hospital re-admission and hospital day-use rate, requirement for oral steroids, health care costs

Study	Design	Intervention	Outcomes
Muhlhauser et al[36]	Open, 12 month, hospital-based (n = 132)	PEFR and symptom-based plan; Structured inpatient treatment and teaching programme; Specialized nurse educator	Hospital re-admission, days absent from work, severe asthma attacks, nocturnal asthma
Ruffin et al[38]	Open, 2 year, hospital-based (n = 45)	"Crisis" plan for asthmatics with previous near fatal asthma; Extensive follow-up with frequent specialist review	Near fatal asthma episodes, hospital re-admission, FEV_1, bronchial reactivity
D'Souza et al[33]	Open, 6 month, community-based (n = 69)	Combined PEFR and symptom-based ("credit card") plan; Specialist community-based clinics; Educational package	Pre-bronchodilator PEFR, nights woken, days "out of action", requirement for nebulized medications
D'Souza et al[35]	Open, 6 month, hospital-based (n = 30)	Combined PEFR and symptom-based ("credit card") plan; "High-risk" patients attending the emergency department	Visits to hospital emergency department, nights woken, days "out of action"
D'Souza et al. community-based[34]	Open, 2 year, community-based (n = 58)	Combined PEFR and symptom-based ("credit card") plan; Minimal long-term medical intervention	Emergency and non-emergency visits to general practitioner, visits to hospital emergency department, nights woken

FVC, forced vital capacity; FEV_1, forced expiratory volume in 1 second; PEFR, peak expiratory flow rate.

a step-wise approach to asthma therapy based on the classification of asthma severity is proposed.[2,6] Its incorporation into a self-management plan represents one way in which the recommendations for acute severe and chronic persistent asthma can be brought together within the framework of one system. At this and all other stages, inhaled bronchodilator therapy is recommended for use as required to relieve symptoms, and not according to a regular scheduled regimen.

Severe Asthma

Systemic corticosteroids, frequent inhaled bronchodilator use and medical practitioner review are the main components of the management plan for severe asthma. High doses of orally administered corticosteroid (30–40 mg daily), begun early in this way, can prevent a protracted or progressive course and reduce the requirement for emergency care or hospitalization.[27,28] It is not possible to predict at this stage the likely rate of recovery from the attack and, as a result, how long the patient will need to continue oral corticosteroid therapy.[29] Therefore, the therapeutic response to oral corticosteroids should be used to determine the duration of treatment, with the patient continuing on a high dose until the peak flow returns to normal values. According to physician and patient preference the patient would then take either half the dose for the same number of days before stopping, or the dose could be tapered more gradually.

With respect to the frequent use of bronchodilators by patients in the situation of severe asthma, the patient needs to recognize that this is undertaken while medical attention is being sought but should not be considered a substitute for medical assessment and treatment. Should asthma deteriorate further, the patient should be instructed to call the emergency doctor or phone for an ambulance. Other resources such as the availability of oxygen in the patient's home and a nebulizer to administer high doses of a β_2 agonist may be helpful for patients with a previous life-threatening attacks, as discussed later. The facility for self-referral and admission to hospital[30] may be organized as part of the self-management programme.

CLINICAL EFFICACY AND PRACTICAL FEATURES OF SELF-MANAGEMENT PLANS

It is disappointing that, despite the consensus on both the necessity and the principles underlying the development of asthma self-management plans, few studies have assessed their clinical efficacy. The clinical studies that have been undertaken have, in general, reported positive results with respect to improvements in asthma morbidity, lung function and requirements for acute medical treatment and hospital admission (summarized in Table 24.2). However, in many of these studies, the introduction of the self-management plans has been in an uncontrolled manner, predominantly in small "high risk" groups, with many factors being potentially responsible for the improvements noted. It is difficult, therefore, to ascertain what proportion of the beneficial effect to attribute to the self-management plans, when a number of other factors (such as education, changes in medication use and follow-up) have been introduced in combination. With these limitations in mind, we will review the self-management plan studies to discuss their evolution and some of the practical features relating to their use.

One of the first self-management plans to be assessed was based on the educated interpretation of peak flow recordings linked to four self-management steps.[31] This approach provided a step-wise system for the long-term management of asthma integrated with a method for self-managing severe attacks. Although the study was limited by its open design and lack of a control group, it did suggest that such written patient guidelines could have a major beneficial effect on asthma morbidity. The study did not attempt to identify which features of the self-management plan were responsible for the improved control of asthma. However, the regular assessment of lung function, adequate maintenance inhaled corticosteroids, early treatment of deteriorating asthma and severe attacks, education of the patients, regular specialist clinical attendance and better compliance were some of the features considered likely to have contributed to the overall improvement observed.

Subsequently Charlton et al.[32] compared this peak flow plan with a "symptom-based" one in which similar management guidelines were based on the educated interpretation of symptoms. Both plans led to a similar reduction in the requirement for acute medical treatment, suggesting that peak flow monitoring in itself may not be a crucial component of an asthma self-management plan. Rather, it stressed the importance of written guidelines coupled with rigorous self-management training and follow-up. This study also demonstrated that a nurse practitioner may be a sensible alternative to a general practitioner for undertaking an asthma management programme.

In response to these findings, an adult "credit card" asthma self-management plan was developed, which incorporated the essential features of both these "peak flow" and "symptom" based plans (Table 24.3). Management guidelines, based on both methods of assessment of asthma severity, are printed on a small plastic card, the size of a standard credit card, making this plan easy to carry in a wallet or purse (Figure 24.1). For both methods of assessment, there are four general stages in which treatment guidelines are recommended. In a series of studies, this credit card self-management plan has been shown to be both an effective and acceptable system for self-managing asthma when introduced in a formal programme of community[33,34] or hospital outpatient[35] clinics.

TABLE 24.3: *Adult "credit card" asthma self-management plan.*

Step	Peak flow	Symptoms	Action
1	80–100% best	Intermittent/few	Continue regular inhaled anti-inflammatory treatment; take bronchodilator for relief of symptoms
2	60–80% best	Waking at night with asthma or coughing	Double the dose of inhaled anti-inflammatory treatment or start if not currently taking
3	40–60% best	Increasing breathlessness or poor response to bronchodilator	Start oral corticosteroids and contact a doctor
4	< 40% best	Severe attack	Call emergency doctor or ambulance urgently

At all stages, take inhaled bronchodilator for relief of symptoms.

In these studies, the participants expressed a preference that the plan should not be bigger or present more detail, suggesting that more complicated plans may not necessarily be more suitable for general use. In the situation of an attack of asthma, most patients preferred using both PEFR and symptom sides of the card (rather than one side alone), suggesting that patients should be offered both peak flow and symptom-based methods of assessment. It was also interesting to observe the way in which the asthmatic subjects used the self-management plan system 2 years after its introduction.[34] Only 35% of patients monitored their peak flow more than once a week when stable, whereas 81% recorded their peak flow during a severe attack. The corresponding proportion of patients who referred to their plan in these situations was 13% and 58% respectively. These findings would suggest that once asthma control has been achieved, and patients are familiar with the management plan, they may be encouraged simply to monitor their peak flow, and refer to the plan primarily during exacerbations. This pragmatic approach may be more realistic than the

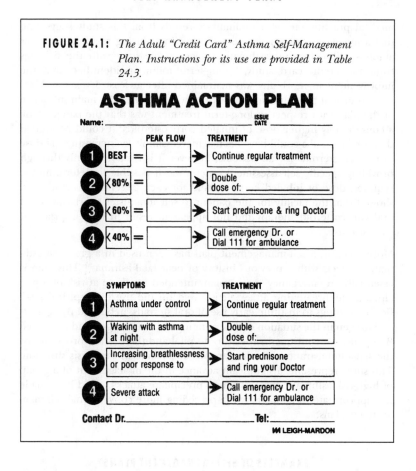

FIGURE 24.1: *The Adult "Credit Card" Asthma Self-Management Plan. Instructions for its use are provided in Table 24.3.*

twice-daily PEFR monitoring and more frequent management plan use currently advocated.

There were significant differences in the way in which therapy was recommended in the self-management plan promoted by Muhlhauser *et al.*[36] compared with the preceding plans. However, this approach also resulted in significant reductions in asthma morbidity and the study demonstrated that most patients could gain the ability and confidence to make the recommended changes in their drug regimens without consultation with their physicians.

In a controlled study, Mayo *et al.*[37] demonstrated the importance of accessibility of medical care and frequent review when management plans are introduced. A feature of this and other studies has been the emphasis on individual self-management skills, rather than the general acquisition of knowledge. This process does not necessarily need to be undertaken by a medical practitioner, with preliminary results from this study suggesting that a nurse practitioner was also effective in reducing re-admission rates amongst difficult adult asthmatic subjects. Consistent with the findings from the credit card study,[34] long-term follow-up identified that the improvement in morbidity was maintained after at least 3 years and was not a transient phenomenon. As with previous studies, the main influence of the plan with respect to long-term treatment was that the patient took a considerably higher dose of inhaled corticosteroids. It could be argued that similar results could have been achieved simply by increasing the dose of inhaled steroids for all patients; however it is likely that only through providing specific self-assessment criteria was it possible to determine the required dose of inhaled corticosteroid for each patient. This study also showed that the facility for the patient to self-administer short courses of oral corticosteroid therapy did not appear to result in inappropriate or excessive use.

More recently, a self-management plan has been used in a group of asthmatic subjects with a previous history of near fatal asthma.[37] This plan is essentially an emergency "crisis" plan, intended for those at risk of a precipitate life-threatening attack. It is based on the use of empirical peak flow recordings to institute early use of oral steroids, nebulized β_2 agonists and oxygen in the situation of deteriorating asthma. Oxygen and nebulized β_2 agonist are continued *en route* to hospital and there is the provision for the self-administration of subcutaneous adrenaline in this crisis situation. This study represents a significant advance in the management of a group of high-risk asthmatic subjects whose precipitate attacks would have made it inappropriate to manage by the preceding more conventional self-management plans.

EXAMPLES OF SELF-MANAGEMENT PLANS

Many different systems of asthma self-management have now been developed reflecting different management and educational practices. Perhaps the major differences in the design of these plans relate to the number of stages, the PEFR percentages that are recommended and their relationship to symptoms, and the amount of detail that is included. It is evident that the needs of all patients cannot be met through the use of one particular version and that different plans will suit different patients. In the following section, two international models are briefly presented to provide examples of different self-management plans that have been recommended for use.

NATIONAL ASTHMA CAMPAIGN: BRITISH PLAN (Fig. 24.2)

This system includes both a detailed and brief (credit card) version of a four-step management plan. The detailed version provides considerable

FIGURE 24.2a: *Asthma self-management plan promoted by National Asthma Campaign (UK). Booklet 7: "Self-management and peak flow measurement".*

For your doctor or nurse to complete

Zone 1

Your asthma is under control if:

- Your peak flow readings are above

  and
- it does not disturb your sleep

  and
- it does not restrict your activities

Action

Continue your normal medicines

Zone 2
(Your doctor or nurse may decide not to use this zone)

Your asthma is getting worse if:

- Your peak flow readings have fallen to between

  and
- You are needing to use your

  (reliever inhaler) more than usual
- You are waking at night with asthma symptoms

Action

- Increase your

  (preventer inhaler) to

- Continue to take your

  (reliever inhaler) to relieve your asthma symptoms

3 Your own asthma management plan

This plan helps you to adjust your treatment according to the measurements on your peak flow chart. If you take quick action, you can usually prevent severe attacks.

These instructions are only a guide, so you and your doctor or nurse may need to change them. Although the plan has four 'zones', some doctors prefer to use three and may wish you to ignore Zone 2.

Your doctor will write the ranges of peak flow which relate to each action below.

Your best (target) peak flow is

FIGURE 24.2b:

For your doctor to complete

Zone 3

Your asthma is severe if:

- Your peak flow readings have fallen to between
  _____ and _____

- You are getting increasingly breathless

- You are needing to use your
  (reliever inhaler) every
  _____ hours or more often

Action

Ring your doctor or nurse

- Take _____ prednisolone (steroid)
  tablets (_____ mgs each) and then
  _____
  _____

- Discuss with your doctor how to stop taking the tablets

- Continue to take your
  _____
  (reliever inhaler) as required

Zone 4

Medical alert/emergency if:

- Your peak flow readings have fallen to below

- You continue to get worse

Action

Get help immediately

- Ring your doctor immediately
  (Telephone _____)
  or call an ambulance

- Continue to take your
  _____
  (reliever inhaler) as needed

Do not be afraid of causing a fuss. Your doctor will want to see you urgently.

4 Update your management plan

- Because your asthma may change as time goes by, your doctor may need to change your plan accordingly. You should visit your doctor or nurse at least twice a year.

- If you often find yourself in Zones 2 or 3, let your doctor know because your medicines may need to be increased or changed.

- If you are in Zone 1 all the time it may be possible for your doctor to reduce your medicines.

- We recommend that a month or so after you start your self-management plan you should review it with your doctor or nurse.

The mini asthma management plan

You might find it helpful to carry this 'credit card' version of your plan with you at all times. It can act as a reminder in case you have unexpected symptoms.

NATIONAL **ASTHMA** CAMPAIGN
getting your breath back
Peak Flow

Name _____

Best peak flow _____

	Treatment
1	Continue regular treatment
2	Increase dose of
3	Start oral steroids and ring doctor
4	Call emergency medical help

Asthma Helpline 0345 01 02 03. Monday to Friday, 9am to 9pm

information for the patient with respect to guidelines for recognizing deteriorating asthma and the appropriate therapeutic response. No fixed PEFR percentages are recommended, to enable doctors to vary the levels at each stage for which treatment guidelines are made according to the requirements of individual patients.

One of the real strengths of this plan is the method of delivery. This system is part of a comprehensive educational booklet that is being promoted to both medical and nursing practitioners in general practice. The booklet explains how to undertake PEFR monitoring, the use of medication for chronic and acute asthma and the system of self-management, with the facility for the patient and doctor to work through the booklet and fill in the details of the self-management plan together. The booklet also includes a brief credit card version of the plan, which can be removed from the main book of instructions and carried by the patient or kept with a peak flow meter.

INTERNATIONAL ASTHMA MANAGEMENT PLAN "ZONE SYSTEM"
(Fig. 24.3)
This system probably represents the most complex plan available and, as with other systems, uses a step-wise approach in which the recognition of deteriorating asthma is undertaken by reduction in peak flow from best, increasingly severe symptoms, as well as the response to treatment itself. In this way, three "zones" of asthma severity are defined for the patient. The zones have been adapted to a traffic light system to make it simpler for patients to use and remember.[39,40] The recognition of trigger factors is also encouraged through this system. Initiation of oral corticosteroids is more flexible and can be introduced at an earlier level (in the yellow zone). Clinical studies assessing the efficacy of this comprehensive system of self-management are awaited with interest.

CONCLUSION

The development of self-management plans arose as clinicians tried to design better methods by which they could deliver asthma care and reduce the significant mortality and morbidity associated with this disease. The basic management principles that resulted have been widely endorsed, with self-management plans now being considered essential in the long-term management of adult asthma.

Self-management plans essentially focus on the early recognition of unstable or deteriorating asthma, by monitoring PEFR or symptoms. Through the use of written guidelines, patients are then able to determine when it is necessary to adjust therapy or obtain medical assistance.

It is generally acknowledged that more research is still needed in many areas to determine the ideal number of stages necessary for a plan, the

FIGURE 24.3a: *Asthma self-management plan adapted from the National Asthma Education Program "Clinician's Guide: Teaching Your Patients About Asthma", National Heart, Lung and Blood Institute, National Institutes of Health, USA.*

ASTHMA CONTROL PLAN FOR_____
(name of patient)

PREPARED BY _____ M.D.

This plan will help you control your asthma and do the right thing if you have an asthma episode. Keeping your asthma under control will help you:

- Be active without having asthma symptoms. This includes being active in exercise or sports.
- Sleep through the night without having asthma symptoms.
- Prevent asthma episodes (attacks).
- Have the best possible peak flow rate.
- Avoid side effects from medicines.

Here are three ways to control your asthma:

■ Follow your medicine plan (see the next page).
  –Follow your Green Zone plan every day to keep most asthma symptoms from starting.
  –Recognize your symptoms of an asthma episode. Act quickly to stop them.
  –Follow the Yellow Zone plan to stop asthma symptoms and to keep an asthma episode from getting serious.
  –Follow the Red Zone plan to take care of a serious episode. This is an emergency plan!

■ Whenever possible, stay away from things that bring on your asthma symptoms. Follow your asthma trigger control plan to reduce the number of things in your home, workplace, or classroom that bother your asthma.

■ See your doctor regularly. Review this plan with your doctor when you visit him/her. Your doctor will write on the plan what you should do.

Your plan has these medicines:

_____

_____

_____

_____

_____

_____

Important Information:

Doctor_____   Hospital _____

Telephone_____   Telephone_____

Address_____   Address_____

_____   _____

Ambulance or Emergency Rescue Squad_____   **Friend to Call**_____

Telephone _____   Telephone_____

Taxi_____

For more information on Asthma:
National Asthma Education Program
Information Center
P.O. Box 30105
Bethesda, MD 20824-0105
(301) 951-3260

Adapted from National Asthma Education Program "Clinician's Guide: Teaching Your Patients About Asthma," National Heart, Lung, and Blood Institute, National Institutes of Health, United States.

FIGURE 24.3b:

ASTHMA CONTROL PLAN FOR _____
(name of patient)

PREPARED BY _____ , M.D.

Green Zone: All Clear

This is where you should be every day.

Peak flow between _____
(80-100% of personal best)*

No symptoms of an asthma episode. You are able to do your usual activities and sleep without having symptoms.

The doctor will check which applies to you.

☐ Take these medicines.

Medicine	How much to take	When to take it

☐ Follow your asthma trigger control plan to avoid things that bring on your asthma.

☐ Take _____ before exercise.
(medicine)

Yellow Zone: Caution

This is not where you should be every day. Take action to get your asthma under control.

Peak flow between _____
(50-80% of personal best)*

You may be coughing, wheezing, feel short of breath, or feel like your chest is tight. These symptoms may keep you from your usual activities or keep you from sleeping.

☐ *First,* take this medicine:

Medicine	How much to take	When to take it

☐ *Next,* if you feel better in 20 to 60 minutes and your peak flow is over _____, then:
(70% of personal best)

☐ Take this medicine

Medicine	How much to take	When to take it

☐ Keep taking your green zone medicine(s).

☐ *But,* if you DO NOT feel better in 20-60 minutes or your peak flow is under _____, **follow the Red Zone Plan.**
(70% of personal best)

Let the doctor know if you keep going into the Yellow Zone. Your Green Zone medicine may need to be changed to keep other episodes from starting.

Red Zone: Medical Alert

This is an emergency! Get help.

Peak flow under _____
(50% of personal best)*

You may be coughing, very short of breath, and/or the skin between your ribs and your neck may be pulled in tight. You may have trouble walking or talking. You may not be wheezing because not enough air can move out of your airways.

This is a general guideline only. Some people have asthma that gets worse very fast. They may need to have a yellow zone at 90-100% of personal best.

☐ *First,* take this medicine:

Medicine	How much to take	When to take it

☐ *Next,* **call the doctor** to talk about what you should do next.

☐ *But,* see the doctor RIGHT AWAY or go to the hospital if *any* of these things are happening:

–Lips or fingernails are blue

–You are struggling to breathe

–You do not feel any better 20 to 30 minutes after taking the extra medicine and your peak flow is still under _____.
50% of personal best

–Six hours after you take the extra medicine, you still need an inhaled beta$_2$-agonist medicine every 1 to 3 hours and your peak flow is under _____.
70% of personal best

---

exact level of symptoms or PEFR requiring a specific therapeutic response, and the relationship (if any) between the different therapeutic responses and outcome (for example, does increasing the dose of inhaled steroids in the "early" stages of an exacerbation prevent further deterioration). It will also be necessary to determine which patients are most likely to benefit from this system of management.

Many different systems of asthma self-management have now been developed, reflecting different management and educational practices. It is apparent that the needs of all patients cannot be met through the use of one particular version. Whatever plan is employed, the written guidelines need to reflect the health care system and cultural needs of the respective community in which it is introduced and must be tailored to meet the specific needs of individual patients.

REFERENCES

1   Avery CH, March J, Book RH. An assessment of the adequacy of self-care by adult asthmatics. *J Community Health* 1980; 5: 167–81.

2   British Thoracic Society, Research Unit of the Royal College of Physicians, Kings Fund Centre, National Asthma Campaign. Guidelines for management of asthma in adults: I. Chronic persistent asthma. *BMJ* 1990; 301: 651–3.

3   Thoracic Society of Australia and New Zealand. Consensus on asthma: Asthma management plan, 1989. *Med J Aust* 1989; 18: 650–8.

4   Hargreave FE, Dolvich J, Newhouse MT (eds). The assessment and treatment of asthma: A conference report. *J Allergy Clin Immunol* 1990; 85: 1098–111.

5   Hargreave FE. The drug treatment of asthma: how can it be better applied? *Postgrad Med J* 1989; 64: 74–81.

6   Lenfant C. International Consensus Report on Diagnosis and Management of Asthma. National Heart, Lung and Blood Institute, National Institutes of Health. *US Department of Health and Human Services, Bethesda, USA, 1992.*

7   Wilson-Pessano SR, Mellins RB. Workshop on asthma self-management: summary of workshop discussion. *J Allergy Clin Immunol* 1987; 80: 487–90.

8   MacDonald JB, Seaton A, Williams DA. Asthma deaths in Cardiff 1963–74: 90 deaths outside hospital. *BMJ* 1976; iii: 1493–5.

9   British Thoracic Association. Death from asthma in two regions of England. *BMJ* 1982; 285: 1251–5.

10 Rea HH, Sears MR, Beaglehole R *et al.* Lessons from the national asthma mortality study: circumstances surrounding death. *N Z Med J* 1987; 100: 10–3.

11 Rubinfield AR, Pain MCF. Perception of asthma. *Lancet* 1975; ii: 822–4.

12 McFadden ER, Kiser R, De Groot WJ. Acute bronchial asthma. Relations between clinical and physiological manifestations. *N Engl J Med* 1973; 288: 221–5.

13 Burdon JGW, Juniper EF, Killian KJ, Hargreave FE, Campbell EJM. The perception of breathlessness in asthma. *Am Rev Respir Dis* 1982; 126: 825–8.

14 Suissa S, Erust P, Boivin J-F *et al.* A cohort analysis of excess mortality in asthma and the use of inhaled β-agonists. *Am J Respir Crit Care Med* 1994; 149: 604–10.

15 Wright BM, McKerrow CB. Maximum forced expiratory flow rate as a measure of ventilatory capacity: with a description of a new portable instrument for measuring it. *BMJ* 1959; 2: 1041–7.

16 Lal S, Ferguson AD, Campbell EJM. Forced expiratory time: a simple test for airways obstruction. *BMJ* 1964; 1: 814–7.

17 Gregg I, Nunn AJ. Peak expiratory flow in normal subjects. *BMJ* 1973; 3: 282–4.

18 Lebowitz MJ. The use of peak expiratory flow rate measurements in respiratory diseases. *Pediatr Pneumol* 1991; 11: 166–74.

19 Quackenboss JJ, Lebowitz MD, Krzyzanowski M. The normal range of diurnal changes in peak expiratory flow rates: relationship to symptoms and respiratory diseases. *Am Rev Respir Dis* 1991; 143: 323–30.

20 Corrao WM, Braman SS, Irwin RS. Chronic cough as the sole presenting manifestation of bronchial asthma. *N Engl J Med* 1979; 300: 633–7.

21 Turner-Warwick M. On observing patterns of airflow obstruction in chronic asthma. *Br J Dis Chest* 1977; 71: 73–86.

22 Partridge MR. Self-care plans for asthmatics. *Practitioner* 1991; 235: 715–21.

23 Pattemore PK, Johnston SL, Bardin PG. Viruses as precipitants of asthma symptoms. I. Epidemiology. *Clin Exp Allergy* 1992; 22: 325–30.

24 Bateman JRM, Clarke SW. Sudden death in asthma. *Thorax* 1979; 34: 40–4.

25 Windom HH, Burgess CD, Crane J, Pearce N, Kwong T, Beasley R. The self-administration of inhaled beta agonist drugs during severe asthma. *N Z Med J* 1990; 103: 205–7.

26 Sears MR, Taylor DR, Print CG *et al.* Regular inhaled beta agonist treatment in bronchial asthma. *Lancet* 1990; 336: 1391–6.

27 Webb JR. Dose response of patients to oral corticosteroid treatment during exacerbations of asthma. *BMJ* 1986; 292: 1046–7.

28 Fiel SB, Swartz MA, Glanz K, Francis ME. Efficacy of short term corticosteroid therapy in outpatient treatment of acute bronchial asthma. *Am J Med* 1983; 75: 259–62.

29 Smith AP. Patterns of recovery from acute severe asthma. *Br J Dis Chest* 1981; 75: 132–40.

30 Crompton GK, Grant IWB. Edinburgh emergency asthma admission service. *BMJ* 1975; 4: 680–2.

31 Beasley R, Cushley M, Holgate ST. A self-management plan in the treatment of adult asthma. *Thorax* 1989; 44: 200–4.

32 Charlton I, Charlton G, Broomfield J, Mullee MA. Evaluation of peak flow and symptoms only self-management plans for control of asthma in general practice. *BMJ* 1990; 301: 1355–9.

33. D'Souza W, Crane J, Burgess C *et al*. Community-based asthma care: trial of a "credit card" asthma self-management plan. *Eur Respir J* 1994; 7: 1260–5.

34. Te Reo o te Ora: The Wairarapa Maori Asthma Project. Wairarapa Maori Executive/Taiwhenua o Ngati Kahunguna ki Wairarapa and the Wellington Asthma Research Group, September 1992.

35. D'Souza W, Burgess C, Crane J *et al*. Trial of a credit card asthma self-management plan in a "high risk" group of asthmatics. *Eur Respir J* 1993; 17: 145s.

36. Muhlhauser I, Richter B, Kraut D, Weske G, Worth H, Berger M. Evaluation of a structured treatment and teaching programme on asthma. *J Intern Med* 1991; 230: 157–64.

37. Mayo PH, Richman J, Harris W. Results of a program to reduce admissions for adult asthma. *Ann Intern Med* 1990; 112: 864–71.

38. Ruffin RE, Latimer K, Schembri DA. Longitudinal study of near fatal asthma. *Chest* 1991; 99: 77–83.

39. Lewis CE, Rachelefsky G, Lewis MA, de la Sota A, Kaplan M. A randomised trial of ACT (asthma care training for kids). *Pediatrics* 1984; 74: 478–86.

40. Mendoza GR, Sander N, Scherrer A. *A User's Guide to Peak Flow Monitoring.* Mothers of Asthmatics Inc., 1988.

KEY POINTS

1   Asthma is an inflammatory disease, with the therapeutic implications:
- (a)   inhaled anti-inflammatory drugs represent the basis of long-term treatment;
- (b)   systemic corticosteroids are essential in the treatment of severe asthma.

2   Requirement for objective assessment of asthma severity, with the educated interpretation of:
- (a)   key symptoms such as nocturnal waking and requirement/response to bronchodilator treatment;
- (b)   peak flow meter recordings.

3   Integration of self-assessment and self-management with written guidelines for both:
- (a)   long-term treatment of asthma;
- (b)   treatment of acute severe asthma.

25

ASSESSMENT OF COMPLIANCE

G.M. Cochrane

INTRODUCTION

Non-compliance or poor adherence to medical advice is a significant problem and may account in part for the failure to improve morbidity in treatment of patients with asthma.[1] Studies over the last 20 years, mainly in diseases other than asthma, have suggested that 40–50% of patients do not use medicines as prescribed[2] and compliance is not associated with age, sex, educational levels, economic status and diagnosis (except mental illness and alcohol addiction).[3] The role of non-compliance with therapy in patients with asthma, particularly with inhaled therapy, has been virtually ignored in both clinical trials and in the community at large.[4]

The extent of non-compliance with treatment and medical advice in patients with asthma is not known, although some insight is now being obtained by assessing and auditing educational programmes for patients with asthma (see Chapter 24) but few trials define end-points for compliance.

Compliance is defined as the extent to which a patient's behaviour coincides with medical advice. Full compliance occurs when the patient follows meticulously the advice stated. Partial compliance can either be that the patient fails to take the total number of doses of prescribed drug each day but completes the course of therapy or has the full number of doses of drug but fails to complete the prescribed course. The biological effects of partial compliance may therefore differ, particularly in asthma where more than one preparation is frequently prescribed. Full compliance with bronchodilator "rescue" therapy but partial compliance with inhaled corticosteroid "preventer" therapy is likely to lead to a differing biological outcome to that where patients take most of their "preventer" therapy but fail to carry their rescue bronchodilator inhaler.

METHODS OF ASSESSMENT OF COMPLIANCE

Assessment of patient compliance can either be by direct or indirect methods (Table 25.1).

DIRECT METHODS OF ASSESSMENT

Direct estimations of blood or urine levels to ascertain compliance with therapy are susceptible to error as they only estimate drug consumption in the previous few hours or days and may be anticipated by the patient if used in regular follow-up appointments. Many of the anti-asthma drugs taken by the inhaled route will be undetectable in biological fluids. Even with serum theophylline estimation, which is cheap and readily available, studies indicate that the patient is either taking too much or none at all.[5] Salbutamol usage has been shown to be both under-used and over-used using a technique measuring urine salbutamol[6] but this is a complex and expensive estimation and only measures compliance on the day of estimation.

INDIRECT METHODS OF ASSESSMENT OF COMPLIANCE

Comparison of direct questioning of patients about their compliance with direct biological fluid drug levels produces variable results depending on the population and disease studied. A recent study[7] in general practice using questionnaires correlated to prescription identified that only one-third of patients with airflow obstruction took more than 50% of their prescribed medication. The situation may be even more complex as there is up to 35% non-agreement between patient interview and direct measurement, particularly in patients on oral theophyllines.[8] When assessed against direct and indirect methods physicians are poor at determining which patients are, or are not, complying.[9] Electronic pill counting is usually less

---

TABLE 25.1: *Traditional methods of assessment of compliance*

Direct
Blood: single observation
Urine: affected by patient pre-knowledge

Indirect
Patient interview: inaccurate
Doctor belief: very inaccurate
Pill counting: rarely applicable in asthma
Aerosol weighing/dry disc counting: errors due to "dumping"
Therapeutic outcome: can be affected by variation in asthma severity

relevant in asthmatic patients but pill-counting studies suggest that only 75% of patients fully comply;[10] others partially comply. As a measure of longitudinal compliance such techniques are open to doubt, since compliance may be affected by patients being aware that they are under scrutiny and involved in a clinical trial.[11] Canister weighing, although accurate in assessing the number of puffs expelled from the canister, tends to be unreliable because patients are aware of being under scrutiny and therefore "dump", but do not inhale, the medication before returning the inhaler.[12]

Therapeutic response remains the commonest form of assessment of compliance, using diary cards with scoring systems for cough, wheeze and nocturnal wakening, in addition to home peak flow monitoring. The development of electronic diary cards that record the time the diary card symptoms and peak flow measurements were actually made, as well as recording the data, has shown that records may suffer falsification and unless objective techniques are used therapeutic outcome may not be as accurate an assessment of compliance as is often suggested. In a 1-week study using such an electronic diary card more than 10% of the diary card entries and peak flow measurements were either mistimed or invented in 17 of 30 patients.[13] Some patients were clearly mainly compliant and occasionally just forgot, but one-third of patients had invented 25% of the times and measurements invalidating any clinical trial. A comparison of a written diary record compared with a hand-held computer[14] that did not include peak flow measurements again showed that approximately 20% of entries were mistimed and potentially invented. The patients in these studies were not directly aware of the timing device. Therapeutic outcome as an index of compliance assumes drug efficacy and therefore is invalid in prospective trials of new drugs. Traditional methods of assessing compliance with therapy, particularly in patients with asthma, tend to be inaccurate, overestimate compliance and, in new drug trials, testing dose relationship may lead to potential errors.[15]

OBJECTIVE ASSESSMENT OF COMPLIANCE WITH INHALED THERAPY

Canister weighing and rotacapsule and disc counting have been suggested but are inherently inaccurate, all overestimating actual drug use and not taking account of deliberate "dumping"[16] when patients believe they may be under surveillance.[12] The development of electronic recording devices, which record actuation,[17] the time of actuation ("Chronolog")[18] and even whether the drug is inhaled (TIC Turbohaler),[19] has allowed considerably greater insight into the magnitude of non-compliance with inhaled therapy in asthma.

The initial study by Spector *et al.*[18] using the "Chronolog" demonstrated the effectiveness of the device, which revealed less than 50% compliance to a four times a day regimen. Mawhinney and co-workers[20] examined compliance in clinical trials of two non-bronchodilator drugs. These workers identified poor compliance even in the clinical trial situation; the level of compliance was adequate in only 6 of 34 patients such that drug efficacy could be determined. They also showed that one-third of their patients had periods of "multiple simultaneous use" of 10 or more actuations, i.e. "dumping", so that the canister weight would be nearer the anticipated weight if the patient had been fully compliant.

Similar non-compliance was found with ipratropium bromide, a bronchodilator prescribed as two inhalations three times a day.[16] The Chronolog data showed that self-reporting and inhaler canister weighing overestimate adherence and again confirmed that a substantial number of monitored patients deliberately "dump" medication prior to follow-up visits.

The prescribing of regular twice-daily inhaled corticosteroids for the treatment of moderate asthma is now generally accepted, but there have been few studies looking at their actual use compared with prescription in the community. A 9-month study by Horn and co-workers[21] supported the effectiveness of inhaled corticosteroids in the treatment of asthma but noted that their efficacy was not as great as anticipated. Using a combination of peak flow response, rotacapsule counting, canister weighing and spot biochemical validation, these authors[22] identified considerable non-compliance but were unable to define whether compliance was greater with β agonist or inhaled corticosteroid. Dompeling and colleagues[23] compared compliance with an inhaled corticosteroid and a bronchodilator using capsule counting; they found compliance with the corticosteroid was less than with the bronchodilator but the two were highly correlated, suggesting compliance was patient dependent rather than drug dependent. In an attempt to see whether there was greater compliance with regularly prescribed inhaled bronchodilator, Bosley and co-workers,[19] in conjunction with the research department of Draco, Sweden, developed the Turbohaler inhalation computer (TIC), which recorded the time and date of each inhalation. The inhalations were recorded using a microphone to identify the rotational click and inspiratory flow noise, which had to be sustained for approximately one-third of a second. Thus only "true" inhalations were recorded and "dumping" or multiple simultaneous rotations without inhalation were not recorded but identified using the number of grip turns on the mechanical counter on the device. This study compared patient compliance with an inhaled corticosteroid (budesonide) and a short-acting inhaled β agonist (terbutaline sulphate) to a Turbohaler inhaler containing a combination of the two drugs.

In this open multicentre parallel group study 102 asthmatic patients were randomly divided into two groups, either receiving the two drugs in separate Turbohalers or combined into one Turbohaler. A dose of one or two inhalations daily was prescribed and a pre-weighed metered-dose inhaler (MDI) of salbutamol was provided for rescue use. Compliance was measured using the TIC, which recorded the time and date of each inhalation over a 12-week period. Forced expiratory volume in 1 s (FEV_1) and forced vital capacity (FVC) measurements were done at 0, 6 and 12 weeks.

A number of patients were lost to follow-up and TIC failure meant results from only 72 patients were analysed. There was no significant difference between the inhalers in the level of compliance, the average compliance being between 60 and 70%. Treatment was taken as prescribed on 30–40% of the study days, and over-usage occurred on less than 10% of days. Only 15% of patients took the drugs as prescribed for more than 80% of the days.

The combination of inhaled corticosteroid and bronchodilator was not associated with significantly greater compliance. A number of patterns of compliance were identified, some patients taking both drugs only once a day, others having full compliance on and off during the study in a sort of "holiday" pattern, while others tended to be compliant just before and just after clinic visits.

PSYCHOLOGY OF NON-COMPLIANCE WITH MEDICAL ADVICE

The same group[24] also studied whether psychological factors such as anxiety, depression, interpersonal problems, attitudes towards asthma and its treatment were related to patient compliance with inhaled medication. As a part of the TIC inhaler study[19] patients underwent prospective psychological assessment using the Hospital Anxiety and Depression Scale, the Inventory of Personal Problems and the semi-structured interview formulary on patient attitudes and treatment beliefs. Of the evaluable 72 patients 37 took less than 70% of the prescribed therapy or had omitted doses for greater than 1 week and were defined as non-compliant. This non-compliant group had higher depression scores than compliant patients. The whole study population had a higher mean anxiety than in non-asthmatic patients but there was no significant difference in anxiety between the non-compliant and compliant asthmatic subjects. Patient self-reporting and clinician's impressions of compliance were again shown to be only weakly associated with actual compliance. Using discriminant analysis, a model was obtained that correctly classified 79% of the patients as compliant or non-compliant. Non-compliance tended to be associated with depression, but was also found in personalities who found it hard to be assertive and take control of their lives, in females and in those younger at age of diagnosis. Non-compliant patients also tended to rationalize harmful activities such as smoking or keeping pets. Compliance was associated with loneliness and obsessional characteristics, satisfaction with treatment, increasing age and support from partners and others. Increased anxiety tended also to improve compliance but only in conjunction with good general self-care and avoidance of harmful activities.

IMPROVING COMPLIANCE WITH MEDICAL ADVICE

Non-compliance with medical advice, like all human behaviour, results from a complex interaction of many different factors.[25] Educational programmes about the disease, particularly aerosol technique and individual drugs, undoubtedly help (see Chapter 23). Simple drug regimens are essential, in particular keeping drug-taking frequency to a maximum of twice a day, and are associated with improved compliance.[12,19] Side-effects, either real or feared, are associated with poorer compliance while treatment regimens that lead to improved morbidity are associated with greater compliance.

Combination therapy, particularly in view of the potential hazards of regular β agonists and the impression that they are no more effective in improving compliance,[19] are not recommended. The timing and frequency of consultations are associated with increased compliance if these are also associated with good doctor–nurse–patient relationships.

However further improvements in compliance and disease management must be associated with patients being actively involved in the process of determining the "therapeutic plan". Recognition that a physician–patient partnership is required rather than the previous authoritarian or paternalistic mode of behaviour is important. This partnership must recognize the patient's own goals, fears, health beliefs and personal circumstances if greater compliance with medical advice is to be obtained, with hopefully a reduction in morbidity and possibly mortality from asthma.

REFERENCES

1 Anon. Are you taking the medicines? *Lancet* 1990; 335: 262–3.

2 Ley P. (ed.) The problem of patient non-compliance. In: *Communicating with Patients: Improving Communication, Satisfaction and Compliance.* London: Croom Helm, 1988; 61–3.

3 Sackett DL, Snow JC. The magnitude of compliance and non-compliance. In: Haynes RB, Taylor DW, Sackett DL (eds) *Compliance in Health Care.* Baltimore: Johns Hopkins University Press, 1979; 11–22.

4. Cochrane GM, Horn CR. The management of asthma in the community: Problems of compliance with treatment. Q J Med 1991; 81: 797–8.

5. Dirks JF, Kinsman RA. Non-dichotomous patterns of medication usage, the yes and no fallacy. Clin Pharmacol Ther 1982; 31: 413–7.

6. Horn CR, Essex E, Hill P, Cochrane GM. Does urinary salbutamol reflect compliance with aerosol regimen in patients with asthma? Respir Med 1989; 83: 15–8.

7. Dekker FW, Dieleman FE, Kaptein AA, Mulder JD. Compliance with pulmonary medication in general practice. Eur Respir J 1993; 6: 886–90.

8. Glanz K, Fiel SB, Swatz MA, Francis ME. Compliance with an experimental drug regimen for treatment of asthma: its magnitude importance and correlates. J Chron Dis 1984; 37: 815–24.

9. Muslim AI, Appel FA. Diagnosing patient non-compliance. Arch Intern Med 1977; 137: 318–21.

10. Cramer JS, Mattson RH, Prevey ML, Scheyer RD, Ouellette VL. How often is medication taken as prescribed? A novel assessment technique. JAMA 1989; 261: 3273–7.

11. Reiser J, Warner JO. The value of participating in an asthma trial. Lancet 1985; i: 206–7.

12. Spector SL. Is your asthmatic really complying. Ann Allergy 1985; 55: 552–6.

13. Chowienczyk PJ, Lawson CP, Morris J, Kermani A, Cochrane GM. Electronic diary card to record physiological measurements. Lancet 1992; 339: 251.

14. Hyland ME, Kenyon CAP, Allen R, Howarth P. Diary keeping in asthma: comparison of written and electronic methods. BMJ 1993; 306: 487–9.

15. Goldsmith CH. The effects of compliance distribution on therapeutics trials. In: Haynes RB, Taylor DW, Sackett DL (eds) Compliance in Health Care. Baltimore: Johns Hopkins Press, 1979, 297–308.

16. Rand CS, Wise RA, Nides M et al. Metered dose inhaler adherence in a clinical trial. Am Rev Respir Dis 1992; 146: 1559–64.

17. Yeung M, O'Connor SA, Parry DT, Cochrane GM. Compliance with drug therapy and the management of asthma. Respir Med 1994; 88: 31–5.

18. Spector SL, Kinsman RA, Mawhinney M et al. Compliance of patients with asthma with an experimental aerosolized medication. Implications for controlled trials. J Allergy Clin Immunol 1986; 77: 65–70.

19. Bosley CM, Parry DT, Cochrane GM. Patient compliance with inhaled medication. Does combining beta agonists with corticosteroids improve compliance? Eur Respir J 1994; 7: 504–9.

20. Mawhinney M, Spector SL, Kinsman RA et al. Compliance in clinical trials of two non-bronchodilator anti-asthma medications. Ann Allergy 1991; 66: 294–9.

21 Horn CR, Clark TJH, Cochrane GM. Can the morbidity of asthma be reduced by high dose inhaled therapy? A prospective study. *Respir Med* 1990; 84: 61–6.

22 Horn CR, Clark TJH, Cochrane GM. Compliance with inhaled therapy and morbidity from asthma. *Respir Med* 1990; 84: 67–70.

23 Dompeling E, Vangrunsven PM, Van Schayckn CP, Folgering H, Molema J, Van Weel C. Treatment with inhaled steroids in asthma and chronic bronchitis. Long term compliance with inhaler technique. *Fam Pract* 1992; 912: 161–6.

24 Bosley CM, Fosbury JA, Cochrane GM. The psychological problems associated with poor compliance with treatment in asthma. *Eur Respir J* 1994 submitted for publication.

25 Mellins RB, Evans D, Zimmerman B, Clark NM. Patient compliance – are we wasting our time and don't know it? *Am Rev Respir Dis* 1992; 146: 1376–7.

KEY POINTS

1   Non-compliance with medical advice is common and underestimated in clinical trials. It is difficult to assess accurately in asthma as direct assessment with inhaled therapy is complicated. New techniques using electronic devices to record inhaler therapy and peak flow longitudinally are required.

2   Causes of non-compliance: these are multifactorial but inappropriate and complex drug regimens are important factors. Depression, shorter duration of illness and lack of family support will all lead to lower levels of compliance with medical advice.

3   Improving compliance: clear written advice with simple drug regimens allied to educational asthma programmes will improve compliance. Consistent advice from doctor and nurse developing a trusting patient relationship should also help.

Management of Asthma

26
GENERAL PRINCIPLES
T.J.H. Clark

The traditional approach to asthma management has been to enable patients to cope with the condition. This essentially means an approach based upon relief of symptoms and the avoidance of precipitating or trigger factors. In the past much attention was paid to the emotional state of patients but it is now accepted that the best way to provide emotional contentment for a patient with asthma is to treat the underlying causes of it effectively rather than rely on treatment of the emotional disturbance itself. Relief of symptoms has traditionally relied on bronchodilators, which in part was conditioned by the view that the cause for symptoms was bronchoconstriction. Other aspects of pathogenesis were either conveniently ignored or not targeted by therapy. The avoidance of trigger factors meant that many patients led a sheltered life and this was often combined with the use of desensitization if there was an obvious allergic cause.

This traditional approach to asthma management has been largely supplanted by treatment directed towards the causes of asthma and its associated bronchoconstriction and by more direct and targeted environmental control in preference to modifying the patient's immune defences.

CONTROL OF ASTHMA

The aims of treatment are now to control asthma. By this is meant a strategy to prevent asthma symptoms arising and to keep symptoms suppressed should they break through the preventive measures.[1] Control of asthma is now made explicit with absence of symptoms, or their minimization if present, being a prime aim. This aim needs to be associated with a normal quality of life as some patients can avoid symptoms simply by not doing anything. Thus freedom from symptoms needs to be accompanied by the patient carrying out normal recreational and social activities like going to work or school and playing games.

In addition to suppression of symptoms, lung function needs to be restored to normal or as near normal as possible. As well as improving daytime lung function it is important to control the diurnal variability of asthma so as to eliminate sleep disturbance, which is an important aim of therapy. Patients who wake at night with asthma are at risk.[2]

The suppression of symptoms, a normal life-style and restoration of lung function should be achieved without adverse side-effects. As total elimination of symptoms is unusual and total freedom from side-effects of treatment is rare, the physician aims to strike a reasonable balance between medication to suppress asthma and the side-effects from treatment itself. Thus oral corticosteroid therapy can achieve excellent control of asthma in the majority of patients but at an unacceptable level of systemic side-effects. It is for this reason that inhaled therapy is generally preferred to oral or parenteral medication as inhaled delivery of drugs enables a small but effective dose to be delivered to the airway, thus minimizing the risks of systemic absorption and side-effects.[3]

Thus control of asthma is outcome related and can be measured for purposes of audit. The importance of these goals of treatment is discussed in greater detail in Chapter 29.

COMPLIANCE

The primary aim of asthma control requires adequate education of both patients, their families and the doctor supervising management. This has been discussed at some length in the preceding chapters, which emphasize the seminal importance of education and communication in achieving control of asthma. Unfortunately this does not always result in improved control.[4]

COST-EFFECTIVENESS

The management of asthma is based largely on the individual patient but those responsible for treatment have a wider obligation to society at large. The prevalence and severity of asthma appear to be increasing and this, combined with the chronic nature of asthma, makes it a costly condition. In general asthma costs about 1% of most countries' health budgets and this applies whether the country is very poor or very wealthy. Asthma medications are usually amongst the most common prescribed drugs and, as asthma leads to many emergency room visits and inpatient admissions, the direct medical costs are very high in addition to the costs of medication.[5]

In the USA, the costs of asthma have been estimated to be just over $6 billion per annum and asthma accounts for 1% of expenditure on health.[6] The majority of these costs are attributable to direct medical expenditure but a substantial minority is expended on indirect costs such as social security payments and lost productivity with time off work. If loss of schooling is added as a further indirect cost then the burden of asthma on society is seen to be very great.[7] In view of this, physicians need to recognize the importance of providing effective therapy to minimize costs. In essence, by achieving asthma control direct medical costs can be substantially reduced as well as the indirect costs referred to above. Thus medication or other interventions can more than repay their cost if they reduce hospital admissions, emergency room visits and social security payments.[8] One of the further aims of management must therefore be to provide the most cost-effective therapy with demonstration of effectiveness in terms of not only the individual patient but also the cost to society.

ENVIRONMENTAL CONTROL

Most asthma management consists of pharmacotherapy. Desensitization or immunotherapy has a diminishing place in asthma management as it has proved difficult safely to modify the immune defence of patients to allergens. Immunotherapy can be successful but carries with it significant risks so its place is limited in asthma, and it is generally reserved for patients who fail to benefit from pharmacotherapy or achieve benefit with unacceptable side-effects.[9]

Over the past few years a new strategy for allergen-induced asthma has become popular. Avoidance of allergens and other causes for asthma might be of very considerable benefit both to individual patients and society. The rising prevalence of asthma may reflect an increasing allergen load associated with increasing urbanization and wealth within societies.[10] This suggests that external and environmental factors are fuelling the increase in asthma prevalence and offers scope for reducing this trend.[11]

A number of especially important candidates are now being examined for environmental control. The role of maternal smoking in increasing the risk of asthma in the newborn and in the neonatal period provides one main avenue for environmental control.[12] The other is to target the commonest allergens of childhood asthma and reduce this exposure in the environment of the newborn child and infant.[13] This might both delay the onset of asthma and reduce its severity and might be achieved by fairly simple measures.

In some countries the intervention to reduce significantly the aeroallergen load might prove very costly and all forms of environmental control to provide primary prevention of asthma need to be rigorously examined in terms of their cost-effectiveness. If demonstrated to be effective and at an acceptable cost the prevention of asthma should be an important aim of treatment.

GUIDELINES

The increasing burden of asthma on both the individual patient and society has led to the development of guidelines for asthma management. This has been based upon the goals of treatment as set out above in which control of asthma is the aim. Guidelines recommend standards of care to achieve these goals based upon best practice.[14] Unfortunately, best practice is often based upon custom rather than a rigorous proof of the effectiveness of the treatment being recommended but over the past few years increasing evidence has been obtained to support the guidelines that are now in current use.[15]

Guidelines must be seen as providing the best advice to physicians and patients concerning the achievement of control of asthma. Asthma itself is extremely diverse in its manifestation and severity so asthma control needs to be made individual for each patient. The guidelines therefore offer advice and cannot be implemented in an inflexible way.

Guidelines for chronic asthma are based on the current view that broncho-constriction and symptoms of asthma are primarily the result of airway inflammation caused by allergens or other unknown factors.[16] Airway inflammation is found in all grades of severity and in all types of asthma and its effective treatment appears to achieve control of asthma and be associated with a decrease in evidence for airway inflammation.[17,18] Based upon this understanding of pathogenesis, control of asthma can be achieved by preventing inflammation with the use of anti-inflammatory medications. The best established of these is inhaled corticosteroids, which have the additional merit of minimizing systemic side-effects by using the inhaled route.

Guidelines began to appear at the end of the 1980s and were first formulated in Australia and spread to other countries.[19] Subsequently attempts were made on an international basis to agree on guidelines, which culminated in an international consensus document produced by the National Institutes of Health.[20] The international consensus was based on the opinions of a limited number of physicians from a limited part of the world largely sharing a similar view on asthma management. The report has stimulated considerable discussion at a national level and revealed substantial differences of opinion between countries but, nonetheless, has helped stimulate debate about how best to achieve good control of asthma. National guidelines are now being drawn up that often use the international consensus report as a template. For each individual nation best practice needs to be related to the affordability of interventions and the nature of the health care provision for each country. These considerations are being incorporated into a WHO Study Group Report on "Global Strategy for Asthma Management".

The WHO Study Group has identified the requirement for asthma to become a public health issue for each country. In addition to the individual treatment of each patient by physicians and nurses, there is a need for each country to determine the scale of the asthma burden and the most cost-effective way of coping with it. The high relative costs of asthma to the individual and to society makes it important to achieve a collective response through public health mechanisms as well as the traditional individual contract between patient and physician.

INTERNATIONAL VARIATIONS IN MANAGEMENT

The growing debate about the suitability and role of guidelines in different countries has identified a very substantial variation in asthma treatment between them. This is largely seen with respect to medication and has a number of explanations. At the simplest level the major difference between countries is based upon socio-economic factors. For example, the pricing mechanisms in some countries favour the use of oral therapy as opposed to inhaled or lead to the use of cheap bronchodilators as opposed to more expensive inhaled treatments. The balance between public and private medical care may also influence the national guidelines with the risk of producing a two-tier system with guidelines for public provision differing from private treatment.

Cultural differences also account for the international variations in asthma management. In many countries traditional medicines are still employed as first-line therapy with more conventional treatment only being used if traditional medicines fail. Partly for reasons of cost but also for cultural ones oral medication is often more popular than the inhaled route. Inhaled therapy is both conspicuous and often more expensive and is therefore diminished in importance. In some countries asthma is seen as an important social weakness; for example, it might diminish the marriageability of young women and as such it is often not diagnosed and treatment is given for some other label such as recurrent bronchitis.

A major cause for variations in treatment in individual countries stems from the teaching of physicians. Traditional treatment patterns are hard to change and the evidence for better control of asthma by treatment given in one country often fails to convince the physicians providing treatment in another. Until good scientific evidence is provided for the benefits of a particular form of treatment in controlling asthma, variations will exist between countries. Once it is self-evident which treatment is best then these differences will largely be eliminated.

FUTURE PROSPECTS

Much of the future requires us to consolidate the past. There is good evidence that many of the modern medications given as recommended in the majority of guidelines can achieve effective control of asthma. Unfortunately this treatment is still only used in the minority of the world's population of asthmatic patients, so the first aim would be to bring everyone up to a similar standard of care once there is general agreement that it is better than traditional therapies. This means there is likely to be a progressive switch from oral to inhaled medication and from bronchodilators to anti-inflammatory treatments.

The effective prevention of airway inflammation and the symptoms produced by it should achieve good control in the majority of patients. However a minority remain poorly controlled by this treatment and there will be a continuing search for additional therapy for these patients. At present, methotrexate and cyclosporin are under investigation but it is possible that the use of lung transplantation might play an important role. The intriguing report recently that the transplantation of healthy lungs into an asthmatic patient led to the disappearance of asthma suggests that the host asthmatic patient may not cause asthma in the transplanted lungs.[21] If this proves to be the case and lung transplantation becomes more widespread and easily available, this treatment might be used for the very few patients who cannot be managed effectively with current medication.

Effective preventive therapy with anti-inflammatory medication is likely to be improved by a better understanding of the effectiveness of corticosteroids. By targeting the main corticosteroid activity with non-steroidal agents more effective and safer prevention of asthma might be achieved. There is currently great interest in the role of cytokines and their antagonism.[22]

Treatment of asthma will always remain second best to preventing its induction. In the absence of gene therapy many patients will continue to be born with a predisposition to asthma, which is likely to be induced if the patient is also atopic. Control of allergen exposure *in utero* and in early life may provide good prospects for reducing the prevalence of asthma and its later severity. Such environmental control should be given as great a priority as the search for newer medications to suppress asthma once it has been induced in the individual patient.

REFERENCES

1. Hargreave FE, Dolovich J, Newhouse MT (eds). The assessment and treatment of asthma: a conference report. *J Allergy Clin Immunol* 1990; 85: 1098–111.

2. Hetzel MR, Clark TJH, Branthwaite MA. Asthma: analysis of sudden deaths and ventilatory arrests in hospital. *BMJ* 1977; 1: 808–11.

3. Newhouse MT, Dolovich MB. Control of asthma by aerosols. *N Engl J Med* 1986; 315: 870–4.

4. Hilton S, Sibbald B, Anderson HR, Freeling P. Controlled evaluation of the effect of patient education on asthma morbidity in general practice. *Lancet* 1986; i: 26–9.

5. Mellis CM, Peat JK, Bauman AE, Woolcock AJ. The cost of asthma in New South Wales. *Med J Aust* 1991; 155: 522–8.

6. Weiss KB, Gergen PJ, Hodgson TA. An economic evaluation of asthma in the United States. *N Engl J Med* 1992; 326: 862–6.

7. Vance VJ, Taylor WF. The financial cost of chronic child asthma. *Ann Allergy* 1971; 29: 455–60.

8. Adelroth E, Thompson S. High dosage inhalation steroids in asthma – analysis of costs and use in health care. *Lakartidningen* 1984; 81: 4285–8.

9. Bousquet J, Hejjaoue A, Michel FB. Specific immunotherapy in asthma. *J Allergy Clin Immunol* 1990; 86: 292–306.

10. Keeley DJ, Neill P, Gallivan S. Comparison of the prevalence of reversible airways obstruction in rural and urban Zimbabwean children. *Thorax* 1991; 46: 549–53.

11. Sporik R, Holgate ST, Platts-Mills TAE, Cogswell JJ. Exposure to house-dust mite allergen and the development of asthma in childhood: A prospective study. *N Engl J Med* 1990; 323: 502–7.

12. Weitzman M, Gortmaker S, Walker DK, Sobol A. Maternal smoking and childhood asthma. *Pediatrics* 1990; 85: 505–11.

13. Arshad SH, Matthews S, Grant C, Hide D. Effect of allergen avoidance on developments of allergic disorders in infancy. *Lancet* 1992; 339: 1494–7.

14. National Asthma Education Programme. Expert Panel on the Management of Asthma, National Heart, Lung and Blood Institute. Guidelines for the Diagnosis and Management of Asthma. *J Allergy Clin Immunol* 1991; 88: 425–534.

15. Kerstjens HAM *et al.* and the Dutch Chronic Non-specific Lung Disease Study Group. A comparison of bronchodilator therapy with or without inhaled corticosteroid therapy for obstructive airway disease. *N Engl J Med* 1992; 327: 1413–9.

16. Barnes PJ. A new approach to the treatment of asthma. *N Engl J Med* 1989; 321: 1517-27.

17. Laitenen LA, Laitenen A, Haahtela T. A comparative study of the effects of an inhaled corticosteroid, budesonide, and a beta$_2$-agonist, terbutaline, on airway inflammation in newly diagnosed asthma: A randomised, double blind, parallel-group controlled trial. *J Allergy Clin Immunol* 1992; 90: 32–42.

18. Jeffery PK, Godfrey RW, Adelroth E, Nelson F, Rogers A, Johansson, SA. Effects of treatment on airway inflammation and thickening of basement membrane reticular collagen in asthma – a quantitative light and electron microscopic study. *Am Rev Respir Dis* 1992; 145: 890–9.

19. British Thoracic Society, Research Unit of Royal College of Physicians, Kings Fund Centre, National Asthma Campaign. Guidelines for management of asthma in adults. I: Chronic persistent asthma. *BMJ* 1990; 301: 651–3.

20. International Asthma Management Project. International Consensus Report on Diagnosis and Treatment of Asthma. US Department of Health and Human Services. Public Health Service. *National Institutes of Health, Bethesda, 1992.*

21. Corris PA, Dark JH. Aetiology of asthma: Lessons from lung transplantation. *Lancet* 1993; 341: 1369–71.

22. Holgate S. Mediator and cytokine mechanisms in asthma. *Thorax* 1993; 48: 103–9.

KEY POINTS

1   *Asthma Control*
   (a) Control of asthma or achievement of best result guides management.
   (b) Freedom from symptoms with restoration of lung function by treatment that does not cause unnecessary side-effects are criteria for asthma control.

2   *Cost of Illness*
   (a) Untreated asthma is a major burden for both patients and society.
   (b) Cost-of-illness studies enable therapeutic interventions to be judged with respect to cost and effectiveness.

3 *Environmental Control*
  (a) The rising prevalence and severity of asthma suggests an external cause.
  (b) Avoidance or reduction of external factors might enable asthma prevalence to be checked and medication minimized.

4 *Guidelines*
  (a) Guidelines are based on best practice and evidence from clinical trials.
  (b) Guidelines need to be flexible and tailored to individual patients.

27

MANAGEMENT OF CHRONIC ASTHMA IN CHILDREN

James Y. Paton

INTRODUCTION

Asthma is the commonest chronic childhood disease in developed countries. For children, asthma causes significant sleep disturbance, loss of time from school,[1] interference with activities[2] and hospitalization.[1-4] For their parents, the consequences are significant time off work, restriction of social activities[5] and anxiety, fear and guilt.[3] The economic costs are huge. Although the morbidity is considerable, asthma mortality is rare in children, but the death rate for asthma has fallen very little over a decade when other causes of childhood mortality have declined.[3]

The prevalence of childhood asthma appears to be increasing, although the extent of the increase has been debated.[6] The reasons for the increase are not known but are thought most probably to be due to environmental factors.[7] There have also been concerns that the severity of asthma has been increasing. Nevertheless, in the UK there is some evidence that the number of severe attacks and chronic disability has fallen[8] and the number of admissions with acute asthma has levelled off.[4] These encouraging signs may be due to more effective treatment of children with recognized asthma. The willingness of doctors to make the diagnosis is probably one of the most significant factors in improving treatment. Correct diagnosis is likely to lead to appropriate management and treatment.[9] A diagnosis of asthma can relieve parental anxiety rather than cause it.

In the last 10–15 years, understanding of asthma has increased greatly. The use of fibreoptic bronchoscopy to obtain mucosal lavage and biopsy material to investigate the pathology of asthma during life has led to a picture of asthma as a chronic inflammatory disease of the airways.[10,11] The consequences of this inflammatory process are bronchoconstriction, oedema, mucous hypersecretion and stimulation of neural reflexes within the airways and, in time, fixed airway obstruction – all the features that comprise the clinical syndrome recognized as asthma.[12] Inflammation may also have a key role in the development of bronchial hyperreactivity,[13] which is present in up to 90% of children with frequent wheezing in the previous year, particularly those with atopy.[14,15]

Because of technical difficulties investigating children, and ethical constraints, there is less information on the pathology of asthma in children. The studies available suggest that airways inflammation is important[16] but there is also increasing recognition that many wheezing illnesses in infants and young children are more closely related to viral infections (Table 27.1).[17,18] Whether the inflammatory response in these circumstances is different is not yet known. Despite some reservations, the concept of asthma as an inflammatory disease has led to a fundamental shift in approach to the treatment of asthma in children. The strategy now aims to control or prevent the underlying inflammation. Where possible, prevention is achieved by avoidance of factors that induce inflammation ("inducers"), such as known allergens. Currently, avoidance strategies are

TABLE 27.1: *Features of the main wheezing disorders of childhood. (From Ref. 17 with permission)*

	Recurrent wheezy LRI in pre-school children	Asthma in school-children
Pattern	Episodic	Interval symptoms and episodic
Peak prevalence	6–36 months	5–10 years
Aetiology	Viral infection	Atopic sensitivity (plus viral episodes)
Bronchial responsiveness	Normal	Increased
Prognosis		
Child/young adult	Symptoms largely confined to pre-school era; minor anomalies in early adult life	Persistent
Later life	?Associated with COPD	No relation to COPD

LRI, lower respiratory illness; COPD, chronic obstructive pulmonary disease.

often ineffective, and control is achieved using anti-inflammatory medication ("preventers"). Bronchodilators ("relievers") are then used as required for the relief of symptoms.

Despite encouraging signs, there is evidence that asthma remains underdiagnosed and inadequately treated.[2,19] The principles of diagnosis and treatment are clear and have been set out in a number of international guidelines.[20–23] This chapter focuses on the practical aspects of diagnosis and management of asthma in childhood.

DIAGNOSIS OF ASTHMA IN CHILDHOOD (see Chapter 5)

The diagnosis of asthma in children is essentially clinical. Lung function testing to demonstrate reversible airways obstruction is not usually possible in young children below 4–5 years of age, except in specialist laboratories, and histological demonstration of inflammation is the subject of active clinical research.

HISTORY

A careful, detailed history is the key to diagnosis (Table 27.2). Such a history is likely to be of more value in planning the management than all other investigations.

The cardinal clinical features are cough, wheeze and breathlessness. As similar symptoms may occur with viral infections in normal children, a pattern of recurrent episodes or exacerbations is important. Children with three or more episodes of cough, wheeze and/or breathlessness should be considered as having asthma.[25]

Wheeze is often described as a whistling noise coming from the chest. Occasionally, parents use wheezing as a descriptive term for any respiratory noise, so it is important to ensure they are not describing another respiratory noise such as stridor. Breathlessness may be obvious in older children but can be more difficult to recognize in younger children. A small child may be unable to keep up with their peers, may become tired more easily, may want to be carried or at worst may be reluctant to take part in any activity. In about 5–6% of children with asthma, cough is the presenting feature.[26] The cough is usually non-productive, and is often worse at night and after exercise. Most of these children will have pulmonary function studies consistent with asthma.

When questioned directly, children often report other sensations such as a feeling of tightness in the chest, discomfort or pain. Sometimes the descriptions are quite graphic, for example "like an elephant sitting on my chest".

The diagnosis of asthma is more likely if the cardinal symptoms occur after exposure to certain typical triggers (Table 27.3). Viral infections

TABLE 27.2: *Important areas of inquiry when taking the history. (Adapted from Ref. 24)*

Age at onset

Nature of symptoms (wheeze, cough, breathlessness, chest tightness)

Triggers (viral infections, exercise, allergens, cigarette smoking)

Pattern of symptoms (frequency, seasonal and diurnal variation)

Severity of symptoms (previous admissions to hospital or intensive care unit admissions)

Environmental hazards and their effects on disease (cigarette smoking, active and passive; housing; exposure to house-dust mite; pets)

Drug therapy (past and present therapy including drugs, dose, devices, response and side-effects)

Impact of disease on child and family (sleep disturbance, school performance and attendance, exercise and activity)

Family history (asthma and atopic illnesses in first and second degree relatives)

Past illness (bronchiolitis, other significant respiratory infections)

TABLE 27.3: *Triggers of asthma*

Viral infections

Exercise

Exposure to allergens: cats, dogs, house-dust mite, grass

Environmental factors: tobacco smoke, pollution, weather changes

Others: emotional stress

(particularly with rhinoviruses) and exercise are the most important in children.

Another important and diagnostic feature of asthma is the variation with time, both in the short and long term. Diurnal variation, with symptoms and lung function being worse during the night and first thing in the morning, is characteristic.[27,28] Often there is longer term variation with acute episodes of respiratory morbidity either superimposed upon perennial symptoms or as the sole manifestation of asthma. Sometimes there are lengthy symptom-free periods between attacks, which may only occur at particular times of year, most commonly in the winter.[18] These patterns of disease are important since the most appropriate treatment may depend on them.

Asthma in children can cause significant morbidity[3] and it is important to inquire specifically about the impact on the child and family. Are they frequently absent from school?[1] Is academic progress satisfactory? Is asthma interfering with activity or stopping the child doing things they would like to do?

Previous treatments, their effectiveness and side-effects should be reviewed. All too often, a history is given of recurrent episodes of coughing and wheezing unresponsive to courses of antibiotics. What drugs and devices has the child had? Were they effective? If not, are the parents able to offer possible reasons for their failure? What do parents understand about the purpose of the medications and the times when they should be used? Has the child experienced side-effects from the medicines? Have any other steps such as house-dust mite avoidance been taken in an attempt to modify the condition?

CLINICAL EXAMINATION

Abnormalities on clinical examination do not confirm a diagnosis of asthma. As asthma is episodic (and modern treatments now so effective) physical examination is often normal. Clinical features of airway obstruction such as hyperinflation and evidence of chest deformity may indicate chronic, poorly controlled asthma but are not diagnostic. There may be evidence of other atopic diseases, particularly eczema and rhinitis. Drug-related side-effects such as tremor due to bronchodilators or oral candidiasis related to inhaled corticosteroids should always be looked for.

Both asthma, especially when poorly controlled,[29] and its therapy may cause slowing of linear growth.[30] Unfortunately, the inaccuracy of height measuring equipment has confounded the effects of asthma and its treatment on linear growth.[22] It is therefore particularly important to measure height accurately using a properly functioning and regularly calibrated device such as a stadiometer. It should always be borne in mind that poor growth may point to another disease such as cystic fibrosis.

Physical examination is particularly useful when specific features such as finger clubbing, which point to an alternative diagnosis, are present. Physical abnormalities in asthma should be generalized; recurrent or persistent focal features may point to alternative diagnoses. In infants and young children it is especially important to remember that there are other important causes of wheezing and cough and to recognize clinical features that point to diagnoses other than asthma (Table 27.4). Further investigations (e.g. sweat test, lower oesophageal pH study) may be necessary.

TABLE 27.4: *Features that should alert the clinician to diagnoses other than asthma*

History
Persistent wheeze not responding to appropriate treatment
Wheeze associated with feeding or vomiting
Neonatal onset or wheeze following neonatal lung disease
Acute onset of wheezing/coughing (suggesting foreign body)
Stridor
Productive cough
Steatorrhoea

Examination
Failure to thrive
Finger clubbing
Focal signs

Investigations
Lack of reversibility of airflow obstruction with bronchodilators
Persistent or focal chest X-ray changes

AIDS TO DIAGNOSIS

When diagnosis is difficult, additional information about the pattern and severity of attacks can be important. There are several useful diagnostic aids.

Diary Cards

Symptom diary cards have been widely used to record the severity and pattern of symptoms over time. In children aged 5 years or over, peak flow can be recorded either alone or in conjunction with symptoms. Unfortunately, diary recording is often inaccurate[31,32] and completion poor. To be valid, diaries should be completed at the time rather than retrospectively. Diaries completed in blocks of unicoloured ink with unvarying similar neat handwriting should arouse suspicions. Electronic diaries that include a date stamp are becoming available and may be a useful, if expensive, improvement.[33,34]

Lung Function Testing

Simple lung function tests, particularly the peak expiratory flow rate (PEFR), have become an increasingly important aspect of asthma management in children old enough to cooperate. More sophisticated lung function tests often provide little additional useful information.

Peak expiratory flow rate Relatively inexpensive portable PEFR meters are now widely available and measurement of PEFR in children over 5 years is reasonably reproducible.[35] Recent studies have found that many portable PEFR meters are non-linear, overreading by 40–80 l min^{-1} in the mid-range peaking around 300 l min^{-1}, and underreading by 30–80 l min^{-1} in the high range. This non-linearity is large and of potential clinical relevance in children. It is possible to correct for non-linearity by changing the scale but such linearized PEFR meters are not yet widely available.[36]

Many children aged between 3 and 5 years can be persuaded to blow into PEFR meters, although the results are less reproducible.[37] Unfortunately, PEFR meters able to record in the range 20–200 l min^{-1} are not now readily available.

The principal problem with PEFR is that the measurement is effort dependent. Poor effort leads to falsely low values. Fortunately, children often enjoy PEFR measurement and try very hard to get the best possible value. Occasionally they even become dispirited if more active asthma leads to levels lower than their best. Older children, particularly boys, can learn to trick the meter by spitting into it and can produce artificially high values.[38] Such cheating can be overcome by using a larger mouthpiece placed well into the mouth, and encouraging the child to huff.

A single reading is usually of little value unless it is clearly abnormal. Home measurements plotted on a chart can provide evidence of variability and severity of airways obstruction over a period of time (Fig. 27.1). Usually, readings are made twice daily before, and if possible after, bronchodilator, with the best of a number of attempts being noted. There are a variety of charts available to allow the values to be recorded for future review.

Predicted values in children are related to height.[39] Where possible the best peak flow rather than the predicted should be used as a guide. An exception is those children who have significant persistent airways obstruction where the aim should be to improve them to the predicted level. Whether diurnal variability in children with asthma is less than that in adults is not clear.[28,40]

Spirometry Spirometry with flow–volume loops may occasionally provide additional information. In particular, the maximum expiratory flows from the flow–volume loop are more sensitive to lesser degrees of airways obstruction.[41] However, the test is only practical in children who can perform a forced vital capacity manoeuvre, usually those aged over 5 years. Measurement of functional residual capacity is possible in some pre-school children who may have hyperinflation even when symptoms are controlled.[42]

Reversibility with bronchodilator In the presence of airways obstruction, an increase in PEFR or forced expiratory volume in 1 s (FEV$_1$) of 15–20% after inhalation of a β$_2$ agonist confirms bronchodilator responsiveness and is typical of asthma. The most appropriate value for reversibility in children is still not clear, and there is no accepted value that can be applied in all

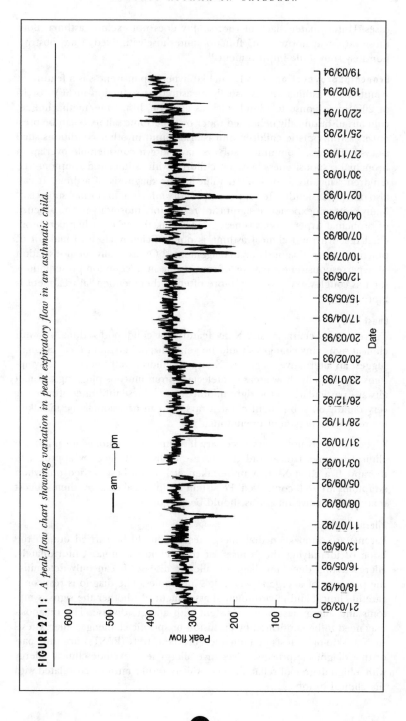

FIGURE 27.1: *A peak flow chart showing variation in peak expiratory flow in an asthmatic child.*

cases. Unfortunately, lack of reversibility does not exclude asthma. Both those with near normal lung function and those with fixed airway obstruction may show little improvement.[41]

Bronchial provocation tests Bronchial hyperresponsiveness is a feature of symptomatic asthma and is usually measured as reduction in FEV_1 of 15 or 20% in response to stimuli such as exercise, histamine/methacholine, cold air, ultrasonically nebulized water or hypertonic saline. It can be present in asymptomatic children and is also found in other conditions such as cystic fibrosis. Community surveys have shown considerable overlap in bronchial responsiveness between children with asthma and symptom-free children[43] making it of limited value in the diagnosis of asthma. It can also occur transiently after upper respiratory infection in normal subjects.[44] Many children experience significant respiratory morbidity in the absence of bronchial hyperresponsiveness.[19,45] Overall, the relation between bronchial reactivity and clinical asthma is not sufficiently close to make it of practical use in diagnosis or management.[46] Occasionally, demonstration of hyperresponsiveness may be of some value in uncommon presentations such as cough-variant asthma; more often, a therapeutic trial treatment is more useful.

Chest X-ray

There are no characteristic X-ray features of childhood asthma. As with clinical signs, any changes should be generalized. Persistent focal changes suggest an alternative diagnosis. X-rays of children with more acute symptoms occasionally show areas of atelectasis from mucous plugging of small airways, particularly in the right middle lobe.[47] These infiltrates often clear very rapidly on subsequent chest X-rays but can occasionally be mistaken for recurrent/persistent pneumonia.[48]

A chest X-ray is not always necessary if asthmatic symptoms are mild, the clinical features typical and the disease easily controlled by appropriate therapy. If a chest X-ray is undertaken, it is often best carried out when symptoms are well controlled. Persistent radiological changes then suggest that an alternative diagnosis should be sought.

Allergy Testing

Parents are often keen that allergy testing should be carried out, in the hope of identifying the "cause" of their child's asthma. Unfortunately, allergy testing does not diagnose allergic disease. It can only determine the presence of allergen-specific IgE antibodies. The diagnosis rests on a careful clinical and environmental assessment of whether the signs, symptoms and allergy tests are consistent with allergic disease. The diagnosis may need to be confirmed by exclusion or specific challenge. Allergy tests such as skin-prick tests or radioallergosorbent tests (RASTs) are only part of that diagnostic process.[49] Negative allergy tests exclude clinical allergy with a high degree of reliability but positive results must be correlated with the clinical history.

Skin-prick testing is most commonly used. It is easy to perform, cheap and quick. Usually a limited panel of antigens (house-dust mite, grass pollen, cat or dog dander and moulds, usually *Alternaria*) is all that is required to confirm atopy. Positive and negative controls (saline and histamine) should always be included. Unfortunately, atopy is virtually universal in asthmatic children by school age.[50,51] In the UK, almost all asthmatic children will react to one or more of house-dust mite extract, mixed grass pollen or cat dander.

RASTs measure the specific quantity of IgE antibodies and are available for a wide range of common antigens. Values correlate well with the size of skin test weals. However, there is no major group of allergens (e.g. pollens, moulds, danders, foods or venoms) in which RAST results are better than those provided by skin tests.[52] RASTs may be useful in the presence of skin disease such as eczema or where there is a risk of anaphylaxis.

Children find both skin-prick testing and RASTs painful and they are not popular.

Direct bronchial challenge with aeroallergen can be undertaken, but because of the possibility of provoking significant asthmatic reactions is limited to clinical research. Indirect challenge, where a change in bronchial reactivity is measured after controlled challenge to a natural dose of a suspected allergen, may be useful particularly in the investigation of food intolerance.[53]

MANAGEMENT OF CHRONIC ASTHMA IN CHILDHOOD

Once a diagnosis has been reached, an appropriate plan of management can be instituted. In the absence of suitable markers of inflammation, decisions on treatment have to be made on clinical grounds based on the frequency and severity of symptoms. In children over 5 years, lung function tests may provide additional objective information.

The general aims (Table 27.5) of asthma management have been clearly set out in published guidelines. Treatment can be broken down into a number of more specific interrelated objectives[21] (Table 27.6) designed to achieve these aims.

Most childhood asthma can be managed satisfactorily in the community.[54] More severe cases and cases where problems develop may require specialist referral (Table 27.7).

EDUCATE TO DEVELOP A PARTNERSHIP IN ASTHMA MANAGEMENT (see also Chapter 23)

Education in asthma is an important and continuing process. Good parental understanding is likely to lead to increased satisfaction with therapy,

TABLE 27.5: *Asthma management once a diagnosis has been made: general aims and desirable outcomes. (From Refs 21 and 22 with permission)*

Aims	Mild/moderate asthma (BTS guidelines steps 1–3) Outcome: control of asthma	Severe asthma (BTS guidelines steps 4–5) Outcome: best possible result
Achieve and maintain control of symptoms	Minimally (ideally) no symptoms during the day No nocturnal disturbance Minimal need for relief bronchodilator	Least possible symptoms during the day Minimal nocturnal disturbance Least possible need for relief bronchodilator
Prevent asthma exacerbations	Minimal (infrequent) exacerbations No hospital admissions or emergency room visits	Least possible exacerbations Minimal hospital admissions
Maintain normal levels of activity, including no exercise limitation	No limitation on activities or exercise Normal school or nursery attendance	Least possible limitation of activity Least possible time off school or nursery
Maintain normal growth	Normal growth	Least possible growth slowing
Avoid adverse effects from medications	Minimal (or no) adverse effects	Least adverse effects
Maintain pulmonary function as close to normal as possible	PEFR $\geq$ 80% of predicted or best Circadian variation < 20%	Best PEFR
Prevent asthma mortality		Least possible circadian variation

BTS, British Thoracic Society.

TABLE 27.6: *Objectives of asthma management. (From Ref. 21 with permission)*

Educate and instruct to develop a partnership in asthma
  management
Monitor asthma severity by:
  Clinical assessment
  Objective measures of lung function
Avoid or control asthma triggers
Establish medication plans for chronic management
Establish plans for managing exacerbations
Provide regular follow-up care

TABLE 27.7: *Suggested indications for hospital referral of children with asthma*

Referral to a general paediatrician	Referral to respiratory paediatrician
Diagnosis is in doubt	After a life-threatening episode or admission to an intensive care unit
Asthma is unstable	Brittle asthma
Asthma interferes with normal life despite treatment	Asthma causing severe restriction in normal activity despite treatment
Parents or family practitioners want support	When special investigations are required
More than 400 μg daily inhaled steroids needed to control asthma	More than 800 μg daily inhaled steroid needed to control asthma

improved compliance and hopefully to decreased morbidity.[55] Initially,
parents may have a poor understanding of the condition and its treatment
but are keen to know more. The aim is to provide sufficient knowledge
and training to enable them to keep their child well. As the children get
older, the emphasis shifts to ensuring that they themselves know about
their asthma and take increasing responsibility for their treatment.

Anxieties about asthma are common, yet often poorly dealt with. Partridge reported on a poll of members of the UK National Asthma Campaign as to their reactions when they or their children were first diagnosed as having asthma: 38% were relieved to have a diagnosis, 32% extremely worried, 23% frightened, 16% bewildered and 10% angry. Only 22% felt that they had had a good discussion with their doctor. Such failures of communication can be costly and may interfere with effective treatment.[56] Fears about the side-effects of inhaled steroids are particularly common and may lead to poor compliance. Appropriate changes in behaviour are only likely when parents and children are given the opportunity to express any fears or concerns and the chance to discuss their expectations of the condition and its treatment. Sometimes parents' expectations may be inappropriately low and it may be up to the clinician to raise the parents' level of expectations.

There is also increasing recognition that, by providing parents and children with skills enabling them to vary treatment with changes in asthma severity, morbidity may be reduced[57–59] and mortality avoided.[60] The development of an individual "guided self-management plan" is therefore an important part of the educational process.

Verbal information should be supplemented by written information. National patient support groups often produce excellent action cards for this purpose. These should include details of both preventative and relieving treatment, instructions on recognizing deterioration of asthma, steps to take in managing an acute episode and guidance on when to seek emergency care. This written plan should be brought to each review so that it can be revised and updated. Over time plans can be fine-tuned, for example by noting particular symptoms or peak flow levels that occurred during an exacerbation.

Asthmatic children and their families should be told of any asthma societies, self-help and support groups, or helplines available. National societies often produce excellent educational material in the form of leaflets, audio-tapes and videos that reinforce the physician's message.[61,62] Foreign language material may be particularly useful for ethnic minorities. Schools should be informed and their cooperation enlisted to ensure that the child's attendance and participation in activities is interrupted as little as possible.

Each clinic visit provides an opportunity for further education. It may be helpful to encourage parents to note down any questions or concerns and to bring their notes to the consultation for discussion. It may also be useful if the parents bring a record of symptoms, and PEFR, recorded for at least 2 weeks before the consultation. Consistency is important if the best possible outcome is to be achieved. Clinics should be organized so that, as far as possible, parents and children do not see a succession of different doctors or nurses.

ASSESS AND MONITOR ASTHMA SEVERITY WITH OBJECTIVE MEASURES OF LUNG FUNCTION (see also Chapters 11-13)

An important part of the assessment is making a judgement about asthma severity using symptoms, objective measures of lung function (Table 27.8) and medication requirements. For children below 5 years the judgement will, of necessity, be based on clinical information alone. Where possible, objective measures are desirable because parental or child assessments of symptoms of airways obstruction may be poor.[63] PEFR measurements, for example, may identify airway narrowing before symptoms develop or wheeze is heard on auscultation.[64] In this way, PEFR monitoring can have a useful educational role in teaching parents about the variations in asthma control and their relationship to symptoms in an individual child.

One of the goals of recent guidelines on the management of asthma has been to promote the use of objective measures[21,22] in a manner analogous to other chronic diseases such as diabetes. Just as a single blood sugar would be regarded as of little value unless clearly abnormal, so a single PEFR measurement is of little value in isolation. Serial measurements are much more useful with the results noted in a diary card or plotted on one of the available charts. Measured in this way, PEFR monitoring can provide objective evidence about the severity of airways obstruction (Fig. 27.1) and can be useful in monitoring the response to treatment, detecting exacerbations or facilitating changes in medication.

For most children with mild or moderate asthma, long-term PEFR recording is an unreasonable expectation. It is usually best confined to those with severe asthma, poor asthma control or previous life-threatening episodes. A practical compromise may be to ask parents to record the PEFR for a period of 2–4 weeks before a clinic visit.

AVOID OR CONTROL ASTHMA TRIGGER FACTORS (see also Chapter 14)

If specific trigger factors (Table 27.3) have been identified, there is the potential for controlling or preventing asthma by manipulating the child's environment. Studies where allergic children have been sent to school at high altitude where house-dust mites, pet allergens and pollens were undetectable, and exposure to tobacco smoke absent show that such avoidance can be very effective at reducing evidence of allergy, bronchial reactivity, symptoms of asthma and medication usage.[65]

There are a number of areas where environmental avoidance approaches have been considered important.

House-dust Mite

While a causal relationship between domestic mites and atopic asthma has not been definitively proved, the close association between mite exposure, mite sensitivity and asthma makes it likely that domestic mites are a major contributor to the development and expression of symptoms in atopic

TABLE 27.8: *National Heart, Lung and Blood Institute's classification of asthma severity*

Characteristics	Mild	Moderate	Severe
Clinical features			
Frequency of symptoms	Intermittent brief symptoms < 1–2 times per week	Symptoms > 1–2 times per week More severe exacerbation < 3 times per year	Symptoms continuously Frequent exacerbations
Interval symptoms	Asymptomatic between symptoms or exacerbations	Cough and wheeze often present	Cough and wheeze almost always present
Nocturnal asthma	Nocturnal asthma < 2/month	Nocturnal asthma > 2–3 times/week	Nightly disturbance with early morning symptoms
Exercise tolerance	Limitation only on vigorous exercise	Diminished exercise tolerance	Marked limitation of activity
School attendance	Good attendance	Attendance may be affected	Frequent loss of time from school
Lung function			
PEFR	PEFR > 80% predicted at baseline PEFR variability < 20%	PEFR 60–80% PEFR variability 20–30%	PEFR < 60% PEFR variability > 30%
Spirometry	Minimal or no airway obstruction	Mild airway obstruction present	Severe airway obstruction

TABLE 27.8: *Continued*

Characteristics	Mild	Moderate	Severe
Spirometry	May be little improvement in already normal flows after bronchodilator	Reversibility to normal after bronchodilator	Incomplete reversibility to bronchodilator, i.e. fixed obstruction
Methacholine sensitivity	Methacholine $PC_{20} > 20$ mg ml^{-1}	Methacholine PC_{20} between 2 and 20 mg ml^{-1}	Methacholine $PC_{20} < 2.0$ mg ml^{-1}

asthma.[51,66] The relationship between exposure, sensitization and symptoms has not always been clear due in part to difficulties in measuring mite exposure. It is also not yet known whether long-term average exposure to airborne allergen is more important than intermittent exposure to high dust levels of the type that can occur when beds, carpets or soft furnishings are disturbed.[67]

The two most common mites found in domestic house dust, *Dermatophagoides pteronyssinus* and *Dermatophagoides farinae*, thrive at 80% relative humidity and 25 °C. As the humidity falls, however, they stop reproducing and become immobile, and below 50% relative humidity they are likely to die.[68] Modern energy-efficient housing with reduced ventilation and heating may have provided ideal conditions for the growth and reproduction of house-dust mites. In addition to their preference for humidity, mites are photophobic; hence, their common habitats in mattresses, bedding, soft furnishings or toys and at the base of carpets.

There are many mite allergens, but five or six predominate. Most mite allergens are water-soluble proteins and are found in the faecal pellets of mites. For example, the common Group 1 allergens (*Der p* I, *Der f* I) are cysteine proteases associated with mite faecal particles. They become airborne for brief periods during domestic activity, with measurable quantities in the air disappearing within minutes.[69]

Mite sensitivity should be suspected if symptoms coincide with sweeping, vacuuming or dusting.[70] Sensitivity can be detected by skin-prick tests or

RAST tests. Up to 85% of atopic asthmatic subjects have skin-prick sensitivity to mites in contrast to 5–30% of the non-asthmatic population.[71] Sensitivity to the house-dust mite is the commonest immediate allergic skin-prick reaction in asthmatic children[72] and also the commonest in school-children in general.[73]

While avoidance of mites either at high altitude[65,74] or in hospital[75] has been shown to reduce asthmatic symptoms and bronchial reactivity, achieving lower levels of dust mite in the home has proved demanding, time-consuming and expensive. Further, it appears that only the most stringent measures produce effective results.[76]

There have been two main approaches to mite avoidance. In the first, attempts have been made to reduce the number of mites in areas most heavily colonized (Table 27.9). Stringent measures such as removing carpets and curtains, increasing the frequency of bed-linen laundering, removing soft toys and mite-containing clothing have shown successful results.[76] Newer bed coverings that effectively contain allergen may prevent mite allergen accumulation and reduce bronchial hyperreactivity in mite-sensitive patients,[77] particularly when combined with frequent hot washing of bed linen. However, the coverings are expensive and the duvet, mattress and pillow all have to be covered to achieve a significant reduction in allergen. Simple cleaning and vacuuming alone reduces the allergen load but has been shown to be of negligible clinical benefit.[78] Acaricides can reduce mite numbers but have not yet been clearly shown to be of benefit in reducing symptoms in asthmatic children.[71] Liquid nitrogen on bedding also reduces mite numbers substantially and airway reactivity to histamine when used in the homes of adult asthmatic subjects[79] but, at present, is not a practical proposition for clinical use. Ionizers, which clean the air electrostatically, can lead to a significant reduction in airborne allergen

TABLE 27.9: *Suggested measures to reduce allergic child's exposure to house-dust mites. (From Ref. 21 with permission)*

Encase the mattress in an allergen non-permeable cover
Either encase the pillow or wash it weekly
Wash the bedding in water of a temperature greater than 55 °C (130 °F)
Avoid sleeping or lying on furniture upholstered with fabric
Remove carpets that are laid on concrete floors
Reduce indoor humidity to less than 50%
Use chemical agents (acaricides) to kill mites or to alter the mite antigens in the house

concentrations but lead to an increase in night-time cough in asthmatic children[67] and cannot therefore be recommended at present.

The alternative approach is to alter the overall home environment to make it less conducive to mite colonization. This can be achieved by reducing humidity, which one Danish study has shown leads to significant improvement in PEFR.[80] However, increased ventilation usually results in heat loss. The consequent increase in heating bills necessary to maintain the indoor temperature makes this option unaffordable for many.

In practice, the costs and the rigorous nature of the multiple measures necessary to remove house-dust mite mean that, at present, such measures are usually reserved for those with severe asthma and definite sensitivity to house-dust mite.

Pets

Pets are the second most common cause of domestic allergen. Over 50% of asthmatic children become sensitive to cat or dog allergens.[81] All warm-blooded pets, including small rodents and birds, produce dander, hair, urine and saliva that can contain allergens. In a household with pets, these allergens become widely distributed.

Exposure to pets can often trigger symptoms. Where there is a clear history of symptoms following exposure and positive allergen tests (skin prick or RAST) it may be appropriate to suggest removing the animal. Unfortunately, animal danders are cleared only slowly from the environment and it can take up to 6 months before beneficial results are seen.[82] For cats, de Blay et al.[83] found that washing the cat regularly reduced the amount of Fel d I allergen present. Weekly washings combined with removing carpets, minimizing upholstered furnishings, vacuum cleaning with a high-efficiency particulate air filter and air filtration could allow a cat-sensitive patient to live with the cat.

Because of these problems, the introduction of furry or feathered pets into the homes of families with asthma is best discouraged. If pets are present, parents should at the very least exclude the pet from their child's bedroom.

Pollens and Moulds

Common allergens such as outdoor pollens or moulds are impossible to avoid completely. Indoor levels can be reduced by closing windows and doors, and using air conditioners during peak pollen or mould seasons.[84]

Unfortunately, not all moulds are external. Damp and mouldy housing has been shown to be associated with an increased prevalence and severity of respiratory illnesses in children. Whether this is due to the effects of moulds and fungi or to high levels of house-dust mite is not yet clear. However, home dampness is common and affects up to 30% or more of the housing stock in some parts of the UK.[85]

Ingested Allergens

Foods and dietary additives do not commonly trigger asthmatic symptoms in children. Definite confirmation that an ingested allergen is responsible requires double-blind challenge. This may not always be necessary before embarking on avoidance (see Chapter 40). Drugs such as aspirin and other non-steroidal anti-inflammatory agents, which can cause severe exacerbations in adults, are fortunately rarely used in children.

Other Air Pollutants Including Cigarette Smoke

Children seem to be very sensitive to respiratory effects from both indoor and outdoor pollutants.[86,87] A number of irritants such as wood smoke or volatile organic substances (e.g. paints and polishes) can cause worsening of asthma. Pollution from road traffic may also be important.[86]

However, by far the most ubiquitous and important pollutant is cigarette smoke. A number of studies have shown that maternal smoking has a substantial effect on wheezing lower respiratory illnesses in infants and young children, increasing the frequency of such illnesses[88] and lowering the age at first presentation.[88,89] Passive smoking also increases both the frequency and severity of asthma symptoms. In pre-school children, maternal smoking has been associated with a higher rate of asthma, an earlier onset of asthma and an increased use of asthma medication.[90] Other studies have shown that maternal smoking is associated with increased asthma symptoms, lower lung function and increased bronchial reactivity.[91] Boys[92] and children with eczema [93] are particularly affected, and the effects are greater in older children and increase with the length of exposure to smoking.

Passive smoking has additional effects on allergic diseases. Children of mothers who smoked during pregnancy have an increased prevalence of allergic disease.[94] Maternal smoking may also lead to higher cord blood IgE levels[95] raising the possibility that maternal smoking may have an adverse effect on the fetal immune system.

Unfortunately, passive smoking is not the sole problem. Active smoking is also common in teenagers with asthma.[96]

All this leaves no doubt that asthmatic children from the intrauterine period onwards should not be exposed to cigarette smoke.

General Points about Avoidance Measures

Unfortunately, the home is not the only environment where children are exposed to measurable aeroallergens or pollutants. Norwegian studies[97] have shown that children are exposed to measurable levels of domestic allergen at school (house-dust mite, cat, dog). There are also data showing that children not exposed at home to smoking had low salivary cotinine concentrations whose level depended on the prevalence of smoking in the community.[98]

The practical difficulties surrounding avoidance strategies mean that for most children they do not represent, at present, particularly productive approaches to asthma control. Either environmental triggers cannot be identified or it is difficult to avoid them completely. In general, suppressive therapy with preventative anti-inflammatory agents is both less demanding and more effective.

Immunotherapy (see also Chapter 21)

The role of immunotherapy as a means of reducing the effects of environmental allergens is controversial. Because of concerns about acute fatal anaphylaxis after allergen injection, immunotherapy is no longer used in the UK. Indeed, the British Thoracic Society Guidelines state that immunotherapy is not indicated in the management of asthma.[22] It remains widely used in other countries.

The results of clinical trials in asthma are variable and conflicting. For example, in controlled trials with dust mite extracts, symptomatic improvement has been shown to occur.[99] However, no significant difference in lung function between control and placebo groups has been demonstrated and variable effects on bronchial hyperreactivity have occurred.[100,101] Similarly, conflicting results have been noted with other allergens such as pollens and animal extracts.

If immunotherapy is considered it should be probably restricted to selected children with severe asthma triggered by one or a very few specific aeroallergens and poorly responsive to pharmacological and avoidance therapies. It is essential to have an accurate diagnosis based on a convincing history that natural exposure to aeroallergens induces clinically significant symptoms combined with detectable immediate hypersensitivity (skin or RAST testing) to relevant environmental allergen(s). The parents should be fully informed of the nature of the treatment – the need for regular injections, the possibility of reactions to injections, the likelihood of success, the need to continue injections for a protracted period and the costs. In clinical trials, a high incidence of systemic anaphylactic reactions is usually reported. These are usually mild and not life-threatening but may require adrenaline therapy.[101] However, as more severe reactions can occur, those using immunotherapy should be trained, equipped and ready to manage major systemic anaphylactic reactions. The child should be observed for at least 30 min after the treatment. Injections should only be given when the child is asymptomatic since lethal reactions are found more often in asthmatic subjects with severe airway obstruction.[21]

Whatever the present role of immunotherapy, it seems likely that the developments in allergen preparation and a better understanding of the immunology of asthma may lead to a re-evaluation of its role in the future.

ESTABLISH MEDICATION PLANS FOR CHRONIC MANAGEMENT

At present, drug treatment is the mainstay of the management of childhood asthma. Establishing a medication plan for an individual child can be broken down into a number of steps:[21]

(1) choosing the drugs to be used;

(2) choosing the route of administration, and for inhaled therapy the appropriate device;

(3) choosing the appropriate drug combinations and doses using a step-wise approach.

Choosing the Drugs

The understanding of asthma as a chronic inflammatory disorder of the airways has led to a more clearly defined therapeutic strategy, with the emphasis on preventing or controlling the underlying inflammatory process. Usually symptom control is brought about using anti-inflammatory medications ("preventers"). Bronchodilators ("relievers") are then used as required for the relief of symptoms. The drugs commonly prescribed in children are discussed below.

Bronchodilators (see also Chapter 19)

β Agonists β Agonists produce bronchodilation by directly stimulating β_2 receptors in airway smooth muscle leading to relaxation. The selective β_2 agonists are the most potent and widely used bronchodilators available for the treatment of asthma. They have a number of other potentially beneficial actions including enhanced mucociliary clearance, decreased vascular permeability and modulation of mediator release from mast cells and basophils. The clinical relevance of these actions in childhood asthma is not known at present.

Most of the selective β_2 agonists currently prescribed for children have a relatively short duration of action (4–6 hours). In the various inhaled formulations they are effective in small doses, rapid in onset and have a relatively low incidence of adverse effects. They are the preferred treatment for the relief of asthma symptoms, for the prophylaxis of exercise-induced asthma and for the treatment of acute exacerbations.

Longer acting inhaled β_2 agonists (salmeterol, formoterol) with a duration of action of over 12 hours are becoming available but, at present, are used mainly for children with more severe asthma who are already receiving corticosteroids. Longer acting β_2 agonists may be particularly useful for persistent nocturnal symptoms[21] or as once-daily prophylaxis against exercise-induced asthma.[23]

Side-effects of β_2 agonists are mainly related to stimulation of extra-pulmonary β_2 receptors (Table 27.10). The side-effects are dose related and are commoner with the larger doses used in oral or intravenous therapy. If side-effects such as over-activity or tremor are troublesome, reducing the dosage may be helpful.

There has been vigorous debate as to whether β_2 agonists cause a deterioration in asthma control and lead to increased asthma mortality and morbidity ("the β-agonist controversy"). Although available studies have not

---

TABLE 27.10: *Side-effects of β_2 agonists. (From Ref. 102 with permission)*

Muscle tremor
Tachycardia
Hypokalaemia
Restlessness, agitation and over-activity
Hypoxaemia due to increased $\dot{V}/\dot{Q}$ mismatching
?Worsening of asthma control

---

directly focused on children,[103] they suggest that heavy use of inhaled β_2 agonists, particularly fenoterol, may be associated with an increased risk of death or near-death from asthma.[104,105] There is also some evidence that regular use of β_2 agonists may be associated with decreased control of asthma.[106,107] Because of these concerns, present advice for children as well as adults is that the regular use of short-acting inhaled β_2 agonists should be minimized:[21,23] they should be used on an "as-needed" basis rather than regularly. Increased use (more than one or two doses per day) is then a mark of deteriorating asthma control, and points to the need to institute or intensify anti-inflammatory therapy. Tolerance (tachyphylaxis) can occur with chronic β_2 agonist use but does not appear to be of major clinical importance.

Theophyllines While theophyllines have been widely used in treatment of both acute and chronic asthma in children for many years, their role has been increasingly questioned.[108,109] Strategies involving the earlier use of inhaled prophylactic treatment (especially inhaled corticosteroids) and the introduction of effective long-acting inhaled bronchodilators, such as salmeterol, have substantially replaced theophylline's traditional role in the treatment of chronic asthma.

Despite extensive studies, the molecular mechanisms responsible for theophylline's therapeutic activity remain poorly defined. Beneficial effects have usually been attributed to bronchodilator action[108] but more recently there has been interest in possible anti-inflammatory effects. Several groups have shown a significant suppression of the late-phase response to allergen at modest serum levels of theophylline.[110,111] Importantly, these anti-inflammatory effects were achieved at doses that are not associated with unacceptable side-effects and where, in appropriate cases, serum monitoring may not be required.[112]

In children, theophylline now tends to be used later in the therapeutic plan when β_2 agonists and inhaled steroids are proving inadequate. Theophylline is also used in certain well-defined situations such as children with nocturnal asthma[113] or children who will not take inhaled medications. In corticosteroid-dependent asthma, theophylline, unlike sodium cromoglycate, can provide clinically useful benefit with a "steroid-sparing" effect.[114] The need to use blood samples for monitoring drug levels is a significant disadvantage for most children.

The variable clearance, narrow therapeutic index, high incidence of side-effects and recognized potential for severe toxic reactions mean that close attention to the details of dosing and monitoring are important when prescribing theophylline for children. Recent evidence suggests that theophylline does not usually cause cognitive or behavioural effects in most children although those with pre-existing attention or achievement problems may be more vulnerable.[115]

If theophyllines are prescribed for children, slow-release preparations have been found to be convenient, usually requiring only twice-daily administration resulting in less fluctuation in serum concentrations. Caffeine-like side-effects such as nausea, nervousness or insomnia occur when initial doses are too high, and can be minimized by starting at a lower dose of around one-half to two-thirds of the expected dose. The dose should be slowly increased at 3-day intervals, only if tolerated, until average doses for age are attained (Fig. 27.2). A peak serum level no higher than the middle of the therapeutic range should be the target (5–15 mg l^{-1}). Parents should be told to stop any dosage that causes adverse side-effects, withholding the drug until the symptoms have disappeared and then resuming at a lower, previously tolerated dose. The final dose should be individualized and should be informed by measurement of peak serum concentration when the dosage has been regular and constant for at least 3 days.

Once the dose is stable, it usually remains stable. If asthma is well controlled and there are no side-effects, follow-up levels can be checked infrequently, at 6–12-monthly intervals. Because of the risks of serious toxicity, parents and children should be able to recognize the early symptoms of intoxication such as nausea and vomiting, and also factors that might alter the drug level (e.g. prolonged fever or the use of other drugs, particularly erythromycin). If their child has a sustained fever, they should decrease the dose by 50% as a precaution, and they should not administer other medications without obtaining medical advice.

Anticholinergics Ipratropium bromide is a topically active quaternary ammonium derivative of atropine that acts as a bronchodilator. It is available both as a metered dose aerosol, which can be used with a large-volume spacer, and as a nebulizing solution. It achieves its bronchodilating effect by blocking reflex cholinergic bronchoconstriction and has no significant blocking effect on the direct effects of inflammatory mediators. It has a slower onset of action than β_2 agonists but may have a longer action of up to 8 hours.

FIGURE 27.2: *Revised algorithm for slow clinical titration of theophylline dosage and guide for final dosage adjustment based on the results of a serum concentration measurement. To provide greater assurance of tolerance and an even wider margin of safety, this algorithm is more conservative than those previously published or than current FDA guidelines in manufacturer's package inserts. For infants < 1 year of age, the initial daily dosage can be calculated by the following regression equation: Dose (in milligrams per kilogram per day) = (0.2) (Age in weeks) + 5.0; subsequent dosage increases in this age group should be based on a peak serum concentration measurement at least 3 days after the start of therapy.* Whenever side effects occur, dosage should be reduced to a previously tolerated lower dose. *In the presence of risk factors for toxic effects (e.g. fever, erythromycin therapy, or oral contraceptive therapy), the "initial dose" should not be exceeded without first documenting that a reliably measured steady-state peak concentration is < 10 μg ml. In patients without risk factors, the subsequent dosage increases are made if judged to be clinically indicated. (From Ref. 116 with permission.)*

Initial dosage
Adults and children >1 year of age:
12–14 mg kg⁻¹ daily up to a maximum of 300 mg daily

↓

After 3 days, *if tolerated,* increase dose to:

Incremental increase
Adults and children ≥45 kg: 400 mg daily
Children <45 kg: 16 mg kg⁻¹ daily up to a maximum of 400 mg daily

↓

After 3 days, *if tolerated,* increase dose to:

Final dosage before serum concentration measurement
Adults and children ≥45 kg: 600 mg daily
Children <45 kg: 20 mg kg⁻¹ daily up to a maximum of 600 mg daily

↓

(*continued overpage*)

FIGURE 27.2: *Continued*

Check serum concentration ⌐4 hours after a morning dose of most slow-release products or 8 hours after a dose of a very slowly absorbed product given once every 24 hours, when no doses have been missed, added, or taken at unequal intervals for 3 days.

↓

Dosage adjustment based on serum concentration

Peak serum concentration	Directions
< 7.5 μg ml^{-1}	Increase dose about 25%. *Recheck serum theophylline concentration for guidance in further dosage adjustment*
7.5–9.9 μg ml^{-1}	If tolerated, increase dose ⌐25%
10–14.9 μg ml^{-1}	If tolerated, maintain dose. *Recheck serum theophylline concentration at 6–12-month intervals[a]*
15–19.9 μg ml^{-1}	Consider 10% decrease in dose to provide greater margin of safety[a]
20–24.9 μg ml^{-1}	Decrease dose 10% to 25%. Recheck serum concentration after 3 days
25–30 μg ml^{-1}	Skip next dose and decrease subsequent doses at least 25%. Recheck serum concentration after 3 days
>30 μg ml^{-1}	Skip next two doses and decrease subsequent doses 50%. *Recheck serum theophylline concentration for guidance in further dosage adjustment[b]*

[a]Dosage reduction or serum concentration measurement is indicated whever adverse effects are present, physiological abnormalities that can reduce theophylline clearance occur (e.g. persistent fever), or a drug that interacts with theophylline is added or discontinued (e.g. erythromycin, carbamazepine).
[b]Administer activated charcoal in water, 0.5 g kg^{-1} every 2 hours until serum concentration <20 μg ml^{-1}. Consider intravenously administered phenobarbital, 20 mg kg^{-1} to prevent seizures if excessive serum concentration has resulted from multiple doses. Consult a regional poison control centre for additional advice.

It is not a mainstream bronchodilator for asthmatic children. It may be useful as an alternative bronchodilator for those children who have significant side-effects to β_2 agonists or theophyllines, or it may be useful as an additional bronchodilator in children with very severe chronic asthma. There has been some evidence that it may be particularly useful in treating wheezy babies where β_2 agonists are often not very effective.[117] Side-effects are uncommon because there is virtually no systemic absorption. Paradoxical bronchoconstriction was reported with the nebulized preparation, but was largely explained by the hypotonicity of the nebulizer solution and by the presence of antibacterial additives in the original product.[118]

Anti-inflammatory drugs (see also Chapters 15 and 16)

Inhaled corticosteroids There is no doubt that in the inhaled form, corticosteroids are the most effective treatment for asthma currently available. A number of properly controlled long-term studies (12–22 months) of both children and adults have shown that regular treatment with inhaled corticosteroids diminishes asthma symptoms, decreases asthma exacerbations and decreases the need for bronchodilator use.[119–122] After long-term use, inhaled corticosteroids decrease bronchial reactivity and improve airway calibre in most, although not to normal.[123] Inhaled steroids are effective in children of all ages and even in younger children improve symptom scores, reduce the need for oral steroids and reduce exacerbations.[124–126]

Unfortunately, corticosteroids do not appear to cure asthma. In one series of asthmatic children, 28–36 months of treatment with inhaled corticosteroids and regular bronchodilator improved both symptoms and objective measures of lung function in children.[123] Tapering-off the steroids after that time, while continuing regular bronchodilator, led to deterioration in asthma control over the next 4–6 months.[127] This suggests that the underlying inflammatory process is still active even after years on inhaled corticosteroids. Treatment with inhaled corticosteroids is therefore principally aimed at bringing about symptomatic remission.

Several inhaled steroids are available, although availability varies from country to country (e.g. beclomethasone, dipropionate (BDP), budesonide (BUD), flunisolide, fluticasone propionate). There are differences between steroids in their binding affinity to the glucocorticoid receptor and in their relative potency in skin blanching.[128] Most experience in children has been with inhaled BDP and BUD. While many studies have addressed the individual efficacy of inhaled steroids, there are relatively few comparative studies (and no long-term comparisons) of inhaled steroids in the same patients. The available evidence suggests that there is no difference in asthma control using similar doses of BDP or BUD.[129]

The steroid dose required depends on the severity of the disease. In children with mild asthma, substantial improvement in symptoms, lung function and airway responsiveness is seen at doses of inhaled budesonide as low as 100 μg daily. There is evidence of a dose–response relationship, with 400 μg daily producing better results than 100 μg daily.[130] Many children will have no additional benefit with doses above 400 μg daily. However, the plateau on the dose–response curve differs from patient to patient, and according to which response is studied.[131] Some children with severe asthma responding poorly to conventional doses of inhaled corticosteroids may benefit from doses of 800 μg or above.

Several studies have shown that twice-daily use is as effective in controlling stable asthma as four times daily administration for both BDP and BUD, although in severe or poorly controlled asthma four times daily adminis-tration may be better.[128] Twice-daily administration is likely to be associated with better compliance.

Side-effects Although inhaled steroids for childhood asthma have been used for over 30 years, anxieties about their side-effects continue, especially as they may be required for quite long periods. Inhaled corticosteroids cause systemic effects to the extent that they are absorbed from the gastro-intestinal tract and the airways. The amount of steroid absorbed varies with the dose, with the site of deposition and with the metabolism of the parti-cular drug. Drugs that are inactivated by first-pass hepatic metabolism are likely to have fewer systemic effects.[128]

The type of inhaler device used is also important because it influences the amount deposited in different sites and therefore changes the amount available for absorption. For example, with metered dose inhalers (MDI) about 80% of the drug is deposited in the oropharynx and can be swal-lowed and absorbed. The use of a spacer with an MDI results in the larger propellant/drug particles becoming smaller and more slow moving as the propellant evaporates. The net result is to reduce the amount impacting in the oropharynx but to maintain or increase the amount reaching the lung. As a consequence the side-effects from systemic absorption can be reduced while the clinical effects, which depend on intra-pulmonary depo-sition, are unaltered. With dry powder inhalers the great majority of the dose is deposited in the oropharynx. The systemic effects can be reduced or abolished by manoeuvres such as mouth-washing that remove drug deposited in the oropharynx.[128]

The major concerns about inhaled steroids, particularly in the long term, have centred on their impact on growth. A number of factors have made it difficult to measure the impact of inhaled steroids on growth. Asthma itself is clearly associated with effects on growth.[30] Children with moderate to severe asthma appear gradually to fall away from their predicted height centile as they approach puberty. The onset of sexual maturation is delayed, and this delay appears to be independent of asthma severity. How-ever, as a result, growth continues for a longer time during the second decade.[132] For the most part, asthmatic children ultimately attain their pre-dicted adult height.[133] The cause of this pattern of growth has been the subject of much speculation but remains unknown. Controlling chronic asthma, even with inhaled corticosteroids, can improve growth.[29]

Reassuringly, the longitudinal data available suggest that doses up to 800 μg daily of inhaled corticosteroids over 1–5 years do not influence long-term linear growth in asthmatic children. At higher doses, data are more limited. A decrease in height centile was noted in 6 of 50 children receiving 750–1500 μg BDP for an average of 19 months, although four were 10–15 years, an age when the pre-pubertal growth slowing is most marked. In pre-pubertal children, Ninan and Russel found normal growth rates in children taking up to 1600 μg BPD or BUD daily, provided that their symptoms were well controlled.[29] Longitudinal data on younger children are limited but also reassuring. Two small studies in children aged 3–7 years who took inhaled BUD 200 μg daily and doses of 200–1100 μg m^{-2} daily for at least 1 year did not detect any adverse effect on height velocity.[134] More recently, a number of studies using knemometry have found a reduction in mean growth velocity of the lower leg in children receiving inhaled BPD 400 μg daily via a Diskhaler[135] and in children on BUD 800 μg daily via a Nebuhaler.[136] As yet, it is not possible to reconcile the short-term knemometry data with data from longitudinal studies, and the long-term implications are unclear.[128]

There is evidence of a significant reduction in physiological cortisol secretion measured at frequent intervals in children taking 400–1000 μg BDP during the night or during a 24-hour period.[137] This is a very sensitive test of the hypothalamic–pituitary axis, however. There is also evidence of a dose-dependent suppression of 24-hour urinary cortisol secretion significant at doses greater than 400 μg daily. Most studies have not observed significant changes in the (less sensitive) urinary cortisol excretion in children taking up to 400 μg daily of BDP.[128] There are at present no reports of a reduced hypothalamic–pituitary axis response to stimulation in children treated with inhaled steroids only. Perhaps most importantly, in adults or children treated with inhaled steroids alone, clinical adrenal insufficiency has not been reported.

Multiple vertebral fractures and generalized osteoporosis are well-recognized effects of long-term oral steroid use, both in children and adults. To date, there is no evidence that inhaled corticosteroids are associated with similar effects. In adults, newer methods of studying bone metabolism have suggested that inhaled steroids can affect biochemical markers of bone turnover. In children, the available data suggest that doses up to 800 μg of BDP or BUD or 200 μg of fluticasone do not affect markers of bone formation or resorption.[128]

Central nervous system effects of inhaled corticosteroids have been reported but are in the main rare and confined to case reports. Connet and Lenney reported four young children who developed acute behaviour disturbance, especially hyperactivity and temper tantrums, on BUD via

Nebuhaler in doses of 400 μg two or three times daily.[138] Usually, the reported effects came on rapidly and subsided completely when the dose was reduced or the drug was stopped.

While posterior subcapsular cataracts are a specific and well-recognized complication of long-term oral glucocorticoids, a recent Canadian study found no evidence that they were associated with the long-term use (median 5 years; range 1–15 years) of inhaled BDP or BUD in moderate to high doses (median 750 μg; range 300–2000 μg) in children and young adults.[139]

At present, while several metabolic effects have been reported after inhaled steroids there is little evidence that such effects are clinically relevant at therapeutic doses in children. In particular, there do not appear to be significant effects on glucose or lipid metabolism. Easy bruising occurs in adults taking inhaled steroids and seems to increase with age and with dose and duration of inhaled steroid, but this does not seem to be a problem in children.

In adults, local effects from deposition of inhaled steroid on the upper airway are among the most frequently reported side-effects but similar effects tend to be rare in children. In the largest study of children (229 with asthma, 129 taking BDP) clinical candidiasis occurred in only one child. Colonization was found in 40–50% of children taking inhaled steroids compared with 29% of the asthmatic control subjects. The rate of colonization was not affected by the device used (MDI vs. Rotahaler), nor by the dose (high vs. low). In the same study, sore throat and hoarseness occurred rarely and were not related to the presence of *Candida* or to treatment with inhaled steroids.[140]

The fact that corticosteroid side-effects have been detected with more sensitive tests and at higher doses is perhaps not especially surprising. It is a testimony to the efficacy and safety of inhaled steroids that any effects detected are rarely of clinical significance.

Systemic steroids Short courses of oral steroid (prednisolone 1–2 mg kg^{-1} for 5–7 days) are an important component of the treatment of acute exacerbations and may reduce the need for hospital admission.[141–143] While short courses may cause adrenal suppression, rapid recovery in adrenal function occurs.[144] Children receiving more than four courses per year may develop more prolonged adrenal suppression.[145]

Nowadays, oral steroids are rarely used in the chronic treatment of childhood asthma. If they are used, the smallest possible dose compatible with control of symptoms should be used and should be given as a single morning dose. Alternate-day use, while preferable, is often not sufficient to control severe asthma and daily use is often necessary. Inhaled steroids should always be continued for their systemic steroid-sparing effect. Apparent (relative) "steroid resistance" is recognized in children with difficult-to-control asthma, and has been shown to be associated with abnormal glucocorticoid pharmacokinetics and glucocorticoid receptor binding.[146]

Cromoglycate Sodium cromoglycate (SCG) is a non-steroidal anti-inflammatory agent with no significant bronchodilator action. Despite much research, the precise mode of action remains unclear. Given prophylactically, SCG inhibits both early- and late-phase allergen-induced airway narrowing. It also blocks acute airway narrowing to exercise and methacholine. There is evidence of a dose–response effect, at least for exercise-induced asthma.[147]

SCG is used for the prophylactic therapy of moderate asthma in children. Because of its wide safety margin it continues to have a role as a first-line prophylactic agent. The individual response to SCG in children is unpredictable. Where it works, it can be very effective indeed. A 4–8-week trial may be necessary to be certain of efficacy.

At the start of treatment, SCG is usually given four times a day but, if effective, it may be possible to reduce the dosage to three times a day. It is available as a nebulizer solution, a dry powder and a metered-dose aerosol. Its major attraction is the very low incidence of side-effects. Occasional coughing due to airway irritation can occur after inhaling the dry powder but may be reduced by pre-treatment with β_2 agonist. Because of this irritant effect SCG is usually stopped during any acute exacerbations. Transient rashes have also been reported.

Nedocromil Nedocromil sodium is a prophylactic drug with a very similar profile of activity to SCG.[148,149] It has not been widely used in children with asthma[150] and its place remains to be clearly established. Nedocromil has been shown to improve daily asthma symptoms and lung function, and to reduce concurrent bronchodilator use, in children with mild to moderately severe disease.[150] It appears to have a fairly rapid onset of action with most of the improvement occurring in the first 4 weeks. The usual dose has been 4 mg two to four times per day. Side-effects of nedocromil are uncommon but headache, sore throat, nausea and a bitter taste have all been reported.

Ketotifen Ketotifen is a potent antihistamine with strong *in vitro* mast-cell stabilizing characteristics. As it is taken orally and lasts for 12 hours, it was hoped that it would be valuable as a long-acting, orally active, anti-asthma compound. A minimum of 8–12 weeks are necessary before any beneficial effects are fully realized. It has been used in doses of 1 mg twice daily for children over 3 years, and 0.5 mg twice daily for children below 3 years. It appears to be a safe drug, although weight gain and sedation are potential problems.[151] Unfortunately, it has not lived up to its original promise and a long-term placebo-controlled trial in children with mild asthma found that it had no clinical benefit.[152] It has no effect on exercise-induced asthma.[153]

Other agents Immunosuppressive therapy (in addition to corticosteroids) has been used on an experimental basis in severe steroid-dependent asthma in adults, but is not, at present, recommended for use in children.

Choosing the Routes of Administration and Appropriate Inhalation Devices (see also Chapter 20)

Since asthma is a disease of airways, treatment via inhalation is generally preferred. The advantages of selective delivery, rapid onset of action, reduced dosage and minimal side-effects are important to both doctors and parents. The respiratory tract, however, has a series of mechanisms to protect it from particle entry and deposition. While devices suitable for use in childhood are now available, careful training and attention to technique is essential. Unfortunately, because of the range of ages and intelligence no single device at present is appropriate for all ages (Table 27.11).

Failure of inhalation treatment is usually due to inadequate device technique or inappropriate device for that age.[154] Young children, particularly, often cooperate poorly with inhaled therapy. It is then not surprising that choosing the appropriate device and making sure parents and children are properly educated in its use can be as important as the choice of drug.

With development of devices for inhaled therapy, systemic therapy is much less used. Intravenous therapy is now confined to acute asthma. Oral therapy remains an attractive option particularly for some groups such as very young children. However, there are no oral prophylactic agents as effective and free from side-effects as those used via the inhaled route. Oral bronchodilators can be useful in very young children but are associated with a slower duration of onset and greater systemic side-effects.

Inhalation devices There is now a substantial body of evidence about device use in children, providing information about the most effective techniques (Table 27.12) and the associated problems.

TABLE 27.11: *Drug inhalation devices for regular use in children*

Age	Appropriate inhaled device
< 2.5 years	Nebulizer
< 2.5 years	Spacer device plus face mask
2–5 years	Spacer device alone
> 4.5–5 years	Dry powder inhaler
> 6 years	Breath-actuated device
> 10 years	Metered dose inhaler

TABLE 27.12: *Techniques of using main inhaled device types in children*

Device	Step	Action	Reason
Nebulizer	1	Fill the nebulizer to 4 ml; set flow rate to 6–8 l min^{-1}	Optimal conditions for generating particles of appropriate size
	2	Inhale using tidal breaths	
Dry powder inhaler	1	Prime the device	
	2	For Rotahaler and Turbohaler hold vertically	Avoids powder falling out
	3	Inhale as quickly as possible	Provide energy to break up the powder into particles of size suitable for inhalation
MDI	1	Remove the cap	
	2	Shake the canister	Disperses drug particles uniformly in the propellant
	3	Hold the canister upright	Metering chamber only fills when upright
	4	Breathe out as far as is comfortable	Conflicting evidence
	5	Place the inhaler between the lips	
	6	Fire the inhaler at the beginning of a slow inspiration	Slow steady inspiration (< 30 l min^{-1}) decreases oropharyngeal deposition

TABLE 27.12: *Continued*

Device	Step	Action	Reason
	7	Hold the breath for 10 s, or as long as is comfortable	Allows particles to settle on the airways by gravitational sedimentation
	8	If repeating keep upright	Allows the canister to return to thermal equilibrium and the metering chamber to fill
MDI plus large volume-spacer	1	Shake the canister and spacer	Disperses drug particles uniformly in the propellant
	2	Actuate the MDI and fill the large-volume spacer	
	3	Inhale from the spacer using five tidal breaths	Child breathes in the aerosol. Lung volume at inhalation and breath-holding technique not necessary

MDI, metered dose inhaler.

Metered dose inhalers In children under 6 years, more than 50% were noted to have faulty and inefficient MDI technique (Table 27.13).[155] Particularly significant were coordination difficulties, cessation of inhalation when cold particles hit the soft palate ("freon" effect), oral actuation but nasal inspiration and rapid inhalation. Use of a small-volume tube spacer significantly improved problems with coordination. Parents coordinating the firing of an MDI alone or with a tube spacer did not improve the situation.

With careful tuition children older than 6 years can be taught to use MDIs successfully. However, as a practical rule they are probably best confined

TABLE 27.13: *Frequency of the most common mistakes observed in 256 children demonstrating the use of an inhaler. (From Ref. 155 with permission)*

	MDI inhaler ($n = 132$)	Tube spacer ($n = 85$)
Forgetting to shake the canister	49%	34%
Forgetting to exhale before firing	45%	51%
Neck flexed during inhalation	12%	14%
Coordination problems	55%	17%
Fast inhalation	67%	28%
Breath-holding ≤ 7 s	42%	39%
Stopping inspiration when firing aerosol	38%	6%
Inspiration through the nose	24%	32%
Submaximal inspiration	23%	19%
Help from the parents	5%	6%

to children older than 10 years. If used, the inhalation technique needs to be reviewed at every visit.

Breath-actuated MDI devices (Autohaler) can remove the coordination difficulties but again do not affect other problems associated with MDI use, such as rapid inhalation. In a series of over 100 children, Pedersen and Mortensen have shown that even with careful instruction provided by videos and a nurse, only 2 of 10 under 5 years old could master the device reliably.[156] Consequently, they cannot be recommended for pre-school children at present.

Spacers An MDI with a spacer attached has become an increasingly attractive method of administering inhaled medication to children. The spacer allows the propellant to evaporate leaving smaller, slow-moving respirable particles suitable for inhalation. The amount of drug deposited in the oropharynx is reduced, thus decreasing the consequent systemic absorption and increasing lung deposition. This feature makes them particularly suitable when high-dose inhaled corticosteroids are required.

The ideal spacer design volume is not known. Less drug is available for inhalation in smaller spacer devices due to impaction on the walls of the device but the drug is in a smaller space and hence is more concentrated. At lower tidal volumes, the higher inhaled drug concentration from smaller devices may enhance drug delivery. Thus a smaller device may be appropriate for infants while a larger device is better for older children.[157] Other problems, such as the static charge on the device, introduce further complications.[158]

Simple spacers such as a paper cup[159] have been shown to be effective and may be useful in emergencies. However, because of the absence of a valve if the child exhales during the actuation then no drug will be inhaled. Valved spacers (Nebuhaler, Volumatic, Aerochamber, Babyhaler), which provide a reservoir from which the child can inhale, avoid this problem and are easy for most children to use.

Large-volume spacers have proved particularly useful for prophylactic medication administration in children between 1 and 4 years of age. For both prophylactic medication and bronchodilator treatment, there is evidence of improvement in symptom scores and lung function, with fewer side-effects.[125,126,160–162] Small children, and infants, and those with severe airway obstruction, may have difficulties triggering the valve of some spacers[163] because they cannot produce sufficient flow. However, measurements have found the valve of both the Nebuhaler and Volumatic opens at flows achievable even by obstructed infants.[164] Tilting the device to allow gravity to keep the valve open may assist. Young children may be unable to seal their lips around the mouthpiece of the device. A spacer with a close-sealing mask (either an attached mask such as a Laerdal mask or one built into the device such as an Aerochamber) allows multiple breaths to be taken with less aerosol escape and can provide effective therapy for children under 3 years.[165]

The usual manufacturer's instructions for a large-volume spacer (slow, deep, inhalation followed by a 5–10 s breath-hold) are not practical for young children. Gleeson and Price found that five tidal breaths from a Nebuhaler with no breath-hold resulted in greater bronchodilation than a more conventional inhalation technique.[166] This "five breath technique" is much more practical for young children. Only one actuation per five breaths is recommended[157] because multiple actuations decrease the final dose available for inhalation. Inhalation should also take place as soon after firing as possible since a delay allows the drug to settle on the spacer walls, and again decreases the dose.[158]

Large-volume spacers are bulky and difficult to carry making them unsuitable for self-administration in school-age children. The physical size of some spacers (Nebuhaler, Volumatic) can make it difficult to use the device in a struggling toddler. In this situation, smaller spacers such as the Aerochamber may be easier for a parent to handle.[157]

Small-volume ("tube") spacers are also available. They have been shown to lead to greater bronchodilation than an MDI alone. They reduce, but do not abolish, the numbers of inhalation errors that occur with MDIs (Table 27.13).[167]

Dry powder inhalers Dry powder inhalers are now the mainstay of asthma treatment in schoolchildren. They are particularly useful in this age group because they are discreet and easy to carry around.

The effectiveness of dry powder inhalers increases with inspiratory flow rate. While the flow rate required to generate an optimum effect varies from one device to another, most require the child to develop an inspiratory flow rate of approximately 20–60 l min^{-1}. On average, peak inspiratory flow rate is about one-third of PEFR.[168] Since an average 4 year old has a mean PEFR of 100 l min^{-1}, it is obvious that pre-school children, particularly if wheezy, may have difficulty generating sufficient inspiratory flow to gain full benefit from a dry powder device.[168] An important advantage of the newer "second generation" multidose devices such as the Turbohaler and the Diskhaler is that they require much lower peak inspiratory flow rates to be effective. Indeed, the Turbohaler retains about 33% of its effect at flow rates around 13 l min^{-1}.[169]

The optimum technique for a dry powder inhaler is to inhale as rapidly as possible. Breath-holding or tilting the head back do not assist.[168,169] This technique is simple and easily taught and aids, such as inspiratory whistles, can simplify the process.

With dry powder inhalers the vast majority of the drug is deposited in the oropharynx; only a small proportion enters the lung. Parents and children sometimes need to be reassured that the drug will be effective, even when most of it seems to be deposited in the mouth. With inhaled corticosteroids, mouth-washing after use can reduce the systemic effects.[128] One practical suggestion is to take the medication just before tooth-brushing and mouth-rinsing. Agertoft and Pedersen found a higher intra-bronchial deposition of BUD from a Turbohaler than from an MDI and Nebuhaler and thus in some cases an increase in systemic effect with dry powder inhalers may actually arise because of increased deposition in the airways.[170]

Since young children and older children during exacerbations may not be able to generate sufficient inspiratory flow rates, dry powder inhalers are not recommended for children much below 5 years and when first used are likely to be better for the administration of prophylactic medication. If prescribing dry powder bronchodilator in younger children, it may be sensible to anticipate the fact that some may need an alternative device during acute wheezing.

Nebulizers Nebulizers allow the delivery of large concentrations of medication and avoid problems with coordination. As a result, they are suitable for the very young and the acutely ill. They are the mainstay of hospital treatment for children with acute asthma. In the home, nebulizers are useful for the delivery of prophylactic medication in young children unable to use other devices because of their age or their intelligence. They are also useful in the severely asthmatic child or in those with frequent severe asthma attacks where they may reduce the need for hospital admission.[171] Unfortunately, compressors suitable for home use are bulky, expensive and time-consuming and need a power source. There is no doubt they are overused, particularly with the development of effective alternatives. All too frequently, a request for a home nebulizer arises because of the failure to treat chronic asthma properly.

Two main types are available. The commonest are jet nebulizers, which work by using the Bernoulli effect to draw drug solution into a gas stream, forcing it onto an impaction plate and forming aerosol droplets by impaction and gas turbulence. Optimal drug delivery using a jet nebulizer has been shown to require a flow rate of 6–8 $l \, min^{-1}$ and dilution of the drug to a fill volume of 4 ml. Minor changes in the details of administration can have dramatic effects on drug output. For example, a close fitting mask is often used. A gap of only 2 cm between mask and face may result in an 85% reduction in the dose delivered.[172]

Before starting nebulizer treatment, parents should be given clear, and preferably written, instructions in the use of the nebulizer. Parents should have a clear understanding that they should seek medical help if their child fails to respond to nebulized bronchodilator.[171]

General points about inhaler device use It is becoming clear that the device and patient factors influencing intra-pulmonary drug deposition can be complex and vary greatly depending on the child's age, the device used and the inhalation technique. There is often surprisingly little clinical or scientific information about such factors. Uncritical introduction of new devices into clinical practice should be avoided until their effects, and side-effects, have been clearly established in the target population.

Whatever device is chosen, careful education in its use and repeated checks on technique are important. Technique should be checked every time an asthmatic child is reviewed. If the technique is poor and cannot be improved, then the device should be changed to one that can be used reliably. Regrettably, the education of clinical staff in the use of inhalers has often been neglected. Clinical staff should know which device is likely to be appropriate for a particular child and how to instruct the child in the use of the chosen device. Nowadays, asthmatic children often know about different inhaler devices. Allowing children to choose the one they like best may help to ensure compliance. Failure to observe these simple rules frequently compromises the therapeutic effectiveness of inhalation treatment in children.

Choosing the Appropriate Drug Combinations and Doses Using a Step-wise Approach [22,23]

The choice of pharmacological treatment should take account of the severity of the disease and the child's current treatment. Successful drug management aims to reduce or abolish symptoms (Table 27.5) with minimum therapy.[22] Whether it is better to give maximum treatment at the outset in order to achieve control of asthma or to begin with moderate therapy that is then increased in a gradual step-up manner is not yet clear. An initial "rescue" course of oral corticosteroids can be useful in bringing about rapid control of symptoms, which may be important in gaining the confidence of the family and encouraging future adherence to treatment. As against this, many parents are concerned about drug side-effects particularly from inhaled corticosteroids. Whichever approach is adopted, therapy should start at a level broadly in keeping with the severity of the asthma.

Thereafter treatment is usually altered using a graded or stepped approach in which the medication is changed when asthma remains uncontrolled despite correct use of the prescribed medication. Since asthma is dynamic as well as chronic, treatment should change to accommodate the variations that occur over time.

The current approach to treatment of childhood asthma is well summarized in a number of national and international consensus statements.[20-23] These give guidelines about treatments appropriate for different severities of asthma. However, the appropriate treatment should then be tailored for each particular child. If control is not achieved with the chosen step, treatment should be increased to the next appropriate step. Before increasing treatment it is essential to check that the child is using the inhaled device properly, and that the present prescription has been understood and correctly taken. Once satisfactory control has been sustained for a period of weeks or months, consideration can be given to a cautious reduction in therapy ("step-down") to the minimum necessary to maintain control.

Mild infrequent asthma: step 1 (Table 27.8) Sixty per cent of children have mild, infrequent symptoms of coughing and wheezing. For such children, bronchodilator to be used as required when symptoms are present is usually sufficient. Bronchodilator delivery by inhalation is preferable. For children between the ages of 2 and 5 years, an MDI with large-volume spacer (and mask, if necessary) is effective. School-age children usually find a dry powder inhaler more convenient. Oral bronchodilators are less effective and have more systemic side-effects but may be useful for younger children with mild infrequent symptoms. Oral bronchodilators may occasionally be sufficient in slightly older children with mild asthma where the infrequent use of bronchodilator makes inhalation skills difficult to maintain.

Some pre-school children may be symptom-free most of the time, but develop occasional acute exacerbations following viral respiratory infections. The parents often recognize a clear pattern of deterioration that can alert them to the need to start medication (Table 27.14). Bronchodilators alone are often insufficient: a short course of oral steroids started early may help to bring the symptoms under control.[142] Intermittent inhalation of high-dose corticosteroids from a large-volume spacer has been tried, but the benefits have been modest.[174,175]

SCG on a seasonal basis may be useful for some children. For pollen-related problems, treatment should be commenced 4–6 weeks before the pollen season and then continued throughout the season. SCG may also be helpful to children with animal-sensitive asthma when taken 15–30 min before exposure to the animal(s).

Moderate asthma: steps 2 and 3 (Table 27.8) About 30% of children suffer more frequent and troublesome symptoms. These children may require daily inhaled prophylactic anti-inflammatory treatments (Table 27.15). Despite much debate, most paediatricians continue to start with a 4–8-week

TABLE 27.14: *Initial prodromal symptoms of asthma and their time-relation to an overt attack of asthma. (From Ref. 173 with permission)*

Symptom	No. of patients	Interval (hours) between initial symptom and onset of overt attack	
		Mean (SD)	Range
Rhinorrhoea	39	26.76 (12.0)	6–60
Cough	23	20.73 (0.42)	6–48
Irritability	7	28.28 (4.53)	12–36
Apathy	7	28.28 (4.13)	12–36
Anxiety	3	30	24–36
Sleep disorders	2	18	12–24
Fever (above 38 °C)	5	16.2 (4.0)	6–24
Abdominal pain	2	13.5 (6.4)	6–24
Loss of appetite	2	18	12–24
Itching	3	9	6–12
Skin eruption	1	9	6–12
Toothache	1	9	6–12

TABLE 27.15: *Indications for prophylactic asthma therapy*

Symptoms of coughing or wheezing more than once or twice a
   week
Nocturnal disturbance with cough or wheeze more than one or
   two nights a week
Bronchodilator use required more than once or twice a day
Persistent airway obstruction on peak flow recording
Frequent acute attacks lasting more than 24 hours (more than
   one every 4–6 weeks)
Frequent hospital admissions

---

trial of SCG, administered either via MDI with large-volume spacer (10 mg four times per day) or, for older children, via a dry powder inhaler (Spincaps 20 mg four times per day). SCG has the advantage of virtually no side-effects.

Prior to starting any prophylactic treatment, it is necessary to explain the plan clearly to the parents so that they appreciate the need for regular treatment. Parents should know that 4–6 weeks may be necessary for the treatment to become effective. Some children will respond well to SCG, but it is not possible to predict beforehand who will respond best. Clinically, children with mild symptoms but a particularly prominent cough often seem to benefit most. Long-term studies suggest that SCG may be effective in about two-thirds of children whose symptoms are not adequately controlled by bronchodilator.[176] If SCG is successful, it may be possible to reduce the frequency of administration to three times a day.

If, after 4–8 weeks of SCG, the response to treatment is inadequate, then an inhaled steroid (BDP or BUD) should be started, usually in a dose of 100–200 μg twice daily. At this point, there is generally no benefit in continuing SCG.

As in earlier steps, β_2 agonists should again be used as required for symptom treatment.

Severe asthma: steps 4 and 5 (Table 27.8) Fewer than 10% of children with asthma fall into the most severe category. With continuing symptoms, or a continuing requirement for a bronchodilator two or three times daily, the next step is usually a further increase in steroid dose to 400–800 μg daily.

Additional long-acting bronchodilators, oral or inhaled, and theophylline preparations may also be useful, particularly for controlling nocturnal symptoms. There is still debate about the precise role of long-acting medications and the best time to introduce them.[177]

If increased steroids (with or without long-acting medications) fail to control symptoms, even higher doses of inhaled corticosteroids (up to 1600–2000 μg daily) may be tried. Before using such high doses, it is important to check the device technique, to ensure, as far as possible, that the child is actually receiving, or taking, the prescribed medicine and to address any factors that may be contributing to poor compliance (Table 27.16) (see also Chapter 25). If possible, the PEFR should be monitored regularly. Close attention should be paid to environmental factors, such as parental smoking, pets or psychosocial problems that may compromise the effectiveness of treatment. Inhaled short-acting bronchodilators should continue to be used as needed for symptom control, although, by this stage, quite high doses are frequently being used regularly.

With doses of inhaled corticosteroids above 800 μg daily, the use of a spacer device to decrease oropharyngeal deposition and systemic absorption[125] may be appropriate; both BDP via a spacer (Volumatic) and BUD via spacer (Nebuhaler) have less systemic activity than the same dose delivered from an MDI or dry powder inhaler (Diskhaler or Turbohaler), although mouth-rinsing after the Turbohaler seems to reduce or abolish this difference. Whatever device is used, it would seem advisable to rinse out the mouth after administration to remove any corticosteroid remaining in the oropharynx.

If control remains poor, the administration of inhaled corticosteroids four times per day may help.[179] The use of high-dose nebulized BUD (up to 2000 μg daily) is also worth considering. If control still remains poor despite maximum doses of inhaled corticosteroids and bronchodilators, oral corticosteroids may be necessary. Often prednisolone 5–10 mg daily will be sufficient and should be used concurrently with high-dose inhaled steroid. Where possible, oral corticosteroids should be administered on

TABLE 27.16: *Possible reasons for non-compliance. (From Ref. 178 with permission)*

Misunderstanding
Lack of confidence in efficacy of the drug
Fear of side-effects/dislike of drugs
Complacency
Rebellion
Difficulties with method of administration
Difficulties with the timing of administration

alternate days to diminish side-effects, but daily administration is often required for asthma control.

When oral steroids are taken, side-effects are likely and families should be warned to expect them. Early dietary advice may avoid some of the weight gain that should be expected. Careful monitoring of height and weight, blood pressure, urine for glucose and eyes for cataract development is necessary. A steroid card containing instructions to increase the steroid dose with intercurrent medical problems should be issued.

It is a rare child whose asthma genuinely cannot be controlled. Where there is apparent continuing inability to control asthma, the diagnosis should be carefully reviewed. Poor compliance is often at the root of the problem.[180] Relative "steroid resistance" can occur[146] but is uncommon. Careful education and meticulous attention to all aspects of asthma care by one experienced clinician can often lead to improved control. The clinician should aim to provide consistent support and to keep the therapeutic plan as simple as possible. Periods of inpatient care may help to re-establish control.

Step-down When satisfactory asthma control is achieved, the treatment can be reduced. This should be done slowly in 4–6 monthly steps. With older children, a period of PEFR monitoring over the period of the reduction of dose may be helpful. If control deteriorates, the patients should return to the previous treatment.

ESTABLISH PLANS FOR DEALING WITH VARIATIONS IN THE DISEASE AND MANAGING EXACERBATIONS (see also Chapter 24)

Devising a strategy to cope with exacerbations is an important element in any treatment plan. The parents must be able to monitor the disease, recognize deterioration early and change the medicine quickly, without necessarily involving their doctor. The aim is to abort any exacerbation before it becomes severe, and in so doing avoid hospital admission.

To achieve such an aim, both parents and children have to be well educated about asthma. They must have a clear understanding of the role of the various medicines, and be fully competent in the use of any inhalation device. They should be able to identify early signs of loss of control, such as more frequent nocturnal waking or increased need for relievers. The necessary education and training are the responsibility of the clinician but can often be successfully delegated to nurses and physiotherapists. The education and advice should be consistent, repeated and reinforced by written guidelines.

For children under 5 years, plans are solely symptom-based. Fortunately, exacerbations do not usually happen without warning. In up to 70% of children a sequence of prodromal findings, which is constant in a particular child, is present for approximately 24 hours before the onset of wheezing (Table 27.14).[173] Recognition of such patterns facilitates the early introduction of treatment. In children over 5 years, these early findings can be combined with PEFR monitoring.

A number of zone or colour coded ("traffic light") systems have been developed to make management plans easier to use; one example is outlined in Table 27.17. Studies of children show that such approaches are effective in improving asthma control and decreasing morbidity, and enhance the likelihood of a correct response to an exacerbation.[58] In some approaches the essence of the plan is written on a small asthma "credit card", which can be carried around with the patient or parent.[181]

The levels of PEFR at which certain interventions should be initiated have not been validated.[22] For example, Charlton et al. instructed their patients to increase treatment at a PEFR of 70% of best, but thought the effect might have been better if 80% of best PEFR had been used.[58] There is also debate about most effective amount of instruction[57,182] and the optimal intensity of follow-up.[183,184]

As part of the emergency plan, parents should be provided with a course of oral corticosteroids. Oral corticosteroids have been shown to be effective in accelerating the recovery and preventing dangerous deterioration in acute exacerbations.[141,185] Parents should be instructed to initiate a course if the attack fails to respond to the usual treatment.[59] For those using PEFR meters, steroids are usually started at a PEFR of 50%[60] to 60% of best.[22] An oral steroid course begun at home by parents at the onset of an exacerbation triggered by a viral upper respiratory tract infection has also been shown to be effective.[142,143]

There is greater uncertainty about the benefits of starting or altering inhaled corticosteroids. Research in adults has demonstrated that doubling twice-daily inhaled steroids if asthma deteriorates can be effective.[57,186] Charlton et al. found a trend towards improvement in children who doubled their inhaled steroid at 70% of best PEFR compared with those who only used bronchodilators, but the numbers studied were small.[58] In pre-school children with wheezing triggered only by viral upper respiratory tract infections, two studies where high-dose inhaled corticosteroids were begun at the onset of symptoms showed modification of symptoms, although the effects were modest.[174,175] More research is needed to establish whether treatment in this way is generally beneficial, particularly for those already on prophylactic treatment.

The other essential treatment during an exacerbation is increased repetitive administration of inhaled short acting β_2 agonists. With more severe exacerbations, higher doses of β_2 agonists will usually be needed. In acute asthma in children, large-volume spacers have been shown to be as effective as nebulizers.[187,188] Ten to twenty puffs may be needed to produce appropriate bronchodilation. It should be remembered that one nebule of 2.5 mg salbutamol contains the equivalent of 25 puffs from an MDI. In

TABLE 27.17: *An example of a colour-coded asthma zone plan. (From Ref. 58 with permission)*

Green zone
Your peak flow is above 70% of normal or your symptoms score is under 6:

... continue "maintenance therapy" of ...

Yellow zone
Your peak flow is less than 70% of normal or your symptoms score is between 6 and 9:

    (a) Double your dose of ... until you return to your highest reading

    (b) Continue on this dose for the same number of days

    (c) Return to the previous dose of "maintenance therapy"

Amber zone
Your peak flow is less than 50% of normal or your symptoms score is less than 9:

    (a) Start oral prednisolone immediately ... mg daily and contact GP within 24 hours

    (b) Continue on this dose until you return to your highest reading

    (c) Reduce oral prednisolone to ... mg daily for the same number of days

    (d) Stop prednisolone

Red zone
Your peak flow is less than 30% of normal or your symptoms score is over 12:

    (a) Call GP urgently, or if unavailable

    (b) Go directly to hospital or if unable

    (c) Call ambulance

an emergency, a coffee cup can be used as a spacer.[159] If the child improves, treatment can be continued at home. Full recovery may be gradual and increased medication may be required for several days.

A plan for managing exacerbations should also set limits so that parents know clearly when treatment is failing and when medical advice should be sought (Table 27.18). It is easier to treat a severe exacerbation successfully at an early stage. A brief hospital admission for frequent inhaled bronchodilators and oral steroids is much less stressful than a period of ventilation in an intensive care unit.

PROVIDE REGULAR FOLLOW-UP CARE

Children with asthma need regular supervision and support by a physician who is knowledgeable about asthma and its treatment. The management plan for children should be subject to a "process of continuing but orderly review" in which they play an active part.[22] There is no doubt that parents prefer to see one doctor or nurse. Wherever possible clinics should be organized to achieve this goal.

There are a number of specific tasks to be completed at any review session (Table 27.19). The central task is to assess whether a child's asthma is well controlled. General open-ended questions such as "How have you been?" rarely produce the necessary information. Questions should be directed to specific symptoms, such as nocturnal disturbance, loss of time from school, problems with exercise, and any exacerbations that have occurred. If a PEFR record is available, it can be a useful basis for discussion and is particularly helpful when discussing the triggers for, and management of, any exacerbations. Useful insights into parent and child perceptions of the disease can be obtained and an individual child's management plan can be fine tuned.

TABLE 27.18: *Indications for seeking early medical help in an exacerbation*

High-risk patient (see Table 27.24)
Severe exacerbation (e.g. PEFR less than 50% of predicted or personal best)
Response to bronchodilator lasts less than 3 hours
β_2 Agonists every 3–4 hours are needed for more than 24–48 hours
No improvement within 2–6 hours of starting oral corticosteroids
Further deterioration

TABLE 27.19: *A checklist of points to cover at clinic review. (From Ref. 22 with permission)*

Points to review	Possible questions
Asthma: severity and control	How does asthma interfere with your/your child's activities?
Trigger factors and their avoidance	What makes the asthma worse?
Drugs: effects and side-effects, compliance, fears	What medicines are you taking?
	Can you explain to me what the drugs do?
	How often do you take your drugs?
	Do you ever miss any doses?
	Can I see your asthma card?
	Some people think steroids are harmful, what do you think?
Devices: correct technique	Show me how you use your inhaler
Monitoring: symptom diary cards, peak flow charts	Can I look at your diary card/peak flow charts?
Acute exacerbations: recognition, treatment, when to get help	When would you call your doctor?
Specific anxieties	What do you expect from asthma treatment?

The drug therapy being used should be ascertained and noted, in particular the specific drugs, their doses and the actual devices. All too frequently parents (or other medical carers), for whatever reason, have changed the drugs or the dosages. It may be appropriate to reinforce the understanding of the purpose of a particular drug. It is also necessary to gauge whether the treatment is being taken appropriately.

Inhalation skills should be reviewed at every visit. If they are inadequate and cannot be improved, a change in device may be indicated. The most appropriate device for a child will change with time, e.g. when a child reaches school age, a more easily portable device such as a dry powder inhaler may be better. Children may have friends with asthma who are using different inhalers, and as a result may have clear ideas about which device they would prefer. Where appropriate, such preferences should be met.

In follow-up, examination usually plays only a limited role. Children with severe asthma taking larger doses of inhaled or oral steroids should be accurately measured, and their height plotted on an appropriate centile chart. Other signs of corticosteroid side-effects should be looked for (Table 27.20). With modern treatments, the chest should usually be clear on auscultation. Both chronic chest deformity and interval wheezing are important signs of more severe asthma and should be noted.[190] Most clinicians caring for children with asthma will be aware of an occasional child with respiratory symptoms due to a disorder other than asthma, so it is always worth checking for signs such as finger clubbing, which point to an alternative diagnosis. Anxieties, particularly about corticosteroids and their side-effects, are common and should be specifically brought up and fully aired, since latent anxieties may compromise management. Finally, it is important to update the action to be taken in the event of an acute deterioration.

Most children with asthma can be managed without referral to a specialist but referral may be necessary when asthma is severe, or when the parents need reassurance (Table 27.7).

SPECIAL PROBLEMS AND COMMON QUESTIONS

ASTHMA IN INFANTS AND YOUNG CHILDREN

Wheezing in young children is very common: 15% of infants in the first year of life, and up to 25% of under-fives, attend their family practitioners with wheezing lower respiratory illnesses. Many more have milder symptoms.[191] Admissions to hospital are common. Indeed, much of the increase in asthma admissions between 1979 and 1985 has been in children under the age of 4 years.[4,192]

Despite the frequency of wheezing in young children, the diagnosis of asthma in infants and young children remains difficult. In recent years, all wheezing in early childhood has tended to be labelled as "asthma". This practice arose because of the failure to demonstrate significant differences between populations of children with "classic" asthma and those with "wheezy bronchitis"[193,194] and in an attempt to act upon the under-diagnosis and under-treatment of asthma.[2] There is increasing evidence challenging this approach (Table 27.1).[17] In particular in infants, there is evidence that lower levels of lung function predispose to wheezing lower respiratory illness.[195] Thus, factors associated with diminished lung function (such as maternal smoking during pregnancy[196,197] and low birth weight[198]) increase the risk of a child developing a wheezing lower respiratory tract infection. Wheezing in this situation is very commonly triggered by viral respiratory infections:[199] allergic triggers are relatively unimportant. Nearly 20% of wheezy children will only have one attack[200] and almost

TABLE 27.20: *Potential side-effects of inhaled corticosteroids to look for when examining children at follow-up. In addition to specific points below, it is important always to keep the dose as low as possible (preferably < 800 µg of budesonide (BUD) or beclomethasone (BDP) daily. (From Ref. 189 with permission)*

Potential problem	Conclusion	Clinical advice
Growth	No evidence from longitudinal studies of impact on long-term growth	Monitor linear growth carefully and regularly at higher inhaled corticosteroid doses
Hypothalamic–pituitary effects	Effects of inhaled steroids can be found but do not appear to be clinically relevant	
Bones	Below 800 µg of BUD or BDP and 200 µg fluticasone, there does not appear to be an effect on bones	
Psychiatric effects	Acute behavioural disturbances (hyperactivity or temper tantrums) reported	Ask about any change in behaviour. May need to reduce dose or discontinue
Eyes	No association with subcapsular cataracts on long-term use	
Metabolic effects	No evidence of clinically relevant effects	
Connective tissues	Easy bruising does not appear to be a problem in children	Check skin for any signs of unusual bruising

TABLE 27.20: *Continued*

Potential problem	Conclusion	Clinical advice
Oral candidiasis	Uncommon in children, but does occur	Check mouth for oral candidiasis. Using large-volume spacers and changing dosage to four times daily may help
Sore throat and hoarseness	Rare in children	Ask about (and listen for) any change in voice or occurrence of sore throats. May be less of a problem with dry powder inhalers

all wheezy infants will have outgrown their symptoms between the ages of 6 and 11 years.[201] Attacks can be frequent, however, with 20% or more of wheezy children having five episodes or more of wheeze in the preceding year.[3]

The likelihood of a doctor diagnosing asthma increases with an increase in the number of episodes per year and with the severity of shortness of breath suffered during attacks. Asthma is also more likely to be diagnosed where the episodes are triggered by factors other than colds.[200] Finally a diagnosis of asthma is to some extent dependent on a child's age, being more likely to be made in older children. Failure to diagnose asthma remains common. Many infants still arrive at paediatric clinics with a history of recurrent "colds", with coughing and wheezing, which have proved unresponsive to antibiotics. Bronchodilators may never have been tried.

Quite apart from the difficulty in diagnosis, management of wheezing is also troublesome (Table 27.21). The response to treatments, particularly bronchodilators, is often variable especially in the first year of life though there is strong evidence that functional β_2 adrenoreceptors are present in the infant airway.[202–205] The unpredictable and often limited effects of β_2 agonists are thought to relate more to airflow limitation due to inflammatory oedema and excess mucous production.[206] In general, anti-asthmatic medications are likely to be more effective than other treatments. Antibiotics, in particular, are not effective.

TABLE 27.21: *Problems in the management of infants and very young children with wheezing. (From Ref. 22 with permission)*

Recurrent wheeze and cough are associated with viral respiratory infections, often without a family history of asthma or atopy

Diagnosis rests almost entirely on symptoms that may be variable, rather than on objective lung function tests

Paucity of suitable designed and tested inhaler devices specific for this age group

Few controlled trials of treatment have been carried out

Bronchodilator response is variable in the first year of life but bronchodilators should still be tried

The younger the child the more other disorders may mimic asthma

Inhalation therapy in very young children is also difficult. Spacer devices with face masks[165] are increasingly used but nebulizers may still be necessary in very young children. For children unable to tolerate a face mask, an MDI with a polystyrene coffee cup is effective and may be particularly useful in emergencies.[159]

Treatment of chronic or recurrent symptoms in young children has tended to follow a step treatment plan similar to that adopted for older children. Oral β_2 agonists may suffice for the treatment of very mild and infrequent symptoms. Nebulized β_2 agonists may be required for more acute wheezing. There is some suggestion that ipratropium bromide may be a more effective bronchodilator in children under 1 year.[117] For recurrent or chronic symptoms, prophylactic medication is appropriate. SCG, either nebulized or via a large-volume spacer, will usually be the first step.[207] Slow-release theophylline preparations may be useful where inhaled therapy proves impractical; however, compliance is poor and side-effects are common.[208] When the response to these treatments is inadequate, inhaled steroids, either nebulized or via a large-volume spacer, are the next step. Nebulized BDP proved very disappointing in practice[209] and is no longer available in the UK; nebulized BUD has been more successful.[210] Inhaled steroids via a large-volume spacer are effective and increasingly used. The most appropriate dose levels are not clearly established but available data suggest that doses in the range of 200–400 µg per day are effective[210–212] and not associated with side-effects.[213] Regular oral steroids may occasionally be indicated.

ADOLESCENTS AND ASTHMA

Asthma usually improves during puberty.[214] For many, symptoms will disappear completely. However, those with more severe asthma may continue to suffer symptoms throughout adolescence. For these children, the teenage years may be particularly difficult. The normal features of adolescence such as growth of autonomy, indifference to risk and peer group identification may all conspire to make management of asthma particularly difficult. Rebellion against the restrictions of the disease, a denial of symptoms and non-compliance with medication are all common. Identification with peers frequently leads to a high incidence of teenage smoking. Conflict with authority may result in a perception that the physician is siding with the parents thus placing the doctor–patient relationship under strain.

The delivery of medical care may also cause problems. Teenage asthmatic patients require services that recognize their autonomy and address their specific needs. This may be best achieved by having separate clinics for teenagers where they can be seen alone. It is important for physicians to gain and keep their young patients' trust. To do so, physicians should be consistent, reasonable and realistic in their therapeutic goals.

EXERCISE-INDUCED ASTHMA (see also Chapter 34)

Exercise-induced asthma (EIA) is most commonly seen in children, as their high levels of physical activity cause high levels of ventilation that, in children with heightened airway reactivity, triggers acute airway narrowing.[215] EIA is not a separate disorder but merely one of the commoner stimuli leading to airflow limitation in children.[216]

Children with EIA can usually undertake and finish vigorous activity, because the brief, intense bursts of exercise typical of childhood produce fewer problems than sustained exercise. Usually, airways obstruction begins shortly after exercise, peaks in 5–10 min and then remits spontaneously and completely within 30–60 min. The more strenuous the effort, the greater the ventilation and the more intense the resultant asthma attack. Running causes more severe airways limitation than jogging, and jogging more than walking (Fig. 27.3). Airways obstruction is also greater when the inspired air is dry and cold, and less when the air is warm and moist. Thus exercise on cold, foggy, winter days will cause symptoms when similar activity on warm, humid, summer days will not. The asthma attacks precipitated by exercise appear no different from those caused by other triggers. However, exercise does not cause prolonged or intense airway obstruction. The problem is not so much the severity of attacks as the limitation of activity that results.

Usually, EIA is easy to recognize. A careful history should elicit the fact that symptoms typically occur not during exercise but when the workload decreases at the end of exercise. Sometimes cough may be the only presenting feature. The diagnosis can be confirmed by a fall in PEFR or FEV_1 of $\geq 15\%$ after exercise. In children, treadmill or free running tests are

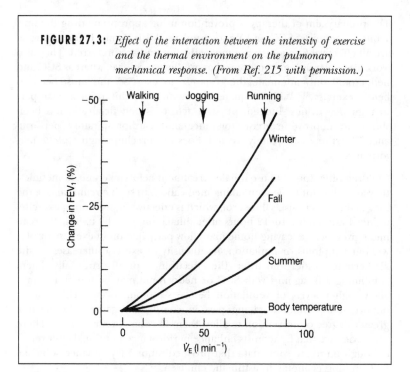

FIGURE 27.3: *Effect of the interaction between the intensity of exercise and the thermal environment on the pulmonary mechanical response. (From Ref. 215 with permission.)*

most widely used[217] but the type of exercise is immaterial as long as the workload is sufficiently high to cause an adequate level of ventilation. In pre-school children, the history may be less obvious. The child may be reluctant to take exercise or want to be carried. Formal exercise testing may not be possible, and a therapeutic trial may be necessary to confirm the diagnosis.

Exercise does not induce increased airway reactivity[218] or long-term deterioration in lung function. Accordingly, continuous therapy is not needed to treat it. However, the sensitivity to exercise and the intensity of symptoms induced by exercise are related to the underlying airway reactivity.[219] Prophylactic therapy may be beneficial by decreasing bronchial hyperreactivity and allowing a greater degree of exercise to occur before airway obstruction develops. Exercise is unique in that it is the only natural trigger that induces tachyphylaxis so that with bouts of exercise performed repeatedly within a period of 40 min or less, the bronchial narrowing progressively decreases ("refractory period").[220] This is of practical importance for children, especially those taking part in competitive games, because they can limit the inevitable airways obstruction by a short warm-up period before planned physical activity.

The primary aim of therapy is prevention using appropriate drug therapy. While β_2 agonists, SCG and nedocromil used 10–15 min before exercise are all effective, β_2 agonists are most effective and are preferred. They also work after exercise on symptoms that are slow to resolve, whereas SCG and nedocromil only attenuate the response to exercise and must be used before exercise.[215] With adequate treatment, most children can take part in regular activities. Indeed, physical activity is beneficial and has been shown to improve exercise tolerance and cardiorespiratory perform-ance.[221] Asthma, adequately treated, does not preclude high athletic per-formance.

Children often forget to use inhaled treatment before exercise. Sometimes, they are reluctant to be seen taking medication. In such circumstances, the long acting β_2 agonist, salmeterol, which is effective in preventing exercise-induced asthma for 10–12 hours after inhalation, may be useful.[147] Treat-ment given before leaving home may allow participation in exercise or play without symptoms or limitation. As intensity of exercise increases or the air becomes colder and drier, the effectiveness of all drugs falls. Then, combining a β_2 agonist with SCG or nedocromil may be useful and may allow higher levels of ventilation before symptoms occur. This can be important for children taking part in competitive games who need a greater degree of prevention to allow them to compete successfully. There is no evidence that β_2 agonists enhance performance in normal children[222] although there are some data that pre-medication may enhance submaxi-mal running economy in asthmatic children.[223]

COUGH-VARIANT ASTHMA

Recurrent wheeze and/or cough are typical of asthma, and often occur together. For example, parents frequently describe coughing and wheezing after exercise in asthmatic children. Coughing may also lead to wheez-ing.[224] However, there is evidence from epidemiological studies,[25] blocking studies[225] and from measurement of the time of occurrence of coughing[226] that, while the mechanisms of cough and wheezing are related, they may be triggered independently.

About 5–6% of children with asthma present with cough as the sole symp-tom.[227] Most of these children also have evidence of abnormal pulmonary function tests in keeping with asthma. For those without abnormal func-tion, the diagnosis is based on a positive response to a therapeutic trial of bronchodilators.

While cough is a common symptom, it has been difficult to assess objec-tively. Diary cards have proved unreliable.[31] More objective cough counting systems used in research studies are likely to lead to better understanding of cough and its treatment.[228]

Cough caused by asthma will usually respond quickly to relatively straight-forward asthma medications; if it does not, then the diagnosis of asthma should be reconsidered and further investigations undertaken. Cough as the only symptom in infants should be comprehensively investigated.

NOCTURNAL DISTURBANCE AND WAKING WITH ASTHMA (See also Chapter 35)

Nocturnal disturbance is common in asthmatic children. About three-quarters of asthmatic children are affected, one-third on a regular basis and a small proportion nearly every night. Such disturbance has a substantial impact on well-being and functioning. Many children feel sleepy in school the next day, or stay at home because they are too tired.[3] Nocturnal disturbance is also frequently disruptive for parents and sibs. During acute exacerbations children frequently deteriorate in the early hours of the morning, leading to contact with family practitioners or attendance at emergency departments.

It is important, therefore, to ask specifically about nocturnal symptoms, medication use during the night and the impact of nocturnal disturbance on both child and family. PEFR monitoring may show excessive diurnal variation. However, diary cards may not accurately reflect nocturnal symptoms.[31]

Continuing nocturnal symptoms generally indicate more severe asthma[229] and poor asthmatic control.[230] In mild cases, a nocturnal bronchodilator may be sufficient. However, usually it will be necessary to increase prophylactic treatment, often by means of inhaled corticosteroids.[231] If high-dose inhaled steroids do not control the symptoms, then a long-acting bronchodilator should be introduced. Long-acting inhaled β_2 agonists such as salmeterol are probably the best choice, and have been shown to improve the nocturnal symptoms of children with mild-to-moderate asthma.[232] Oral long-acting bronchodilators are an alternative, but may have a high incidence of side-effects[233] and do not improve objective sleep quality in adults; indeed theophyllines may even worsen it.[234]

With appropriate treatment it is usually possible to improve a child's nocturnal asthma. Unfortunately, nocturnal cough – often the most troublesome symptom[235] – can be difficult to settle. Generally, it is not necessary to look for other diagnoses. However, where nocturnal symptoms respond poorly to asthma treatment other possible diagnoses such as pertussis should be considered. Improving nasal symptoms due to allergic rhinitis may help.

IS IT DUE TO SOMETHING IN THE DIET? (see also Chapter 40)

Ingested substances can occasionally affect airway function (Table 27.22)[236] and may be identified by parents and children as exacerbating asthma.

Typically, two situations arise. In the first, the parents or child spontaneously give a clear history that a particular ingestant has precipitated asthmatic symptoms, often accompanied with other acute allergic features such as urticaria. The child may have other atopic features such as eczema.

TABLE 27.22: *Dietary ingestants causing diet-related asthma. (Adapted from Ref. 236)*

Type	Examples
Ingested protein allergens	Eggs, milk, fish, wheat, nuts
Food additives	
Metabisulphite and sulphur dioxide	
Artificial colourings and other preservatives	Tartrazine, sodium benzoate
Aspirin and acetylsalicylic acid	
Physical agents	Cold drinks
	Fizzy drinks with low pH (e.g. cola)

Ethnic differences occur, Asian children being more sensitive to cola drinks, ice and fried foods.[53] The parents may already have carried out simple food challenges, and may already have instituted dietary avoidance, especially if the substance is not a common dietary constituent. In these situations, further objective confirmation is usually unnecessary, and the parents should continue to avoid the substance.

A second more difficult situation arises where parents worry that food is a factor in their child's symptoms, but cannot identify any particular culprit. In this situation, a link between asthmatic symptoms and oral ingestants is often not confirmed objectively.[237]

Immunological markers such as skin tests or RASTs are not particularly useful in diagnosing asthma associated with food allergy. Many asthmatic children are atopic and can have positive responses to foods without any evidence that the food causes asthmatic symptoms. Objective confirmation then depends on a formal food challenge, which should be blind and placebo controlled. Unfortunately, food challenges give rise to a number of problems. Firstly, variations of lung function over time may confound the effect of the ingestant, making it difficult to demonstrate reactions occurring anything more than a few hours after ingestion. Secondly, asthma prophylaxis may attenuate or abolish a response to an ingestant. More difficult problems arise if repeated doses are required or where the response to the substance is enhanced by an additional stimulus such as exercise. In some cases, a change in bronchial responsiveness has been clearly documented without a change in baseline lung function.[53]

Where a particular dietary substance is clearly identified as causing asthmatic symptoms, eliminating the item from the child's diet may be possible. Accidental ingestion, if it occurs, can be treated symptomatically. As children grow out of food allergies, periodic re-testing may be useful, particularly where the substance is a basic or frequently encountered dietary constituent, such as milk or eggs, the exclusion of which makes the diet unduly complicated.

Where children present with mild asthma but no clear history of ingestant-related symptoms, a search for hidden dietary factors is usually not worth while. Even if the symptoms are rather more troublesome, prophylactic asthma treatment may prevent or substantially alleviate the problem without the necessity of resorting to formal food challenges.

Children with more severe asthma that is difficult to control may be considered for an elimination diet to screen for unrecognized food allergies, but only after all other factors have been excluded. Such diets are often very restrictive and unpalatable, and may be nutritionally deficient. They should always be carefully supervised by a dietician. It should be remembered that drugs often have preservatives or colourings which may have to be excluded. If clinical improvement occurs, the diet can be gradually liberalized, preferably one item at a time. If deterioration occurs, the provoking substance can be avoided. If improvement does not occur within a defined period, the diet should be discontinued.

IS IT PSYCHOLOGICAL?

The clear consensus is that childhood asthma is a physical disease. There are nevertheless related psychosocial factors (Table 27.23). Emotions such as anger or excitement can trigger asthmatic symptoms.[238] The asthma itself may have psychological side-effects such as stigma, loss of self-esteem, and strained family relationships. In children who have died from asthma, psychosocial factors, particularly depression, have been more frequent.[239,240] Further, asthma may affect family dynamics: manipulative children may use the illness to get their own way;[241] parents may be overprotective or unwilling to discipline an asthmatic child. Finally, psychological factors such as fear of observing the symptoms or the threat of serious complications may lead to denial of the condition, and may compromise the success of treatment.[242]

Many of these psychosocial factors give rise to poor communication and poor compliance, and are associated with feelings of hopelessness about the illness. Such factors must, therefore, be addressed in order to achieve successful treatment. Clinicians should be particularly wary when high-risk psychological features are present in children with severe asthma (Table 27.24).

Occasionally, a functional laryngeal obstruction causes or aggravates asthmatic symptoms[246] resulting in wheezing that is resistant to treatment. The

TABLE 27.23: *High-risk psychological variables. (From Ref. 239 with permission)*

Wheezing with stress
    Parents and/or physician considered stress a frequent factor
    for acute episodes

Problems of self-care
    Parents and/or physician state that there are regular
    problems
    Child's inability to respond appropriately to asthma
    symptoms
    Child's inability to attend to routine prophylactic care

Disregard of perceived symptoms
    No action taken to recognized asthma symptoms

Conflict between parent and physician, child and physician or
parent and child
    Positive when perceived by either parent or physician
    Ongoing
        Disagreement
        Frustration
        Dissatisfaction with performance of either of identified
        persons involved

Family dysfunction
    Marital discord
    Lack of parental support to child
    Parental drug or alcohol abuse
    Financial stress
    Inappropriate use of resources

Reaction to separation or loss
    Child frequently has excessive and developmentally
    inappropriate responses to separation from parent or carer
    A significant loss from which the child has not recovered,
    e.g. death of a parent

Emotional disturbance
    Severe enough to require referral for psychiatric treatment

Manipulative use of asthma
    Use of asthma symptoms to:
        Avoid unpleasant tasks
        Place pressure on others to respond to child's wishes

Depression
    Specific psychiatric disturbance (diagnosed from symptoms,
    affect and functioning)
    Hopelessness/despair (expressed emotional state and
    direct/indirect references to suicide)

TABLE 27.24: *Factors that point to a high risk for asthma mortality. (From Refs 60, 239, 243–245 with permission)*

Previous history of acute life-threatening attacks
Hospitalization within the previous year
Psychosocial problems
Recent reduction or cessation of corticosteroids
Non-compliance with recommended medical therapy (especially in teenagers)
Socio-economic factors: low income, inner city, poor access to medical care, cultural differences

diagnosis can be difficult, but there may be clinical clues. The child, often an adolescent, may be mostly free of wheeze when asleep at night or during anaesthesia. There may be variable dyspnoea when awake, often increased by stress or anxiety (caused sometimes by the mere approach of the physician). On auscultation, the wheezing may be poorly heard in the lower lung fields, and appears to be localized in the extra-thoracic trachea. Management is likely to involve consultation with a mental health professional.

Effective management of asthma should always recognize the psychosocial adjustment of the child and family, particularly where the child has severe asthma and high-risk psychological features. Such children should have regular follow-up with specific concentration on risk factors. For example, intensive education may help to address poor self-care, and attention to the details of medication may aid compliance. Intervention by a child psychiatrist or social worker may be necessary and can result in improvement in asthma control.[240,247] Behavioural approaches (extending to the child's family) can modify the reaction to emotional triggers, deal with manipulative behaviour and improve compliance. Residential schooling may occasionally be helpful for children with severe asthma who fail to respond to outpatient management and psychosocial care.[248]

WHAT ABOUT HEATING AND HOUSING?

During the last thirty years, substantial changes in indoor environment, including heating and insulation and the more widespread use of fitted carpets, have combined to produce an environment that is ideal for the house-dust mite.

Another significant health hazard that has been recognized in the last 10 years is damp housing. There is now considerable evidence that damp and mouldy housing has a detrimental effect on the respiratory health of children.[85,249,250] There is also evidence that damp and mouldy housing is associated with symptomatic asthma, though whether caused by house-dust mites or some effect of moulds is not yet known. Reducing indoor humidity has been shown to lead to significant improvement in PEFR.[80] However, decreased humidity usually requires increased ventilation, which leads to heat loss and increased fuel bills.

The best type of heating for an asthmatic child is not known. Recent evidence relating to adults suggests that those with moderate to severe asthma should reduce their exposure to indoor sources of combustion such as gas stoves, fireplaces or wood stoves.[250] Evidence relating to children suggests that symptoms of respiratory tract irritation are commoner in homes heated by wood stoves.[251]

Overall, present evidence suggests that asthmatic children are best housed in dry, warm accommodation with some form of closed heating.

WHAT HAPPENS AT SCHOOL?

Asthma is now so common, affecting 1 in 10 children or more, that an average school class is likely to have two or three children with asthma. An asthmatic child may be absent from school as a result of the disease on average 7–10 days per year.[1] In more severe cases, 30 days absence per year is not uncommmon.[252] Help may be needed to allow a child to keep up with school work.

Teachers are responsible for asthmatic children during school hours, and often have to take decisions about physical activities and treatment, both emergency and regular. All too often teachers have a limited understanding of the condition; few receive training and, not surprisingly, many often feel inadequate to cope with an asthmatic child.[253] Teachers should be informed of the stimuli that can precipitate attacks; the standard anti-asthma medicines; and the steps to take if a child has an acute attack.

The school environment may present a problem. Guinea-pigs, hamsters, birds and rabbits may have to be removed from the classroom if there are asthmatic children in the class. Fumes from experiments or glues can also trigger symptoms.

Medications to be taken at school often cause problems. Many children do not like carrying their medication with them, and find it embarrassing to use inhalers at school or in front of their friends.[3] The use of twice-daily prophylactic treatment and long-acting bronchodilators before school[147] may help. Coping with inhaled medication is also a problem for many schools because of anxieties about other children taking the medication inappropriately. Fortunately, the inhaled drugs available today are not toxic in normal children, even in very large doses.

Children with asthma usually know when they need their inhalers and should have easy access to them. Older children (above 7 years) should keep their inhalers with them and be responsible for taking them. Younger children should be supervised by a responsible adult. If there are difficulties, assistance from the school nurse or local community health services should be sought.

Exercise-induced symptoms can interfere with school games and sport. Prolonged outdoor running on a cold, dry winter day is an activity particularly likely to provoke wheezing but even swimming, which is generally well-tolerated, may provoke symptoms.[3] Accordingly, while the use of appropriate warm-up exercises and β_2 agonists before activities may help avoid symptoms, children should carry their medication with them and stop to take it if they become symptomatic.

Minor attacks need not interrupt a child's school day. Rapid use of reliever should help to control the problem and allow the child to continue. If the attack is severe with marked distress or inability to talk, or if the reliever does not work within 5–10 min, or if the child is getting exhausted urgent medical advice must be called. Ten to twenty puffs of bronchodilator via a large-volume spacer may be given while awaiting medical help.

CAN I TAKE MY CHILD ON HOLIDAY?

Parents often worry that asthma exacerbations may occur away from home, and are not sure whether it is safe to go on holiday. Such anxieties restrict their choice of holiday.[3]

Planning ahead is important, particularly where the holiday involves a foreign country. Asthma societies frequently provide useful information pamphlets about going on holiday. Travelling, particularly by air, is not usually a problem, but for long journeys avoiding cigarette smoke can be important.

Unfortunately, there is no guaranteed safe or best place for asthmatic patients to go on holiday. It is sensible to avoid trigger factors but not always possible to predict all possible hazards in advance. Damp or mouldy housing, exposure to unusual aeroallergens such as pollens or animal danders in country areas, house-dust mite in hotel rooms or certain weather conditions can all exacerbate asthma. Air pollution is a problem in some countries. Cigarette smoke can sometimes be difficult to avoid.

A clinic appointment just before a holiday provides an opportunity to review the child's treatment plan. A letter from the physician outlining the diagnosis and treatment may be useful, both for negotiating customs and advising local physicians in the event of an attack. Regular preventive treatment should help to avoid most problems. Stepping-down treatment just before departure should be avoided.

Parents should take sufficient quantities of both routine and emergency medications to cover the period of the holiday. A medical pack for emergencies, including a written emergency action plan, adequate "relieving" treatment and a course of steroids, should be carried. Children aged over

5 years should take their peak flow meter. A full β_2-agonist MDI and a plastic coffee cup can provide effective and portable bronchodilation in an emergency. Parents should be told to use 10–25 puffs of reliever at 10-s intervals. Where the child is dependent on a nebulizer, it is important to check the electrical voltage in the foreign country and to make sure that the nebulizer will work there. Any necessary electrical adapters should be purchased in advance. Some nebulizers can handle multiple voltages; alternatively, a hand or foot pump nebulizer or battery-operated compressor may be used.

Since medical care abroad can be expensive, adequate insurance cover or the appropriate certificate to allow reciprocal health care is essential. If asthma is severe and an exacerbation likely, it is sensible to find out in advance how and where to obtain medical attention. Happily, problems with asthma on holidays are rare.

WILL IT GET BETTER? (see also Chapter 2)

Parents frequently want to know what will happen in the longer term. There are as yet few population-based and longitudinal cohort studies of the natural course of asthma from childhood to adult life. Most of the published studies start at around 7 years of age[54,214,254,255] or later.[256] Most studies have also been based on moderate or severe asthmatic patients and, therefore, provide limited information on the full range of the disease.[257]

Despite these limitations, the evidence is reassuring. Over 20–25 years about two-thirds of children with asthma will outgrow their disease and be symptom-free as adults, especially those with mild disease. About one-third with more severe disease will have persistent symptoms in adult life. Asthma usually improves during the teenage years, although less so for girls than boys.[214] The amount of wheezing in early adolescence seems to be a guide for severity in later life; about 70% of those with few symptoms at age 14 continue to have little or no asthma at age 28 and, conversely, about 70% of those with frequent symptoms at age 14 are still having recurrent symptoms at age 28.[255] Other risk factors have been identified (Table 27.25) and may provide targets for preventive and/or more aggressive treatment strategies in the future. Interestingly, about 1 in 9 children not reported as having asthma at 7 years will have developed asthma by age 30, with female sex, family history of asthma and lower lung function at age 7 being important risk factors.[254]

Other outcomes also seem generally favourable. Although growth may be delayed, particularly during puberty, final height appears to be normal.[132,133,214] The social outcome, too, in terms of education, employment, housing and social class is not greatly affected, at least for mild or moderate asthma.[258,259] One recurrent finding is that smoking is no less common in asthmatic subjects than in the general population, even though asthmatic smokers are more likely to be symptomatic.[256]

TABLE 27.25: *Risk factors for persistence of childhood asthma*

Sex	Conflicting evidence
Age of onset	Yes; early onset
Severity of asthma	Yes; more severe
Eczema	Yes
Family history of atopy	Yes
Smoking (active/passive)	Yes
Level of lung function	Yes; impaired lung function at age 7 predicts asthmatic symptoms
Treatment	Not known

Does treatment influence outcome? In particular, can a prolonged remission from asthma be achieved by long-term use of inhaled cortico-steroids? Evidence from children is limited. Van Essen-Zandvliet *et al.*[123] showed that 28–36 months of treatment with inhaled corticosteroids and regular bronchodilator improved both symptoms and objective measures of lung function in almost all children. Mean PD_{20} histamine stabilized after 20 months but usually did not normalize, and even after 36 months on inhaled corticosteroids airway responsiveness remained abnormal in the majority. Cessation of inhaled corticosteroids was followed by a rapid decrease in lung function and a deterioration in lung function,[127] suggesting that the underlying inflammatory process was still present even after years on inhaled corticosteroids, and thus that the asthma had not been "cured". Treatment should, therefore, be aimed principally at symptomatic remission, i.e. normalization in symptoms, without the need for additional bronchodilator.

The long-term relationship between asthma in children and chronic obstructive lung disease remains unclear.[260]

CONCLUSION

In the main, childhood asthma is a simple and rewarding disease to treat. Effective treatments with a low incidence of side-effects are now available. Most children can be cared for in the community, and their symptoms substantially improved by appropriate treatment. Referral to a hospital pae-diatrician will only be required in certain circumstances. Despite this, under-diagnosis and poor symptom control remain all too common. Com-prehensive guidelines summarizing the best in present practice are avail-able but successful treatment requires careful implementation of what is already known. Problem areas remain. A better understanding of wheezing illnesses in infants and young children is needed, particularly the relationship between asthma and viral respiratory infections. The factors that cause or contribute to asthma must also be better understood if effective preventive measures are to be developed.

REFERENCES

1. Hill RA, Standen PJ, Tattersfield AE. Asthma, wheezing and school absence in primary schools. *Arch Dis Child* 1989; 64: 246–51.

2. Speight ANP, Lee DA, Hey EW. Underdiagnosis and undertreatment of asthma in childhood. *BMJ* 1983; 286: 1253–6.

3. Lenney W, Wells NEJ, O'Neil BA. Burden of paediatric asthma. *Eur Respir Rev* 1994; 4: 49–62.

4. Hyndman SJ, Williams DRR, Merrill SL, Lipscombe JM, Palmer CR. Rates of admission to hospital for asthma. *BMJ* 1994; 308: 1596–600.

5. Nocon A, Booth T. The social impact of asthma. *Fam Pract* 1991; 8: 37–41.

6. Phelan PD. Asthma in childhood: epidemiology. *BMJ* 1994; 308: 1584–5.

7. Cullinan P, Newman Taylor AJ. Asthma in children: environmental factors. *BMJ* 1994; 308 1585–6.

8. Anderson HR, Butland BK, Strachan DP. Trends in prevalence and severity of childhood asthma. *BMJ* 1994; 308: 1600–4.

9. Anderson HR, Bailey PA, Cooper JS, Palmer JC. Influence of morbidity, illness label, and social, family, and health service factors on drug treatment of childhood asthma. *Lancet* 1981; ii: 1030–2.

10. Laitinen LA, Heino M, Laitinen A, Kava T, Haahtela T. Damage of the airway epithelium and bronchial reactivity in patients with asthma. *Am Rev Respir Dis* 1985; 139: 599–606.

11. Djukanovic R, Roche WR, Eilson JW *et al.* State of the art. Mucosal inflammation in asthma. *Am Rev Respir Dis* 1990; 142: 434–57.

12. Barnes PJ. New concepts in asthma and the implications for therapy. In: Mitchell DM (ed) *Recent Advances in Respiratory Medicine No. 5.* London: Longman Group UK, 1991; 45–60.

13. Snapper JR. Inflammation and airway function: the asthma syndrome. *Am Rev Respir Dis* 1990; 141: 531–3.

14. Lee DA, Winslow NR, Speight ANP, Hey EW. Prevalence and spectrum of asthma in childhood. *BMJ* 1983; 286: 1256–8.

15 Clough JB, Williams JD, Holgate ST. Effect of atopy on the natural history of symptoms, peak expiratory flow, and bronchial responsiveness in 7- and 8-year-old children with cough and wheeze. A 12-month longitudinal study. Am Rev Respir Dis 1991; 143: 755–60. [Published erratum appears in Am Rev Respir Dis 1992; 146: 540.]

16 Cutz E, Levison H, Cooper DM. Ultrastructure of airways in children with asthma. Histopathology 1978; 2: 407–21.

17 Silverman M. Out of the mouths of babes and sucklings: lessons from early childhood asthma. Thorax 1993; 48: 1200–4.

18 Clough JB, Holgate ST. Episodes of respiratory morbidity in children with cough and wheeze. Am J Respir Crit Care Med 1994; 150: 48–53.

19 Clifford RD, Radford M, Howell JB, Holgate ST. Prevalence of respiratory symptoms among 7 and 11 year old schoolchildren and association with asthma. Arch Dis Child 1989; 64: 1118–25.

20 Warner JO, Gotz M, Landau LI et al. Management of asthma: a consensus statement. Arch Dis Child 1989; 64: 1065–79.

21 National Heart Lung and Blood Institute. International consensus report on diagnosis and treatment of asthma. Bethesda, Md. Department of Health and Human Services, 1991: 1–72.

22 Anonymous. Guidelines on the management of asthma. Thorax 1993; 48: S1–S24.

23 International Paediatric Consensus Group. Asthma: a follow-up statement from an international paediatric consensus group. Arch Dis Child 1992; 67: 240–8.

24 Milner AD. Childhood Asthma: Diagnosis, Treatment and Management, 2nd edn. London: Martin Dunitz, 1993: 1–155.

25 Luyt DK, Burton PR, Simpson H. Epidemiological study of wheeze, doctor diagnosed asthma, and cough in preschool children in Leicestershire. BMJ 1993; 306: 1386–9.

26 Johnson D, Osborne LM. Cough variant asthma: a review of the clinical literature. J Asthma 1991; 28: 85–90.

27 Hetzel MR, Clark TJH. Comparison of normal and asthmatic circadian rhythms in peak expiratory flow rate. Thorax 1980; 35: 732–8.

28 Henderson AJW, Carswell F. Circadian rhythm of peak expiratory flow rate in asthmatic children. Thorax 1989; 44: 410–4.

29 Ninan TK, Russell G. Asthma, inhaled corticosteroid treatment, and growth. Arch Dis Child 1992; 67: 703–5.

30 Ferguson AC, Murray AB, Wah-Jun T. Short stature and delayed skeletal maturation in children with allergic disease. J Allergy Clin Immunol 1982; 69: 461–6.

31 Archer LNJ, Simpson H. Night coughs and diary card scores in asthma. Arch Dis Child 1985; 60: 473–4.

32 Lister J, Budin-Jones S, Palmer J, Cochrane GM. How accurate are asthma diary cards? Arch Dis Child 1994; 44: 343.

33 Hyland ME, Kenyon CAP, Allen R, Howarth P. Diary keeping in asthma: comparison of written and electronic methods. BMJ 1993; 306: 487-9.

34 Chowienczyk PJ, Lawson CP, Morris J, Kermani A, Cochrane GM. Electronic diary to record physiological measurements. Lancet 1992; 339: 251.

35 Nairn JR, Bennett AJ, Andrew JD, MacArthur P. A study of respiratory function in normal school children; the peak flow rate. Arch Dis Child 1961; 36: 253-6.

36 Burge PS. Peak flow measurement. Thorax 1992; 47: 903.

37 Milner AD, Ingram D. PEFRs in children under 5 years of age. Arch Dis Child 1970; 45: 820-3.

38 Connolly CK. Falsely high peak expiratory flow readings due to acceleration in the mouth. BMJ 1987; 294: 285.

39 Godfrey S, Kamburoff PL, Nairn JR. Spirometry, lung volumes and airway resistance. Br J Dis Chest 1970; 64: 15-24.

40 Sly PD, Hibbert ME, Landau LI. Diurnal variation of peak expiratory flow rate in asthmatic children. Pediatr Pulmonol 1986; 2: 141-6.

41 Landau LI. The value of lung function in guiding drug therapy in childhood asthma. Eur Respir Rev 1994; 4: 10-4.

42 Pool JB, Greenough A, Price JF. Abnormalities of functional residual capacity in symptomatic and asymptomatic young asthmatics. Acta Paediatr Scand 1988; 77: 419-23.

43 Pattemore PK, Innes Asher M, Harrison AC, Mitchell EA, Rea HH, Stewart AW. The interrelationship among bronchial hyperresponsiveness, the diagnosis of asthma, and asthma symptoms. Am Rev Respir Dis 1990; 142: 549-54.

44 Empey DW, Laitinen LA, Jacobs L, Gold WM, Nadel JA. Mechanisms of bronchial hyperreactivity in normal subjects after upper respiratory tract infection. Am Rev Respir Dis 1976; 113: 131-9.

45 Clough JB, Williams JD, Holgate ST. The profile and spectrum of bronchial responsiveness and its relationship to atopy and wheezing in 7 and 8 year old children with respiratory symptoms. Arch Dis Child 1992; 67: 574-9.

46 Josephs LK, Gregg I, Mullee MA, Holgate ST. Nonspecific bronchial reactivity and its relationship to the clinical expression of asthma. A longitudinal study. Am Rev Respir Dis 1989; 140: 350-7.

47 Altamirano HG, McGready SJ, Mansmann HC. Right middle lobe syndromes in asthmatic children. Pediatr Asthma Allergy Immunol 1991; 5: 33-7.

48 Eigen H, Laughlin JJ, Homrighausen J. Recurrent pneumonia in children and its relationship to bronchial hyperreactivity. Pediatrics 1982; 70: 698-704.

49 Ownby DR. Allergy testing: in vivo versus in vitro. Pediatr Clin North Am 1988; 35: 995-1009.

50 Burrows B, Mortimer FD, Halonen M, Barbee RA, Cline MG. Association of asthma with serum IgE levels and skin-test reactivity to allergens. *N Engl J Med* 1989; 320: 271-7.

51 Sporik R, Holgate ST, Platts-Mills TAE, Cogswell JJ. Exposure to house-dust mite allergen (*Der p* 1) and the development of asthma in childhood: A prospective study. *N Engl J Med* 1990; 323: 502-7.

52 Adkinson NF. The radioallergosorbent test in 1981 – limitations and refinements. *J Allergy Clin Immunol* 1981; 67: 87-9.

53 Wilson NM, Silverman M. Diagnosis of food sensitivity in childhood asthma. *J R Soc Med* 1985; 78: 11-6.

54 Oswald H, Phelan PD, Lannigan A, Hibbert ME, Bowes G, Olinsky A. Outcome of childhood asthma in mid-adult life. *BMJ* 1994; 309: 95-6.

55 Conway SP, Littlewood JM. Admission to hospital with asthma. *Arch Dis Child* 1985; 60: 636-9.

56 Korsch BM, Negrete VF. Doctor patient communication. *Sci Am* 1972; 227: 66-72.

57 Beasley CRW, Cushley M, Holgate ST. A self management plan in the treatment of adult asthma. *Thorax* 1989; 44: 200-4.

58 Charlton I, Antoniou AG, Atkinson J *et al.* Asthma at the interface: bridging the gap between general practice and a district general hospital. *Arch Dis Child* 1994; 70: 313-8.

59 Klingelhofer EL, Gershwin ME. Asthma self management programs: Premises, not promises. *J Asthma* 1988; 25: 89-101.

60 Fletcher HJ, Ibrahim SA, Speight ANP. Survey of asthma deaths in the Northern region 1970–1985. *Arch Dis Child* 1990; 65: 163-7.

61 Partridge MR. Asthma education: More reading or more viewing? *J R Soc Med* 1994; 79: 326-8.

62 Mulloy EMT, Albazzaz MK, Warley ARH, Harvey JE. Video education for patients who use inhalers. *Thorax* 1987; 42: 719-20.

63 Sly PD, Landau LI, Weymouth R. Home recording of peak expiratory flow rates and perception of asthma. *Am J Dis Child* 1985; 139: 479-82.

64 Shim CS, Williams H. Relationship of wheezing to the severity of airway obstruction in asthma. *Arch Intern Med* 1992; 1983: 890-2.

65 Peroni DG, Boner AL, Vallone G, Antolini I, Warner JO. Effective allergen avoidance at high altitude reduces allergen-induced bronchial hyperresponsiveness. *Am J Respir Crit Care Med* 1994; 149: 1442-6.

66 Korsgaard J. Mite allergy and residence: a case controlled study on the impact of exposure to house-dust mites in dwellings. *Am Rev Respir Dis* 1983; 128: 231-5.

67 Warner JA, Marchant JL, Warner JO. Double blind trial of ionisers in children with asthma sensitive to the house-dust mite. *Thorax* 1993; 48: 330–3.

68 Anonymous. Report of international workshop. Dust mite allergens and asthma – a worldwide problem. *J Allergy Clin Immunol* 1989; 83: 416–27.

69 Platts-Mills TAE, Heymann PW, Longbottom JL, Wilkins SR. Airborne allergens associated with asthma: particle sizes carrying dust mite and rat allergens measured with a cascade impactor. *J Allergy Clin Immunol* 1986; 77: 850–7.

70 Murray AB, Ferguson AC, Morrison AJ. Diagnosis of house-dust mite allergy in asthmatic children: What constitutes a positive history? *J Allergy Clin Immunol* 1983; 71: 21–8.

71 Feather IH, Warner JA, Holgate ST, Thompson PJ, Stewart GA. Cohabiting with domestic mites. *Thorax* 1993; 48: 5–9.

72 Sarsfield JK, Gowland G, Toy R, Norman ALE. Mite-sensitive asthma of childhood: trial of avoidance measures. *Arch Dis Child* 1974; 49: 716–21.

73 Godfrey RC, Griffiths M. The prevalence of immediate positive skin test to *Dermatophagoides pteronyssinus* and grass pollen in school children. *Clin Allergy* 1976; 6: 79–82.

74 Charpin D, Birnbaum J, Haddi E. Altitude and allergy to house-dust mites. *Am Rev Respir Dis* 1991; 143: 983–6.

75 Platts-Mills TAE, Mitchell EB, Nock P, Tovey ER, Moszoro H, Wilkins SR. Reduction of bronchial hyperreactivity during prolonged allergen avoidance. *Lancet* 1982; ii: 675–8.

76 Murray AB, Ferguson AC. Dust free bedrooms in the treatment of children with house dust mite allergy: a controlled trial. *Pediatrics* 1983; 71: 418–22.

77 Ehnert B, Lau-Schadendorf S, Weber A, Buettner P, Wahn E. Reducing domestic exposure to dust mite allergen reduces bronchial hyperreactivity in sensitive children with asthma. *J Allergy Clin Immunol* 1992; 90: 135–8.

78 Carswell F, Robinson DW, Oliver J, Clark J, Robinson P, Wadsworth J. House dust mites in Bristol. *Clin Allergy* 1982; 12: 533–45.

79 Collof MJ. Use of liquid nitrogen in the control of house dust mite populations. *Clin Allergy* 1986; 16: 411–7.

80 Korsgaard J, Iversen M. Epidemiology of house dust mite allergy. *Allergy* 1991; 46 (suppl 11): 14–8.

81 Warner JA. Environmental changes and asthma control in paediatrics. *Paediatr Respir Med* 1993; 1: 9–13.

82 Wood RA, Chapman MD, Adkinson NF, Eggleston PA. The effect of cat removal on allergen content in household-dust samples. *J Allergy Clin Immunol* 1989; 83: 730–4.

83 de Blay F, Chapman MD, Platts-Mills TAE. Air-borne cat allergen (*Fel d* 1): Environmental control with the cat *in situ*. *Am Rev Respir Dis* 1991; 143: 1334–9.

84 Solomon LOR, Burge HA, Bloise JR. Exclusion of particulate allergens by window air conditioners. *J Allergy Clin Immunol* 1980; 65: 305–8.

85 Strachan DP. Damp housing, mould allergy and childhood asthma. *Proc R Coll Physicians Edinb* 1991; 21: 140–6.

86 Wjst M, Reitmeir P, Dold S *et al.* Road traffic and adverse effects on respiratory health. *BMJ* 1993; 307: 596–600.

87 Samet JM. Learning about air pollution and asthma. *Am J Respir Crit Care Med* 1994; 149: 1398–9.

88 Ferusson DM, Horwood LJ, Corkhill RT. Parental smoking and respiratory illness in infancy. *Arch Dis Child* 1980; 55: 358–61.

89 Wright AL, Holberg C, Martinez FD, Taussig LM. Group Health Medical Associates. Relationship of parental smoking to wheezing and non-wheezing lower respiratory tract illnesses in infancy. *J Pediatr* 1991; 118: 207–14.

90 Weitzman M, Gortmacher SL, Walker DK, Sobol A. Maternal smoking and childhood asthma. *Pediatrics* 1990; 85: 505–11.

91 Murray AB, Morrison BJ. The effect of cigarette smoke on bronchial hyper-responsiveness and severity of symptoms in children with asthma. *J Allergy Clin Immunol* 1986; 77: 575–81.

92 Murray AB, Morrison BJ. Passive smoking by asthmatics: its greater effect on boys than on girls and on older than younger children. *Pediatrics* 1989; 84: 451–9.

93 Murray AB, Morrison BJ. It is children with atopic dermatitis who develop asthma more frequently if the mother smokes. *J Allergy Clin Immunol* 1990; 86: 732–9.

94 Magnusson CGM. Maternal smoking influences cord serum IgE and IgD levels and increases the risk for subsequent infant allergy. *J Allergy Clin Immunol* 1986; 78: 898–904.

95 Kjellman NIM. Effect of parental smoking on IgE levels in children. *Lancet* 1994; i: 993–4.

96 Gergen PJ, Mullally DI, Evans R. National survey of prevalence of asthma in the United States. *Pediatrics* 1990; 81: 1–7.

97 Dybendal T, Hetland T, Vik H, Apold J, Elsayed S. Comparative measurements of antigenic and allergic proteins in dust vacuumed from carpeted and non-carpeted classrooms in Norwegian schools. *Clin Exp Allergy* 1989; 19: 217–24.

98 Cook DG, Whincup PH, Jarvis MJ, Strachan DP, Papacosta DP, Bryant A. Passive exposure to tobacco smoke in children aged 5–7 years: individual, family, and community factors. *BMJ* 1994; 308: 384–9.

99 Norman PS, Van Metre TE. The safety of allergenic immunotherapy. *J Allergy Clin Immunol* 1990; 85: 522–5.

100 Eggleston PA. Immunotherapy for allergic respiratory disease. *Pediatr Clin North Am* 1988; 35: 1103–14.

101 Ostergaard PA, Kaad PN, Kristensen T. A prospective study on the safety of immunotherapy in children with severe therapy. *Allergy* 1986; 41: 588–93.

102 Barnes PJ. General pharmacologic principles. In: Murray JF, Nadel JA (eds) *Textbook of Respiratory Medicine*, 2nd edn. Philadelphia: W.B. Saunders, 1994: 1–2739.

103 Warner JO. The beta$_2$-agonist controversy and its relevance to the treatment of children. *Eur Respir Rev* 1994; 4: 21–6.

104 Spitzer WO, Suissa S, Ernst P *et al.* The use of β-agonists and the risk of death and near death from asthma. *N Engl J Med* 1992; 326: 501–6.

105 Ernst P, Habbick B, Suissa S *et al.* Is the association between inhaled beta-agonist use and life-threatening asthma because of confounding by severity? *Am Rev Respir Dis* 1993; 148: 75–9.

106 Sears MR, Taylor DR, Print CG *et al.* Regular inhaled beta-agonist treatment in bronchial asthma. *Lancet* 1990; 336: 1391–6.

107 Van Schayck CP, Dompeling E, Van Herwaarden CLA. Bronchodilator treatment in moderate asthma or chronic bronchitis: continuous or demand. A randomized control trial. *BMJ* 1991; 303: 1426–31.

108 Milgrom H, Bender B. Current issues in the use of theophylline. *Am Rev Respir Dis* 1993; 147: S33–S9.

109 Weinberger M. Theophylline: when should it be used? *J Pediatr* 1993; 122: 403–5.

110 Pauwels R, van Renterghem D, van der Straeten M, Johannesson N, Persson CGA. The effects of theophylline and enprophylline on allergen-induced bronchoconstriction. *J Allergy Clin Immunol* 1985; 76: 583–90.

111 Ward AJM, McKenniff M, Evans JM, Page CP, Costello JF. Theophylline – an immunomodulatory role in asthma? *Am Rev Respir Dis* 1993; 147: 518–23.

112 Sullivan P, Bekir S, Jaffar Z, Jeffery P, Costello J. Anti-inflammatory effects of low-dose oral theophylline in atopic asthma. *Lancet* 1994; 343: 1006–8.

113 Barnes PJ, Greening AP, Neville L, Timmers J, Poole GW. Single-dose slow-release aminophylline at night prevents nocturnal asthma. *Lancet* 1982; i: 299–301.

114 Brenner M, Berkowitz R, Marshall N, Strunk RC. Need for theophylline in severe steroid-requiring asthmatics. *Clin Allergy* 1988; 18: 143–50.

115 Schlieper A, Alcock D, Beaudry P, Feldman W, Leikin L. Effect of therapeutic plasma concentrations of theophylline on behavior, cognitive processing, affect in children with asthma. *J Pediatr* 1991; 118: 449–55.

116 Hendles L, Weinberger M, Szefler S, Ellis E. Safety and efficacy of theophylline in children with asthma. *J Pediatr* 1992; 120: 179–83.

117 Hodges IGC, Groggins RC, Milner AD, Stokes GM. Bronchodilator effects of inhaled ipratropium bromide in wheezy toddlers. *Arch Dis Child* 1981; 56: 729–32.

118 Beasley CRW, Rafferty P, Holgate ST. Bronchoconstrictor properties of preservatives in ipratropium bromide (Atrovent) nebuliser solution. *BMJ* 1987; 294: 1197–8.

119 Juniper EF, Kline PA, Vanzieleghem MA, Ramsdale EH, O'Byrne PM, Hargreave FE. Effect of long-term treatment with an inhaled corticosteroid (budesonide) on airway hyperresponsiveness and clinical asthma in non-steroid-dependent asthmatics. *Am Rev Respir Dis* 1990; 142: 832–6.

120 Juniper EF, Kline PA, Vanzieleghem MA, Ramsdale EH, O'Byrne PM, Hargreave FE. Long-term effects of budesonide on airway responsiveness and clinical asthma severity in inhaled-steroid dependent asthmatics. *Eur Respir J* 1990; 3: 1122–7.

121 Haahtela T, Jarvinen M, Kava T *et al.* Comparison of a β_2-agonist, terbutaline, with an inhaled corticosteroid, budesonide, in newly detected asthma. *N Engl J Med* 1991; 325: 388–92.

122 van Essen-Zandvliet EE, Hughes MD, Waalkens HJ *et al.* Effects of 22 months treatment with inhaled corticosteroid and/or beta-2-agonist on lung function, airway responsiveness and symptoms in children with asthma. *Am Rev Respir Dis* 1992; 146: 547–54.

123 van Essen-Zandvliet EE, Hughes MD, Waalkens HJ, Duiverman EJ, Kerrebijn KF. Dutch CNSLD study group. Remission of childhood asthma after long-term treatment with an inhaled corticosteroid (budesonide): Can it be achieved? *Eur Respir J* 1994; 7: 63–8.

124 Ilangovan P, Pedersen S, Godfrey S, Nikander K, Novisky N, Warner JO. Treatment of severe steroid dependent preschool asthma with nebulised budesonide suspension. *Arch Dis Child* 1993; 68: 356–9.

125 Bisgaard H, Munck SL, Nielsen JP, Peterson W, Ohlsson SV. Inhaled budesonide for treatment of recurrent wheezing in early childhood. *Lancet* 1990; 336: 649–51.

126 Gleeson JGA, Price JF. Controlled trial of budesonide given by the Nebuhaler in preschool children with asthma. *BMJ* 1988; 297: 163–6.

127 Waalkens HJ, van Essen-Zandvliet EE, Hughes MD *et al.* Cessation of long-term treatment with inhaled corticosteroid (budesonide) in children with asthma results in deterioration. *Am Rev Respir Dis* 1993; 148: 1252–7.

128 Barnes PJ, Pedersen S. Efficacy and safety of inhaled corticosteroids in asthma. *Am Rev Respir Dis* 1993; 148: S1–S26.

129 Baran D. A comparison of inhaled budesonide and beclomethasone dipropionate in childhood asthma. *Br J Dis Chest* 1987; 81: 170–5.

130 Pedersen S, Hansen OR. Budesonide treatment of asthma in children: a dose response study. *Eur J Respir Dis* 1993; 6 (suppl 17): 358s.

131 Geddes DM. Inhaled corticosteroids: benefits and risks. *Thorax* 1992; 47: 404–7.

132 Balfour-Lynn L. Growth and childhood asthma. *Arch Dis Child* 1986; 61: 1049–55.

133 Shohat M, Shohat T, Kedem R, Mimouni M, Danon YL. Childhood asthma and growth outcome. *Arch Dis Child* 1987; 62: 63–5.

134 Price JF. Growth, asthma and treatment with inhaled corticosteroids. *Paediatr Respir Med* 1993; 1: 19–21.

135 Wolthers O, Pedersen S. Short term growth during treatment with inhaled fluticasone dipropionate and beclomethasone dipropionate. *Arch Dis Child* 1993; 68: 673–6.

136 Wolthers O, Pedersen S. Growth of asthmatic children during treatment with budesonide: a double blind trial. *BMJ* 1991; 303: 163–5.

137 Law CM, Marchant JL, Honour JW, Preece MA, Warner JO. Nocturnal adrenal suppression in asthmatic children taking inhaled beclomethasone dipropionate. *Lancet* 1986; i: 942–4. [Published erratum appears in *Lancet* 1987; i: 1321.]

138 Connett GJ, Lenney W. Inhaled budesonide and behavioural disturbances. *Lancet* 1991; 338: 634.

139 Simons FE, Persaud MP, Gillespie CA, Cheang M, Shuckett EP. Absence of posterior subcapsular cataracts in young patients treated with inhaled glucocorticoids. *Lancet* 1993; 342: 776–8.

140 Shaw NJ, Edmunds AT. Inhaled beclomethasone and oral candidiasis. *Arch Dis Child* 1986; 61: 788–90.

141 Deshpande A, McKenzie SA. Short course of steroids in home treatment of children with acute asthma. *BMJ* 1986; 293: 169–71.

142 Harris JB, Weinberger MM, Nassif E, Smith G, Milavetz G, Stillerman A. Early intervention with short courses of prednisone to prevent progression of asthma in ambulatory patients incompletely responsive to bronchodilators. *J Pediatr* 1987; 110: 627–33.

143 Brunette MG, Lands L, Thibodeau LP. Childhood asthma: prevention of attacks with short-term corticosteroid treatment of upper respiratory tract infection. *Pediatrics* 1988; 81: 624–9.

144 Zora JA, Zimmerman D, Carey TL, O'Connell EJ, Yunginger JW. Hypothalamic–pituitary–adrenal axis suppression after short-term, high-dose glucocorticoid therapy in children with asthma. *J Allergy Clin Immunol* 1986; 77: 9–13.

145 Dolan LM, Kesarwala HH, Holroyde JC, Fischer TJ. Short-term, high-dose, systemic steroids in children with asthma: the effect on the hypothalamic–pituitary–adrenal axis. *J Allergy Clin Immunol* 1987; 80: 81–7.

146 Kamada AK, Spahn JD, Surs W, Brown E, Leung DYM, Szefler SJ. Coexistence of glucocorticoid receptor and pharmacokinetic abnormalities: factors that contribute to a poor response to treatment with glucocorticoids in children with asthma. *J Pediatr* 1994; 124: 984–6.

147 Green CP, Price JF. Prevention of exercise induced asthma by inhaled salmeterol xinafoate. *Arch Dis Child* 1992; 67: 1014–7.

148 Chudry N, Correa F, Silverman M. Nedocromil sodium and exercise induced asthma. *Arch Dis Child* 1987; 62: 412–4.

149 Comis A, Valletta EA, Sette L, Andreoli A, Boner AL. Comparison of nedocromil sodium and sodium cromoglycate administered by pressurized aerosol, with and without a spacer device in exercise-induced asthma in children. *Eur Respir J* 1993; 6: 523–6.

150 Armenio L, Baldini G, Bardare M *et al.* Double blind, placebo controlled study of nedocromil sodium in asthma. *Arch Dis Child* 1993; 68: 193–7.

151 Maclay WP, Crowder D, Spiro S, Turner P. Post-marketing surveillance: Practical experience with ketotifen. *BMJ* 1984; 288: 911–4.

152 Loftus BG, Price JF. Long-term, placebo-controlled trial of ketotifen in the management of pre-school children with asthma. *J Allergy Clin Immunol* 1987; 79: 350–5.

153 Kennedy JD, Hasham F, Clay MJD, Jones RS. Comparison of action of disodium cromoglycate and ketotifen on exercise-induced bronchoconstriction in childhood asthma. *BMJ* 1980; 281: 1458.

154 Reiser J, Warner JO. Inhalation treatment for asthma. *Arch Dis Child* 1986; 61: 88–94.

155 Pedersen S, Frost L, Arnfred T. Errors in inhalation technique and efficiency in inhaler use in asthmatic children. *Allergy* 1986; 41: 118–24.

156 Pedersen S, Mortensen S. Use of different inhalation devices in children. *Lung* 1990; 168 (suppl): 653–7.

157 Everard ML, Clark AR, Milner AD. Drug delivery from holding chambers with attached facemask. *Arch Dis Child* 1992; 67: 580–5.

158 O'Callaghan C, Lynch J, Cant M, Robertson C. Improvement in sodium cromoglycate delivery from a spacer device by use of an antistatic lining, immediate inhalation, and avoiding multiple actuations of drug. *Thorax* 1993; 48: 603–6.

159 Henry RL, Milner AD. Simple drug delivery system for use by young asthmatics. *BMJ* 1983; 286: 2021–2.

160 Rivlin J, Mindorff C, Reilly P, Levison H. Pulmonary response to a bronchodilator delivered from three inhalation devices. *J Pediatr* 1984; 104: 470–3.

161 Brown PH, Blundell G, Greening AP *et al.* Do large volume spacer devices reduce the systemic effects of high dose inhaled corticosteroids? *Thorax* 1990; 45: 736–9.

162 Prahl P, Jensen T. Decreased adreno-cortical suppression utilizing the Nebuhaler for inhalation of steroid aerosols. *Clin Allergy* 1987; 17: 393–8.

163 Freelander M, Van Asperen PP. Nebuhaler versus nebuliser in children with acute asthma. *BMJ* 1984; 288: 1873–4.

164 Sennhauser FM, Sly PD. Pressure flow characteristics of the valve in spacer devices. *Arch Dis Child* 1989; 64: 1305-7.

165 O'Callaghan C, Milner AD, Swarbrick A. Spacer device with face mask attachment for giving bronchodilators to infants with asthma. *BMJ* 1989; 298: 160-1.

166 Gleeson JGA, Price JF. Nebuhaler technique. *Br J Dis Chest* 1988; 82: 172-4.

167 Pedersen S. Aerosol treatment of bronchoconstriction in children, with or without a tube spacer. *N Engl J Med* 1983; 308: 1328-30.

168 Pedersen S. How to use a rotahaler. *Arch Dis Child* 1986; 61: 11-4.

169 Pedersen S, Hansen OR, Fuglsang G. Influence of inspiratory flow upon the effect of a turbohaler. *Arch Dis Child* 1990; 65: 308-19.

170 Agertoft L, Pedersen S. The importance of the inhalation device on the effects of budesonide. *Arch Dis Child* 1993; 69: 130-3.

171 Bendefy IM. Home nebulisers in childhood asthma: survey of hospital supervised use. *BMJ* 1991; 302: 1180-1.

172 Everard ML, Clark AR, Milner AD. Drug delivery from jet nebulisers. *Arch Dis Child* 1992; 67: 586-92.

173 Beer S, Laver J, Karpuch J, Chabut S, Aladjem M. Prodromal features of asthma. *Arch Dis Child* 1987; 62: 345-8.

174 Wilson NM, Silverman M. Treatment of acute, episodic asthma in pre-school children using intermittent high dose inhaled steroids at home. *Arch Dis Child* 1990; 65: 407-10.

175 Connett G, Lenney W. Prevention of viral induced asthma attacks using inhaled budesonide. *Arch Dis Child* 1993; 68: 85-7.

176 Godfrey S, Balfour-Lynn L, Konig P. The place of cromolyn sodium in the long-term management of childhood asthma based on a 3-5 year follow-up. *J Pediatr* 1974; 87: 465-73.

177 Greening AP, Ind PW, Northfield M, Shaw G, on behalf of Allen & Han-burys Limited UK Study Group. Added salmeterol versus higher-dose corticosteroid in asthma patients with symptoms on existing inhaled corticosteroid. *Lancet* 1994; 344: 219-24.

178 Partridge MR. Problems with asthma care delivery. In: Mitchell DM (ed) *Recent Advances in Respiratory Medicine*, No. 5. London: Churchill Livingstone, 1991; 61-78.

179 Malo J-L, Cartier A, Merland N *et al.* Four-times-a-day dosing frequency is better than twice-a-day regimen in subjects requiring a high-dose inhaled steroid budesonide, to control moderate to severe asthma. *Am Rev Respir Dis* 1989; 140: 624-48.

180 Coutts JAP, Gibson NA, Paton JY. Measuring compliance with inhaled medication in asthma. *Arch Dis Child* 1994; 67: 332-3.

181 D'Souza W, Crane J, Burgess C *et al*. Community-based asthma care: trial of a "credit card" asthma self-management plan. *Eur J Respir Dis* 1994; 7: 1260–5.

182 Bailey WC, Richards JN, Brooks N, Seng Jaw Soong, Windsor RA, Nanzelle BA. A randomised trial to improve the self management practices of adults with asthma. *Arch Intern Med* 1994; 150: 1664–8.

183 Hughes DM, McLeod M, Garner B, Goldbloom RB. Controlled trial of a home management and ambulatory programme for asthmatic children. *Pediatrics* 1991; 87: 54–61.

184 Zeiger RS, Heller S, Mellon MH, Wald J, Falkoff R, Schatz M. Facilitated referral to asthma specialist reduces the relapses in asthma emergency room visits. *J Allergy Clin Immunol* 1991; 87: 1160–8.

185 Storr JE, Barrell E, Lenney W, Hatcher G. Effect of a single oral dose of prednisolone in acute childhood asthma. *Lancet* 1987; i: 879–82.

186 Charlton I, Charlton G, Broomfield J, Mullee MA. Evaluation of peak flow and symptoms only self management plans for control of asthma in general practice. *BMJ* 1990; 301: 1355–9.

187 Benton G, Thomas RC, Nickerson BG, McQuitty JC, Okikawa J. Experience with a metered dose inhaler with a spacer in the pediatric emergency department. *Am J Dis Child* 1989; 143: 678–81.

188 Fuglsang G, Pedersen S. Comparison of nebuhaler and nebuliser treatment of acute severe asthma in children. *Eur J Respir Dis* 1986; 69: 109–13.

189 Paton JY. The safety of inhaled steroids in childhood asthma. *Practitioner* 1994; 238: 322–6.

190 McNicol KN, Williams HE. Spectrum of asthma in childhood. I. Clinical and physiological components. *BMJ* 1973; 4: 7–11.

191 Strachan DP. The prevalence and natural history of wheezing in early childhood. *J R Coll Gen Pract* 1985; 35: 182–4.

192 Tattersfield AE. Asthma – where now? In: Lawson DH (ed) *Current Medicine*, 4th edn. Edinburgh: Churchill Livingstone, 1994: 29–49.

193 Williams HE, McNicol KN. Prevalence, natural history and relationship of wheezy bronchitis and asthma in children: an epidemiological study. *BMJ* 1969; 4: 321–5.

194 Clifford RD, Radford M, Howell JB, Holgate ST. Associations between respiratory symptoms, bronchial responsiveness to methacholine and atopy in two age groups of school children. *Arch Dis Child* 1989; 64: 1133–9.

195 Martinez FD, Morgan WJ, Wright AL, Holberg CJ, Taussig LM. Diminished lung function as a predisposing factor for wheezing respiratory illness in infants. *N Engl J Med* 1988; 319: 1112–7.

196 Taylor B, Wadsworth J. Maternal smoking during pregnancy and lower respiratory tract illness in early life. *Arch Dis Child* 1987; 62: 786–91.

197 Tager IB, Hanrahan JP, Tostesan TD *et al.* Lung function, pre- and post-natal smoke exposure, and wheezing in the first year of life. *Am Rev Respir Dis* 1993; 147: 811–7.

198 Chan KN, Wong YC, Silverman M. Relationship between infant lung mechanics and childhood lung function in children of very low birthweight. *Pediatr Pulmonol* 1990; 8: 74–81.

199 Horn MEC, Gregg I, Brain EA, Inglis JM, Yealland SJ, Taylor P. Respiratory viral infection and wheezy bronchitis in childhood. *Thorax* 1979; 34: 23–8.

200 Luyt DK, Burton P, Brooke AM, Simpson H. Wheeze in preschool children and its relation with doctor diagnosed asthma. *Arch Dis Child* 1994; 71: 24–30.

201 Selander P. Asthmatic symptoms in the first year of life. *Acta Paediatr Scand* 1960; 49: 265–9.

202 O'Callaghan C, Milner AD, Swarbrick A. Nebulised salbutamol does have a protective effect on airways in children under 1 year old. *Arch Dis Child* 1988; 63: 479–83.

203 Tepper RS. Airway reactivity in infants: a positive response to methacholine and metaproterenol. *J Appl Physiol* 1987; 62: 1155–9.

204 Henderson AJW, Young S, Stick S, Landau LI, Le Soeuf PN. Effect of salbutamol on histamine induced bronchoconstriction in healthy infants. *Thorax* 1993; 48: 317–23.

205 Prendiville A, Green S, Silverman M. Paradoxical response to salbutamol in wheezy infants. *Arch Dis Child* 1987; 42: 86–91.

206 Clough JB. Bronchodilators in infancy. *Thorax* 1993; 48: 308.

207 Cogswell JJ, Simpkiss MJ. Nebulised sodium cromoglycate in recurrently wheezy preschool children. *Arch Dis Child* 1985; 60: 736–8.

208 Loftus BG, Price JF. Treatment of asthma in preschool children with slow release theophylline. *Arch Dis Child* 1985; 60: 770–2.

209 Webb MS, Milner AD, Hiller EJ, Henry RL. Nebulised beclomethasone dipropionate suspension. *Arch Dis Child* 1986; 61: 1108–10.

210 Ilangovan P, Pedersen S, Godfrey S, Nikander K, Novisksi N, Warner JO. Treatment of severe steroid dependent preschool asthma with nebulised budesonide suspension. *Arch Dis Child* 1993; 68: 356–9.

211 Gleeson JG, Price JF. Controlled trial of budesonide given by the nebuhaler in preschool children with asthma. *BMJ* 1988; 297: 163–6.

212 Varsano I, Volovitz B, Malik H, Amir Y. Safety of 1 year of treatment with budesonide in young children with asthma. *J Allergy Clin Immunol* 1909; 85: 914–20.

213 Freigang B, Ashford DR. Adrenal cortical function after long-term beclomethasone aerosol therapy in early childhood. *Ann Allergy* 1990; 64: 342–4.

214 Martin AJ, McLennan LA, Landau LI, Phelan PD. The natural history of childhood asthma to adult life. *BMJ* 1980; 280: 1397–400.

215 McFadden ER Jr, Gilbert IA. Exercise-induced asthma. *N Engl J Med* 1994; 330: 1362-7.

216 Jones RS, Buston MH, Wharton MJ. The effect of exercise on ventilatory function in children with asthma. *Br J Dis Chest* 1962; 56: 78-86.

217 Anderson SD, Silverman M, Konig P, Godfrey S. Exercise-induced asthma. *Br J Dis Chest* 1975; 69: 1-39.

218 Zawadski DK, Lenner KA, McFadden ER Jr. Effect of exercise on nonspecific airway reactivity in asthmatics. *J Appl Physiol* 1988; 64: 812-6.

219 Mussaffi H, Springer C, Godfrey S. Increased bronchial responsiveness to exercise and histamine after allergen challenge in children with asthma. *J Allergy Clin Immunol* 1986; 77: 48-52.

220 Edmunds AT, Tooley M, Godfrey S. The refractory period after exercise-induced asthma: its duration and relation to severity of exercise. *Am Rev Respir Dis* 1978; 117: 247-54.

221 Orenstein DM, Reed ME, Grogan FT, Crawford LV. Exercise conditioning in children with asthma. *J Pediatr* 1985; 106: 556-60.

222 Unnithan VB, Thomson KJ, Aitchison TC, Paton JY. β_2-Agonists and running economy in prepubertal boys. *Pediatr Pulmonol* 1994; 17: 378-82.

223 Zanconato S, Baraldi E, Santuz P, Magagnin G, Zacchello F. Effect of inhaled disodium cromoglycate and albuterol on energy cost of running in asthmatic children. *Pediatr Pulmonol* 1990; 8: 240-4.

224 Young S, Bitsaku H, Caric D, McHardy GJR. Coughing can relieve or exacerbate symptoms in asthmatic patients. *Respir Med* 1991; 85: 7-12.

225 Sheppard D, Rizk NW, Boushey HA, Bethel RA. Mechanism of cough and bronchoconstriction caused by distilled water. *Am Rev Respir Dis* 1983; 127: 691-4.

226 Thomson A, Pratt C, Simpson H. Nocturnal cough in asthma. *Arch Dis Child* 1987; 62: 1001-4.

227 McKenzie S. Cough – but is it asthma? *Arch Dis Child* 1994; 70: 3-4.

228 Hsu JY, Stone RA, Logan-Sinclair RB, Wordsell M, Busst CM, Chung KF. Coughing frequency in patients with persisting cough: assessment using a 24 hour ambulatory recorder. *Eur J Respir Dis* 1994; 7: 1246-53.

229 Martin RJ, Cicutto LC, Ballard RD. Factors related to the nocturnal worsening of asthma. *Am Rev Respir Dis* 1990; 140: 33-8.

230 van Aalderen WM, Postma DS, Koeter GH, Knol K. The effect of reduction of maintenance treatment on circadian variation in peak expiratory flow rates in asthmatic children. *Acta Paediatr Scand* 1988; 77: 269-74.

231 Horn CR, Clark TJH, Cochrane GM. Inhaled therapy reduces morning dips in asthma. *Lancet* 1984; i: 1143-5.

232　Verberne A, Lenney W, Kerrebijn KF. A 3 way crossover study comparing twice daily dosing of salmeterol 25 mcg and 50 mcg with placebo in children with mild to moderate reversible airways disease. *Am Rev Respir Dis* 1991; 143: A20.

233　Zeitlin S, Rolles C, Antolainen I *et al.* An open, multicentre, cross-over comparison of albuterol controlled release tablets and individually titrated slow release theophylline in the treatment of childhood asthma. *Am Rev Respir Dis* 1988; 137: 33A.

234　Douglas NJ. Nocturnal asthma. *Thorax* 1993; 48: 100–2.

235　Hoskyns EW, Thomson AH, Decker E, Hutchins A, Simpson H. Effect of controlled release salbutamol on nocturnal cough in asthma. *Arch Dis Child* 1191; 66: 1209–1212.

236　Wilson NM. Diet related asthma in children. *Paediatr Respir Med* 1993; 1: 14–20.

237　May CD. Objective clinical and laboratory studies of immediate reactions to foods in asthmatic children. *J Allergy Clin Immunol* 1976; 58: 500–15.

238　Matus I. Assessing the nature and clinical significance of psychological contributions to childhood asthma. *Am J Orthopsychiatry* 1981; 51: 327–41.

239　Strunk RC. Identification of the fatality-prone subject with asthma. *J Allergy Clin Immunol* 1989; 83: 477–85.

240　Miller BD. Depression and asthma: a potentially lethal mixture. *J Allergy Clin Immunol* 1987; 80: 481–6.

241　Quinn CM. Children's asthma: new approaches, new understandings. *Ann Allergy* 1988; 60: 283–92.

242　Nocon A. Social and emotional impact of childhood asthma (editorial). *Arch Dis Child* 1991; 66: 458–60.

243　Robertson CF, Rubinfeld AR, Bowes G. Pediatric asthma deaths in Victoria: the mild are at risk. *Pediatr Pulmonol* 1992; 13: 95–100.

244　Weiss KB, Wagener DK. Changing patterns of asthma mortality – Identifying target populations at high risk. *JAMA* 1990; 264: 1683–7.

245　Newcomb RW, Akhter J. Respiratory failure from asthma: a marker for children with high morbidity and mortality. *Am J Dis Child* 1988; 142: 1041–8.

246　Barnes SD, Grob CS, Lachman BS, Marsh BR, Loughlin GM. Psychogenic upper airway obstruction presenting as refractory wheezing. *J Pediatr* 1986; 109: 1067–70.

247　Lask B, Matthew D. Childhood asthma. A controlled trial of family psychotherapy. *Arch Dis Child* 1979; 54: 116–9.

248　Strunk RC, Fukuhara JT, LaBrecque JL, Mrazek DA. Outcome of long-term hospitalisation for asthma in children. *J Allergy Clin Immunol* 1989; 83: 17–25.

249　Brunekreef B, Dockery DW, Speizer FE, Ware JH, Spengler JD, Ferris BG. Home dampness and respiratory morbidity in children. *Am Rev Respir Dis* 1989; 140: 1363–7.

250 Dales RE, Zwanenburg H, Burnett R, Franklin CA. Respiratory effects of home dampness and molds among Canadian children. *Am J Epidemiol* 1991; 134: 196–203.

251 Williamson IJ, Martin CJ, McGill G, Monie RDH, Fennerty AG. Is there an association between asthma and damp housing? *Am J Respir Crit Care Med* 1994; 149: A68.

252 Anderson HR, Bailey PA, Cooper JS, Palmer JC, West S. Morbidity and school absence caused by asthma and wheezing illness. *Arch Dis Child* 1983; 58: 777–84.

253 Bevis M, Taylor B. What do school teachers know about asthma? *Arch Dis Child* 1990; 65: 622–5.

254 Jenkins MA, Hopper JL, Bowes G, Carlin JB, Flander LB, Giles GG. Factors in childhood as predictors of asthma in adult life. *BMJ* 1994; 309: 90–3.

255 Kelly WJW, Hudson I, Phelan PD, Pain MC, Olinsky A. Childhood asthma in adult life: a further study at 28 years of age. *BMJ* 1987; 294: 1059–62.

256 Godden DJ, Ross S, Abdalla MI *et al.* Outcome of wheeze in childhood: symptoms and pulmonary function 25 years later. *Am Rev Respir Dis* 1994; 149: 106–12.

257 Blair H. Natural history of childhood asthma. *Arch Dis Child* 1977; 52: 613–9.

258 Ross S, Godden DJ, McMurray D *et al.* Social effects of wheeze in childhood: a 25 year follow-up. *BMJ* 1992; 305: 545–8.

259 Sibbald B, Anderson HR, McGuigan S. Asthma and employment in young adults. *Thorax* 1992; 47: 19–24.

260 Strachan DP. Do chesty children become chesty adults? *Arch Dis Child* 1990; 65: 161–2.

KEY POINTS

1 *Diagnosis*
   (a) Diagnosis depends on a detailed history.
   (b) Recurrent episodes of cough, wheeze and breathlessness are the key symptoms.
   (c) Viral infections and exercise are the main triggers.
   (d) Physical signs should be generalized, not focal, and are not essential to diagnosis.
   (e) Be careful when diagnosing asthma in children under one year, especially if cough is the only symptom or growth is poor.

2   *Management*

    (a) Effective management requires an informed partnership between parents, children and doctors.

    (b) Avoid trigger factors, particularly passive cigarette smoking, where possible.

    (c) Plan ahead – establish clear written plans for treating chronic asthma and managing acute exacerbations.

    (d) Devices are critical to the success of inhaled therapy in children – choose carefully and check frequently.

    (e) Attainment of final height may be delayed but is usually normal.

3   *Special Problems*

    (a) Treating children under two with asthma is often difficult – for everyone.

    (b) Expect poor compliance with medication in adolescents.

    (c) Aim to achieve normal exercise performance.

    (d) Nocturnal disturbance is common and can be difficult to prevent completely.

    (e) Beware of asthmatic children with depression.

    (f) Asthma usually improves around puberty, particularly for boys – it may recur in the twenties.

    (g) Current evidence suggests that asthma can be controlled but not cured.

28

MANAGEMENT OF ACUTE ASTHMA IN CHILDREN

S. Pedersen

The number of hospitalizations due to acute asthma has been increasing,[1,2] probably because of an increase in asthma prevalence or severity, but other factors including poor patient understanding, inadequate recognition and under-treatment also seem to have contributed substantially.[2,3] An acute severe asthma attack is a potentially life-threatening event, which should always be treated effectively without delay. The aims of the treatment are:

- to prevent death,

- to relieve hypoxaemia and normalize lung functions as quickly as possible, and

- to avoid future relapses.

The principles and modalities of the treatment are the same as in adults. However, there are differences in dosages of medication and clinical assessment. A precondition for achieving the aims without unnecessary delay is a detailed knowledge about the optimal doses and mode of administration of the drugs used in the treatment of the condition and the ability to recognize severe attacks.[4] This will be discussed with special emphasis on the results from controlled trials in different age groups. This information will then form the basis for some suggestions for management strategies at home and in hospital. Table 28.1 summarizes the recommended doses of the various drugs used to treat acute severe asthma.

β_2 AGONISTS

The value of inhaled β_2 agonists in the treatment of acute asthma in school and pre-school children has been demonstrated in several controlled trials.[5–19] Such treatment is superior to treatment with all other bronchodilators since it works effectively within minutes of administration. In

TABLE 28.1: *Recommended average doses of the various drugs used to treat acute severe asthma in all age groups of children. Only the most commonly used drugs are mentioned. Individual dose adjustments should be made based upon the clinical response and occurrence of side effects*

β_2 *Agonists*

Nebulizer	0.2 mg kg^{-1} salbutamol or 0.4 mg kg^{-1} terbutaline (maximum = 10 mg) Volume-fill = 4 ml Mouthpiece or tightly fitting face mask May be repeated at frequent intervals in doses of 0.3 mg per kg hour^{-1} salbutamol or 0.6 mg per kg hour^{-1} terbutaline
Spacer device or other inhalers	One puff every minute until satisfactory response Maximum dose: 50 μg salbutamol or 100 μg kg^{-1} terbutaline
Subcutaneous or intramuscular	10 μg kg^{-1} salbutamol or terbutaline
Intravenous (salbutamol/terbutaline)	Loading dose: 2–5 μg kg^{-1} over 5 min Continuous: 5 μg kg^{-1} hour^{-1}

Ipratropium bromide

Nebulizer	250 μg in a volume-fill of 4 ml to all age groups May be repeated 4–6-hourly

Corticosteroids

Prednisolone	Loading dose: 1–2 mg kg^{-1} (maximum 60 mg) Continuous: 2 mg kg^{-1} daily divided into two doses
Intravenous methylprednisolone	Loading dose: 1–2 mg kg^{-1} Continuous: 1 mg kg^{-1} 6-hourly
Intravenous hydrocortisone	Loading dose: 10 mg kg^{-1} Continuous: 5 mg kg^{-1} 6-hourly

TABLE 28.1: *Continued*

Theophylline (for patients not receiving theophylline prior to treatment)

Intravenous	Loading dose: 6 mg kg^{-1} lean body weight over 10 min
Oral or rectal administration	Loading dose: 8–9 mg kg^{-1} lean body weight
Continuous treatment (oral or intravenous). Measurement of serum levels required	< 1 year: (0.3)*(age in weeks) + 8 mg kg^{-1} per 24 hours
	1–9 years: 24 mg kg^{-1} per 24 hours
	9–12 years: 20 mg kg^{-1} per 24 hours
	12–16 years: 18 mg kg^{-1} per 24 hours
	Over 16 years: 14 mg kg^{-1} per 24 hours

addition, subcutaneous, intramuscular or intravenous administration is associated with a significant effect.[20,21]

MODES OF ADMINISTRATION OF β₂ AGONISTS

No direct comparisons between inhaled and systemic administration of β₂ agonists have been performed in children. However, in general the inhaled route provides a better clinical effect to side-effect ratio than the systemic route in adults with severe acute symptoms.[22] Furthermore, the inhaled route appears to be less affected by the pre-treatment given prior to admission.[23] For these reasons inhalations are the best way to administer β₂ agonists to children with acute asthma attacks.

CHOICE OF INHALATION SYSTEM

Nebulizers are simple to use and in the acute situation it is advantageous that oxygen can be administered through the nebulizer at the same time as the β₂ agonist. Therefore, nebulizers are still the delivery system of choice in the treatment of acute severe asthma in all age groups of hospitalized children, even though most studies show that the same results can be obtained with other inhalation systems in schoolchildren.[5,6,14,15]

Simply varying the choice of compressor, jet nebulizer and volume-fill has been shown to modify the mass of drug in respirable particles over a tenfold range.[24] Therefore, conclusions from one nebulizer may not be transferred to other nebulizers or to other inhalers. It is also important to realize that inhalations should take place through a tightly fitting face mask or a mouthpiece. Inhalation through a face mask 2–3 cm from the face, which often happens, will reduce drug delivery to the patient by approximately 50% in schoolchildren, with a corresponding increase in release of aerosol to the environment. In agreement with this, *in vitro* studies have reported an 85% reduction in the inhaled dose of respirable particles when the face mask was moved 2 cm from the inspiratory orifice.[25] The effect appears to be the same in schoolchildren whether the inhalation takes place through a mouthpiece or a face mask.[15]

After 1 year of age the quantity of aerosol inspired from a jet nebulizer is largely independent of age due to entrainment, which occurs when inspiratory flow exceeds jet-nebulized flow;[26] therefore the same dose ($\mu g\ kg^{-1}$) can be used from that age.

Spacers are also easy to use[27] and virtually all schoolchildren can learn to use these devices; children can also use them effectively during attacks of acute bronchoconstriction when they are as effective as nebulizers.[5,6,14,15,17,28] Because of the enormous variation in nebulizer output it is not possible to define exact equi-effective doses between nebulizers and spacers. Normally, lower doses are required from spacers to produce the same response as a nebulizer.[17,28–30]

It is also possible to train most pre-school children to use spacers, particularly with a valve system and a face mask.[31–37] During episodes of acute wheeze, however, many young children may not be able to open or close the valve system properly and therefore do not gain optimal benefit. Problems with opening and closing the valve of some spacers like Nebuhaler and Volumatic may also occur in some younger children not suffering from acute wheeze. These difficulties may be reduced by tilting the spacer inhaler upwards during the inhalation so that the valve opens by gravity.[35]

Fast inhalations are required to produce a maximum effect from *dry powder inhalers*[27,38–41] and therefore it is sometimes suggested that dry powder inhalers are ineffective during acute attacks of wheeze. However, the majority of schoolchildren can generate sufficient inspiratory flow rate during episodes of acute wheeze[40,42] and therefore dry powder inhalers can be used in such situations in schoolchildren.[42] However, many pre-school children may not be able to generate sufficiently high inspiratory flow rates during acute episodes of bronchoconstriction[27,40,43] and therefore dry powder inhalers should be reserved for children older than 5 years. The same is true for *conventional metered dose inhalers*, which can normally only be used effectively in schoolchildren after careful tuition[27,44] but often not during episodes of acute wheeze.[45]

DOSE RECOMMENDATIONS

It is always dangerous to recommend doses for acute severe asthma. This is because the dose required depends upon the response. The correct strategy is to administer enough drug for each individual patient while carefully monitoring for adverse effects and clinical response. Therefore, the dose recommendations detailed here should be considered as suggestions for an average patient. Furthermore, not all selective β_2 agonists have been extensively studied in children. When conclusions from studies with one drug are transferred to the others it must be remembered that some differences exist between the various agents.

Nebulized Therapy

The optimal dose of nebulized β_2 agonists for acute asthma depends upon not only the nebulizer brand but also volume-fill: more drug will be delivered if the same concentration of drug is given in 4 ml than 2 ml. However, high doses of salbutamol ($0.3\,\text{mg kg}^{-1}$) were better than low doses ($0.15\,\text{mg kg}^{-1}$) when given at 3-hourly intervals.[12] No significant difference was observed on heart rate or potassium levels between the two treatments. Furthermore, continuous nebulization of salbutamol at a dose of $0.3\,\text{mg kg}^{-1}\,\text{hour}^{-1}$ produced better results than the same dose nebulized intermittently over 20 min every hour.[46] The value of continuous or frequent administration has also been emphasized by other investigators.[47–49] Finally, a study on less severe asthma attacks questioned the importance of administering salbutamol on a per kilogram body weight basis ($0.1\,\text{mg kg}^{-1}$), since a fixed dose of 2.5 mg to all children produced similar results.[50]

A dose–response study found that 5–10 mg nebulized metaproterenol seems to be the optimal bronchodilating dose for acute asthma in school-children.[51]

Inhalation of high doses of β_2 agonists causes significant systemic absorption so that after some inhalations plasma drug levels are in the same range as after continuous systemic administration. As a consequence the same side-effects may be seen.[28,52,53] Therefore, this treatment combines the effects of local and systemic administration.

Spacers

The optimal dose from a spacer is not known. Doses from 2 to 6 mg and doses around $0.1\,\text{mg kg}^{-1}$ have been used without unacceptable side-effects.[5,6,14,15,17,28,29] In agreement with the nebulizer studies frequent administration seems to be better than single high-dose administration. A single dose of six puffs terbutaline (1500 µg) from a spacer was less effective than three puffs given twice at 15-min intervals;[8] in addition, one dose of 500 µg terbutaline was less effective than two doses of 250 µg given 5 min apart.[54]

Systemic Administration

A significant correlation is seen between plasma drug levels and bronchodilating effect after systemic administration of a β agonist.[20,55] However, considerable inter-individual variations exist in plasma levels obtained after a given dose.[20,55] Therefore, standard doses are not feasible for effective therapy. Dosing should be individualized with monitoring of therapeutic response and for the occurrence of side-effects.[56]

In a dose–response trial an intravenous loading dose of 2 μg kg^{-1} terbutaline followed by a continuous infusion of 5 μg kg^{-1} hour^{-1} was optimal for the majority of children not receiving other therapy.[20] Furthermore, inhalation of 1 mg terbutaline from a Nebuhaler did not further improve bronchodilation, indicating that maximum effect in these children could be achieved by systemic administration of the drug. The same intravenous doses seem to be effective when salbutamol is used.[57–59] When systemic administration is combined with high-dose inhaled therapy the systemic doses should probably be reduced.

Finally, doses around 10 μg kg^{-1} of terbutaline or salbutamol given subcutaneously or intramuscularly have produced significant clinical effect without unacceptable side-effects.[21,60] In one of these studies 12 μg kg^{-1} was better than 3 and 6 μg kg^{-1}.[60]

Adrenaline has both α and β activity. Although it is an effective bronchodilator, the side-effects caused by its α and $β_1$ actions – anxiety, tremor, hypertension, tachycardia, palpitations and cardiac arrhythmias – are undesirable. It is sometimes suggested that adrenaline, with its α-adrenoceptor vasoconstricting activity, would be better than other drugs at decreasing bronchial oedema because of its constrictor effect on arterioles. However, it also causes venous vasoconstriction and this effect could negate or even supersede any beneficial effect on arterial constriction. Controlled clinical trials do not demonstrate any advantages of adrenaline over the modern adrenoceptor agonists in relieving airway obstruction in children.[10,16,18,19,21,61–63] As a consequence its use in modern asthma treatment is obsolete. However, the α-stimulating action makes adrenaline the drug of choice for the treatment of anaphylactic shock.

Special Considerations in Infants

Several early studies failed to find any bronchodilator response to nebulized $β_2$ agonists in infants[64–67] and for many years it was believed that β agonists were ineffective in this age group, though functioning β adrenoceptors are present. In agreement with these observations, two recent studies assessing transcutaneous oxygen pressure and/or oxygen saturation found a fall in these parameters after treatment of acute wheeze in infants with nebulized salbutamol.[68,69] One of these studies suggested that some of the fall in Po_2 might be caused by the acidity of the aerosol.[68] In contrast, another study found an increase in tcPo_2 after nebulized salbutamol in children aged 11–30 months.[70] In accordance with this, recent placebo-controlled double-blind studies have demonstrated significant bronchodilator effects,[71–77] protective effects against bronchoconstrictor agents[69,78,79] and clinical improvement in infants treated with $β_2$ agonists either alone or in combination with steroids.[67,80] The reason for this discrepancy is not clear. The various studies have differed with respect to dose, inhaler (spacer, nebulizer), baseline lung function, duration of symptoms and method of lung function measurement. The discrepancy is only seen in studies assessing bronchodilator effects. All studies find a significant protection against bronchoconstriction induced by various challenges. Thus, it seems that infants have functioning β_2 receptors from birth and that stimulation of these receptors can produce the same effects as in older children. However, often the response is rather small and marked interindividual differences are seen. As a consequence, further studies are needed to assess optimal use during episodes of acute wheeze.

SIDE-EFFECTS

Generally, treatment of children with β_2 agonists is very safe. The occurrence of side-effects is directly proportional to the plasma concentration of drug and therefore mainly depends on route of administration as well as on selectivity. Skeletal muscle tremor, headache, palpitations and some agitation are the most common complaints when high doses are used. After systemic administration, the occurrence of side-effects can be used as an indication that the top of the bronchodilatory dose–response curve has been reached.[20] Tolerance to the side-effects seems to develop easily so that they will disappear with continued use of the drug.[81,82]

A small drop in blood pressure and a compensatory increase in pulse rate is seen after systemic use or administration of high doses of inhaled drug.[20] Furthermore, hyperglycaemia, hypokalaemia and an increase in free fatty acids are common under these conditions.[81,82] The hypokalaemia is more pronounced when concomitant high doses of steroids are used. The clinical importance of this remains to be elucidated since it is due to an increased transport of potassium into skeletal muscles. Thus there is no decrease in total body potassium level.

Asthma is associated with considerable ventilation–perfusion imbalance. This may result in low P_aO_2. β Agonists have two pharmacological actions that may affect P_aO_2 in different directions. Firstly, they may decrease P_aO_2 by causing pulmonary vasodilatation, which increases perfusion of the poorly ventilated areas and thus increases the shunt effect. Secondly, β agonists increase cardiac output, decrease peripheral resistance and cause bronchodilation, which will all increase P_aO_2. The net effect on P_aO_2 will be the balance of these effects. The significance of any β agonist-induced fall in P_aO_2 will depend on the initial oxygen tension of the patient, but normally it is without any clinical importance and often occurs in patients with relatively high pre-treatment P_aO_2.

Concomitant use of theophylline seems to enhance most of the side-effects of β agonists.

STEROIDS

The beneficial effects of systemic steroids in the management of acute severe asthma has been shown in several controlled trials in all age groups except infants[83–91] and the value of such therapy has only rarely been questioned, though some studies have found minimal or no benefit.[92,93] The optimal dose of steroid and route of administration have not been carefully evaluated, so the recommendations for this condition are rather empirical being based upon personal experience and the dose regimens used in studies evaluating the treatment. Undoubtedly, oral prednisolone is sufficient in the majority of children, especially when used early during the exacerbation,[86] when it has been shown to reduce the severity of virally induced asthma attacks and hospital admissions. Oral prednisolone is rapidly and reliably absorbed and therefore normally to be preferred. However, in some patients intravenous hydrocortisone or methylprednisolone may be necessary in case of gastrointestinal problems. Theoretically, methylprednisolone is preferable to hydrocortisone because of less mineralocorticoid effect and a better penetration into the lung tissue,[94] but no clinical differences in efficacy have been demonstrated. Very high doses of steroids are probably not necessary and may cause hypokalaemia, fluid retention and an acute myopathy.[95] Normally recommended steroid doses, which have produced significant effects in controlled trials, are given below.

- *Prednisolone*: loading dose 1–2 mg kg^{-1} (maximum 60 mg). This should be followed by 2 mg kg^{-1} per 24 hours divided into two doses.

- *Methylprednisolone*: loading dose 1–2 mg kg^{-1}. This should be followed by 1 mg kg^{-1} every 6 hours.

- *Hydrocortisone*: loading dose 10 mg kg^{-1}, followed by 5 mg kg^{-1} every 6 hours.[49]

Systemic dexamethasone or oral prednisolone were of little benefit in infants with acute wheeze in two studies[67,96] but of significant benefit in another.[97] Therefore, further studies are needed in this age group.

Controlled trials have found that nebulized beclomethasone reduced the frequency (but not the severity) of respiratory symptoms and improved lung function in infants with post-bronchiolitis wheezing.[98,99]

High doses of inhaled corticosteroids are sometimes recommended for the treatment of exacerbations. However, at present there are no studies to support this except for a recent study that did find a significant additional effect of nebulized budesonide in acute wheeze in children up to 18 months of age.[97] However, it seems that if given early to children with asthma provoked by viral upper respiratory tract infection such treatment can reduce the severity of asthma attacks, though probably not the incidence of hospital admissions.[100,101]

METHYLXANTHINES

Xanthine derivates (aminophylline or theophylline) have been used for many years in the treatment of acute severe asthma in children. The number of placebo-controlled studies assessing the acute effect are relatively sparse. It has been demonstrated that a bolus dose of theophylline causes significant increases in lung functions in schoolchildren with acute wheeze.[102–104] However, only one double-blind controlled trial has supported its use in hospitalized children with severe asthma[105] who were receiving other treatment but not aggressive treatment with inhaled β_2 agonists.

No formal dose–response studies have been conducted in children with acute wheeze, but the bronchodilating effect seems to correlate with the plasma theophylline level.[104] Therefore, it is normally recommended that the therapeutic strategy in such situations is to aim at plasma levels between 55 and 110 μmol l^{-1}. This can be achieved in all age groups by giving an intravenous bolus of 6 mg kg^{-1} lean body weight over 5 min to a child who has not received any theophylline for 12 hours prior to the treatment, and then continue with the theophylline infusion rates or oral therapy shown in Table 28.1. Since the volume of distribution is around 0.5 l kg^{-1} a bolus of 6 mg kg^{-1} will result in a mean serum level of 12 μg ml^{-1} (66 μmol l^{-1}). Gastrointestinal and rectal absorption of an aqueous solution is almost complete, with peak serum theophylline levels being measured within 1 hour of administration; somewhat higher loading doses are required when these administration forms are used (8–9 mg kg^{-1}).[104,106] If the child is already receiving treatment with theophylline, additional theophylline therapy should only be given while monitoring plasma theophylline levels.

Though significant bronchodilating effects have been demonstrated in children the role of theophylline in the acute management of asthma has been questioned based on the findings in a recent study,[107] which did not find any additional benefit of theophylline in children treated with steroids and frequent inhalation of β_2 agonists, probably because theophylline is a weaker bronchodilator than inhaled β_2 agonists.[108,109] In accordance with this, a recent meta-analysis of 13 double-blind controlled studies on the treatment of acute asthma in children and adults did not find convincing evidence of any clinical benefit of adding theophylline to treatment with steroids and sympathomimetics.[110]

Theophylline has not been thoroughly studied in pre-school children and infants with wheeze.

Some knowledge about theophylline pharmacokinetics is important for effective safe therapy. This has been thoroughly described in an excellent review.[111] Generally, children metabolize theophylline much more rapidly than adults, and in the child population the elimination rate also varies with age so that young children have a much higher clearance than older children. The normally recommended theophylline doses for continuous therapy in different age groups are shown in Table 28.1. These dose recommendations are based upon lean body weight and they aim at plasma theophylline levels between 55 and 110 μmol l^{-1}. Within each group there may be up to tenfold inter-individual variation in theophylline half-life and, in addition, other drugs and viral infections may also affect theophylline metabolism (β_2 agonists increase clearance so that higher doses are required; viral infections reduce clearance). Therefore, theophylline dose must always be individualized and if high doses are used, as in the treatment of acute asthma, plasma theophylline levels must be measured. When dose adjustments are made upon the basis of serum theophylline determinations it is important to remember that theophylline often shows dose-dependent kinetics so that on average the percentage change in serum concentration is about 50% greater than the percentage change in dose.[112]

SIDE-EFFECTS

Theophylline has a narrow therapeutic window and potentially lethal side-effects when excessive doses are given.[113–115] During the last decade 63 deaths have been reported in studies with theophylline.[116] The most common side-effects are anorexia, nausea, vomiting and headache.[114,115,117] These symptoms are quite common. Mild central nervous stimulation, palpitations, tachycardia, arrhythmias, abdominal pain, diarrhoea and, rarely, gastric bleeding may also occur.

The most serious toxicity is the risk of seizures, which have been associated with a mortality rate as high as 50%. However, seizures appear to be rare at serum levels less than 220 μmol l^{-1}. In theophylline-induced seizures higher than normal doses of benzodiazepines should be used as theophylline antagonizes the effect of benzodiazepines on γ-aminobutyric acid (GABA) receptors in the brain.[118] If modern kinetic principles are used seizures should not occur.[111]

ANTI-MUSCARINIC AGENTS

Virtually all pharmacodynamic data in children refer to one drug: ipratropium bromide. The dose-ranging studies in schoolchildren have all used a nebulizer for the delivery so the optimal dose is only known for this administration. It would be expected, however, to be lower if a metered dose inhaler with a spacer is used.[119] Normally, increasing the ipratropium bromide dose above 250 μg adds no extra benefit in protection against exercise-induced asthma,[120] cold air hyperventilation or in bronchodilation.[121] This dose (250 μg) has also been used in most studies on preschool children. No formal dose–response studies have been performed in infants but a dose of 25 μg kg^{-1} has produced beneficial effects in one study.[72] The optimal dose frequency and optimal dose in acute severe wheeze remain unknown.

Generally, maximum bronchodilation from these doses of ipratropium bromide seems to be slower and the duration of action similar to that of an inhaled β_2 agonist.

Anti-cholinergics result in less bronchodilation than inhaled β_2 agonists[122] and administered alone these drugs have no role in the management of acute severe asthma in schoolchildren.[7] However, controlled studies have found that the combination of β_2 agonist and an anti-cholinergic produces somewhat better results than either drug used alone[7,123–126] without an increase in side-effects. Though statistically highly significant, the advantages of the combination therapy were rather small in most studies. This may be the reason why other studies failed to find any benefit of such combined therapy.[64,127–129]

It has been argued that the augmented effects elicited by the combination of adrenergic and anti-cholinergic agents might simply be a consequence of under-dosing with the adrenergic drug. However, the additional effect has also been reported in studies using quite high doses of β_2 agonists. Furthermore, in one study frequent nebulized doses of salbutamol were administered to children until a plateau in the response was seen. The children were then randomized to receive either ipratropium bromide or placebo. A significant additional increase in lung function of around 20% was observed after 2 hours in the ipratropium bromide group as compared with placebo (5%).[125]

A clinical study in acute viral bronchiolitis in infants did not find any beneficial effects of ipratropium bromide,[130] though other studies suggest some benefit in this condition.[72,124]

Although the findings have not been consistent, the data do suggest that ipratropium bromide has a role as an adjunct to inhaled β_2 agonists in the treatment of acute asthma in children older than 1 year.

SIDE-EFFECTS

Paradoxical bronchoconstriction after inhalation and dryness of the mouth may be a problem in some patients.[131,132] Some of these incidents seemed to be due to benzalkonium chloride, which has now been removed from the nebulizer solution. Otherwise, no important side-effects are associated with treatment with anti-cholinergics.

ASSESSMENT OF SEVERITY

Asthma severity in children is often underestimated by physicians. The child may appear deceptively well and yet suffer from quite marked airway obstruction (peak expiratory flow rate (PEFR) around 50–60% predicted normal or personal best value). Even in the presence of wheeze many children still want to participate in other children's activities. Therefore, objective measurements are important and necessary for a correct assessment. Even trained doctors may not be good at predicting a patient's lung function.[133] Table 28.2 provides some parameters that are normally used in the assessment. Since these are guidelines only, all features in one category need not be present. When in doubt about whether the condition should be categorized as moderate or severe it is normally severe.

Absolute criteria for admission or a particular treatment recommendation are difficult to formulate and depend upon several factors including past history, availability of treatment, social circumstances (parental understanding and capability of accurate monitoring) and geographic isolation. Unfortunately, there is no identifiable factor that can be used to predict which children will respond to treatment.[84,133] In light of this, the value of some of the parameters in Table 28.2 will be briefly discussed.

SPECIAL CONSIDERATIONS IN INFANTS AND YOUNG CHILDREN
Differences in lung anatomy and physiology and a poorer response to treatment place infants at greater risk than older children. Marked hyperinflation is often prevalent in young children with wheeze.[134] As a consequence, respiratory work is increased and these age groups are prone to develop hypercapnia (hypoventilation) and respiratory failure more readily than older children. It is more common to underestimate severity in infants and, in general, young children are more severely obstructed and have higher Pco_2 than older children.[135] Therefore, measurement of time trends in Pco_2, Po_2 or oxygen saturation is usually indicated in addition to the clinical observations in severe wheeze in these age groups.

HISTORY
History should always include likely triggers (infection, allergy, compliance), duration, treatment prior to admission (dose, drug, response) and other lung diseases.

OBJECTIVE FINDINGS
Symptom scores assessing degree of auscultatory findings, respiratory rate, patient distress, respiratory effort (retractions) and pallor have been used to assess severity and the efficacy of drugs in the treatment of acute asthma.[50,133,135–138] The various scores correlate weakly with oxygen saturation and lung function,[133] though not all studies have found this.[135] Furthermore, findings of a quiet chest on auscultation, inability to talk and cyanosis or a high score strongly suggest hypercapnia and severe bronchoconstriction.[136,139] However, in the individual patient it cannot be used as a single criterion to predict outcome. It is important to remember that respiratory muscle fatigue may result in slowing of the respiration rate, disappearance of retractions and appearance of paradoxical thoraco-

TABLE 28.2: *Assessment of severity of asthma exacerbations in children. Patients exhibiting moderate symptoms should be considered for admission*

	Mild	Moderate	Severe
Treatment place	Home/out-patient	Home/out-patient	Hospitalization
Wheeze	Only end-expiratory	Loud	Loud or absent
Breathless			
Old child	Playing	Walking	Talks in single words
Infant	Crying	Difficult feeding	Stops feeding
Accessory muscle retractions	Usually not	Moderate	Marked
Respiratory rate			
< 3 months	< 60 min^{-1}	60–70 min^{-1}	> 70 min^{-1}
3–12 months	< 50 min^{-1}	50–60 min^{-1}	> 60 min^{-1}
1–6 years	< 40 min^{-1}	40–50 min^{-1}	> 50 min^{-1}
> 6 years	< 30 min^{-1}	30–40 min^{-1}	> 40 min^{-1}
Pulse rate			
< 1 year	< 150 min^{-1}	150–170 min^{-1}	> 170 min^{-1}
1–2 years	< 120 min^{-1}	120–140 min^{-1}	> 140 min^{-1}
> 2 years	< 110 min^{-1}	110–130 min^{-1}	> 130 min^{-1}
Pre-treatment PEFR	> 70%	50–70%	< 50%
Response to β_2 agonist	> 3 hours	2–3 hours	< 2 hours
$P_a co_2$	< 35 mmHg	< 40 mmHg	> 40 mmHg
$S_a o_2$ (on air)	> 94%	92–94%	< 92%

Life-threatening features
PEFR < 40% of best
Cyanosis
Bradycardia
Fatigue/exhaustion/reduced consciousness
Silent chest
Paradoxical thoraco–abdominal movement

(*continued overpage*)

TABLE 28.2: *Continued*

	Mild	Moderate	Severe

Life-threatening features
Disappearance of retractions without concomitant clinical
  improvement

High-risk patient:[155] *low admission threshold*
Recent withdrawal of oral steroids
Hospitalization for asthma in past year
Earlier catastrophic attacks
Psychiatric disease/psychosocial problems
Poor compliance
Young children (develop respiratory failure more readily and
  are difficult to assess)

abdominal movement. Remember that anxiety and confusion may be due to hypoxaemia! Therefore, anxiety should never be treated with sedatives.

PULSUS PARADOXUS

The pulsus paradoxus of acute severe asthma is an exaggeration of the normal fall in systolic blood pressure during inspiration. Its size is thought to relate to the severity of the attack. However, pulsus paradoxus is difficult to measure in children and the association between worsening obstruction and increase in pulsus paradoxus is weak.[133] The sign is not present in one-third of patients with severe obstruction and only a severe paradox (> 20 mmHg) is a reliable indicator of a severe attack.[140]

BRONCHODILATOR RESPONSE

It is normally suggested that the duration of effect following the administration of β_2 agonists is a useful guide to the severity. Those with a low or short effect (< 2 hours) following inhalation of a β_2 agonist tend to be prone to a slower recovery. Clinically this has not been thoroughly assessed in children, though some studies suggest that it is probably true.[135,141]

BLOOD GASES

$P\text{co}_2$ can be reliably measured on capillary blood, which makes this parameter very useful particularly in young children. It may also be monitored transcutaneously together with $P\text{o}_2$. Normally, $P\text{co}_2$ is low due to hyperventilation and a slight respiratory alkalosis is common.[136] When airway obstruction becomes excessive the low $P\text{co}_2$ and high pH return to normal and severe respiratory failure may soon develop. Therefore, normal or elevated $P\text{co}_2$ values should always be considered a sign of danger. High values that increase in spite of aggressive treatment are one of the indications for assisted ventilation. One paper found that blood gas measurement was the only satisfactory method to assess severity in children.[135]

OXYGEN SATURATION

The initial arterial oxygen saturation has been evaluated as a criterion to decide to admit or discharge a child with acute asthmatic symptoms. An oxygen saturation level $\leq 91\%$ was found predictive of a very severe condition requiring admission; saturation levels of 92–93% were borderline cases and $\geq 94\%$ indicated moderate and mild attacks, respectively.[142] In that study post-bronchodilator saturation was not predictive of the outcome.[142] At variance with this, other studies have found that a post-bronchodilator oxygen saturation $< 91\%$ was the best predictor for a severe attack.[133,143] Whilst arterial oxygen saturation is a useful tool in the evaluation and surveillance of acute asthma, the correlation with lung function is weak and this parameter has not been shown to be sufficiently sensitive to be used as a single criterion for the admission to hospital of an acutely ill child.

LUNG FUNCTIONS

Most children ≥ 5 years can make reproducible measurements. Remember, however, that in the acute situation it is better to treat children than to use the time training them in lung function measurements. Furthermore, forced expiratory manoeuvres may provoke/increase bronchoconstriction when the airways are very hyperreactive. The best way of assessing lung function is the measured value as a percentage of the child's personal best. If that is not known the percentage of predicted normal can be used. It is worth while remembering that normally the percentage predicted forced expiratory volume in 1 s (FEV_1) or forced expiratory flow 25–75% ($FEF_{25-75\%}$) is lower than the percentage predicted PEFR. Though lung functions correlate to the various clinical signs and objective measurements, the correlation is always weak and therefore these parameters are not good predictors in the individual patient. Lung functions are still the best measurement of the degree of airway obstruction and there is a highly significant association between low PEFR ($< 25\%$ and $< 50\%$) as well as the percentage improvement after β_2-agonist treatment and need for intensive treatment.[141] Therefore, PEFR (or FEV_1, $FEF_{25-75\%}$ and FVC if the equipment is available) should be measured whenever possible. These measurements are the most valuable of all parameters for assessing the response to treatment and for decisions about stepping down treatment and discharging the patient. As for the other parameters, lung function may not be used as a single criterion for admission, though one study suggested that children with PEFR $> 25\%$ predicted normal or personal best could be managed outside hospital.[135] It is my opinion that 25% is too low a value. Therefore somewhat higher values are suggested in Table 28.2.

CHEST X-RAYS

Chest X-rays are rarely helpful in acute asthma in children. It can be reserved for cases when the initial progression in clinical improvement is poor, or objective findings or history suggest that complicating factors or differential diagnoses may be important.

INFECTIONS

Viral infections are frequent causes of exacerbations; nasopharyngeal swabs and sputum for viral and bacterial culture should be taken if infection is suspected as a precipitating cause.

TREATMENT AND MONITORING

There is more than one way to manage an acute asthma exacerbation in a child. No two patients or situations are alike and many excellent reviews have suggested various management plans.[144–151] The following is my suggestion of a protocol for treating acute asthma in various age groups of children. It is based upon the controlled studies mentioned earlier, personal experience and the fact that the primary factors leading to obstruction are bronchoconstriction, inflammation, mucous plugging and oedema.

First of all it is important to ensure that the correct treatment has been applied and that it is improving the condition satisfactorily. Careful monitoring is therefore mandatory. It should include the assessment of the parameters in Table 28.2. It is recommended to carry out regular recordings of respiration rate, pulse rate, PEFR, use of auxiliary muscles and retractions, colour, duration of effect of nebulized β_2 agonist, blood gases (especially $P\text{co}_2$), oxygen saturation and the general clinical condition, including occurrence of side-effects (measurement of electrolytes (potassium), see pp. 517 and 520). The frequency of assessment depends upon severity, but generally more frequent monitoring (every 30 min) is required at the beginning of treatment and in the more severe cases.

GENERAL PRACTICE

The child should be seen without delay. It is important to assess the child both before, during and after treatment to get an accurate perception of the severity.

IMMEDIATE TREATMENT

All Children

Independent of the initial assessment of severity of the acute attack, a short-acting β_2 agonist should be given, preferably via a metered dose inhaler (MDI) and a spacer device. Use a face mask in pre-school children. If a spacer is not available other inhalers may be used (see Chapter 20). Give one puff every minute until satisfactory improvement occurs, i.e. the clinical condition is changed into mild severity (Table 28.2). Maximum dose is equivalent to 50 μg kg^{-1} salbutamol or 100 μg kg^{-1} terbutaline.

If inhaled treatment cannot for some reason be given or taken by the child, salbutamol or terbutaline 10 μg kg^{-1} can be administered subcutaneously or intramuscularly.

SUBSEQUENT TREATMENT

Mild Attacks

Continue with regular inhaled β_2 agonist (every 3–6 hours) as long as it is required and consider doubling the normally taken dose or adding high-dose (800 μg daily) inhaled corticosteroid until the condition has been stable for 1 week. If 3–4 hourly treatments are still required after 24 hours the attack should be considered as moderate and treated accordingly.

Moderate Attacks

If the response to initial treatment is good and the dose of β_2 agonist required to achieve the response is less than 50% of the maximum dose (50 μg kg^{-1} salbutamol or 100 μg kg^{-1} terbutaline), then continue with regular inhaled β_2 agonist (every 2–4 hours) as long as it is required and double the normally taken dose or add high dose (800 μg daily) inhaled corticosteroid until the condition has been stable for 1–2 weeks. If 3-hourly β_2 agonist is still required after 24 hours, add a short course of oral prednisolone.

If the response to the initial treatment is good but high β_2-agonist doses are required to achieve the response, add a short course of oral prednisolone 2 mg kg^{-1} daily (maximum dose 60 mg) divided into two doses per day for 3–5 days to the suggested treatment.

If the response to the initial treatment is poor or of short duration (< 2 hours), consider hospitalization and give 1–2 mg kg^{-1} of oral prednisolone (maximum dose 60 mg).

Severe Attacks

Admit the patient to hospital without delay after the initial treatment. Give 1–2 mg kg^{-1} of oral prednisolone (maximum dose 60 mg).

The various treatments may be supplemented by continuous oral theophylline or oral β_2-agonist treatment for some days as suggested in Table 28.1.

All parents should be instructed in monitoring procedures and encouraged to call the doctor again if the resolution of the exacerbation is not progressing satisfactorily (individual criteria and a written action plan (see later) should be given according to the global assessment of the situation).

HOSPITAL MANAGEMENT

IMMEDIATE TREATMENT
All Children

- Oxygen (8–10 l min^{-1}) via a face mask or nasal cannula.

- Salbutamol or terbutaline 0.2 or 0.4 mg kg^{-1} respectively (maximum 10 mg) in a volume-fill of 4 ml via oxygen-driven nebulizer. If a face mask is used it should fit tightly to the child's face.

- Prednisolone 1–2 mg kg^{-1} body weight orally (maximum 60 mg).

- If the child is critically ill or vomits, oral prednisolone should be replaced by intravenous methylprednisolone 2 mg kg^{-1}.

SUBSEQUENT TREATMENT
In many children the immediate treatment produces significant and marked improvement. Subsequent management in these cases may only require repeated nebulized β_2 agonist 2–4-hourly and continued treatment with oral prednisolone 2 mg kg^{-1} daily.[86]

In those with more severe asthma (the response to the initial treatment is poor or the duration less than 2 hours) the following should be tried in addition to continued prednisolone.

- Repeat nebulized β_2-agonist treatment and add 0.25 mg ipratropium bromide to the solution in the chamber.

- This can be followed by frequent or continuous nebulized β_2 agonist (equivalent to 0.3 mg kg^{-1} salbutamol hourly given in divided doses at 20–30-min intervals or as continuous nebulization if the equipment is available). Ipratropium bromide 0.25 mg can be repeated 4–6-hourly.

- If the improvement is still not satisfactory consider intravenous β_2 agonists or theophylline as outlined in Table 28.1. These doses are average doses and should be adjusted on the basis of the clinical effect, side-effects and (for theophylline) serum drug concentrations. If the child is already receiving oral theophyllines, systemic β_2 agonists are preferred. In such patients, serum theophylline concentration should be monitored before theophylline treatment is initiated. If the child is receiving systemic β_2 agonists the initial loading theophylline dose should be halved to minimize side-effects.

Additional Treatment

- Give supplemental oxygen to maintain saturation above 90%.

- Assess the need for intravenous fluids but do not overhydrate.

- Antibiotics should not be given routinely but only to patients suspected of bacterial pneumonia or other bacterial infections.

- Acute asthma is a frightening condition and the child needs psychological support.

Useless or Dangerous Treatments

Cough medicine is useless and never indicated in acute severe asthma. Sedatives are dangerous and may induce respiratory failure or apnoea. Therefore, these drugs should only be given in the intensive care unit when facilities for intubation and assisted ventilation are available and ready.

Indications for Intensive Care

Children with acute severe asthma require intensive monitoring by experienced staff; all patients with life-threatening features (Table 28.2) not responding convincingly to treatment require intensive care.

Indications for Assisted Ventilation

Not all children admitted to the intensive care unit need ventilation, but it may be necessary in a small number of patients as a life-saving procedure. In general, it is accepted that this procedure is necessary in those patients who fulfil the following criteria:

- $P_a CO_2$ of > 8.6 kPa and rising,

- $P_a O_2$ of < 6.6 kPa and falling,

- pH of 7.25 or less and falling,

- apnoea,

- respiratory arrest,

- cardiorespiratory arrest.

STEPPING DOWN TREATMENT

- *Step 1.* When the condition has been stable for 12 hours the intensive treatment can be gradually reduced, starting with systemic β_2 agonists and theophylline. Some may want to continue with these treatments for some time. In this case intravenous treatment can be stopped and oral maintenance treatment started with the doses given in Table 28.1.

- *Step 2.* The next step is less frequent β_2-agonist inhalations.

- *Step 3.* Finally, the patient is switched to inhaled therapy with cortico-steroids and β_2 agonist with the inhaler that is going to be used at home. Oral prednisolone continues unchanged.

The duration of oral prednisolone treatment is individual depending upon severity of the attack and response. A rule of thumb is to continue after the condition is brought back to "mild" for twice as many days as it took to bring it there, but never less than 3 days. The dose may be gradually reduced or simply stopped based upon individual assessments.

RECOVERY AND DISCHARGE

An acute attack must always be considered a failure of prophylaxis and before discharge measures must be taken to prevent relapse, which has been reported to occur at a rate of 20–30% within the first 2 weeks after presentation.[146,150,160] Therefore, patients should not normally be discharged until the following have occurred:

- symptoms have disappeared;

- lung function has stabilized (diurnal variability < 25%) and returned to its normal or best level (PEFR > 75% of the predicted or personal best);

- the child should be stabilized on maintenance treatment, which should *always* include inhaled corticosteroids at a higher than pre-admission dosage;

- it must be ensured that the child is able to comply with the regimen.

The treatment with inhaled steroids should preferably be started 24–48 hours before discharge if the attack was severe. Nebulizers should be replaced by standard inhaler devices 24–48 hours before discharge unless the patient requires a nebulizer at home. Inhaled β_2 agonist should preferably be prescribed for use "as necessary". The inhalation technique should be checked and performance recorded. In patients requiring oral xanthines blood theophylline concentrations should be monitored.

Recovery after acute asthma is often very slow. Children can remain vulnerable despite appearing well; the airways can remain hyperresponsive and small airways lung function compromised for many weeks after an acute asthmatic attack. Therefore, inhaled corticosteroids should continue throughout the recovery phase, which is often of 4–8 weeks' duration.

Investigation of the Circumstances of Admission

It is important to address the following questions, which relate to avoidable factors.

- Was there an avoidable precipitating cause? An allergy history should be taken.

- Was this a catastrophic sudden attack or was there a period of recognizable deterioration before the "acute" attack?

- Did the patient (or relatives) react appropriately when the asthma got worse?

- Was the patient complying with regular treatment, and, if not, can anything be done to help?

- Was medical management appropriate?

The admission to hospital provides an opportunity to educate patients about their asthma and train them to respond to changes in symptoms and peak flow. Children ≥ 5 years should have a PEFR meter and be taught how to use it. PEFR should be recorded and the results brought to the first follow-up visit.

Self-Management Plan

All patients should have a written self-management plan. The child and its parents:

- should know at what values of PEFR or level of symptoms to increase the treatment,

- how treatment should be increased and for how long,

- when to call their doctor, or re-admit themselves to hospital.

In this respect it is important to remember that overuse of a β_2 agonist is a marker for uncontrolled asthma. Physicians should be alert for children who require frequent use (more than twice daily) of a β_2 agonist. Such patients should be prescribed an inhaled steroid or have their inhaled steroid treatment modified to achieve symptom control. Furthermore, the patient should be instructed not to rely too much on the inhaled β_2 agonist during periods of worsening symptoms.

Contact with a General Practitioner

Good communication with the patient's general practitioner is essential. Discharge letters should include the PEFR on admission and at discharge (recorded on the patient's meter) and details of treatment to be continued at home and the self-management plan.

Follow-up Arrangements

All children require follow-up. The initial outpatient appointment should be within a month. Clinical assessment including lung function and discussion of the home recordings with the child and its parents should be performed and a further management plan should be made to enable the patient to lead a normal life and to prevent further severe attacks. It is also important to evaluate if the patient has read and understood the information given at discharge, particularly the action plan.

Many of the measures suggested after the hospital treatment have not been thoroughly evaluated in controlled trials. However, studies do suggest that use of steroids, good instructions, self-management plans and use of prophylactic medication markedly reduce morbidity and the occurrence of relapses.[153,154]

REFERENCES

1. Mitchell EA, Anderson HR, Freeling P, White PT. Why are hospital admission and mortality rates for childhood asthma higher in New Zealand than in the United Kingdom? *Thorax* 1990; 45: 176–82.

2. Anderson HR. Increase in hospital admissions for childhood asthma: Trends in referral, severity, and readmissions from 1970 to 1985 in a health region in the United Kingdom. *Thorax* 1989; 44: 614–9.

3. Fletcher HJ, Ibrahim SA, Speight N. Survey of asthma deaths in the Northern region, 1970–85. *Arch Dis Child* 1990; 65: 163–7.

4. Webb LZ, Kuykendall DH, Zeiger RS *et al.* The impact of status asthmaticus practice guidelines on patient outcome and physician behavior. *QRB Qual Rev Bull* 1992; 18: 471–6.

5. Pendergast J, Hopkins J, Timms B, Van Asperen PP. Comparative efficacy of terbutaline administered by Nebuhaler and by nebulizer in young children with acute asthma. *Med J Aust* 1989; 151: 406–8.

6. Fuglsang G, Pedersen S. Comparison of a new multidose powder inhaler with a pressurized aerosol in children with asthma. *Pediatr Pulmonol* 1989; 7: 112–5.

7. Watson WT, Becker AB, Simons FE. Comparison of ipratropium solution, fenoterol solution, and their combination administered by nebulizer and face mask to children with acute asthma. *J Allergy Clin Immunol* 1988; 82: 1012–8.

8. Phanichyakarn P, Kraisarin C, Sasisakulporn C, Kittikool J. A comparison of different intervals of administration of inhaled terbutaline in children with acute asthma. *Asian Pac J Allergy Immunol* 1992; 10: 89–94.

9. Kelly HW, McWilliams BC, Katz R, Murphy S. Safety of frequent high dose nebulized terbutaline in children with acute severe asthma. *Ann Allergy* 1990; 64: 229–33.

10. Victoria MS, Battista CJ, Nangia BS. Comparison between epinephrine and terbutaline injections in the acute management of asthma. *J Asthma* 1989; 26: 287–90.

11 Portnoy J, Aggarwal J. Continuous terbutaline nebulization for the treatment of severe exacerbations of asthma in children. *Ann Allergy* 1988; 60: 368–71.

12 Schuh S, Reider MJ, Canny G *et al.* Nebulized albuterol in acute childhood asthma: comparison of two doses. *Pediatrics* 1990; 86: 509–13.

13 Pool JB, Greenough A, Price JF. Abnormalities of functional residual capacity in symptomatic and asymptomatic young asthmatics. *Acta Paediatr Scand* 1988; 77: 419–23.

14 Scalabrin DM, Naspitz CK. Efficacy and side effects of salbutamol in acute asthma in children: comparison of oral route and two different nebulizer systems. *J Asthma* 1993; 30: 51–9.

15 Lowenthal D, Kattan M. Facemasks versus mouthpieces for aerosol treatment of asthmatic children. *Pediatr Pulmonol* 1992; 14: 192–6.

16 Ben-Zvi Z, Lam C, Hoffman J, Teets-Grimm KC, Kattan M. An evaluation of the initial treatment of acute asthma. *Pediatrics* 1982; 70 (suppl 3): 348–53.

17 Kerem E, Levison H, Schuh S *et al.* Efficacy of albuterol administered by nebulizer versus spacer device in children with acute asthma. *J Pediatr* 1993; 123: 313–7.

18 Turpeinen M, Kuokkanen J, Backman A. Adrenaline and nebulized salbutamol in acute asthma. *Arch Dis Child* 1984; 59: 666–8.

19 Becker AB, Nelson NA, Simons FER. Inhaled salbutamol (albuterol) vs injected epinephrine in treatment of acute asthma in children. *J Pediatr* 1983; 102: 465–9.

20 Fuglsang G, Pedersen S, Borgstrom L. Dose–response relationships of intravenously administered terbutaline in children with asthma. *J Pediatr* 1989; 114: 315–20.

21 Davis WJ, Pang LM, Chernack WJ, Mellins RB. Terbutaline in the treatment of acute asthma in childhood. *Chest* 1977; 72: 614–7.

22 Janson C. The role of adrenergics in the management of severe, acute asthma. *Res Clin Forums* 1993; 15: 9–14.

23 Swedish Society of Chest Medicine. High dose inhaled versus intravenous salbutamol combined with theophylline in acute severe asthma. *Eur Respir J* 1990; 3: 163–70.

24 Newman SP, Pellow PGD, Clay MM, Clarke SW. Evaluation of jet nebulizers for use with gentamycin solution. *Thorax* 1985; 40: 671–6.

25 Everard ML, Clark AR, Milner AD. Drug delivery from holding chambers with attached facemask. *Arch Dis Child* 1992; 67: 580–5.

26 Collis GG, Cole CH, Le Souëf PN. Dilution of nebulised aerosols by air entrainment in children. *Lancet* 1990; 336: 341–3.

27 Pedersen S. Inhaler use in children with asthma. *Danish Med Bull* 1987; 34: 234–49.

28 Fuglsang G, Pedersen S. Comparison of Nebuhaler and Nebulizer treatment of acute severe asthma in children. *Eur J Respir Dis* 1986; 69: 109-13.

29 Blackhall MI, O'Donnell SR. A dose–response study of inhaled terbutaline administered via nebuhaler or nebuliser to asthmatic children. *Eur J Respir Dis* 1987; 71: 96-101.

30 Freelander M, Van Asperen PP. Nebuhaler versus nebuliser in children with acute asthma. *BMJ* 1984; 288: 1873-4.

31 Noble V, Ruggins NR, Everad ML, Milner AD. Inhaled budesonide via a modified Nebuhaler for chronic wheezing in infants. *Arch Dis Child* 1992; 67: 285-8.

32 Connett GJ, Warde C, Wooler E, Lenney W. Use of budesonide in severe asthmatics aged 1–3 years. *Arch Dis Child* 1993; 69: 351-5.

33 Greenough A, Pool J, Gleeson JG, Price JF. Effect of budesonide on pulmonary hyperinflation in young asthmatic children. *Thorax* 1988; 43: 937-8.

34 Bisgaard H, Munck SL, Nielsen JP, Petersen W, Ohlsson SV. Inhaled budesonide for treatment of recurrent wheezing in early childhood. *Lancet* 1990; 336: 649-51.

35 Bisgaard H, Ohlsson S. PEP-spacer: an adaption for administration of MDI to infants. *Allergy* 1989; 44: 363-4.

36 Gleeson JG, Price JF. Controlled trial of budesonide given by the nebuhaler in preschool children with asthma. *BMJ* 1988; 297: 163-6.

37 Pool JB, Greenough A, Gleeson JG, Price JF. Inhaled bronchodilator treatment via the nebuhaler in young asthmatic patients. *Arch Dis Child* 1988; 63: 288-91.

38 Pedersen S. How to use a rotahaler. *Arch Dis Child* 1986; 61: 11-4.

39 Pedersen S, Steffensen G. Fenoterol powder inhalator technique in children: Influence of inspiratory flow rate and breath-holding. *Eur J Respir Dis* 1986; 68: 207-14.

40 Pedersen S, Hansen OR, Fuglsang G. Influence of inspiratory flow rate upon the effect of a Turbuhaler. *Arch Dis Child* 1990; 65: 308-10.

41 Richards R, Dickson CR, Renwick AG, Lewis RA, Holgate ST. Absorption and disposition kinetics of cromolyn sodium and the influence of inhalation technique. *J Pharmacol Exp Ther* 1987; 241: 1028-32.

42 Rufin P, Benoist MR, de Blic J, Braunstein G, Scheinmann P. Terbutaline powder in asthma exacerbations. *Arch Dis Child* 1991; 66: 1465-6.

43 Bisgaard H, Pedersen S, Nikander K. Use of budesonide Turbuhaler in young children suspected of asthma. *Eur Respir J* 1994; 7: (in press).

44 Pedersen S, Frost L, Arnfred T. Errors in inhalation technique and efficacy of inhaler use in asthmatic children. *Allergy* 1986; 41: 118-24.

45 Pedersen S. Aerosol treatment of bronchoconstriction in children, with or without a tube spacer. *N Engl J Med* 1983; 308: 1328–30.

46 Papo MC, Frank J, Thompson AE. A prospective, randomized study of continuous versus intermittent nebulized albuterol for severe status asthmaticus in children. *Crit Care Med* 1993; 21: 1479–86.

47 Robertson CF, Smith F, Beck R, Levison H. Response to frequent low doses of nebulized salbutamol in acute asthma. *J Pediatr* 1985; 106: 672–4.

48 Portnoy J, Nadel G, Amado M, Willsie-Ediger S. Continuous nebulization for status asthmaticus. *Ann Allergy* 1992; 69: 71–9.

49 Singh M, Kumar L. Continuous nebulized salbutamol and oral once a day prednisolone in status asthmaticus. *Arch Dis Child* 1993; 69: 416–9.

50 Oberklaid F, Mellis CM, Souëf PN, Geelhoed GC, Maccarrone AL. A comparison of a bodyweight dose versus a fixed dose of nebulised salbutamol in acute asthma in children. *Med J Aust* 1993; 158: 751–3.

51 Shapiro GG, Furukawa CT, Pierson WE, Chapko MK, Sharpe M, Bierman CW. Double-blind, dose–response study of metaproterenol inhalant solution in children with acute asthma. *J Allergy Clin Immunol* 1987; 79: 378–86.

52 Janson C, Herala M. Plasma terbutaline levels in nebulisation treatment of acute asthma. *Pulmon Pharmacol* 1991; 4: 135–9.

53 Pedersen S. Treatment strategies for acute asthma in infants and children. *Res Clin Forums* 1993; 15: 55–61.

54 Pedersen S. The importance of a pause between the inhalation of two puffs of terbutaline from a pressurized aerosol with a tube spacer. *J Allergy Clin Immunol* 1986; 77: 505–9.

55 Lonnerholm G, Foucard T, Lindstrom B. Oral terbutaline in chronic childhood asthma; effects related to plasma concentrations. *Eur J Respir Dis* 1984; 65 (suppl 134): 205–10.

56 Morgan DJ. Clinical pharmacokinetics of beta-agonists. *Clin Pharmacokinet* 1990; 18: 270–94.

57 Bohn D, Kalloghlian A, Jenkins J, Edmunds J, Barker G. Intravenous salbutamol in the treatment of status asthmaticus in children. *Crit Care Med* 1984; 12: 892–6.

58 Ahlström H, Svenonius E, Svensson M. Treatment of asthma in children with inhalation of terbutaline Turbuhaler compared with Nebuhaler. *Allergy* 1989; 44: 515–8.

59 Edmunds AT, Godfrey S. Cardiovascular response during severe acute asthma and its treatment in children. *Thorax* 1981; 36: 534–40.

60 Estelle F, Simons R, Gillies JD. Dose response of subcutaneous terbutaline and epinephrine in children with acute asthma. *Am J Dis Child* 1981; 135: 214–7.

61　Ting CK, Liao MH. [A comparative study of epinephrine injection and beta 2-agonist inhalation in the treatment of childhood asthma]. *Acta Paediatr Sin* 1991; 32: 372–81.

62　Kornberg AE, Zuckerman S, Welliver JR, Mezzadri F, Aquino N. Effect of injected long-acting epinephrine in addition to aerosolized albuterol in the treatment of acute asthma in children. *Pediatr Emerg Care* 1991; 7: 1–3.

63　Uden DL, Goetz DR, Kohen DP, Fifield GC. Comparison of nebulized terbutaline and subcutaneous epinephrine in the treatment of acute asthma. *Ann Emerg Med* 1985; 14: 229–32.

64　Lenney W, Evans NAP. Nebulised salbutamol and ipratropium bromide in asthmatic children. *Br J Dis Chest* 1986; 80: 59–65.

65　Lenney W, Milner AD. At what age do bronchodilator drugs work? *Arch Dis Child* 1978; 53: 532–5.

66　O'Callaghan C, Milner AD, Swardbrick A. Paradoxical deterioration in lung function after nebulised salbutamol in wheezy infants. *Lancet* 1986; ii: 1424–5.

67　Tal A, Bavilski C, Yohai D, Bearman JE, Gorodischer R, Moses SW. Dexamethasone and salbutamol in the treatment of acute wheezing in infants. *Pediatrics* 1983; 71: 13–8.

68　Seidenberg J, Mir Y, Von der Hardt H. Hypoxaemia after nebulized salbutamol in wheezy infants: the importance of aerosol acidity. *Arch Dis Child* 1991; 66: 672–5.

69　Ho L, Collis G, Landau LI, Le Souef PN. Effect of salbutamol on oxygen saturation in bronchiolitis. *Arch Dis Child* 1981; 66: 1061–4.

70　Holmgren D, Bjure J, Engstrom I, Sixt R, Sten G, Wennergren G. Transcutaneous blood gas monitoring during salbutamol inhalations in young children with acute asthmatic symptoms. *Pediatr Pulmonol* 1992; 14: 75–9.

71　Yuksel B, Greenough A. Effect of nebulized salbutamol in preterm infants during the first year of life. *Eur Respir J* 1991; 4: 1088–92.

72　Wilkie RA, Bryan MH. Effect of bronchodilator on airway resistance in ventilator-dependent neonates with chronic lung disease. *J Pediatr* 1987; 111: 278–82.

73　Sosulski R, Abbasi S, Bhutani V, Fox W. Physiological effects of terbutaline on pulmonary function of infants with bronchopulmonary dysplasia. *Pediatr Pulmonol* 1986; 2: 269–73.

74　Kao LC, Durand DJ, Nickerson GB. Effects of inhaled metraproterenol and atropine on the pulmonary mechanics of infants with bronchopulmonary dysplasia. *Pediatr Pulmonol* 1989; 7: 74–80.

75　Cabal LA, Lanazabal C, Ramanathan R *et al.* Effects of metraproterenol on pulmonary mechanics, oxygenation and ventilation in infants with chronic lung disease. *J Pediatr* 1987; 110: 116–9.

76 Yuksel B, Greenough A. Effect of nebulized salbutamol in preterm infants during the first year of life. *Eur Respir J* 1991; 4: 1088–92.

77 Kraemer R, Frey U, Sommer CW, Russi E. Short term effect of albuterol, delivered via a new auxiliary device, in wheezy infants. *Am Rev Respir Dis* 1991; 144: 347–51.

78 Prendiville A, Green S, Silverman M. Airway responsiveness in wheezy infants: evidence for functional beta adrenergic receptors. *Thorax* 1987; 42: 100–4.

79 O'Callaghan C, Milner AD, Swarbrick A. Nebulised salbutamol does have a protective effect on airways in children under one year old. *Arch Dis Child* 1988; 63: 479–83.

80 Daugbjerg P, Brenoe E, Forchammer H *et al.* A comparison between nebulized terbutaline, nebulized corticosteroid and systemic corticosteroid for acute wheezing in children up to 18 months of age. *Acta Paediatr* 1993; 82: 547–51.

81 Larsson S, Svedmyr N, Thiringer G. Lack of bronchial beta adrenoceptor resistance in asthmatic patients during long term treatment with terbutaline. *J Allergy Clin Immunol* 1977; 59: 93–100.

82 Bengtsson B, Fagerström PO. Extrapulmonary effects of terbutaline during prolonged administration. *Clin Pharmacol Ther* 1982; 31: 726–32.

83 Deshpande A, McKenzie SA. Short course of steroids in home treatment of children with acute asthma. *BMJ* 1986; 293: 169–71.

84 Connett GJ, Warde C, Wooler E, Lenney W. Prednisolone and salbutamol in the hospital treatment of acute asthma. *Arch Dis Child* 1994; 70: 170–3.

85 Shapiro G, Furukawa CT, Pierson EE, Gardinier R, Bierman CW. Double blind evaluation of methylprednisolone versus placebo for acute asthma episodes. *Pediatrics* 1983; 71: 510–4.

86 Brunette MG, Lands L, Thibidou LP. Childhood asthma: prevention of attacks with short-term corticosteroid treatment of upper respiratory tract infection. *Pediatrics* 1988; 81: 624–9.

87 Tal A, Levy N, Bearman JE. Methylprednisolone therapy for acute asthma in infants and toddlers: a controlled clinical trial. *Pediatrics* 1990; 86: 350–6.

88 Storr J, Barry W, Barrell E, Lenney W, Hatcher G. Effect of a single dose of prednisolone in acute childhood asthma. *Lancet* 1987; i: 879–82.

89 Younger RE, Gerber PS, Herrod HG, Cohen RM, Crawford LV. Intravenous methylprednisolone efficacy in status asthmaticus of childhood. *Pediatrics* 1987; 80: 225–30.

90 Gleeson JG, Loftus BG, Price JF. Placebo controlled trial of systemic corticosteroids in acute childhood asthma. *Acta Paediatr Scand* 1990; 79: 1052–8.

91 FitzGerald JM, Kearon MC. Corticosteroids in acute asthma: results of a meta-analysis. *Am Rev Respir Dis* 1991; 143: 624.

92 Kattan M, Gurwitz D, Levison H. Corticosteroids in status asthmaticus. *Pediatrics* 1980; 96: 596–9.

93 Pierson WE, Bierman CW, Kelly WC. A double blind trial of corticosteroid therapy in status asthmaticus. *Pediatrics* 1974; 54: 282–8.

94 Vichyanond P, Irvin CG, Larsen GL, Szefler SJ, Hill MR. Penetration of corticosteroids into the lung: Evidence for a difference between methylprednisolone and prednisolone. *J Allergy Clin Immunol* 1989; 84: 867–73.

95 Shee CD. Risk factors for hydrocortisone myopathy in acute severe asthma. *Respir Med* 1990; 84: 229–33.

96 Webb MSC, Henry RL, Milner AD. Oral corticosteroids for wheezing attacks under 18 months. *Arch Dis Child* 1986; 61: 15–9.

97 Daugbjerg P, Brenøe E, Forchammer H. A comparison between nebulized terbutaline, nebulized corticosteroid and systemic corticosteroid for acute wheezing in children up to 18 months of age. *Acta Paediatr* 1993; 82: 547–51.

98 Maayan C, Itzhaki T, Bar-Yishay E, Gross S, Tal A, Godfrey S. The functional response of infants with persistent wheezing to nebulized beclomethasone dipropionate. *Pediatr Pulmonol* 1986; 2: 9–14.

99 Carlsen KH, Leegard J, Larsen S, Orstravik I. Nebulised beclomethasone dipropionate in recurrent obstructive episodes after acute bronchiolitis. *Arch Dis Child* 1988; 63: 1428–33.

100 Wilson NM, Silverman M. Treatment of acute episodic asthma in preschool children using intermittent high dose inhaled steroids at home. *Arch Dis Child* 1990; 65: 407–10.

101 Connett G, Lenney W. Prevention of viral-induced asthma attacks using inhaled budesonide. *Arch Dis Child* 1990; 65: 407–10.

102 Ishizaki T, Minegishi A, Morishita M *et al.* Plasma catecholamine concentrations during a 72-hours aminophylline infusion in children with acute asthma. *J Allergy Clin Immunol* 1988; 82: 146–54.

103 Roddick LG, South RT, Mellis CM. Value of combining an oral sympathomimetic agent with oral theophylline in asthmatic children. *Med J Aust* 1979; 118: 153–4.

104 Pedersen S, Sommer B, Nissen P. Treatment of acute asthma in children with a solution of aminophylline given rectally. *Eur J Respir Dis* 1984; 65: 354–61.

105 Pierson W, Bierman C, Stamm S, Van Arsdel P. Double-blind trial of aminophylline in status asthmaticus. *Pediatrics* 1971; 48: 642–6.

106 Pedersen S, Sommer B. Rectal administration of theophylline in aqueous solution. *Acta Paediatr Scand* 1981; 70: 243–6.

107 Carter E, Cruz M, Chesrown S, Shieh G, Reilly K, Hendeles L. Efficacy of intravenously administered theophylline in children hospitalized with severe asthma. *J Pediatr* 1993; 122: 470–6.

108 Barclay J, Whiting P, Mickey M, Addis G. Theophylline–salbutamol interaction: bronchodilator response to salbutamol at maximally effective plasma theophylline concentrations. Br J Clin Pharmacol 1981; 11: 203–8.

109 Fanta C, Rossing T, McRadden E. Treatment of acute asthma: is combination therapy with sympathomimetics and methylxanthines indicated? Am J Med 1986; 80: 5–10.

110 Littenberg B. Aminophylline treatment in severe, acute asthma. JAMA 1988; 259: 1678–84.

111 Hendeles L, Iafrate R, Weinberger M. A clinical and pharmacokinetic basis for the selection and use of slow release theophylline products. Clin Pharmacokinet 1984; 9: 95–135.

112 Sarrazin E, Hendeles L, Weinberger M, Muir K, Riegelman S. Dose-dependent kinetics for theophylline: Observations among ambulatory asthmatic children. J Pediatr 1980; 97: 825–8.

113 Hendeles L, Bighley L, Richardson RH, Hepler CD, Carmichael J. Frequent toxicity from IV aminophylline infusions in critically ill patients. Drug Intell Clin Pharm 1977; 11: 12–8.

114 Barker D. Theophylline toxicity in children. J Pediatr 1986; 109: 538–42.

115 Hendeles L, Weinberger M, Szefler S, Ellis E. Safety and efficacy of theophylline in children with asthma. J Pediatr 1992; 120: 177–83.

116 Tsiu SJ, Self TH, Burns R. Theophylline toxicity: update. Ann Allergy 1990; 64: 241–57.

117 Ellis EF. Theophylline toxicity. Anti-asthma Xanthines and Adenosine. 1985; 352–60.

118 Niemand D, Martiness S, Arvidsson S. Adenosine in the inhibition of diazepam sedation by aminophylline. Acta Anaesthet 1986; 30: 493–5.

119 Gross NJ, Petty TL, Friedman M, Skorodkin MS, Silvers GW, Donohue JF. Dose response to ipratropium as a nebulised solution in patients with chronic obstructive pulmonary disease. A three-center study. Am Rev Respir Dis 1989; 139: 1188–91.

120 Boner AL, Vallone G, De Stefano G. Effect of inhaled ipratropium bromide on methacholine and exercise provocation in asthmatic children. Pediatr Pulmonol 1989; 6: 81–5.

121 Anonymous. Determination of dose–response relationship for nebulised ipratropium bromide in asthmatic children. J Pediatr 1984; 105: 1002–5.

122 Svenonius E, Arborelius M, Wiberg R, Ekberg P. Prevention of exercise-induced asthma by drugs inhaled from metered aerosols. Allergy 1988; 43: 252–7.

123 Reisman J, Galdes-Sebalt M, Kazim F, Canny G, Levison H. Frequent administration by inhalation of salbutamol and ipratropium bromide in the initial management of severe acute asthma in children. J Allergy Clin Immunol 1988; 81: 10–20.

124 Stokes GM, Milner AD, Hodges IGC, Elphick MC, Henry RI. Nebulised therapy in acute severe bronchitis in infancy. *Arch Dis Child* 1983; 58: 279–82.

125 Beck R, Robertson C, Galdès-Sebaldt M, Levison H. Combined salbutamol and ipratropium bromide by inhalation in the treatment of severe acute asthma. *J Pediatr* 1985; 107: 605–8.

126 Phanichyakarn P, Kraisarin C, Sasisakulporn C. Comparison of inhaled terbutaline and inhaled terbutaline plus ipratropium bromide in acute asthmatic children. *Asian Pac J Allergy Immunol* 1990; 8: 45–58.

127 Storr J, Lenney W. Nebulised ipratropium and salbutamol in asthma. *Arch Dis Child* 1986; 61: 602–3.

128 Summers OA, Tarala RA. Bronchodilator efficacy of nebulized ipratropium sequentially and in combination in acute asthma. *Thorax* 1987; 42: 731.

129 Rayner RJ, Cartlidge PHT, Upton CJ. Salbutamol and ipratropium in acute asthma. *Arch Dis Child* 1987; 62: 840–1.

130 Henry RC, Milner AD, Stokes GM. Ineffectiveness of ipratropium bromide in acute bronchiolitis. *Arch Dis Child* 1983; 58: 925–6.

131 Beasley CRW, Rafferty P, Holgate ST. Bronchoconstrictor properties of preservatives in ipratropium bromide (Atrovent) nebuliser solution. *BMJ* 1987; 294: 1197–8.

132 Mann JS, Howarth PH, Holgate ST. Bronchoconstriction induced by ipratropium bromide in asthma: relation to hypotonicity. *BMJ* 1984; 289: 469.

133 Connett GJ, Lenney W. Use of pulse oximetry in the hospital management of acute asthma in childhood. *Pediatr Pulmonol* 1993; 15: 345–9.

134 Greenough A, Pool J, Gleeson JG, Price JF. Effect of budesonide on pulmonary hyperinflation in young asthmatic children. *Thorax* 1988; 43: 937–8.

135 McKenzie SA, Edmunds AT, Godfrey S. Status asthmaticus in children. *Arch Dis Child* 1979; 54: 581–6.

136 Moler FW, Hurwitz ME, Custer JR. Improvement in clinical asthma score and P_aCO_2 in children with severe asthma treated with continuously nebulized terbutaline. *J Allergy Clin Immunol* 1988; 81: 1101–9.

137 Bentur L, Kerem E, Canny G *et al.* Response of acute asthma to a beta-2 agonist in children less than two years of age. *Ann Allergy* 1990; 65: 122–6.

138 Bishop J, Carlin J, Nolan T. Evaluation of the properties and reliability of clinical severity scale for acute asthma in children. *J Clin Epidemiol* 1992; 45: 71–6.

139 Mountain RD, Sahn SA. Clinical features and outcome in patients with acute asthma presenting with hypercapnia. *Am Rev Respir Dis* 1988; 138: 535–9.

140 Pearson MG, Spence DPS, Ryland I, Harrison BD. Value of pulsus paradoxus in assessing acute severe asthma. *BMJ* 1993; 307: 659.

141 Carson JWK, Taylor MRH. Relapse after single dose nebulized salbutamol in children with acute asthma. *Irish Med J* 1985; 78: 93–6.

142 Geelhoed GC, Landau LI, LeSouef PN. Predictive value of oxygen saturation in emergency evaluation of asthmatic children. *BMJ* 1988; 297: 395-6.

143 Bishop J, Nolan T. Pulse oximetry in acute asthma. *Arch Dis Child* 1991; 66: 724-5.

144 Rachelefsky GS, Warner JO. International consensus on the management of pediatric asthma: a summary statement. *Pediatr Pulmonol* 1993; 15: 125-7.

145 Warner JO, Gotz M, Landau LI *et al*. Management of asthma: a consensus statement. *Arch Dis Child* 1989; 64: 1065-79.

146 Nelson DR, Sachs MI, O'Connell EJ. Approaches to acute asthma and status asthmaticus in children. *Mayo Clin Proc* 1989; 64: 1392-402.

147 McWilliams B, Kelly HW, Murphy S. Management of acute severe asthma. *Pediatr Ann* 1989; 18: 774-5, 779.

148 Murphy S, Kelly HW. Management of acute asthma. *Pediatrician* 1991; 18: 287-300.

149 Press S, Lipkind RS. A treatment protocol of the acute asthma patient in a pediatric emergency department. *Clin Pediatr* 1991; 30: 573-7.

150 Henry RL, Robertson CF, Asher I *et al*. Management of acute asthma. Respiratory paediatricians of Australia and New Zealand. *J Paediatr Child Health* 1993; 29: 101-3.

151 Niggemann B, Wahn U. Die Therapie des Status asthmaticus im Kindesalter. *Monatsschr Kinderheilk* 1991; 139: 323-9.

152 Geelhoed GC, Landau LI, LeSouef PN. Oximetry and peak expiratory flow in assessment of acute childhood asthma. *J Pediatr* 1990; 117: 907-9.

153 Zeiger RS, Heller S, Mellon MH, Wald J, Falkoff R, Schatz M. Facilitated referral to asthma specialist reduces relapses in asthma emergency room visits. *J Allergy Clin Immunol* 1991; 87: 1160-8.

154 Chapman KR, Verbeek PR, White JG, Rebuck AS. Effect of short course of prednisone in the prevention of early relapse after the emergency room treatment of acute asthma. *N Engl J Med* 1991; 324: 788-94.

155 Strunk RC. Identification of the fatality-prone subject with asthma. *J Allergy Clin Immunol* 1989; 83: 477-85.

KEY POINTS

1   Acute asthma in children can be managed in many different ways. No two patients or situations are alike and individualization is important.

2   Inhaled β_2 agonists and systemic steroids are the cornerstone in the acute management. Other drugs are additional.

3   It may be difficult clinically to assess the severity of airway obstruction in children. Therefore, objective measurements are important for a correct assessment and monitoring of response to treatment.

4   Young children and infants develop respiratory failure more readily than older children.

5   After initial treatment and stabilization, measures should be taken for preventing future attacks.

29

MANAGEMENT OF CHRONIC ASTHMA IN ADULTS

Frederick E. Hargreave and Romain Pauwels

INTRODUCTION

Under-treatment of asthma has been appreciated for a number of years. It has been evident from unnecessary deaths,[1] hospital admissions[2] and emergency room visits,[3] loss of work[4] or school,[5] disturbance of sleep, limitation of activities and symptoms that should not be present. When treatment has been increased hospital admissions, school absenteeism and clinical abnormalities have decreased.[2,5-7]

Most asthma would appear to be mild as indicated by epidemiological data and by the unimodal distribution of airway hyperresponsiveness.[8] The large majority of asthmatic subjects if appropriately treated should therefore have little or no symptoms, little or no need for inhaled β_2 agonist, no limitation of normal activities, normal or near normal airflow rates at rest, normal flow rates after bronchodilator, normal or near normal diurnal variation of peak expiratory flow rate (PEFR) and no side-effects from medications.

The recognition of under-treatment has resulted in specialists in a number of countries publishing guidelines for the treatment of asthma.[9-12] These cover different aspects of asthma and reflect a consensus opinion. Their aim is to reduce deaths and ill health from asthma and adherence to them has been proposed as a target in practice. While there is general agreement on the principles of treatment, there is some uncertainty and disagreement concerning treatment choices because of gaps in knowledge of how best to monitor the effects of treatment, of the anti-inflammatory actions of commonly used drugs, of what doses of inhaled steroid are most appropriate, of long-term outcomes and of the clinical relevance of side-effects of regular treatment with higher doses of inhaled steroids. None of the existing anti-asthma therapies has yet been shown to modify the natural history of the disease. Recent studies with prolonged use of inhaled steroids demonstrate that this treatment is very effective in suppressing the disease but when stopped, long-lasting remissions are seldom observed.[13]

This chapter reviews the principles of chronic treatment. The approach presented is largely representative of treatment regimens that have been published in the consensus reports. However, it should be remembered that the consensus reports are based on relatively small studies and that the recommended overall approach has never been compared with other therapeutic strategies. Many questions remain unanswered with regard to the rank order of different treatments. Studies on the impact of consensus guidelines on the morbidity and mortality of asthma are ongoing in different parts of the world.

WHAT ARE WE TRYING TO ACHIEVE?

The most widely held view of the pathogenesis of asthma is that it results from an infiltration of the airways with inflammatory cells and this, together with resulting structural changes, cause the clinical features of symptoms, variable airflow obstruction and airway hyperresponsiveness. There is evidence that the inflammation is the primary cause of the clinical condition, is responsible for exacerbations and is an important determinant of both current and future severity.[14] This view implies that optimum treatment must reduce and maintain the inflammatory cell infiltration to a minimum. Such treatment includes the avoidance of causal allergens or chemical sensitizers that cause the inflammation, and the use of medications that prevent or reverse it. If the treatment is successful, symptoms, variable airflow obstruction and airway hyperresponsiveness will be minimal. Furthermore the need for medications that seem only to prevent or reverse airway smooth muscle constriction (or oedema), e.g. bronchodilators, will be least. This view is justified by the demonstration that treatment with anti-inflammatory therapy is more effective than regular bronchodilator therapy[6,15–17] and that this treatment, especially inhaled steroids, reduces both inflammatory cell infiltration in the airways and clinical parameters.[18–20]

OBJECTIVES OF TREATMENT

Success in any sphere of life requires the setting of goals, and the treatment of asthma is no exception. Fortunately, the goals can be limited to three in number and are therefore easy to remember (Table 29.1). The first is to achieve and identify the best results, the second is to maintain this state with a minimum of anti-inflammatory medication, and the third is to treat exacerbations early and effectively to prevent them from becoming severe and to restore best results as quickly as possible. The goals need to be appreciated by both the physician and patient and need to be systematically achieved. If the first goal is not achieved, then the patient will have

TABLE 29.1: *Objectives of treatment*

1. Establish best result
2. Maintain this state with a minimum of medications
3. Treat exacerbations early to prevent them from becoming severe

symptoms, impairment and disability that should not be present. If the second goal is not achieved because too little medication is maintained, then the patient will have recurring exacerbations. If the third goal is not achieved, then exacerbations will be disabling or even fatal.

Best results means least symptoms, least need for inhaled β_2 agonist, best airflow rates, least daily variation of PEFR and least side-effects from medication. The best results achievable differ between patients. However, as most asthma is mild, it seems likely that the best results in most asthmatic patients will be no daily symptoms, no daily need for bronchodilator, normal airflow rates and normal diurnal variation of PEFR. In some people with more severe asthma, however, the best results are not as good. They may still include daily symptoms, daily need for inhaled β_2 agonist, airflow obstruction that is not completely reversed by bronchodilator and abnormal diurnal variation of PEFR. Hence, appreciating the meaning of best results in individual patients is essential to be able to tell when the treatment is sufficient and when to treat exacerbations early and effectively. A trial of a high level of treatment is often needed to characterize the best result.

It is appropriate to emphasize that while symptoms are commonly a sensitive indicator of the presence and severity of asthma, both they and physical examination are imprecise in recognizing the presence and severity of airflow obstruction (see also Chapters 11–13). Measurement of forced expiratory volume in 1 s (FEV_1) or PEFR are required for this purpose[21] and to help identify and maintain the best results from treatment. Guidelines recommend that every physician treating asthma should have, at least, a peak flow meter. There is disagreement about how often a peak flow meter is needed by patients when asthma is mild. However, patients who recognize airflow obstruction poorly, appear to need a lot of medication or have difficulty in achieving the objectives of treatment, including the prevention of severe exacerbations, should own their own peak flow meter. In research, other methods to measure the effects of treatment need investigation. For example, histamine or methacholine airway responsiveness has been recognized to progressively improve when symptoms, FEV_1 and PEFR measurements have plateaued.[6,16] Changes in airway responsiveness are probably an indirect measure of changes in airway inflammatory cell infiltration and progressive improvement may reflect progressive healing. However, these methods can only be used as indirect indices of airway inflammation when the treatments that are used do not have a bronchodilator or functional antagonistic activity. The use of direct and indirect challenging agents may help to discern different mechanisms involved in airway responsiveness.[22] Other more direct markers of airway inflammation also need to be examined in relation to treatment choices. While bronchial biopsies and bronchoalveolar lavage have provided useful information, their invasive nature limits their more widespread application. Relatively non-invasive measurements using peripheral blood and spontaneous or induced sputum are more practical and need further investigation.[23]

ASTHMA TREATMENT PLAN

The treatment plan is directed to achieve the goals of treatment (Table 29.2). The first goal is achieved by avoidance strategies and medications, the second by a trial reduction of anti-inflammatory medication and the third by a written action plan. The patient needs to be educated about treatment. Regular supervision is required initially to achieve the objectives and subsequently at less frequent intervals to check that they are being maintained.

AVOIDANCE STRATEGIES
Allergy to inhaled allergens, especially house-dust mite, is regarded as the commonest cause of asthma (Table 29.3). Occupational chemical sensitizers are also an important cause of asthma in adults. Hence, appropriate investigation by history and allergy skin tests should be part of the investigation of all asthmatic subjects so that avoidance strategies can be introduced appropriately (see Chapter 14). Such avoidance of relevant allergens or occupational sensitizers (see Chapter 31) is the preferred method

---

TABLE 29.2: *Asthma treatment plan*

1. Establish best result by avoidance strategies and medications
2. Maintain this state with minimum of medication. Trial reduction of anti-inflammatory drugs
3. Treat exacerbations early and effectively by a written action plan
4. Educate the patient about treatment
5. Arrange regular supervision

TABLE 29.3: *Asthma: causes of airway inflammation as well as constriction*

Definite	Possible
Allergen	Cigarette smoke
Chemical sensitizer	Gastro-oesophageal reflux
Viral infections	Sinusitis

to reduce symptoms and need for medications and to improve lung functions.[24–27] In persistent asthma the improvement that ensues can be expected to progress over months even when the exposure has been abruptly terminated.

Cigarette smoking is a cause of airway inflammation with different characteristics to asthma and smoking by parents increases asthma symptoms and airway hyperresponsiveness in their children. Parental smoking has also been shown to be associated with a higher prevalence of asthma in high-risk children.[28] If parents are aware that smoke will aggravate their child's asthma, they will be exposed to fewer cigarettes, and the asthma will be less severe.[29] Cessation of smoking should therefore be encouraged in patients and family members in the home of patients.

Asthma is commonly associated with nasal conditions such as rhinitis, nasal polyps and sinusitis. Nasal corticosteroid treatment of rhinitis can improve asthma symptoms and airway hyperresponsiveness.[30] This observation suggests that the optimum treatment of asthma should include appropriate treatment of rhinitis (see also Chapter 39).

Agents that can cause dangerously severe airway constriction (apparently without inflammatory cell infiltration) also need to be carefully avoided when these are relevant (Table 29.4). For example, β blockers should be avoided in all asthmatic subjects, and non-steroidal anti-inflammatory drugs (including acetylsalicylic acid), sulphites and monosodium glutamate when the patient is intolerant to them. Stimuli that cause constriction are usually not dangerous, such as irritant dust or fumes, and can be avoided less stringently. One of these stimuli is exercise, which should *not* be avoided and can be used as an indicator of the effectiveness of treatment (see also Chapter 34). When asthma is optimally treated, exercise should have little or no effect and even vigorous exercise as in sports should not be limited.

TABLE 29.4: *Asthma: causes of constriction only*

Dangerous	Less dangerous
β Blocker	Exercise
Non-steroidal anti-inflammatory drugs	Cold air
	Hyperventilation
Sulphites	Irritants
Monosodium glutamate	Odours
	Pollution
	Emotional upset

AN APPROACH TO THE USE OF MEDICATIONS

Most patients with asthma need treatment with medications as well as by avoidance strategies. The medications currently available to treat asthma can be considered in two groups: those that prevent or reverse the inflammatory cell infiltration of asthma and those that prevent or reverse airway constriction. The former include corticosteroids, cromoglycate and nedocromil (see Chapters 15 and 16) and, of these, corticosteroids are the most effective and have both prevention and reversal effects. Furthermore, corticosteroids are the only drugs demonstrated to reduce inflammatory cell counts in the airways.[18–20] Cromoglycate and nedocromil prevent the allergen-induced late asthmatic response and heightening of methacholine airway responsiveness at 24 hours and, because these are associated with eosinophil infiltration into the airways, they are considered to prevent the inflammatory cell infiltration.[31,32] However, there has been no direct confirmation of this action except for a decrease in airway mucous eosinophils after prolonged treatment with cromoglycate.[33] Cromoglycate and nedocromil also prevent airway constriction to a number of stimuli including allergens, exercise and cold air. Ketotifen is a potent H_1 antagonist with moderate anti-asthma effects.[34] Its inhibitory effect on inflammatory cell infiltration of the airways has only been shown in experimental animals. β Agonists (either short or long acting) and theophylline prevent and reverse airway constriction (see Chapter 19). There is no evidence yet that they prevent or reverse airway inflammatory cell infiltration, although they may influence other components of the inflammation such as oedema.[20,35,36]

Delivery of medications by inhalation is generally preferred because inhaled drugs are more effective, are not absorbed when given orally and cause fewer side-effects (see Chapter 20). Potential side-effects of inhaled steroids need to be minimized by using the smallest effective dose, using a valved spacer when corticosteroids are delivered by pressurized inhaler, and by rinsing the mouth with water and spitting out the water after steroid delivered by a powder inhaler.[37,38]

It is useful to bracket the use of medications into four levels (Table 29.5). Level 1 involves no regular anti-inflammatory medication. Levels 2–4 include regular anti-inflammatory drugs in increasing amounts. In each level an inhaled short-acting β_2 agonist is used for transient symptomatic relief. The use of short-acting β_2 agonists only when needed has three advantages. First, it allows identification of the best result from anti-inflammatory treatment; when this is achieved, the need for β_2 agonists will be the *least*. Second, the as-needed use provides a sensitive early indicator of an exacerbation of inflammation – the usual need for β_2 agonists will increase.[39] Finally, the non-regular use avoids the possible adverse effects of the regular use of β_2 agonists particularly in higher doses, which include aggravation of asthma[40] and a decrease in the protective effect against airway constriction.[41]

Level 1 treatment is only appropriate for the patient in whom the best results are achieved without regular anti-inflammatory medication. Here an inhaled short-acting β_2 agonist can be used to reverse infrequent (not daily) symptoms. This or cromoglycate or nedocromil can be used prophylactically just before non-sensitizing stimuli that cause airway constriction, e.g. more strenuous exercise or cold air. Cromoglycate or nedocromil can also be used prophylactically just before unavoidable exposure to an allergen to which the patient is sensitized. Short- or long-acting β_2 agonists should probably not be used for the latter purpose since their very effective inhibitory effect on the allergen-induced early response may prolong the exposure and result in a more severe late asthmatic response.

The levels of treatment should not be considered as a gradual approach. Rather, the appropriate level of treatment is indicated by the current

---

TABLE 29.5: *Asthma: levels of medication*

Level 1	Inhaled β_2 agonist when needed ± cromoglycate or nedocromil (before provocation only)
Level 2	Add low dose inhaled steroid, or regular cromoglycate or nedocromil
Level 3	High-dose inhaled steroid[a]
Level 4	Add ingested steroid[a]

[a] Consider added cromoglycate, nedocromil, long-acting β_2 agonist, theophylline or ipratropium.

severity of the clinical features and the level of treatment that the patient is already taking. If the patient has symptoms and the best results have not previously been identified, then a trial of additional anti-inflammatory treatment is indicated. Enough anti-inflammatory medication is used initially to achieve the best result. For example, if the patient has been on no regular anti-inflammatory treatment, symptoms are mild and FEV_1 or PEFR are normal or near normal, Level 2 (or 3) treatment can be introduced. On the other hand, if the symptoms are more troublesome or the FEV_1 or PEFR is more severely reduced, it may be appropriate to begin treatment with Level 3 or Level 4. Once the best results have been achieved, then the regular anti-inflammatory drug needs to be reduced to identify the minimum required to maintain the best results for long periods of time. Such regular treatment reduces exacerbations, and produces a progressive decrease in airway hyperresponsiveness.[6,16] The latter usually increases again when the steroid is discontinued; however there is one report of prolonged treatment for 1 year where this did not occur, raising the possibility that the chronic inflammatory process can be switched-off, at least temporarily, in some people.[42] The results of other studies are less affirmative and most patients with asthma relapse after discontinuation of their inhaled steroids.

In using regular anti-inflammatory treatment, possible side-effects have to be considered. Inhaled steroid in low doses are considered to be safe even in young children (see also Chapters 15 and 27). Daily doses of up to 600 µg of budesonide, even given for more than 2 years, do not affect linear growth in children.[13,43] However, doses of 800 µg or more of beclomethasone or budesonide (or an equivalent dose of another inhaled steroid) have systemic effects, although the clinical relevance of these is not clear. High doses of inhaled steroids may cause skin bruising and thinning in adults.[44] It is therefore important to weigh clinical benefit against possible side-effects and ensure that long-term regular treatment is with the lowest needed dose.

The place of cromoglycate, nedocromil or ketotifen in regular treatment is more controversial, particularly when treating children. Cromoglycate and nedocromil have virtually no side-effects, with the exception of transient bronchoconstriction and bad taste respectively (see also Chapters 16 and 27). Ketotifen is an antihistamine and has a mild anti-asthmatic effect; however, the evidence that it influences asthmatic inflammation has not been established.[34,35]

If the minimum treatment falls into Levels 3 or 4, where systemic side-effects from regular steroid treatment are possible, then it is appropriate to consider the addition of a third or fourth drug to see if this will have a steroid-sparing effect. This may be another place for a trial of cromoglycate or nedocromil in such patients, to try to reduce the dose of steroid or to reduce symptoms due to recurring bronchoconstriction. The addition of a long-acting bronchodilator may be required when symptoms due to recurrent airway constriction require an inhaled short-acting β_2 agonist three or four times a day or more. These approaches need evaluation in formal clinical trials, including outcomes of airway inflammatory cell infiltration as well as clinical asthma parameters and steroid side-effects.

EARLY AND EFFECTIVE TREATMENT OF EXACERBATIONS

The third objective of the treatment of asthma is to educate patients to recognize exacerbations early so that they are reversed quickly and do not become severe. A written action plan is useful (see Chapters 23 and 24). This should include when, how, and for how long to increase treatment, when to call or see the doctor, and when to go to the hospital emergency room. If the objectives of treatment are successfully achieved, then an emergency visit should never be required.

The time to treat an exacerbation of asthma is as early as possible. Exacerbations are associated with an increase in airway eosinophil cell infiltration. This is often indicated first by an increase in symptoms and need for β_2 agonist.[39] In many patients, a reduction in FEV_1 or PEFR and an increase in diurnal variation of PEFR follows an increase in symptoms. Presumably, this is why treatment based on symptoms may be better than when it is based on changes in PEFR.[46] Early treatment of such exacerbations is usually successful, by increasing the dose of inhaled steroid two- or four-fold until the patient feels back to their best (or PEFR is within 5% of previous best values, when these measurements are required) for a few days. If the patient is already on a higher dose of inhaled steroid (e.g. 2000–4000 μg), additional prednis(ol)one may be required.[47] If the patient is already taking prednis(ol)one, the dose needs to be doubled or increased to at least 30 mg daily, whichever is the lowest.

PATIENT EDUCATION AND REGULAR SUPERVISION

The objectives of the treatment of asthma will not be achieved without attention to measures known to improve compliance (see also Chapter 25). These include an understanding of the objectives of treatment, the meaning of best results or control and the details of the treatment plan. The patient needs to know that asthma can be severe but that treatment is usually effective. The use of medicines needs to be kept as simple as possible, preferably with the use of only two drugs, and with regular treatment only required twice per day. There needs to be a good patient–clinician relationship. Regular supervision is needed, initially to achieve the objectives and educate the patient and subsequently, at less frequent intervals, to ensure that the objectives are maintained. This will require organization of care in general practice. Perhaps this can be developed by interested chest physicians, paediatricians and general practitioners working together to provide good practice in health promotion or asthma clinics.[48]

FUTURE DEVELOPMENTS

The increasing prevalence and awareness of asthma has stimulated both basic and pharmacological research in asthma. Several new approaches to the diagnosis and treatment of this disease are currently under investigation. The use of indices of inflammation in sputum and/or blood may help in the diagnosis of asthma and the differentiation from other obstructive pulmonary diseases. These parameters, when validated, may also be useful in the evaluation of the therapeutic effects of new anti-asthma therapy.

The basic and pharmacological research will without any doubt contribute to the understanding of asthma and may result in more effective treatment. It seems predictable that treatment directed at the origins of the sensitization process have the highest chance of inducing long-lasting remissions of the disease. Some of the new approaches are listed in Table 29.6. They may be targeted at the allergen-specific sensitization process, inhibit the development of airway inflammation or interfere with the effector mechanisms responsible for the abnormal airway response in asthma. The introduction of these new therapeutic strategies will help to delineate the essential components in the pathogenesis of bronchial asthma.

TABLE 29.6: *New therapeutic approaches in asthma*

Interfering with sensitization
    Allergen-derived peptides
    Interleukin-4 antagonists or synthesis inhibitors
    IgE-receptor antagonists

Interfering with development of inflammation
    Interleukin-5 antagonists or synthesis inhibitors
    Phosphodiesterase IV inhibitors
    Leukotriene B_4 antagonists
    Cyclosporin analogues

Interfering with effector mechanisms
    Leukotriene D_4 antagonists
    5-Lipoxygenase inhibitors
    Phospholipase A_2 inhibitors
    Leukotriene synthetase inhibitors
    Bradykinin antagonists
    Tachykinin antagonists
    Phosphodiesterase III inhibitors
    Potassium channel agonists

REFERENCES

1 Jackson R, Sears MR, Beaglehole R, Rea HH. International trends in asthma mortality: 1970–1985. *Chest* 1988; 94: 914-9.

2 Mayo PH, Richman J, Harris HW. Results of a programme to reduce admissions for adult asthma. *Ann Intern Med* 1990; 112: 864-71.

3 Dales RE, Kerr PE, Schweizer I *et al*. Asthma management preceding an emergency department visit. *Arch Intern Med* 1992; 152: 2041-4.

4 Burney PGJ. Strategy for asthma. *BMJ* 1991; 303: 571-3.

5 Speight ANP, Lee DA, Hey EN. Underdiagnosis and undertreatment of asthma in childhood. *BMJ* 1983; 286: 1253-6.

6 Van Essen Zandvliet EE, Hughes MD, Waalkens HJ, Duiverman EJ, Pocock SJ, Kerrebijn KF. Effects of 22 months of treatment with inhaled corticosteroids and/or beta-2-agonists on lung function, airway responsiveness, and symptoms in children with asthma. *Am Rev Respir Dis* 1992; 146: 547-54.

7 Haahtela T, Jarvinen M, Kava T *et al*. Comparison of beta2-agonist, terbutaline, with an inhaled corticosteroid, budesonide, in newly detected asthma. *N Engl J Med* 1991; 325: 388-92.

8 Cockcroft DW, Berscheid BA, Murdock KY. Unimodal distribution of bronchial responsiveness to inhaled histamine in a random human population. *Chest* 1983; 83: 751-4.

9 Woolcock A, Rubeinfeld AF, Seale JP *et al*. Asthma management plan. *Med J Aust* 1989; 151: 650-3.

10 Hargreave FE, Dolovich J, Newhouse MT. The assessment and treatment of asthma: a conference report. *J Allergy Clin Immunol* 1990; 85: 1098-111.

11 Guidelines on the management of asthma. *Thorax* 1993; 48: S1-S24.

12 Sheffer ALE. International Consensus Report on Diagnosis and Management of Asthma. *Eur Respir J* 1992; 5: 601-41.

13 Van Essen-Zandvliet EEM. *Long-term intervention in childhood asthma.* Erasmus University, Rotterdam, 1993.

14 Hargreave FE, Ramsdale EH, Kirby JG, O'Byrne PM. Asthma and the role of inflammation. *Eur J Respir Dis* 1986; 69 (suppl 147): 16-21.

15 Haahtela T, Jarvinen M, Kava T *et al*. Comparison of a beta2-agonist, terbutaline, with an inhaled corticosteroid, budesonide, in newly detected asthma. *N Engl J Med* 1991; 325: 388-92.

16 Juniper EF, Kline PA, Vanzieleghem MA, Ramsdale EH, O'Byrne PM, Hargreave FE. Effect of long-term treatment with an inhaled corticosteroid on

airway hyperresponsiveness and clinical asthma in non-steroid dependent asthmatics. *Am Rev Respir Dis* 1990; 142: 632–6.

17 Cherniak RM, Wasserman SI, Ramsdell JW *et al.* A double blind multicentre group comparative study of the efficacy and safety of nedocromil sodium in the management of asthma. *Chest* 1990; 97: 1299–306.

18 Djukanovic R, Wilson JEW, Britten KM *et al.* Effect of an inhaled corticosteroid on airway inflammation and symptoms in asthma. *Am Rev Respir Dis* 1992; 22: 669–74.

19 Jeffery PK, Godfrey RW, Adelroth E, Nelson F, Rogers A, Johansson SA. Effects of treatment on airway inflammation and thickening of basement membrane reticular collagen in asthma – a quantitative light and electron microscopic study. *Am Rev Respir Dis* 1992; 145: 890–9.

20 Laitinen LA, Laitinen A, Haahtela T. A comparative study of the effects of an inhaled corticosteroid, budesonide, and a beta2-agonist, terbutaline, on airway inflammation in newly diagnosed asthma: a randomized, double-blind, parallel-group controlled trial. *J Allergy Clin Immunol* 1992; 90: 32–42.

21 Connolly CK. FEV_1 and peak flow: Wright and the mini-meters. *Respir Med* 1992; 86: 451–3.

22 Pauwels R, Joos G, Van Der Straeten M. Bronchial hyperresponsiveness is not bronchial hyperresponsiveness is not bronchial asthma. *Clin Allergy* 1988; 18: 317–21.

23 Hargreave FE, Popov T, Kidney J, Dolovich J. Sputum measurements to assess airway inflammation in asthma. *Allergy* 1993; 48: 81–3.

24 Platts-Mills TAE, Mitchell EB, Nock P, Tovey ER, Moszoro H, Wilkins SR. Reduction of bronchial hyperreactivity during prolonged allergen avoidance. *Lancet* 1982; ii: 675–8.

25 Chan-Yeung M, Lam S. Occupational asthma. *Am Rev Respir Dis* 1986; 133: 686–703.

26 Chan-Yeung M, Leriche J, Maclean L, Lam S. Comparison of cellular and protein changes in bronchial lavage fluid of symptomatic and asymptomatic patients with red cedar asthma on follow-up examination. *Clin Allergy* 1988; 18: 359–65.

27 Malo JL, Cartier A, Ghezzo H, Lafrance M, McCants M, Lehrer S. Patterns of improvement in spirometry, bronchial hyperresponsiveness, specific IgE antibody levels after cessation of exposure in occupational asthma caused by snow crab processing. *Am Rev Respir Dis* 1988; 138: 807–12.

28 Arshad SH, Matthews S, Gant C, Hyde DW. Effect of allergen avoidance on development of allergic disorders in infancy. *Lancet* 1992; 339: 1493–7.

29 Murray AB, Morrison BJ. The decrease of severity of asthma in children of parents who smoke since the parents exposing them to less cigarette smoke. *J Allergy Clin Immunol* 1993; 91: 102–10.

30   Watson WTA, Becker AB, Simons FER. Treatment of allergic rhinitis with intranasal corticosteroids in patients with mild asthma – effect on lower airway responsiveness. J Allergy Clin Immunol 1993; 91: 97-101.

31   Altounyan REC. Review of clinical activity and mode of action of sodium cromoglycate. Clin Allergy 1980; suppl 10: 481-9.

32   Busse WW, Orr TSC, Pauwels R. International symposium on nedocromil sodium. Drugs 1989; 37: 1-137.

33   Diaz P, Galleguillos FR, Gonzalez MC, Pantin CFA, Kay AB. Bronchoalveolar lavage in asthma: the effect of disodium cromoglycate (cromolyn) on leukocyte counts, immunoglobulins, and complement. J Allergy Clin Immunol 1984; 74: 41-8.

34   Medici TC, Radielovic P, Morley J. Ketotifen in the prophylaxis of extrinsic bronchial asthma. Chest 1990; 96: 1252-7.

35   Tattersfield AE. Long-acting beta2-agonists. Clin Exp Allergy 1992; 22: 600-5.

36   Pauwels R. New aspects of the therapeutic potential of theophylline in asthma. J Allergy Clin Immunol 1989; 83: 548-53.

37   Keeley D. Large volume plastic spacers in asthma. BMJ 1992; 305: 598-9.

38   Selroos O, Halme M. Effect of a volumatic spacer and mouth rinsing on systemic absorption of inhaled corticosteroids from a metered dose inhaler and dry powder inhaler. Thorax 1991; 46: 891-4.

39   Gibson PG, Wong BJO, Hepperle MJR et al. A research method to induce and examine a mild exacerbation of asthma by withdrawal of inhaled corticosteroid. Clin Exp Allergy 1992; 22: 525-32.

40   Sears MR, Taylor DR, Pruit CG et al. Regular inhaled beta-agonist treatment in bronchial asthma. Lancet 1990; 336: 1391-6.

41   O'Connor BJ, Aikman SL, Barnes PJ. Tolerance to the non-bronchodilator effects of inhaled beta2-agonists in asthma. N Engl J Med 1992; 327: 1204-8.

42   Juniper EF, Kline PA, Vanzieleghem MA, Hargreave FE. Reduction of budesonide after a year of increased use: a randomised controlled trial to evaluate whether improvements in airway responsiveness and clinical asthma are maintained. J Allergy Clin Immunol 1991; 87: 483-9.

43   Wolthers OD, Pedersen S. Controlled study of linear growth in asthmatic children during treatment with inhaled glucocorticosteroids. Pediatrics 1992; 89: 839-42.

44   Mak VHF, Melchor R, Spiro SG. Easy bruising as a side-effect of inhaled corticosteroids. Eur Respir J 1992; 5: 1068-74.

45   Bousquet J, Godard P, Michel FB. Antihistamines in the treatment of asthma. Eur Respir J 1992; 5: 1137-42.

46   Charlton I, Charlton G, Broomfield J, Mullee MA. Evaluation of peak flow and symptoms only self-management plans for control of asthma in general practice. BMJ 1990; 301: 1355-9.

47 O'Driscoll BR, Kalra S, Wilson M, Pickering CAC, Carroll KB, Woodcock A. Double-blind trial on steroid tapering in acute asthma. *Lancet* 1993; 341: 324–7.

48 Barritt PW. General practitioners and asthma. *Thorax* 1992; 47: 669–70.

KEY POINTS

1   The main asthma guidelines are similar but the methods of assessment and treatment are chiefly based on expert opinion and require validation by clinical trials.

2   The treatment of asthma requires that the physician and patient understand the goals of treatment and how to achieve them.

3   Treatment is primarily directed to reverse and prevent airway inflammation.

4   An important component is avoidance of causes of airway inflammation and constriction.

30

GUIDELINES FOR MANAGEMENT OF ACUTE ASTHMA IN ADULTS

Brian D. W. Harrison

INTRODUCTION

Since 1989 there has been an explosion of national and international guidelines on the management of acute asthma in adults.[1-6] The British Thoracic Society and associated royal colleges and other specialty societies have contributed twice to this explosion, in 1990, when the first "Guidelines on the Management of Asthma in Adults" were published,[2] and in 1993 when the "Revised Guidelines on the Management of Asthma" were published.[5,6] The aims of this chapter are to describe what stimulated the publication of these guidelines and what the various groups hoped to achieve with them; how they were developed and produced; to summarize the important messages contained in the guidelines; and to describe their use for auditing the care of adults developing an acute deterioration of their severe asthma.

REASONS FOR PRODUCING THE GUIDELINES

PREVENTABLE MORTALITY AND MORBIDITY FROM ASTHMA

During the late 1970s and early-to-middle 1980s there was a progressive increase in deaths from asthma seen in all ages[7] (see Chapter 1). Repeated studies during the last two decades[8-17] have consistently shown that there are preventable factors associated with over 80% of these deaths (Table 30.1). Despite asthma being the commonest chronic disease affecting all age groups in developed countries, management of the severe episode far too often remains poor despite the availability of effective anti-inflammatory and bronchodilator medication. Published studies and clinical experience have also shown that it is very rare for patients admitted to hospital for their asthma to die under the care of a respiratory physician and team. Furthermore patients admitted to hospital for treatment of an acute severe

TABLE 30.1: *Preventable factors identified in studies of asthma deaths*

Underestimation of severity by doctor – usually because of
  failure to make objective measurements

Underestimation of severity by patient or relative

Under-treatment with systemic steroids

Psychosocial factors

Inappropriate therapy

Failure to recognize and treat deterioration weeks or months
  before fatal attack

episode of asthma have usually experienced a deterioration in the control of their asthma for days, or even weeks, before the admission.[18-20] Patients discharged from hospital following an episode of asthma that has been treated by a team which includes a respiratory physician have significantly reduced morbidity in the weeks and months after discharge than patients looked after by a team including no respiratory specialist[21] (Table 30.2).

The implications of these observations are that effective anti-inflammatory and bronchodilator drugs are available for managing acute severe asthma and preventing the majority of deaths but they are not being used appropriately. Furthermore none of the new drugs being developed for managing asthma is likely to have any impact whatsoever on the management of acute severe asthma[22-24] (see Chapter 18). As the editor wrote in *Thorax* in 1978: "The major problem in asthma today is the education of the profession about the disease".[25] Up until 1989 there had been no attempts to produce consensus statements or guidelines on the management of asthma aimed at general practitioners and general physicians.

DEFINITIONS AND RECOMMENDATIONS FOR PRODUCING GUIDELINES

Clinical guidelines have been defined as "systematically developed statements which assist in decision making about appropriate health care for specific clinical conditions".[26] This distinguishes guidelines from protocols, which require specific action and cover the detailed development of the principles contained in guidelines for local application.[26-28] Guidelines are thus usually national or international in origin, while protocols are usually produced locally to help clinicians in their day-to-day practice. The Scottish group also state that a multidisciplinary approach to the development and

TABLE 30.2: *Suboptimal management of asthma in non-chest wards. (From Ref. 21 with permission)*

	General ward with respiratory specialist input ($n = 86$) (%)	General ward without respiratory specialist input ($n = 64$) (%)
Treatment with oral steroids	83	67
Regular peak flow recordings made	73	42
Return appointments made	92	56
Regular inhaled therapy increased on discharge	55	28
Sleep disturbance at 13 days after discharge	23	41
Morning chest tightness 13 days after discharge	37	55
Re-admission within 1 year	2	20

dissemination of guidelines is essential and strongly commends it.[26] This means that the group developing the guidelines should include specialists, both academic and non-academic, generalists, both from hospital and general practice, other relevant health care professionals and patients.[29] Guidelines should not be formulated and handed down from on high, solely by academics and experts. Such guidelines will not gain acceptance by doctors looking after the majority of patients, away from the academic departments and centres of excellence.

Debate continues about the level of quality of care that guidelines should aim to achieve: *minimal acceptable*; *optimal*, in which current knowledge and experience are balanced against the constraints of available facilities and resources; or *ideal*, in which constraints are disregarded and ideal conditions assumed. Since most physicians and other health care professionals strive for excellence and aim to achieve the best possible care for their patients and since most recognize that there are finite constraints, guidelines should aim to achieve optimal performance.[26] Obviously, this need not prevent local or national pressure for more resources.

Clinical guidelines are based on research where it is available and accepted best practice where it is not.[27,30] Frequently, guidelines contain more of the latter than the former. This serves to highlight areas for future research and certainly focuses attention on areas where there is disagreement about best practice.[27,30] Therefore, guidelines should stimulate research and not fossilize practice and should always list areas of uncertainty or controversy.[27] The implication of this is that guidelines are relevant to the time when they are produced but may rapidly become outdated. For these reasons clinical guidelines must be revised regularly.[30]

The Institute of Medicine in the USA has given useful recommendations on the format of guidelines.[26] These include:

- a short one to two page summary of the principal recommendations;

- a structure shown by bold type, subheadings, and other highlighting techniques;

- attractive typeface and graphic aids;

- uncluttered layout;

- listing of other sources of information that might be helpful.

Guidelines may be difficult and costly to develop but their implementation is usually even more difficult and more costly. "The measure of a guideline is not the elegance of its logic but by how much it improves patient care."[26] The importance of ownership by the group expected to implement the optimal practice has already been discussed. It is also essential for the development of the guidelines to be, and to be seen to be, independent of commercial organizations, including pharmaceutical companies.

The motivation for producing guidelines includes improving all practice to optimal level, reducing variation in practice and an attempt to reduce the costs of care, particularly the costs of ineffective or inappropriate care.[26,29,31]

There are six ways of changing physicians' practices: education, feedback, participation by physicians in efforts to bring about change, administrative rules, financial incentives and financial penalties.[32] Clinical guidelines, protocols and audit incorporate education, feedback, participation by physicians in efforts to bring about change and administrative rules.

Finally, audit is an essential component of quality assurance and the potential for using guidelines in audit should be an integral part of the development of those guidelines.

COMPARISON OF GUIDELINES FOR MANAGING ACUTE SEVERE ASTHMA IN ADULTS

This is summarized in Table 30.3. The process of producing the British Guidelines has been fully described recently.[33]

CONTENT OF THE REVISED GUIDELINES

ACUTE SEVERE ASTHMA
The charts on acute severe asthma in adults are reproduced in Figs 30.1–30.3.

Management of an acute exacerbation of asthma begins with the recognition of uncontrolled asthma, acute severe asthma or life-threatening asthma (Fig. 30.1). Acute severe asthma is reflected by the presence of one or more of the following: breathlessness that prevents the completion of a sentence in one breath; tachypnoea ($\geq 25\,min^{-1}$); tachycardia ($\geq 110\,min^{-1}$); or peak expiratory flow rate (PEF) of 50% or less of predicted or best. Life-threatening features are indicated by PEF < 33% predicted or best, a silent chest, cyanosis, feeble respiratory effort, bradycardia, hypotension, exhaustion, confusion or coma. Very severe attacks are also suggested by hypoxia ($P_a o_2 < 8\,kPa$), a normal or elevated $P co_2$ or a low pH.

Treatment of uncontrolled asthma is summarized in Fig. 30.1, which includes guidance for nebulized β_2-agonist therapy, use of systemic or increased inhaled steroid medication and criteria for hospital admission. Immediate treatment of acute severe asthma consists of high-flow oxygen, high doses of inhaled β agonists and systemic corticosteroids. If life-threatening features are present, then nebulized ipratropium and/or intravenous bronchodilators are added. Subsequent management (Fig. 30.2) is determined by progress and response to treatment monitored by repeated PEF measurements, repeated oximetry aiming for an oxygen saturation above 92% and, if necessary, repeated blood gas measurements. Indications for transfer to the intensive care unit are given in Fig. 30.2. Not all such patients will require ventilation, but those with worsening hypoxia or hypercapnia, drowsiness or unconsciousness and those who have had a respiratory arrest require intermittent positive pressure ventilation.[5] Intubation in such patients is very difficult and should ideally be performed

TABLE 30.3: *Comparison of groups involved in producing guidelines for management of acute severe asthma.*

	Number of participants	Specialists/ generalists	Journal	Length in pages	Reference
Canadian	30	Specialists	Specialist	14[a]	1
British	36	Both	General	4	2
American	46	Both	Specialist	109[a]	3
International	19	Specialists	Specialist	72[a]	4
British	39	Both	General	24[a] and 4	5, 6

[a] Include guidelines for children and for chronic persistent asthma.

FIGURE 30.1: *Acute severe asthma in adults in general practice. (From Ref. 5 with permission.)*

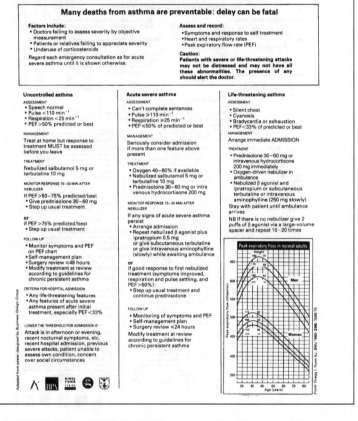

by an experienced anaesthetist.[5] Recommendations for management just before and after discharge from hospital are also given in Fig. 30.2.[5]

COMPARISON BETWEEN THE BRITISH GUIDELINES AND THE INTERNATIONAL CONSENSUS REPORT

The similarities between the British (Figs 30.1–30.3) and the International (Figs 30.4 and 30.5), and indeed the Canadian and US, guidelines[1-6] are

FIGURE 30.2: *Acute severe asthma in adults. (From Ref. 5 with permission.)*

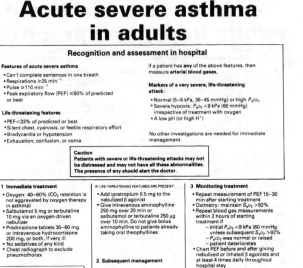
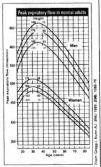

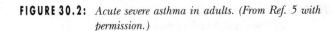

more impressive and more important than their differences. Indeed, the overall agreement is extremely reassuring.

IMPORTANT DIFFERENCES

Participants and Length of the Guidelines

The International Consensus Report was produced by experts in the management of asthma, most of whom were professors or based in academic

FIGURE 30.3: *Asthma in accident and emergency departments. (From Ref. 5 with permission.)*

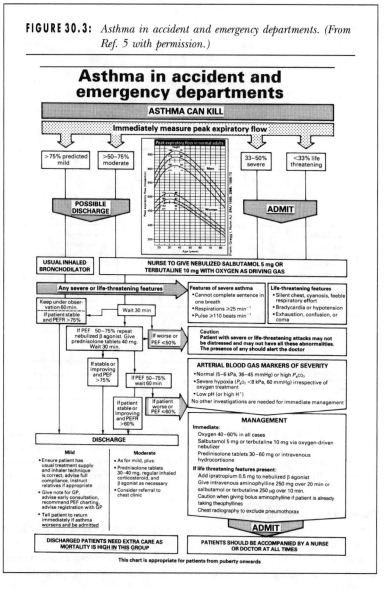

Asthma in accident and emergency departments

ASTHMA CAN KILL

Immediately measure peak expiratory flow

This chart is appropriate for patients from puberty onwards

---

centres. The participants in the British Guidelines covered a much broader spectrum of clinical practice with physicians ranging from academic professors to generalists in hospital and family medicine. The International Report was three times as long as the British Guidelines (Table 30.3) and, although it has been published three times, as a publication of the National Institutes of Health, in *Clinical and Experimental Allergy*[4] and the *European*

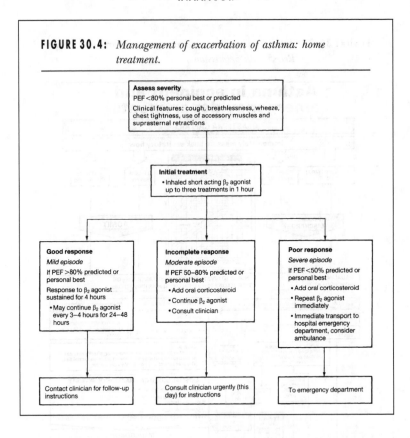

FIGURE 30.4: *Management of exacerbation of asthma: home treatment.*

Respiratory Journal, it is only likely to be read by specialists in the management of asthma. The shorter British Guidelines have been published in a general medical journal,[2,6] they have been posted to every general practitioner in Britain and the summary charts have been developed into plasticised posters that are available from the National Asthma Campaign.

Objective Measurements of Airway Calibre

The British Guidelines concentrate on PEF, giving a chart of predicted normal values. The International Report includes the forced expiratory volume in 1 s (FEV_1) as an alternative to PEF. Spirometry is a measurement that is not available to the majority of physicians treating patients with asthma.

Definition of Severity of Asthma Exacerbations

One figure combining mild, moderate and severe asthma with imminent respiratory arrest severity for both adults and children is included in the International Report. The British Guidelines produced separate charts for acute severe asthma in adults (Fig. 30.2), acute severe asthma in children,

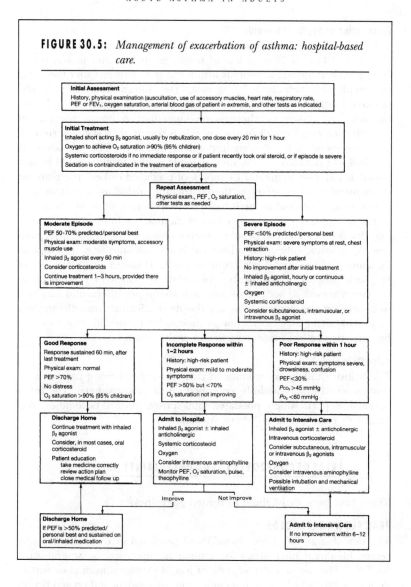

FIGURE 30.5: *Management of exacerbation of asthma: hospital-based care.*

Initial Assessment
History, physical examination (auscultation, use of accessory muscles, heart rate, respiratory rate, PEF or FEV_1, oxygen saturation, arterial blood gas of patient *in extremis*, and other tests as indicated

Initial Treatment
Inhaled short acting β_2 agonist, usually by nebulization, one dose every 20 min for 1 hour
Oxygen to achieve O_2 saturation ≥90% (95% children)
Systemic corticosteroids if no immediate response or if patient recently took oral steroid, or if episode is severe
Sedation is contraindicated in the treatment of exacerbations

Repeat Assessment
Physical exam., PEF , O_2 saturation, other tests as needed

Moderate Episode
PEF 50-70% predicted/personal best
Physical exam: moderate symptoms, accessory muscle use
Inhaled β_2 agonist every 60 min
Consider corticosteroids
Continue treatment 1–3 hours, provided there is improvement

Severe Episode
PEF <50% predicted/personal best
Physical exam: severe symptoms at rest, chest retraction
History: high-risk patient
No improvement after initial treatment
Inhaled β_2 agonist, hourly or continuous ± inhaled anticholinergic
Oxygen
Systemic corticosteroid
Consider subcutaneous, intramuscular, or intravenous β_2 agonist

Good Response
Response sustained 60 min, after last treatment
Physical exam: normal
PEF >70%
No distress
O_2 saturation >90% (95% children)

Incomplete Response within 1–2 hours
History: high-risk patient
Physical exam: mild to moderate symptoms
PEF >50% but <70%
O_2 saturation not improving

Poor Response within 1 hour
History: high-risk patient
Physical exam: symptoms severe, drowsiness, confusion
PEF <30%
P_{CO_2} >45 mmHg
P_{O_2} <60 mmHg

Discharge Home
Continue treatment with inhaled β_2 agonist
Consider, in most cases, oral corticosteroid
Patient education
take medicine correctly
review action plan
close medical follow up

Admit to Hospital
Inhaled β_2 agonist ± inhaled anticholinergic
Systemic corticosteroid
Oxygen
Consider intravenous aminophylline
Monitor PEF, O_2 saturation, pulse, theophylline

Admit to Intensive Care
Inhaled β_2 agonist ± anticholinergic
Intravenous corticosteroid
Consider subcutaneous, intramuscular or intravenous β_2 agonists
Oxygen
Consider intravenous aminophylline
Possible intubation and mechanical ventilation

Improve   Not Improve

Discharge Home
If PEF is >50% predicted/personal best and sustained on oral/inhaled medication

Admit to Intensive Care
If no improvement within 6–12 hours

acute severe asthma in adults in general practice (Fig. 30.1) and asthma in accident and emergency departments (Fig. 30.3) (appropriate for patients from puberty onwards). Each of these charts is much simpler than the International Report chart and designed for use where and when the patient with severe asthma is seen.[26,30]

Prescription of Systemic Steroids

The British Guidelines recommend oral or intravenous steroids in patients seen with a PEF of 50% or less of predicted or best and in less severe "uncontrolled" asthma in patients whose PEF is 75% or less after the initial treatment with nebulized β_2 agonist. The International Report recommends repeated treatment up to three times in 1 hour with high-dose nebulized β_2 agonist. If there is no immediate response, the patient recently took oral steroids or the episode is severe, then systemic steroids are recommended. If following initial nebulization the PEF is between 50 and 70% of predicted or best, then systemic corticosteroids should be *considered*. If PEF rises to greater than 80% of predicted or best, there are no recommendations concerning steroid therapy, including no recommendation to start or double the inhaled steroid therapy dose. Furthermore, in the management of exacerbations of asthma, the International Guidelines list the treatment to be administered concurrently in the order: oxygen, β_2 agonists, ephedrine, additional bronchodilators, e.g. ipratropium or aminophylline, and lastly corticosteroids. These small differences of emphasis may be important when physicians or patients are reluctant to use systemic steroids because of their well-known side-effects and may lead to a delay in the patient receiving the most effective anti-inflammatory treatment during an exacerbation of their asthma. After all, severe exacerbations often reflect inadequate action at the onset.

Pulse Oximetry

The British Guidelines recommend that all wards receiving patients with acute severe asthma should be equipped with a pulse oximeter. The International Report, which pre-dated the revised British Guidelines, recommends pulse oximetry "where available".

AREAS OF CONTROVERSY AND UNCERTAINTY (Table 30.4)

These have been highlighted in revised guidelines.

PEAK FLOW THRESHOLDS

The view that a PEF of less than 33% of predicted or best reflects a very severe life-threatening attack of asthma is supported by several studies.[19,35-38] The use of a PEF of 50% or less of predicted normal or best to define a severe attack, though included in the Canadian and revised British Guidelines,[1,5] is not supported by any clinical scientific study. However, the British audit of 766 patients admitted to hospital with acute severe asthma provides some empirical support for this figure, since the median PEF on admission was 40% of the best achieved by the patient whilst still in hospital.[39] Clearly, using PEF thresholds expressed as a percentage of predicted normal or best is only valid for patients whose best PEF approaches their predicted normal when they are well and in remission. These guidelines,

> **TABLE 30.4:** *Some areas of uncertainty. (From Ref. 5 with permission)*
>
> PEF thresholds for recognizing acute severe asthma, life-
> threatening asthma and for recommending hospital
> admission
> Role of ipratropium bromide
> Role of intravenous aminophylline
> Role of oxygen saturation measurements in reducing need for
> arterial gas measurement
> PEF diurnal variability criterion for appropriateness for
> discharge from hospital

therefore, do not apply to many patients who have a combination of smoking-induced and asthmatic airways obstruction, or to that group of usually elderly patients with asthma who develop a greater or lesser degree of fixed airways narrowing.

ROLE OF IPRATROPIUM BROMIDE

Most[40–43] but not all[44,45] short-term (up to 4 hours) studies have shown measurably faster recovery in patients with severe asthma treated with combined nebulized β_2 agonist and ipratropium than in those treated with nebulized β_2 agonist alone. One study found significantly greater bronchodilation at 6–24 hours and at 48 hours after admission in patients given the combination.[46] Since most patients recover rapidly and satisfactorily with oxygen, systemic steroids and nebulized β_2-agonist treatment alone, the addition of nebulized ipratropium is recommended only in patients whose asthma is very severe or life-threatening when they are first seen or who deteriorate or fail to improve rapidly when treated with the standard regimen.[5]

ROLE OF INTRAVENOUS AMINOPHYLLINE

Some[47] but not all[48] studies seem to show an advantage when intravenous aminophylline is added to subcutaneous or nebulized β_2 agonists in the management of asthma in patients seen in the emergency room. These were both short-term studies and included patients whose pre-treatment function and rapid response to treatment indicates that their asthma was not particularly severe. Some[48] but not all[47,49] studies have shown more adverse effects when aminophylline is added. On the basis of experience and published evidence it seems reasonable to include intravenous aminophylline in the initial treatment of very severe life-threatening asthma and in the patient who has not responded to initial treatment with oxygen, nebulized β_2 agonist and systemic steroid therapy.[5]

ROLE OF OXYGEN SATURATION MEASUREMENTS

The potential for using oxygen saturation measurements to reduce the need for arterial puncture and blood gas measurement has been reported in one study of 89 patients admitted to hospital with acute severe asthma. The authors concluded that blood gases are not required if the patient's arterial saturation measured by pulse oximetry is 92% or higher, since only 5% of patients with saturations in this range had P_aO_2 or P_aCO_2 values in the respiratory failure range, and none of these patients was either severely hypoxaemic or hypercapnic.[50]

DIURNAL VARIABILITY OF PEF

Guidelines recommend that patients should not be discharged from hospital until their PEF is above 75% of their predicted or best and their diurnal variability, i.e.

$$\frac{\text{highest PEF} - \text{lowest PEF}}{\text{highest PEF} \times 100}$$

in each 24 hours is less than 25%.[2,5] This is based on one published report, which concluded that patients should not be discharged until their PEFR variability was less than 20%.[51] It is hoped that such guidance will result in fewer re-admissions but the importance of hospitalization as opposed to therapy in such patients has not been established.

AUDIT

One of the original intentions of the British Guidelines was to use them as a basis for audit. Using the guidelines as a standard against which to measure practice, audit of all patients admitted with acute severe asthma to 36 hospitals in August and September 1990, and in the same two months a year later, was undertaken and the results of the first audit have just been published.[39] One of the most striking results of this first audit was the difference in care of patients admitted under respiratory physicians compared with those admitted under general physicians (Table 30.5). Several studies had shown this difference before.[21,52,53] They had also shown that practice can be improved but that the quality of care provided by respiratory physicians remains at a higher level than that provided by general physicians.[53,54] This should not be surprising, since it would appear to be unreasonable to expect general physicians whose main subspecialty interest is in a different field to remain abreast of all the literature and advances in the field of asthma care. As a consequence of these observations, the following suggestions have been made.[55]

> (1) All patients admitted to hospital with acute severe asthma should be admitted under the care of a respiratory physician

TABLE 30.5: *Differences between respiratory and non-respiratory physicians' care*

	General physicians ($n = 340$) (%)	Respiratory physicians ($n = 426$) (%)	χ^2 (P)
Patients admitted by general practitioner	40	60	$P < 0.01$
Measurement of PEF on admission	83	89	$P < 0.05$
Measurement of arterial blood gases on admission	58	79	$P < 0.01$
No steroid therapy in first 24 hours	12	6	$P < 0.01$
PEF monitored and recorded on the ward	63	83	$P < 0.01$
PEF variability not measured on ward	32	19	16.6 ($P < 0.001$)
Home management plan not given	94	87	7.6 ($P < 0.005$)
No steroids at all on discharge	10	6	3.98 ($P < 0.05$)
No outpatient appointment made	44	9	124.0 ($P < 0.001$)
Not seen in outpatient department within 2 months of discharge	56	27	64.6 ($P < 0.001$)

or managed according to guidelines agreed by the local respiratory physician and transferred to the care of the respiratory physician on the next full working day.

(2) All patients requiring hospital follow-up as outpatients should be attending respiratory medical clinics and not the clinics of general physicians whose specialty interest is not respiratory medicine.[2,4,56]

A further result of the audit concerns systolic paradox. This was measured in fewer than half the 766 patients in the first audit and was found to be abnormal (10 mmHg or greater) in less than half of those. It was the only abnormal sign of those signs used to define a severe attack in under 5% of the patients.[57] Consequently systolic paradox is not included as a useful sign in recognizing severe asthma in the revised guidelines.[5,6]

THE FUTURE

Further revisions of the guidelines will follow publication of evidence addressing areas of controversy already highlighted[5] and other developments in the management of asthma.

LOCAL GUIDELINES

One important use to which national guidelines can be put is the generation of local guidelines or protocols.[30] This has already happened in several parts of Britain, where the national guidelines have been translated into local dialect for local consumption by general practitioners and hospital physicians. National guidelines allow local physicians to resist the charge that "they would say that, wouldn't they". They add strength to what the local physician may have been trying to achieve already. The production of local guidelines or protocols involves local physicians, paediatricians, general practitioners and nurses. This results in local "ownership" and increases the likelihood of the guidelines being accepted and followed.[26] Local protocols can be displayed on boards or walls in the ward or accident and emergency department.[28]

REFERENCES

1   Hargreaves FE, Dolovich J, Newhouse MT (eds) The Assessment and Treatment of Asthma: A Conference Report. *J Allergy Clin Immunol* 1990; 85: 1098-111.

2   Statement by the British Thoracic Society, Research Unit of the Royal College of Physicians of London, King's Fund Centre, National Asthma Campaign. Guidelines for management of asthma in adults: II – acute severe asthma. *BMJ* 1990; 301: 767-800.

3   National Asthma Education Program, Expert Panel on the Management of Asthma, National Heart, Lung and Blood Institute. Bethesda, Maryland, *J Allergy Clin Immunol* 1991; 88: 425-534.

4   International Consensus Report on the Diagnosis and Management of Asthma. *Clin Exp Allergy* 1992; 22 (suppl): 1-72.

5. Statement by the British Thoracic Society and others. Guidelines on the Management of Asthma. *Thorax* 1993; 48: S1–S24.

6. Guidelines for the Management of Asthma: a summary. *BMJ* 1993; 306: 776–82.

7. Lung and Asthma Information Agency. Trends in asthma mortality. *Factsheet* 92/1.

8. Cochrane GM, Clark TJH. A survey of asthma mortality in patients between ages 35 and 64 in the Greater London hospitals. *Thorax* 1975; 30: 300–5.

9. Macdonald JB, Seaton A, Williams JA. Asthma deaths in Cardiff 1963–74: 90 deaths outside hospital. *BMJ* 1976; 1: 1493–5.

10. Macdonald JB, Macdonald ET, Seaton A, Williams DA. Asthma deaths in Cardiff 1963–74: 53 deaths in hospital. *BMJ* 1976; 2: 721–3.

11. Bateman JRM, Clarke SW. Sudden death in asthma. *Thorax* 1979; 34: 40–4.

12. Ormerod LP, Stableforth DE. Asthma mortality in Birmingham 1975–7: 53 deaths. *BMJ* 1980; 280: 687–90.

13. British Thoracic Association. Death from asthma in two regions of England. *BMJ* 1982; 285: 1251–5.

14. Sears MR, Rea HH, Beaglehoe RG *et al*. Asthma mortality in New Zealand: a two year national study. *N Z Med J* 1985; 98: 271–5.

15. Eason J, Markowe HLJ. Controlled investigation of deaths from asthma in hospitals in the North East Thames Region. *BMJ* 1987; 294: 1255–8.

16. Wareham NJ, Harrison BDW, Jenkins PF, Nicholls J, Stableforth DE. A district confidential enquiry into death due to asthma. *Thorax* 1993; 48: 1117–40.

17. Somerville M, Ryland I, Williams EMI, Pearson MG. Asthma deaths in Mersey in 1989–90. *Thorax* 1993; 48: 420P.

18. Bellamy D, Collins JV. "Acute" asthma in adults. *Thorax* 1979; 34: 36–9.

19. Arnold AG, Lane DJ, Zapata E. The speed of onset and severity of acute severe asthma. *Br J Dis Chest* 1982; 76: 157–63.

20. McDonough BJ, Watkin SW, Hind CRK. Community treatment of worsening asthma symptoms in patients requiring hospital admission. *Thorax* 1994; 49: 388P.

21. Bucknall CE, Robertson C, Moran F, Sevenson RD. Differences in hospital asthma management. *Lancet* 1988; i: 748–50.

22. Barnes PJ. New drugs for asthma. *Eur Respir J* 1992; 5: 1126–36.

23. Weinberger SE. Recent advances in pulmonary medicine. *N Engl J Med* 1993; 328: 1389–97.

24. Holgate ST. New treatments for asthma. Horizons in Medicine No. 3. Royal College of Physicians. *Blackwell Scientific Publications* 1992: 264–76.

25 Seaton A. Editorial. *Thorax* 1978; 33: 1.

26 Clinical Resource and Audit Group. *Clinical Guidelines.* Edinburgh: Scottish Office, 1993.

27 Smith A. In search of consensus. *BMJ* 1991; 302: 800.

28 Grimshaw JM, Russell IT. Effect of clinical guidelines on medical practice: a systematic review of rigorous evaluations. *Lancet* 1993; 342: 1317-22.

29 Kassirer JP. The quality of care and the quality of measuring it. *N Engl J Med* 1993; 29: 1263-5.

30 Pearson MG. Asthma guidelines: who is guiding whom and where to? *Thorax* 1993; 48: 197-8.

31 Farmer A. Medical practice guidelines; lessons from the United States. *BMJ* 1993; 307: 313-7.

32 Greco PJ, Eisenberg JM. Changing physicians practices. *N Engl J Med* 1993; 329: 1271-4.

33 Harrison BDW. Guidelines on the management of asthma in adults. Horizons in Medicine No. 6. Royal College of Physicians of London. Blackwell Scientific Publications 1995 (in press).

34 Neville E, Gribbin H, Harrison BDW. Acute severe asthma. *Respir Med* 1991; 85: 463-74.

35 McFadden ER, Lyons HA. Arterial blood gas tension in asthma. *N Engl J Med* 1968; 278: 1027-32.

36 Rebuck AS, Read J. Assessment and management of severe asthma. *Am J Med* 1971; 51: 788-98.

37 Harrison BDW, Swarbrick ET. Peak flow percentage in asthma. *Lancet* 1971; ii: 494.

38 Nowak RM, Tomlanovich MC, Sarkar DD, Kvale PA, Anderson JJ. Arterial blood gases and pulmonary function testing in acute bronchial asthma. *JAMA* 1983; 249: 2043-6.

39 Pearson MG, Ryland I, Harrison BDW. A national audit of acute severe asthma in adults admitted to hospital. *Quality in Health Care* 1995; 4: 24-31.

40 Ward MJ, Fentem PH, Roderick-Smith WH, Davis D. Ipratropium bromide in acute asthma. *BMJ* 1981; 282: 598-600.

41 Leahy BC, Gomm SA, Cullen SC. Comparison of nebulised salbutamol with nebulised ipratropium bromide in acute asthma. *Br J Dis Chest* 1983; 77: 159-63.

42 Rebuck AS, Chapman KR, Abboud R *et al.* Nebulised anti-cholinergic and sympathomimetic treatment of obstructive airways disease in the Emergency Room. *Am J Med* 1987; 82: 59-64.

43 O'Driscoll BR, Taylor RJ, Horsby MG, Chambers DK, Bernstein A. Nebulised salbutamol with and without ipratropium bromide in acute airflow obstruction. *Lancet* 1989; i: 1418-20.

44 Higgins RM, Stradling JR, Lane DJ. Should ipratropium bromide be added to beta-agonists in treatment of acute severe asthma? *Chest* 1988; 94: 718–22.

45 Summers QA, Tarala RA. Nebulised ipratropium in the treatment of acute asthma. *Chest* 1990; 97: 430–4.

46 Bryant DH. Nebulised ipratropium bromide in the treatment of acute asthma. *Chest* 1985; 88: 24–8.

47 Rossing TH, Fanta CH, McFadden ER. A controlled trial of the use of single versus combined drug therapy in the treatment of acute episodes of asthma. *Am Rev Respir Dis* 1981; 123: 190–4.

48 Siegel D, Sheppard D, Gelb A, Weinberg PF. Aminophylline increases the toxicity but not the efficacy of an inhaled beta-adrenergic agonist in the treatment of acute exacerbations of asthma. *Am Rev Respir Dis* 1985; 132: 283–6.

49 Fanta CJ, Rossing TH, McFadden ER. Emergency room treatment of asthma. Relationships among therapeutic combinations, severity of obstruction and time course of response. *Am J Med* 1982; 72: 416–22.

50 Carruthers D, Harrison BDW. Arterial blood gas analysis or oxgyen saturation in the assessment of acute asthma. *Thorax* 1995; 50: 186–8.

51 Udwadia ZF, Harrison BDW. An attempt to determine the optimal duration of hospital stay following a severe attack of asthma. *J Coll Physicians (Lond)* 1990; 24: 112–4.

52 Osman J, Ormerod LP, Stableforth DE. Management of acute asthma: a survey of hospital practice and comparison between thoracic and general physicians in Birmingham and Manchester. *Br J Dis Chest* 1987; 81: 232–41.

53 Bell D, Layton AJ, Gabbay J. Use of a guideline based questionnaire to audit hospital care of acute asthma. *BMJ* 1991; 302: 1440–3.

54 Baldwin DR, Ormerod LP, Mackay AD, Stableforth DE. Changes in hospital management of acute severe asthma by thoracic and general physicians in Birmingham and Manchester during 1978 and 1985. *Thorax* 1990; 4: 130–4.

55 Harrison BDW, Pearson MG. Audit in acute severe asthma – who benefits. *J R Coll Physicians Lond* 1993; 27: 387–90.

56 Statement by the British Thoracic Society, Research Unit of the Royal College of Physicians of London, King's Fund Centre, National Asthma Campaign. Guidelines for management of asthma in adults: I – chronic persistent asthma. *BMJ* 1990; 301: 651–3.

57 Pearson MG, Spence DPS, Ryland I, Harrison BDW. Value of pulsus paradoxus in assessing acute severe asthma. *BMJ* 1993; 307: 659.

KEY POINTS

1   *Reasons for Developing the Guidelines*
    "The major problem in asthma today is the education of the profession about the disease".[25]

2   *Important Points about Guidelines*
    They should be national, involve a multidisciplinary approach, aim for optimal care, always highlight areas of uncertainty or controversy, be dated and then updated regularly, include a short one to two page summary and facilitate audit.

3   *Management of Acute Severe Asthma*
    Requires *recognition* and *assessment* of the severity based on objective clinical measurements; *treatment* with prednisolone tablets, nebulized β_2 agonists and oxygen (augmented if necessary by intravenous bronchodilators); *monitoring* with repeated PEF and oxygen saturation measurements; and appropriate *discharge planning*.

4   *Recommendations*
    Inpatients with asthma should be cared for by respiratory physicians or according to their local protocols. Asthmatic patients requiring hospital follow-up should only attend respiratory medical clinics.

31

SPECIFIC PROBLEMS: OCCUPATIONAL ASTHMA

Jean-Luc Malo and Moira Chan-Yeung

INTRODUCTION AND DEFINITION

Although interest in occupational diseases has focused primarily on conditions that affect the lung parenchyma, referred to as pneumoconiosis (asbestosis and silicosis being the most common), there is now growing interest in conditions that involve the airways. This includes bronchial cancer, chronic bronchitis and fixed airway obstruction, and asthma. Occupational asthma (OA) is now the most common occupational respiratory ailment.[1,2] In a sentinel-based survey conducted in the UK in 1989, it was estimated that OA represented 26% of all cases of occupational respiratory diseases.

OA can be defined as "a disease characterized by variable airflow limitation and/or airway hyperresponsiveness due to causes and conditions attributable to a particular occupational environment and not to stimuli encountered outside the workplace".[3] Two types of OA are distinguishable by whether or not they appear after a latency period. The usual form develops after a latency period that is necessary for "sensitization", although, in many instances of OA due to low molecular weight agents, the mechanism for sensitization is unknown. Some of the agents causing OA with a latency period can be classified as high or low molecular weight (greater or less than 1000–5000). The principal differences between OA caused by high and low molecular weight agents are listed in Table 31.1. The other form of OA occurs without a latency period and follows exposure(s) to high concentrations of an irritant product.

HOW TO DIAGNOSE OCCUPATIONAL ASTHMA

It is important to remove subjects from exposure to an occupational agent that may be the cause of their asthma.[4] OA can lead to permanent

TABLE 31.1: *Characteristics of high and low molecular weight agents*

	High molecular weight	Low molecular weight
Physical		
Size	< 1000–5000	> 1000–5000
Examples of agents	Proteins, enzymes gums, flour	Isocyanates, white and red cedar
Immunological mechanism		
Humoral mechanism	IgE	Non-IgE
Clinical		
Predisposition	Atopy, smoking (?)	Unknown
Interval between onset of exposure and symptoms	Longer	Shorter
Functional		
Temporal patterns of reaction on specific inhalation challenges	Isolated immediate, dual	Late, atypical
Epidemiological		
Prevalence in high-risk populations	< 5%	> 5%
Model	"Extrinsic asthma"	"Intrinsic asthma"

impairment/disability.[5] Several retrospective studies have shown that the earlier affected workers are removed from exposure to a causal agent present at work, the more likely it is they will recover, if this is going to occur.[6,7] Not diagnosing OA can therefore have a significant impact on respiratory health. A diagnosis of OA has serious social consequences. Workers have to leave their job, which implies a diminished quality of life[8] and financial loss.[9–11] For these reasons, objective evidence in confirming the diagnosis is very important. The various means of diagnosing OA have been reviewed in different guidelines and statements.[12,13] They include the following.

MEDICAL QUESTIONNAIRE

All asthmatic subjects should be questioned as to possible exposure to causal agents at their current or previous workplaces. Asthmatic subjects can be left with permanent asthma after removal from the workplace. The current asthma could therefore result from previous exposure to occupational causal agents. Physicians should be aware that certain workplaces are at high risk of exposing subjects to agents that can cause asthma. They should also have ready access to a databank of causal agents. There are national agencies that offer these services. The most successful one is the French MINITEL system, which gives physicians access to a databank listing causes according to workplaces and agents.[14] Safety data sheets on all products used in the workplace should be obtained from employers and/or from local safety committees. Table 31.2 lists the most frequent causes of OA and the most commonly implicated workplaces.

Clinical questionnaires should be sensitive although, in general, they are not very specific tools.[15] Exposure to a known causal agent at work and the presence of asthma should be sufficient to alert the physician to the possibility of OA even though the temporal relationship between exposure at work and symptoms may seem discordant. Subjects with OA may experience improvement in their symptoms on weekends and vacations, but it is our experience that this occurs at the beginning of the illness only. Once OA is well established, it is sometimes difficult for subjects to notice any significant improvement on these occasions. The possibility of the presence of nasal or conjunctival symptoms should be addressed. Ocular and nasal symptoms often accompany or even precede the occurrence of OA.

IMMUNOLOGICAL TESTING

Atopy, defined as the presence of immediate cutaneous reactivity to at least one of a battery of common inhalant allergens (pollens, house dust, moulds, etc.) is a predisposing factor for OA due to high molecular weight agents, but its positive predictive value is weak.[16,17] Allergy skin tests should not be used to exclude atopic subjects from high-risk workplaces. Skin-prick tests can be done with extracts derived from specific high molecular weight agents. However, the presence of immediate skin sensitivity only is an important first step in demonstrating the presence of sensitization and does not confirm the diagnosis of OA. The target organ, the bronchial tubes in this instance, should be shown to be hyperresponsive. This can be done through the assessment of airway responsiveness (see below). The combination of positive skin tests using a relevant occupational allergen and airway hyperresponsiveness in a subject means that there is a ~80% likelihood of OA.[18]

ASSESSMENT OF AIRWAY RESPONSIVENESS

In order to make a diagnosis of OA, it is important to demonstrate the presence of asthma. Airway hyperresponsiveness can be shown either by assessing the response to bronchodilators if there is airway obstruction, or

TABLE 31.2: *Common agents causing occupational asthma and frequently implicated workplaces*

Agent	Workplace
High molecular weight agents	
Cereals	Bakers, millers
Animal-derived allergens	Animal handlers
Enzymes	Detergent, pharmaceutical, bakers
Gums	Carpet, pharmaceutical
Latex	Health professional
Seafoods	Seafoods processors
Low molecular weight agents	
Isocyanates	Spray painters, insulation, plastics and rubbers, foam
Wood-dusts	Forest workers, carpenters, cabinet makers
Anhydrides	Plastics, epoxy resins users
Amines	Shellac and lacquer handlers, solderers
Fluxes	Electronic workers
Chloramine T	Janitor-cleaners
Dyes	Textile industries
Persulphate	Hairdressers
Formaldehyde, glutaraldehyde	Hospital staff
Acrylate	Adhesive handlers
Drugs	Pharmaceutical companies, health professionals
Metals	Solderers, refiners

by estimating the degree of bronchoconstrictive response to a pharmacological agent. If the worker is still employed, airway responsiveness should be evaluated on a working day after a minimum period of 2 weeks at work, as it may be normal when the subject has not been exposed for a period of time[19] although this is not always the rule.[20] The absence of airway hyperresponsiveness in a subject when still working and exposed to the agent(s) suspected of causing OA virtually excludes OA.

ASSESSMENT OF AIRWAY CALIBRE AND ITS FLUCTUATIONS
As for non-occupational asthma, it is important to assess the degree of airway obstruction serially over time. Serial measurement of peak expiratory flow rates (PEFR) in the diagnosis and management of asthma[21,22] has

been used since the late 1970s.[23] In the investigation of OA, workers are asked to measure and register their PEFR at least four times a day and to record their medication, symptoms and whether they are at work or away from work (Fig. 31.1). Although monitoring of PEFR has been found to have satisfactory sensitivity and specificity in the diagnosis of OA[24,25] several aspects of this method of monitoring have yet to be explored: arithmetic indices to assess fluctuations at work and away from work (graph reading still relies on "eye balling" by expert physicians), compliance, comparison with a more suitable functional index such as forced expiratory volume in 1 s (FEV_1), etc. The availability of portable instruments that can assess FEV_1 as well as PEFR and store the data on computer chips will be very useful in future years.

SPECIFIC INHALATION CHALLENGES

Exposing individuals to the potential causal agent(s) in a hospital laboratory or at the workplace under careful supervision is a good method to confirm OA. This method was first proposed in the 1970s by Pepys et al.[26] However, these tests require the expertise of highly trained personnel and

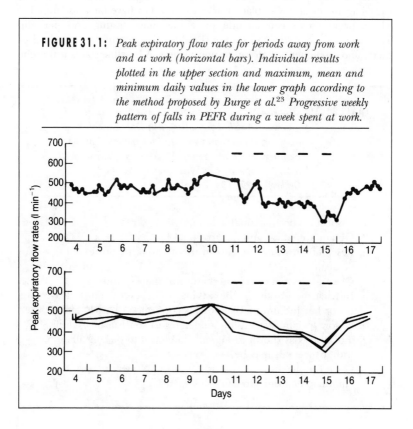

FIGURE 31.1: *Peak expiratory flow rates for periods away from work and at work (horizontal bars). Individual results plotted in the upper section and maximum, mean and minimum daily values in the lower graph according to the method proposed by Burge et al.[23] Progressive weekly pattern of falls in PEFR during a week spent at work.*

can only be done in specialized centres. They should be performed in a dose–response manner, exposing subjects to non-irritant and controlled concentrations of the agent with serial monitoring of FEV_1 in the minutes and hours following exposure.[27] Several patterns of reactions have been described. Isolated immediate and dual reactions occur more commonly after exposure to high molecular weight agents while isolated late reactions or atypical reactions occur as a rule after exposure to low molecular weight agents.[28] These tests have furthered understanding of the mechanism of asthma.

The investigation of OA is a step-wise procedure as shown in Table 31.3 and further illustrated in Fig. 31.2. It can be seen that several methods have to be combined.

SCREENING PROGRAMMES IN HIGH-RISK GROUPS

Physicians may be asked to screen for OA in subjects exposed to known causal agents or at a workplace where cases of OA have been identified.[29] These programmes can include pre-employment testing and periodic assessment. Pre-employment testing should include a questionnaire, spirometry and assessment of airway responsiveness. A baseline status is thereby

---

TABLE 31.3: *Step-wise approach to the assessment of occupational asthma. (Modified from Bernstein DI. Clinical assessment and management of occupational asthma. In: Bernstein IL, Chan-Yeung M, Malo JL, Bernstein DI (eds)* Asthma in the Workplace. *New York: Marcel Dekker, 1993: 103–23)*

1. Suspect an occupational aetiology
2. Obtain a medical and occupational history
3. Research all suspect agents in the medical literature and databank
4. Obtain information on the nature of the exposure
5. Instruct the worker (if the asthma is not severe) not to leave his or her job until a diagnosis is confirmed or excluded
6. Follow specific steps using guidelines to confirm or exclude a diagnosis as shown in Fig. 31.2. Referral to or consultation with a specialist may be necessary
7. Once the diagnosis is confirmed, institute measures to eliminate exposure to causative agent(s)

FIGURE 31.2: *Step-wise scheme for investigating occupational asthma. The white zone corresponds to the investigation that should be carried out in specialized centres whereas the grey zone represents the steps that should be followed by allergologists, pneumologists and internists implicated in the initial step of the investigation. *, Assessed at the end of a working day and after a minimal period of 2 weeks at work. †, The choice depends on the facilities of the investigation centre. (After Ref. 4 with permission.)*

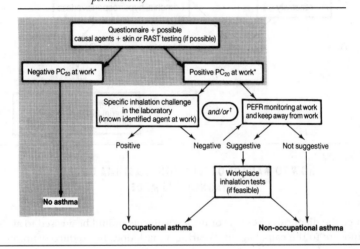

documented. Workers with pre-existing asthma should not be excluded, as there is no reason to believe that asthmatic subjects are more likely to develop OA than anyone else. It is important to measure baseline lung function and the degree of airway responsiveness so that any change can be detected. Figure 31.3 illustrates the steps in the assessment of workers according to the nature of the agent. It is difficult to recommend a frequency for screening assessments. It has been estimated that 40% of subjects with OA due to low molecular weight agents develop their symptoms during the first year of exposure, while the corresponding figure for high molecular weight agents is 20%.[30] After that, there is a progressive reduction in the rate of development of OA. From these findings, it seems advisable to assess subjects in the workplace 1 year after exposure begins and every 2 years thereafter.

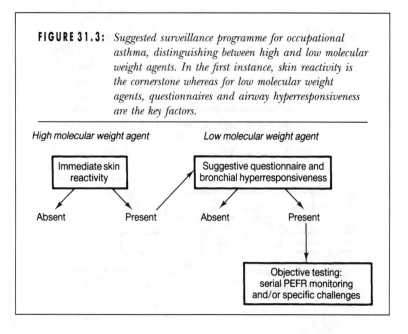

FIGURE 31.3: *Suggested surveillance programme for occupational asthma, distinguishing between high and low molecular weight agents. In the first instance, skin reactivity is the cornerstone whereas for low molecular weight agents, questionnaires and airway hyperresponsiveness are the key factors.*

HOW TO MANAGE OCCUPATIONAL ASTHMA ONCE THE DIAGNOSIS IS MADE

Once the diagnosis of OA is confirmed, subjects should be advised to avoid exposure to the causal agent. Wearing a mask does not reduce symptomatology or functional abnormalities.[31] It is unknown whether treatment with inhaled steroids while keeping the subject at work is justified. On the other hand, in subjects who are unable to leave their job, this measure should be considered. For some, treatment with inhaled steroids coupled with removal from exposure has accelerated recovery.[32] Subjects with OA whose symptoms persist after removal from exposure should be treated in the same way as patients with non-occupational asthma.

Patients with OA should be offered suitable help in finding another job, either with the same employer or another one, provided there is no further exposure to the causal agent (Table 31.4). Subjects aged 55 or over should be offered early retirement, and young subjects should be retrained for a new job, all with financial compensation. Medicolegal agencies should offer these programmes to workers and assess the cost-effectiveness of them. The time needed to make a diagnosis and to instigate a programme is very long, causing hardship to the subjects.[9] Furthermore, it has been estimated that a single case of OA costs approximately C$50 000 in Quebec; such statistics have not been collected to the best of our knowledge in other countries.

TABLE 31.4: *How to manage occupational asthma once the diagnosis is confirmed[a]*

1. Removal from exposure
2. Assess for temporary disability
3. Refer to a rehabilitation programme
   Finding a job with the same employer without exposure to the causal agent
   Finding a job with a different employer without exposure to the causal agent
   Retraining for a new job
   Early retirement
   When a subject cannot change jobs, minimize exposure and treat asthma with anti-inflammatory preparations
4. Treat asthma
5. For those who are unable to change jobs, ensure minimal exposure to the causal agent
6. Assess for permanent disability 2 years after cessation of exposure[b]
   Ensure that asthma is in a stable clinical condition
   Set disability/impairment using the following criteria:
   (a) airway calibre;
   (b) responsiveness to a bronchodilator or a bronchoconstrictive agent;
   (c) need for medication to treat asthma
7. Re-assess periodically if necessary

---

[a] Refer to a medicolegal agency (if not done) or a private insurance programme. The diagnosis should be confirmed as rapidly as possible.
[b] See Ref. 5.

Because OA can lead to permanent impairment/disability, subjects should be re-assessed periodically. The first assessment should take place 2 years after removal from exposure, when a plateau of improvement can occur, as in the case of a high molecular weight agent such as snow-crab.[33] Impairment/disability should be assessed using different tools from those proposed for pneumoconiosis. Impairment is the functional abnormality resulting from a medical condition; disability is the total effect of impairment on a patient's life.[5] The three main criteria for assessing impairment/disability for asthma are: (1) airway calibre; (2) airway responsiveness either to a bronchodilator if airway obstruction is present or a bronchoconstrictor if this is not the case; (3) the need for medication, which is a reflection of the clinical severity of asthma.

A SPECIFIC ENTITY: IRRITANT-INDUCED OA OR REACTIVE AIRWAYS DYSFUNCTION SYNDROME (RADS)

A type of irritant-induced asthma was labelled "RADS" by Brooks et al.[34] It involves the onset of asthma symptoms and the presence of airway hyper-responsiveness in subjects exposed in an acute manner to high concentrations of an occupational irritant product. This can be a single exposure, as proposed by Brooks et al.[34], or multiple exposures, provided that respiratory symptoms occur on each occasion. There seems to be a dose-dependent relationship between exposure and the likelihood of permanent disability/impairment.[35–37] Chlorine and ammonia are common causal agents. Prevention is mandatory in high-risk workplaces where such inhalational accidents can occur. Assessment of methacholine airway responsiveness should also be considered as a pre-employment test so that, if an accident occurs, comparisons are possible.

CONCLUSION

OA is the most common occupational respiratory condition. It is important to diagnose the condition with precision so that proper medical and medicolegal advice can be given. Moreover, screening programmes should be available to workers in high-risk industries. If a worker develops OA, proper compensation, including temporary and permanent impairment/disability through a medicolegal agency or access to private insurance, should be offered.

ACKNOWLEDGEMENTS

The authors wish to thank Katherine Tallman for reviewing the manuscript.

REFERENCES

1. Meredith SK, Taylor VM, McDonald JC. Occupational respiratory disease in the United Kingdom 1989: a report to the British Thoracic Society and the Society of Occupational Medicine by the SWORD project group. Br J Ind Med 1991; 48: 292–8.

2   Lagier F, Cartier A, Malo JL. Statistiques médico-légales sur l'asthme professionnel au Québec de 1986 à 1988. [Medico-legal statistics on occupational asthma in Quebec between 1986 and 1988]. *Rev Mal Respir* 1990; 7: 337-41.

3   Bernstein DI, Bernstein IL, Malo JL, Chan-Yeung M. Definition and classification of asthma. In: Bernstein IL, Chan-Yeung M, Malo JL, Bernstein DI (eds) *Asthma in the Workplace.* New York: Marcel Dekker, 1993: 1-4.

4   Malo JL. The case for confirming occupational asthma: Why, how much, how far? *J Allergy Clin Immunol* 1993; 91: 967-70.

5   American Thoracic Society. Guidelines for the evaluation of impairment/disability in patients with asthma. *Am Rev Respir Dis* 1993; 147: 1056-61.

6   Chan-Yeung M, Lam S, Koener S. Clinical features and natural history of occupational asthma due to western red cedar (*Thuja plicata*). *Am J Med* 1982; 72: 411-5.

7   Hudson P, Cartier A, Pineau L *et al.* Follow-up of occupational asthma caused by crab and various agents. *J Allergy Clin Immunol* 1985; 76: 682-7.

8   Malo JL, Boulet JP, Dewitte JD *et al.* Quality of life of subjects with occupational asthma. *J Allergy Clin Immunol* 1993; 91: 1121-7.

9   Malo JL, Dewitte JD, Cartier A *et al.* Le système québécois d'indemnisation pour asthme professionnel. Description, efficacité et coûts. [The Quebec system of compensation for occupational asthma: description, effectiveness and cost]. *Rev Mal Respir* 1993; 10: 313-23.

10   Marabini A, Dimich-Ward H, Kwan SYL, Kennedy SM, Waxler-Morrison N, Chan-Yeung M. Clinical and socioeconomic features of subjects with red cedar asthma. *Chest* 1993; 104: 821-4.

11   Gannon PFG, Weir DC, Robertson AS, Burge PS. Health, employment, and financial outcomes in workers with occupational asthma. *Br J Ind Med* 1993; 50: 491-6.

12   Bernstein DI, Cohn JR. Guidelines for the diagnosis and evaluation of occupational immunologic lung disease: preface. *J Allergy Clin Immunol* 1989; 84: 791-3.

13   Immunology Subcommittee on Occupational Allergy of the European Academy of Allergology and Clinical Guidelines for the diagnosis of occupational asthma. *Clin Exp Allergy* 1991; 22: 103-8.

14   Perrin B, Dhivert H, Godard P, Bousquet J, Michel FB. The telematic information service (MINITEL) on occupational asthma in France. In: Bernstein IL, Chan-Yeung M, Malo JL, Bernstein DI (eds) *Asthma in the Workplace.* New York: Marcel Dekker, 1993: 635-8.

15   Malo JL, Ghezzo H, L'Archevêque J, Lagier F, Perrin B, Cartier A. Is the clinical history a satisfactory means of diagnosing occupational asthma? *Am Rev Respir Dis* 1991; 143: 528-32.

16　Slovak AJM, Hill RN. Does atopy have any predictive value for laboratory animal allergy? A comparison of different concepts of atopy. Br J Ind Med 1987; 44: 129–32.

17　Venables KM. Epidemiology and the prevention of occupational asthma (editorial). Br J Ind Med 1987; 44: 73–5.

18　Malo JL, Cartier A, L'Archevêque J et al. Prevalence of occupational asthma and immunologic sensitization to psyllium among health personnel in chronic care hospitals. Am Rev Respir Dis 1990; 142: 1359–66.

19　Hargreave FE, Ramsdale EH, Pugsley SO. Occupational asthma without bronchial hyperresponsiveness. Am Rev Respir Dis 1984; 130: 513–5.

20　Chan-Yeung M, Malo JL. Natural history of occupational asthma. In: Bernstein IL, Chan-Yeung M, Malo JL, Bernstein DI (eds) Asthma in the Workplace. New York: Marcel Dekker, 1993: 299–322.

21　Epstein SW, Fletcher CM, Oppenheimer EA. Daily peak flow measurements in the assessment of steroid therapy for airway obstruction. BMJ 1969; 1: 223–5.

22　Turner-Warwick M. On observing patterns of airflow obstruction in chronic asthma. Br J Dis Chest 1977; 71: 73–86.

23　Burge PS, O'Brien IM, Harries MG. Peak flow rate records in the diagnosis of occupational asthma due to colophony. Thorax 1979; 34: 308–16.

24　Côté J, Kennedy S, Chan-Yeung M. Sensitivity and specificity of PC 20 and peak expiratory flow rate in cedar asthma. J Allergy Clin Immunol 1990; 85: 592–8.

25　Perrin B, Lagier F, L'Archevêque J et al. Occupational asthma: validity of monitoring of peak expiratory flow rates and non-allergic bronchial responsiveness as compared to specific inhalation challenge. Eur Respir J 1992; 5: 40–8.

26　Pepys J, Hutchcroft BJ. Bronchial provocation tests in etiologic diagnosis and analysis of asthma. Am Rev Respir Dis 1975; 112: 829–59.

27　Cartier A, Malo JL. Occupational challenge tests. In: Bernstein IL, Chan-Yeung M, Malo JL, Bernstein DI (eds) Asthma in the Workplace. New York: Marcel Dekker, 1993; 215–47.

28　Perrin B, Cartier A, Ghezzo H et al. Reassessment of the temporal patterns of bronchial obstruction after exposure to occupational sensitizing agents. J Allergy Clin Immunol 1991; 87: 630–9.

29　Malo JL. Occupational asthma. In: Hirsch A, Goldberg M, Martin JP, Masse M (eds) Prevention of Respiratory Diseases. Lung Biology in Health and Disease Series, vol. 68. New York: Marcel Dekker, 1993: 117–31.

30　Malo JL, Ghezzo H, D'Aquino C, L'Archevêque J, Cartier A, Chan-Yeung M. Natural history of occupational asthma: Relevance of type of agent and other factors in the rate of development of symptoms in affected subjects. J Allergy Clin Immunol 1992; 90: 937–43.

31 Côté J, Kennedy S, Chan-Yeung M. Outcome of patients with cedar asthma with continuous exposure. *Am Rev Respir Dis* 1990; 141: 373–6.

32 Maestrelli P, Marzo N De, Saetta M, Boscaro M, Fabbri LM, Mapp CE. Effects of inhaled beclomethasone on airway responsiveness in occupational asthma. *Am Rev Respir Dis* 1993; 148: 407–12.

33 Malo JL, Cartier A, Ghezzo H, Lafrance M, Mccants M, Lehrer SB. Patterns of improvement on spirometry, bronchial hyperresponsiveness, and specific IgE antibody levels after cessation of exposure in occupational asthma caused by snow-crab processing. *Am Rev Respir Dis* 1988; 138: 807–12.

34 Brooks SM, Weiss MA, Bernstein IL. Reactive airways dysfunction syndrome (RADS). Persistent asthma syndrome after high level irritant exposures. *Chest* 1985; 88: 376–84.

35 Kennedy SM, Enarson DA, Janssen RG, Chan-Yeung M. Lung health consequences of reported accidental chlorine gas exposures among pulpmill workers. *Am Rev Respir Dis* 1991; 143: 74–9.

36 Kern DG. Outbreak of the reactive airways dysfunction syndrome after a spill of glacial acetic acid. *Am Rev Respir Dis* 1991; 144: 1058–64.

37 Bhérer L, Cushman R, Courteau JP *et al.* A survey of construction workers repeatedly exposed to chlorine over a 3–6 month-period in a pulpmill. II. Follow-up of affected workers with questionnaire, spirometry and assessment of bronchial responsiveness 18 to 24 months after exposure ended. *Occup Environ Med* 1994; 51: 225–8.

KEY POINTS

1 *Occupational Asthma: Definition*
A disease characterized by variable airflow limitation and/or airway hyperresponsiveness due to causes and conditions attributable to a particular occupational environment and not to stimuli encountered outside the workplace.

2 Occupational asthma is the most common occupational respiratory condition. It is important to diagnose the condition with precision so that proper medical and medicolegal advice can be given.

3 Screening programmes for occupational asthma should be available to workers in high-risk industries.

32

SPECIFIC PROBLEMS: ASTHMA INDUCED BY ASPIRIN AND OTHER NON-STEROIDAL ANTI-INFLAMMATORY DRUGS

Barbro Dahlén, Olle Zetterström and
Sven-Erik Dahlén

INTRODUCTION

Aspirin (acetylsalicylic acid) was introduced with considerable success for the treatment of fever and inflammatory disorders in 1899, but a few years later severe intolerance reactions, including life-threatening asthma, were reported among subjects taking therapeutic doses of aspirin.[1-3] Aspirin and other non-steroidal anti-inflammatory drugs (NSAIDs) are today widely used for a number of different indications, from alleviation of common ailments to prevention of cardiovascular fatalities. Therefore, it is important for every physician to be aware of the syndrome of aspirin intolerance. In particular, it is unacceptable that deaths are reported every year to the drug regulatory authorities around the world because of failure to recognize that most NSAIDs may trigger adverse reactions in aspirin-intolerant asthmatic subjects.

CLINICAL MANIFESTATIONS

A typical intolerance reaction occurs within 30 min to 2 hours after intake of an NSAID. Ocular injection, rhinorrhoea and nasal congestion is very common. There may be a heat rash, increased perspiration and flushing on the chest and face. The symptoms from the lower respiratory tract include dry cough and feeling of tightness in the chest. Although auscultation may reveal relatively few rhonchi, the pulmonary function test will generally demonstrate a severe airway obstruction. In addition to the symptoms from the eyes, nose and lungs, the patients often experience fatigue and a general feeling of malaise. The reaction may progress to shock, unconsciousness and respiratory arrest. Sometimes gastrointestinal symptoms including vomiting and diarrhoea occur, and occasionally urticaria or angio-oedema develops. Subjects with chronic urticaria may in addition display isolated intolerance reactions in the skin to ingested NSAIDs, whereas asthmatic subjects preferentially display the more severe respiratory manifestations. However, there is no given sequence of events during an episode of NSAID intolerance; the described symptoms may occur in isolation or combination, and in any order.[4–6]

The first episode of an NSAID intolerance reaction in the airways is often unexpected. However, there is a strong preponderance of rhinitis with recurrent nasal polyposis among those subjects who develop NSAID intolerance, providing the clinical triad of nasal polyposis, asthma and aspirin intolerance.[4,7] Eosinophilia in blood and tissues is often prominent,[8–11] but it can obviously not be considered a specific sign. NSAID intolerance is rare among children, more common among women and usually presents during the second or third decade of life. Typically, intermittent watery rhinitis develops, eventually followed by chronic nasal congestion, recurrent nasal polyposis, sinusitis, loss of ability to smell and finally the appearance of asthma and aspirin intolerance. This course of events may progress during a couple of months or take one or two decades. However, there are also cases where the first intolerance reaction appears to precipitate the onset of asthma and rhinitis. As a further example of the unpredictable nature of this syndrome, there are several patients with an identical clinical picture who apparently never develop aspirin intolerance and, at the opposite end of the spectrum, a few rare patients whose asthma is relieved by aspirin.[12–14]

The prevalence of atopy in aspirin-intolerant patients has been reported to be low[4,15,16] and there are no strong indications of family aggregations of aspirin intolerance,[17] which together with the observation that aspirin intolerance often develops after viral infections[6,18] suggests an acquired disease. Due to the variable clinical picture and the difficulties relating to diagnosis of aspirin intolerance, estimations of the prevalence of aspirin intolerance vary considerably, but most authors have concluded that around 10% of adult asthmatic subjects may belong to this group (reviewed in ref. 6). The information on the epidemiology and natural course of aspirin-induced asthma is incomplete. It is generally agreed that NSAID-intolerant asthmatic subjects display a particularly severe variety of asthma, which often requires chronic treatment with high doses of oral or inhaled glucocorticosteroids (GCS).[5,6,8] However, the association between aspirin intolerance and asthma may not be causal, since desensitization to aspirin appears to have little influence on the clinical course of the airway disease[19] and chronic asthma persists despite careful avoidance of NSAIDs.[4]

DIAGNOSIS

Although NSAID intolerance may be the first presenting symptom, an asthmatic subject with chronic rhinitis and/or recurrent nasal polyposis should always be considered as an individual at risk for development of aspirin intolerance. In the absence of a predictable *in vitro* test, the diagnosis depends upon provocations to demonstrate intolerance towards aspirin and other NSAIDs. Skin tests with aspirin have not been successful[3,15] and may in fact be dangerous if accidental systemic injection occurs.[20] Nasal provocations with lysine-aspirin (a more water-soluble derivative of aspirin) have rather low sensitivity,[21,22] but would be of interest to develop further as an initial screening test. Oral provocations with aspirin have been used for many years to diagnose aspirin-induced asthma,[6,23,24] although the procedure is fairly time-consuming and always associated with significant risk of provoking severe bronchial and/or systemic reactions. In the most cautious protocols, the patient is challenged with increasing doses of aspirin over the course of 3 days,[6] but it has been concluded that oral challenges generally are unsuitable for routine clinical practice. Bronchial provocation with lysine-aspirin was introduced by Bianco *et al.*[25] in 1977 and has been documented to be simpler to perform, less time-consuming and considerably safer than the oral challenge test,[26] presumably because the inhalation challenge produces a reaction limited to the airways.[26] By inhalation of increasing doses of lysine-aspirin, the provocative dose for a 20% decrease (PD_{20}) in forced expiratory volume in 1 s (FEV_1) can be determined in protocols similar to those used for conventional bronchial reactivity testing with histamine or methacholine,[26–28] and the repeatability of the challenge is excellent.[28] Although the reaction to inhaled lysine-aspirin in intolerant individuals in some respects resembles the early reaction to inhaled allergen in atopic asthmatic subjects, it should be noted that the response to aspirin is not followed by a late phase reaction.[27,28]

After a positive provocation response to inhaled or oral aspirin, a state of refractoriness to further doses of aspirin or other NSAIDs follows.[7,25,29,30] The refractory period lasts between 2 and 5 days. As a corollary, desensitization as well as cross-desensitization may be retained provided aspirin is ingested with a maximum interval of 48 hours. Complete sensitivity to aspirin and other NSAIDs reappears about 7 days after the last exposure to these drugs.[29] Therefore, repeated challenges for diagnosis or research purpose should be separated by at least 1 week. Another pitfall that may produce false-negative aspirin provocations is that high doses of GCS may mask aspirin intolerance.[31]

To summarize the diagnostic tests, the inhalation challenge test with lysine-aspirin should be the preferred method to demonstrate aspirin intolerance in the airways. Oral challenge with aspirin should only be used if negative inhalation challenges have been performed but suspicion of extra-pulmonary NSAID intolerance remains. Due to the ability of aspirin intolerance to wax and wane,[5,32,33] it should be remembered that a negative history or challenge test in an asthmatic subject with nasal polyposis never excludes the possibility that the patient in the future will acquire intolerance to NSAIDs.

PATHOPHYSIOLOGY

The mechanisms that create the state of aspirin intolerance in certain individuals remain completely unknown. It is well documented (reviewed in refs 6 and 24) that the common denominator among the NSAIDs that precipitate intolerance reactions is their ability to inhibit the cyclooxygenase enzyme that catalyses the initial step in the formation of prostaglandins (PG) and thromboxane from arachidonic acid (Fig. 32.1). There is no evidence of immunological hypersensitivity reactions towards this large family of structurally unrelated compounds,[15,16] and other alternative hypotheses[7-9] all suffer from a lack of critical experimental support. A great

FIGURE 32.1: *Schematic drawing of the cyclooxygenase (COX) and 5-lipoxygenase (5-LOX) pathways for cellular oxygenation of arachidonic acid. PG, prostaglandin; LT, leukotriene. COX-I and COX-II denote the constitutive and inducible COX isoenzymes, respectively. They catalyse the same reactions, but differ in structure and with respect to kinetics and susceptibility to pharmacologic antagonism (see text and refs 34–36). However, the currently available NSAIDs inhibit both isoenzymes with little practical difference in affinity.*

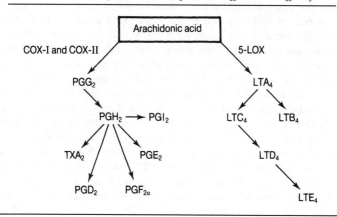

number of findings have firmly established the cyclooxygenase theory orig-inally proposed by Szczeklik et al.[40] Thus, there is a positive correlation between the potency of NSAIDs to induce airway obstruction and the potency of the same drugs as cyclooxygenase inhibitors in vitro.[40,41] In further support of the cyclooxygenase theory, NSAIDs with cyclooxygenase-inhibiting properties always elicit airway obstruction in intolerant subjects, whereas those NSAIDs that do not inhibit cyclooxygenases in therapeutic doses usually are well tolerated.[5,42,43] It was recently shown that the plasma level of acetylsalicylic acid during the development of aspirin-induced bronchoconstriction is in the concentration range known to be required for in vivo inhibition of the cyclooxygenase enzyme.[44] Moreover, after aspirin desensitization, cross-tolerance to other cyclooxygenase inhibitors is also achieved.[29,45]

Although it is clear that cyclooxygenase inhibition is central in the patho-genesis of NSAID intolerance, it is not known which cells are activated during the intolerance reaction to aspirin. In vitro investigations have gen-erally failed to show specific and reproducible metabolic or functional abnormalities in any single population of the great number of different cells that have been collected from aspirin-intolerant asthmatic subjects. In vivo, it has been shown that aspirin challenge is associated with release of histamine,[46] leukotrienes[22,46-50] and, at least during systemic reactions to aspirin, tryptase,[51] together suggesting that the mast cell may be a key effec-tor cell. In this context, it is of considerable interest that a marked over-production of the mast cell metabolite PGD_2, increased histamine excretion and elevated serum tryptase levels were reported in a subset of patients with systemic mastocytosis who had attacks provoked by low doses of aspirin and aspirin-like drugs.[52] The almost anaphylactic nature of the intolerance reactions makes it natural to assume that the mast cell is involved, but its obligatory role has yet to be proved conclusively.

Despite the acknowledged uncertainties concerning several critical steps and the role of different cells in the intolerance reactions to NSAIDs, a number of recent investigations have firmly established that leukotrienes are important mediators of the airway obstruction, and perhaps leukotri-enes mediate also some of the extra-pulmonary manifestations. First, the cysteinyl-leukotrienes (LTC_4, LTD_4 and LTE_4), previously known as the presumed mediator of asthma and hypersensitivity, slow reacting substance of anaphylaxis (SRS-A) (for reviews of biological activities and biochemistry see refs 53–55), are potent inducers of bronchoconstriction in aspirin-intol-erant asthmatic subjects.[56] In fact, there are interesting observations sug-gesting that aspirin-intolerant asthmatic subjects display a specific and unique airway hyperresponsiveness to LTE_4 when compared with other asthmatic subjects.[57] Second, aspirin provocation is associated with increased excretion of cysteinyl-leukotrienes in nasal washings,[22,46] in the urine[47-49] and in bronchoalveolar lavages (BAL).[58] The third, and most definite piece of evidence, is provided by recent investigations which document that pre-treatment with anti-leukotriene drugs provide partial or complete prevention[28,59,60] of the airway obstruction induced by aspirin challenge. Since the leukotriene biosynthesis inhibitor zileuton also attenuated nasal, gastrointestinal and dermal symptoms induced by oral challenge with aspirin,[60] it is possible that leukotrienes also mediate significant components of the extra-pulmonary symptoms in the aspirin-intolerance syndrome.

There are also indications that leukotrienes may be important regulators of baseline bronchomotor tone in aspirin-intolerant asthmatic subjects. First, several independent observations have documented that aspirin-intolerant asthmatic subjects have an over-production of cysteinyl-leukotrienes, expressed as an increased basal (i.e. prior to aspirin challenge) excretion of urinary LTE_4 compared with other asthmatic subjects.[47,48,61] It is known that the basal levels of urinary LTE_4 generally overlap considerably between asthmatic and non-asthmatic subjects,[62] whereas aspirin-sensitive asthmatic subjects have been reported to have basal values of urinary LTE_4 that are significantly (two to five times) higher than those of other asthmatic subjects. Second, the leukotriene receptor antagonist MK-0679 was found to produce a long-lasting baseline bronchodilation in a group of aspirin-intolerant asthmatic subjects[63] (Fig. 32.2). The response varied among the studied individuals, but interestingly correlated directly both with general disease severity and the sensitivity to aspirin in the subjects. More information about the contribution of leukotrienes to the asthma symptoms in aspirin-intolerant subjects will obviously be available when clinical trials with anti-leukotriene drugs have been performed in this group of asthmatic subjects.

The mechanism by which aspirin and other cyclooxygenase inhibitors trigger enhanced dependence upon the leukotriene system remains elusive. It has been speculated that arrested formation of prostaglandin endoperoxides after inhibition of the cyclooxygenase enzyme by NSAIDs would result in shunting of the common substrate arachidonic acid into the leukotriene pathway (Fig. 32.1), but there is no experimental proof of this "shunting hypothesis" and there are theoretical arguments against it. Further, the "shunting hypothesis" does not seem to explain why aspirin-tolerant asthmatic subjects fail to produce more leukotrienes after inhibition of the cyclooxygenase system. One, perhaps more likely, hypothesis assumes that aspirin-intolerant asthmatic subjects are particularly dependent upon one or several continuously produced cyclooxygenase products, which tonically act to inhibit release of mediators from different inflammatory cells. Incidentally, the concentration of PGE_2, which has several anti-inflammatory effects including *in vivo* inhibition of mast cell mediator release,[64] was recently found to be elevated in the airways of aspirin-intolerant asthmatic subjects.[58] The "PGE_2-hypothesis" would thus explain the almost anaphylactic reaction to cyclooxygenase inhibitors as a consequence

FIGURE 32.2: *Basal pulmonary function was followed as FEV_1 in eight ASA-sensitive asthmatic subjects for 12 hours after ingestion of placebo (○) or the leukotriene receptor antagonist MK-0679 (825 mg) (●) on two different occasions in a double-blind cross-over design. Each point represents mean ± SE in the group. The mean maximal improvement in FEV_1 was 18 ± 3.5%, calculated from the peak effect in each individual. For comparison, inhalation of a nebulized solution of salbutamol (2500 μg) produced a 22.8 ± 4.3% improvement of FEV_1 in this group of subjects. Data are expressed as percentage change from baseline FEV_1 (mean of first two recordings upon arrival to clinic) during each study day. The difference between placebo and MK-0679 is significant ($P \leq 0.05$) at all time points except when indicated (ns, not significant, $P > 0.05$). (Modified from Ref. 63 with permission.)*

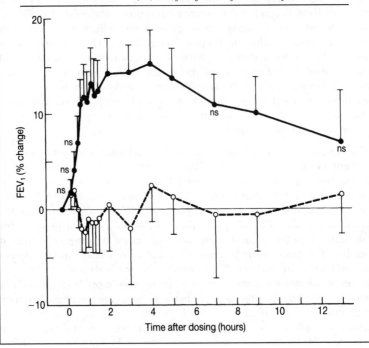

of removal of a brake (PGE_2) that certain individuals (aspirin intolerant) need to control their mediator-producing cells. One could speculate that the induction of the aspirin-intolerant state through viral infections or other factors has altered some key regulatory cell resulting in enhanced production of PGE_2 or increased expression of its receptors. Inhalation of PGE_2 has recently been found to inhibit airway obstruction induced by allergen[65] and exercise,[66] suggesting that the general function of PGE_2 in the airways is to act as a modulator that protects against bronchoconstriction and inflammatory mediators. For unknown reasons, NSAID-intolerant subjects may be especially dependent upon this protection.

Finally in this context, it has recently been discovered[34–36] that there exist at least two cyclooxygenase (COX) isoenzymes, one constitutive (COX-I) that may mediate the physiological functions of the prostaglandins and one (COX-II) that is induced at inflammatory sites and may be the desired target of anti-inflammatory drugs. The present generation of NSAIDs are generally unselective and inhibit both isoenzymes. The findings have created the hypothesis that NSAIDs which are selective for COX-II may have lesser side-effects by preserving gastrointestinal mucosal integrity, platelet and renal function, to mention some of the tissues associated with severe side-effects of NSAIDs in individuals without aspirin idiosyncrasy. It will be of great interest to find out which isoenzyme is involved in aspirin intolerance.

CURRENT TREATMENT STRATEGIES

Treatment of the asthma in NSAID-intolerant individuals follows the general guidelines for treatment of asthma outlined in other chapters. The nasal affliction and in particular the recurrent nasal polyposis requires continuous treatment with topical GCS, and frequently also repeated surgical interventions.

Asthmatic subjects with a history of an episode of unequivocal NSAID intolerance or a previous positive aspirin-provocation test should for the future refrain from using NSAIDs (Table 32.1). It has previously been suggested that there is an association between hypersensitivity to tartrazine and related dyes among aspirin-intolerant subjects, but a large multicentre study showed that this was not the case.[71] Hydrocortisone and in particular its succinate salts have also been reported to elicit adverse reactions among individual aspirin-intolerant asthmatic subjects,[72–75] but a general cross-reactivity between hydrocortisone and NSAIDs could not be confirmed in a recent large population study.[76] Very recently, adverse reactions to biphosphonate was reported among a few aspirin-intolerant asthmatic subjects,[77] but the general importance of this finding remains to be evaluated.

TABLE 32.1: *Effects of some NSAIDs in aspirin-intolerant subjects*

Precipitate intolerance reactions	Well tolerated
Salicylates	Sodium salicylate[a]
Aspirin (acetylsalicylic acid)	Choline salicylate
Diflunisal	Choline magnesium
Salsalate (salicylsalicylic acid)	trisalicylate[a]
Polycyclic acids	Salicylamide
Acetic acids	Dextropropoxyphene
Indomethacin	Benzydamine
Sulindac	Chloroquine
Diclofenac	Paracetamol (acetaminophen)[b]
Tolmetin	
Aryl aliphatic acids	
Naproxen	
Fenoprofen	
Ibuprofen	
Ketoprofen	
Tiaprofenic acid	
Flurbiprofen	
Enolic acids	
Piroxicam	
Tenoxicam	
Fenemates	
Mefenamic acid	
Flufenamic acid	
Cyclofenamic acid	
Pyrazolones	
Aminopyrine	
Noramidopyrine	
Sulphinpyrazone	
Phenylbutazone	
Azapropazone	
Phenazone	
Ketorolac	

[a]Well tolerated in controlled studies, but two cases of bronchoconstriction after sodium salicylate[67,68] and one after choline magnesium trisalicylate[69] have been reported.
[b]Adverse reactions occur in no more than 5% of aspirin-sensitive asthmatic subjeects.[5,70] It is recommended that when beginning therapy, half a tablet should be given under observation for 2–3 hours.

As evident from Table 32.1, when NSAID-intolerant asthmatic subjects need to instil anti-pyretic or analgesic treatment for milder afflictions, paracetamol (acetaminophen), dextropropoxyphene or salicylic acid may be used. (Interestingly, salicylic acid, the immediate metabolite of acetylsalicylic acid is a weak cyclooxygenase inhibitor[78] and is tolerated by NSAID-intolerant subjects.) It has been reported[5,70] that some 5% of NSAID-intolerant asthmatic subjects also react to paracetamol (acetaminophen), but this appears to be a question of dosing, and the likelihood of an intolerance reaction appears insignificant when the dose is less than 1000 mg. In ambiguous cases, it may be advised to give the first doses of paracetamol (acetaminophen) under supervision and to start with a lower than usual dose, e.g. 250 mg. In cases of more severe inflammation, e.g. osteoarthritis or rheumatic diseases, desensitization with aspirin is an alternative that will allow for use of regular NSAIDs. However, this should be performed at specialist centres with considerable experience, and the selected individuals must understand that only a few days of withdrawal of the NSAID may result in a dangerous intolerance reaction if the regular dose is taken again. In severe GCS-resistant inflammation, other alternatives may be treatment with chloroquine, cyclosporin A or methotrexate.

CONCLUSIONS AND PROSPECTS FOR THE FUTURE

By more widespread use of the lysine-aspirin inhalation test, it is hoped that more definite information about the prevalence and clinical course of NSAID intolerance will be obtained in the future. The discovery of cyclooxygenase isoenzymes has the potential to provide further insight into the molecular defects behind the abnormal reaction to NSAIDs in aspirin-intolerant asthmatic subjects and, on a speculative note, perhaps even produce a group of isoenzyme-selective NSAIDs that are tolerated among these patients. The recent indications that cysteinyl-leukotrienes are important and perhaps even the predominant mediators both of spontaneous and aspirin-induced airway obstruction in aspirin-intolerant asthmatic subjects has both diagnostic and therapeutic implications. First, the findings of elevated urinary LTE_4 among NSAID-intolerant asthmatic subjects should be evaluated as a marker to use when screening for NSAID intolerance. Second, since aspirin-sensitive asthmatic subjects as discussed above may display both an over-production and a hyperresponsiveness to cysteinyl-leukotrienes compared with other asthmatic subjects, one could speculate that this subgroup of asthmatic subjects should respond especially well to recently developed anti-leukotriene drugs. It is therefore possible that anti-leukotrienes may provide a new approach in the treatment of aspirin-induced asthma. Irrespective of the outcome of the new exciting basic discoveries relating to NSAID intolerance, it remains important for the practising physician to always remember the clinical triad of rhinitis with nasal polyposis, asthma and aspirin intolerance, and the fact that virtually all NSAIDs produce the sometimes fatal intolerance reactions in the predisposed individuals.

ACKNOWLEDGEMENTS

Barbro Dahlén is supported by grants from the Swedish Heart Lung Foundation and the Swedish Association Against Asthma and Allergy, and Sven-Erik Dahlén's research position is funded by the Swedish Heart Lung Foundation. The research projects from the authors' laboratories have been supported by grants from the Swedish Medical Research Council (project 14X-09071), the Swedish Association Against Chest and Heart Diseases, the Swedish Association Against Asthma and Allergy (RmA), the Swedish National Board for Laboratory Animals (CFN), the Scientific Council of the Swedish Association Against Use of Experimental Animals in Research, the Institute of Environmental Medicine, the Swedish Environment Protection Board (5324069-3), the Swedish Public Health Institute, and Karolinska Institutet.

REFERENCES

1 Hirschberg VGS. Mitteilung über ein Fall von Nebenwirkung des Aspirin. Deutsch Med Wochenschr 1902; 28: 416.

2 Gilbert GB. Unusual idiosyncrasy to aspirin. JAMA 1911; 56: 1262.

3 Cooke RA. Allergy in drug idiosyncrasy. JAMA 1919; 73: 759-60.

4 Samter M, Beers RF. Intolerance to aspirin. Clinical studies and considerations of its pathogenesis. Ann Intern Med 1968; 68: 975-83.

5 Szczeklik A, Gryglewski RJ, Czerniawska-Mysik G. Clinical patterns of hypersensitivity to nonsteroidal anti-inflammatory drugs and their pathogenesis. J Allergy Clin Immunol 1977; 60: 276-84.

6 Stevenson DD, Simon RA. Aspirin sensitivity: Respiratory and cutaneous manifestations. In: Middleton E Jr, Reed CE, Ellis EF, Adkinson NF, Yunginger JW (eds) Allergy, Principles and Practice. St Louis: CV Mosby, 1988: 1537-54.

7 Widal F, Abrami P, Lermoyez J. Anaphylaxie et idiosyncrasie. Presse Med 1922; 30: 189-93.

8 Friedlaender S, Feinberg S. Aspirin allergy: Its relationship to chronic intractable asthma. Ann Intern Med 1947; 26: 734-40.

9 Salén EB, Arner B. Some views on the aspirin-hypersensitive allergy group. *Acta Allergol* 1948; I: 47–84.

10 Godard P, Chaitreull J, Damon M *et al.* Functional assessment of alveolar macrophages: comparison of cells from asthmatics and normal subjects. *J Allergy Clin Immunol* 1982; 70: 88–93.

11 Lumry WR, Curd JG, Zeiger RS, Pleskow WW, Stevenson DD. Aspirin-sensitive rhinosinusitis: the clinical syndrome and effects of aspirin administration. *J Allergy Clin Immunol* 1983; 71: 580–7.

12 Cooke RA. *Allergy in Theory and Practice.* Philadelphia: W.B. Saunders, 1947.

13 Kordansky D, Adkinson F, Norman PS, Rosenthal RR. Asthma improved by non steroidal anti-inflammatory drungs. *Ann Intern Med* 1978; 88: 508–11.

14 Szczeklik A, Nizankowska E. Asthma improved by aspirin-like drugs. *Br J Dis Chest* 1983; 77: 153–8.

15 Schlumberger HD, Löbbecke EA, Kallós P. Acetylsalicylic acid intolerance. Lack of N-acetylsalicylic acid specific, skin-sensitizing antibodies in the serum of intolerant individuals. *Acta Med Scand* 1974; 196: 451–8.

16 Delaney JC, Kay AB. Complement components and IgE in patients with asthma and aspirin idiosyncrasy. *Thorax* 1976; 31: 425–7.

17 Lockey RF, Rucknagel DL, Vanselow NA. Familial occurrence of asthma, nasal polyps and aspirin intolerance. *Ann Intern Med* 1973; 78: 57–63.

18 Szczeklik A. Aspirin-induced asthma as a viral disease. *Clin Allergy* 1988; 18: 15–20.

19 Stevenson DD, Pleskow WW, Simon RA. Aspirin-sensitive rhinosinusitis asthma: a double blind crossover study of treatment with aspirin. *J Allergy Clin Immunol* 1984; 73: 500–7.

20 Storm van Leeuwen W. Pathognomonische Bedeutung der Ueberempfindlichkeit gegen Aspirin bei Asthmatikern. *Münch Med Wschr* 1928; 37: 1588–90.

21 Patriarca G, Nucera E, DiRienzo V, Schiavino D, Pellegrino S, Fais G. Nasal provocation test with lysine acetylsalicylate in aspirin-sensitive patients. *Ann Allergy* 1991; 67: 60–2.

22 Picado C, Ramis I, Rosellò J *et al.* Release of peptide leukotriene into nasal secretions after local instillation of aspirin in aspirin-sensitive asthmatic patients. *Am Rev Respir Dis* 1992; 145: 65–9.

23 Rosenhall L. Evaluation of intolerance to analgesics, preservatives and food colorants with challenge tests. *Eur J Respir Dis* 1982; 63: 410–9.

24 Szczeklik A, Virchow C, Schmitz-Schumann M. Pathophysiology and pharmacology of aspirin-induced asthma. In: Page CP, Barnes PJ (eds) *Handbook of Experimental Pharmacology: Pharmacology of Asthma.* Berlin: Springer-Verlag, 1991: 291–314.

25 Bianco S, Robuschi M, Petrini G. Aspirin-induced tolerance in aspirin-asthma detected by a new challenge test. *IRCS J Med Sci* 1977; 5: 129.

26 Dahlén B, Zetterström O. Comparison of bronchial and per oral provocation with aspirin in aspirin-sensitive asthmatics. *Eur Respir J* 1990; 3: 527–34.

27 Phillips GD, Foord R, Holgate ST. Inhaled lysine-aspirin as a bronchoprovocation procedure in aspirin-sensitive asthma: Its repeatability, absence of late-phase reaction, and the role of histamine. *J Allergy Clin Immunol* 1989; 84: 232–41.

28 Dahlén B, Kumlin M, Margolskee DJ *et al*. The leukotriene-receptor antagonist MK-0679 blocks airway obstruction induced by inhaled lysine-aspirin in aspirin-sensitive asthmatics. *Eur Respir J* 1993; 6: 1018–26.

29 Pleskow WW, Stevenson DD, Mathison DA, Simon RA, Schatz M, Zeiger RS. Aspirin desensitization in aspirin-sensitive asthmatic patients: clinical manifestations and characterization of the refractory period. *J Allergy Clin Immunol* 1982; 69: 11–9.

30 Zeiss CR, Lockey RF. Refractory period to aspirin in a patient with aspirin-induced asthma. *J Allergy Clin Immunol* 1976; 57: 440–8.

31 Nizankowska, E, Szczeklik A. Glucocorticosteroids attenuate aspirin-precipitated adverse reactions in aspirin-intolerant patients with asthma. *Ann Allergy* 1989; 63: 159–62.

32 Pleskow WW, Stevenson DD, Mathison DA, Simon RA, Schatz M, Zeiger RS. Aspirin-sensitive rhinosinusitis/asthma: spectrum of adverse reactions to aspirin. *J Allergy Clin Immunol* 1983; 71: 574–9.

33 Prieto L, Palop J, Castro J, Basomba A. Aspirin-induced asthma in a patient with asthma previously improved by non-steroidal anti-inflammatory drugs. *Clin Allergy* 1988; 18: 629–32.

34 Meade EA, Smith WL, DeWitt DL. Differential inhibition of prostaglandin endoperoxide synthase (cyclooxygenase) isoenzymes by aspirin and other non-steroidal anti-inflammatory drugs. *J Biol Chem* 1993; 268: 6610–4.

35 Masferrer JL, Seibert K, Zweifel B, Needleman P. Endogenous glucocorticoids regulate an inducible cyclooxygenase enzyme. *Proc Natl Acad Sci USA* 1992; 89: 3917–21.

36 O'Neill GP, Ford-Hutchinson AW. Expression of mRNA for cyclooxygenase-1 and cyclooxygenase-2 in human tissues. *FEBS Lett* 1993; 330: 156–60.

37 Capron A, Ameisen JC, Joseph M, Auriault C, Tonnel AB, Caen J. New function for platelets and their pathological implications. *Int Arch Allergy Appl Immunol* 1985; 77: 107–14.

38 Pearson DJ, Suarez-Mendez VJ. Abnormal platelet hydrogen peroxide metabolism in aspirin hypersensitivity. *Clin Exp Allergy* 1990; 20: 157–63.

39 Williams WR, Pawlowicz A, Davies BH. *In vitro* tests for the diagnosis of aspirin-sensitive asthma. *J Allergy Clin Immunol* 1990; 86: 445–51.

40 Szczeklik A, Gryglewski RJ, Czerniawska-Mysik G. Relationship of inhibition of prostaglandin biosynthesis by analgesics to asthma attacks in aspirin-sensitive patients. *BMJ* 1975; 1: 67–9.

41 Stevenson DD, Hougham AJ, Schrank PJ, Goldlust MB, Wilson RR. Salsalate cross-sensitivity in aspirin-sensitive patients with asthma. *J Allergy Clin Immunol* 1990; 86: 749–58.

42 Bianco S, Petrigni G, Felisi E, Robuschi M. Tolerance of guaiacolic ester of acetylsalicylic acid by patients with aspirin-asthma. *Scand J Respir Dis* 1979; 60: 350–4.

43 Szczeklik A, Nizankowska E, Dworski R. Choline magnesium trisalicylate in patients with aspirin-induced asthma. *Eur Respir J* 1990; 3: 535–9.

44 Dahlén B, Boréus LO, Anderson P, Andersson R. Plasma acetylsalicylic acid and salicylic acid levels during aspirin provocation in aspirin-sensitive subjects. *Allergy* 1994; 49: 43–9.

45 Kowalski ML, Grzelewska-Rzymowska I, Rozniecki J, Szmidt M. Aspirin tolerance induced in aspirin-sensitive asthmatics. *Allergy* 1984; 39: 171–8.

46 Ferreri NR, Howland WC, Stevenson DD, Spiegelberg HL. Release of leukotrienes, prostaglandins, and histamine into nasal secretions of aspirin-sensitive asthmatics during reaction to aspirin. *Am Rev Respir Dis* 1988; 137: 847–54.

47 Christie PE, Tagari P, Ford-Hutchinson AW *et al.* Urinary leukotriene E_4 concentrations increase after ASA challenge in ASA-sensitive asthmatic subjects. *Am Rev Respir Dis* 1991; 143: 1025–9.

48 Kumlin M, Dahlén B, Björck T, Zetterström O, Granström E, Dahlén S-E. Urinary excretion of leukotriene E_4 and 11-dehydro-thromboxane B_2 in response to bronchial provocations with allergen, aspirin, leukotriene D_4 and histamine in asthmatics. *Am Rev Respir Dis* 1992; 146: 96–103.

49 Knapp HR, Sladek K, FitzGerald GA. Increased excretion of leukotriene E_4 during aspirin-induced asthma. *J Lab Clin Med* 1992; 119: 48–51.

50 Sladek K, Szczeklik A. Cysteinyl leukotrienes overproduction and mast cell activation in aspirin-provoked bronchospasm in asthma. *Eur Respir J* 1993; 6: 391–9.

51 Bosso JV, Schwartz LB, Stevenson DD. Tryptase and histamine release during aspirin-induced respiratory reactions. *J Allergy Clin Immunol* 1991; 88: 830–7.

52 Roberts LJ II, Sweetman BJ, Lewis RA, Austen KF, Oates JA. Increased production of prostaglandin D_2 in patients with systemic mastocytosis. *N Engl J Med* 1980; 303: 1400–4.

53 Samuelsson B, Dahlén S-E, Lindgren JÅ, Rouzer CA, Serhan CN. Leukotrienes and lipoxins: structures, biosynthesis, and biological effects. *Science* 1987; 237: 1171–6.

54 Lewis RA, Austen KF, Soberman RJ. Leukotrienes and other products of the 5-lipoxygenase pathway. Biochemistry and relation to pathobiology in human diseases. *N Engl J Med* 1990; 323: 645–55.

55　Dahlén S-E. Leukotrienes as mediators of airway obstruction and bronchial hyperresponsiveness. In: Page C, Gardiner PJ (eds) *Airway Hyperresponsiveness: Is it Really Important for Asthma?* Oxford: Blackwell Scientific Publications, 1993: 188–205.

56　Arm JP, O'Hickey SP, Spur BW, Lee TH. Airway responsiveness to histamine and leukotriene E_4 in subjects with ASA-induced asthma. *Am Rev Respir Dis* 1989; 140: 148–53.

57　Christie PE, Schmitz-Schumann, Spur BW, Lee TH. Airway responsiveness to leukotriene C_4 (LTC_4), leukotriene E_4 (LTE_4) and histamine in aspirin-sensitive asthmatic subjects. *Eur Respir J* 1993; 6: 1468–73.

58　Sladek K, Dworski R, Soja J *et al.* Eicosanoids in broncheoalveolar lavage fluid of aspirin-intolerant patients with asthma after aspirin challenge. *Am J Respir Crit Care Med* 1994; 149: 940–6.

59　Christie PE, Smith CM, Lee TH. The potent and selective sulfidopeptide leukotriene antagonist, SK&F 104353, inhibits aspirin-induced asthma. *Am Rev Respir Dis* 1991; 144: 957–8.

60　Israel E, Fischer AR, Rosenberg MA *et al.* The pivotal role of 5-lipoxygenase products in the reaction of aspirin-sensitive asthmatics to aspirin. *Am Rev Respir Dis* 1993; 148: 1447–51.

61　Smith CM, Hawksworth RJ, Thien FCK, Christie PE, Lee TH. Urinary leukotriene E_4 in bronchial asthma. *Eur Respir J* 1992; 5: 693–9.

62　Kumlin M, Stensvad F, Larsson L, Dahlén B, Dahlén S-E. Validation and application of a new simple strategy for measurements of urinary leukotriene E_4 in humans. *Clin Exp Allergy* 1995; 25: 467–79.

63　Dahlén B, Margolskee DJ, Zetterström O, Dahlén S-E. Effect of the leukotriene-antagonist MK-0679 on baseline pulmonary function in aspirin-sensitive asthmatics. *Thorax* 1993; 48: 1205–10.

64　Raud J, Dahlén SE, Sydbom A, Lindbom L, Hedqvist P. Enhancement of acute allergic inflammation by indomethacin is reversed by prostaglandin E_2: Apparent correlation with *in vivo* modulation of mediator release. *Proc Natl Acad Sci USA* 1988; 85: 2315–9.

65　Pavord ID, Wong CS, Williams J, Tattersfield AE. Effect of inhaled prostaglandin E_2 on allergen-induced asthma. *Am Rev Respir Dis* 1993; 148: 87–90.

66　Melillo E, Wooley KL, Manning PJ, Watson RM, O'Byrne PM. Effect of inhaled prostaglandin E_2 on exercise-induced bronchoconstriction in asthmatic subjects. *Am J Respir Crit Care Med* 1994; 149: 1138–41.

67　Park HS, Lim YS, Suh JE, Rhu NS, Cho D III, Kim JW. Sodium salicylate sensitivity in an asthmatic patient with aspirin sensitivity. *J Korean Med Sci* 1991; 6: 113–7.

68　Schäufele A, Schmitz-Schumann M, Virchow JChr Jr, Menz G, Virchow Chr Sr. Eignet sich Natriumsalizylat (NaS) als Protektivum beim Analgetika-asthma-syndrom (AIA)? *Pneumologie* 1990; 44: 371–2.

69 Shudwin DS, Strub M, Golden RE, Frey CDO, Richmond GW, Luskin T. Sensitivity to non acetylated salicylates in a patient with asthma, nasal polyps and rheumatoid arthritis. *Ann Allergy* 1986; 57: 133-4.

70 Settipane RA, Stevenson DD. Cross sensitivity with acetaminophen in aspirin-sensitive subjects with asthma. *J Allergy Clin Immunol* 1989; 84: 26-33.

71 Virchow Ch, Szczeklik A, Bianco S *et al.* Intolerance to tartrazine in aspirin-induced asthma: results of a multicenter study. *Respiration* 1988; 53: 20-3.

72 Partridge MR, Gibson GJ. Adverse bronchial reactions to intravenous hydrocortisone in two aspirin sensitive patients. *BMJ* 1978; 1: 1521-2.

73 Dajani BM, Sliman NA, Shubair KS, Hamzeh YS. Bronchospasm caused by intravenous hydrocortisone sodium succinate (Solu-Cortef) in aspirin-sensitive asthmatics. *J Allergy Clin Immunol* 1981; 68: 201-4.

74 Szczeklik A, Nizankowska E, Czerniawska-Mysik G, Sek S. Hydrocortisone and airflow impairment in aspirin-induced asthma. *J Allergy Clin Immunol* 1985; 76: 530-6.

75 Tanaguchi M, Sato A. Aspirin-induced asthmatics (AIA) have cross-sensitivity with the steroid succinate esters *N Engl Reg Allergy Proc* 1988; 9: 338(A 358).

76 Feigenbaum BA, Stevenson DD, Simon RA. Lack of cross-sensitivity to iv hydrocortisone in subjects with aspirin-sensitive asthma. *ACI News* 1994; suppl 2: 156(A 563).

77 Rolla G, Bucca C, Brussino L. Biphosphonate-induced bronchoconstriction in aspirin-sensitive asthma. *Lancet* 1994; 343: 426-7.

78 Vane JR. Inhibition of prostaglandin synthesis as a mechanism of action for aspirin-like drugs. *Nature New Biol* 1971; 231: 232-5.

KEY POINTS

1 An asthmatic with chronic rhinitis and/or nasal polyposis should always be suspected of being at risk of intolerance to aspirin and other non-steroidal anti-inflammatory drugs.

2 Inhibition of the cyclooxygenase enzyme is the common feature of all drugs that elicit this syndrome and these patients must thus always refrain from using common non-steroidal anti-inflammatory drugs.

3 For treatment of pain, acetaminophen (paracetamol) or dextropropoxyphen, or these in combination should be used.

4   Inhalation challenge with lysine-aspirin, or other non-steroidal anti-inflammatory drugs is the preferred method of confirming a diagnosis of aspirin intolerance. Oral challenge with aspirin is always associated with a risk of severe reactions.

5   Apart from avoidance of NSAIDs, the treatment of subjects with aspirin-induced asthma currently follows the same principles as in aspirin tolerant subjects.

33

SPECIFIC PROBLEMS: ALLERGIC BRONCHOPULMONARY ASPERGILLOSIS

Nicholas Chanarin and Peter H. Howarth

INTRODUCTION

Allergic bronchopulmonary aspergillosis (ABPA) was first reported in 1952.[1] The report described three patients with recurrent episodes of wheezing, eosinophilia, fever and sputum production associated with fleeting shadows on their chest X-ray and bronchial plugging by secretions containing *Aspergillus fumigatus* hyphae. Since then ABPA has become widely recognized with cases reported worldwide. The increase in case recognition appears linked to improved physician awareness, improved diagnostic criteria and to the development of more specific serological techniques.

MYCOLOGY

The fungus *Aspergillus* derives its name from its resemblance to a brush used for sprinkling holy water called an aspergillum.[2] It is a common and widely dispersed organism found in decaying matter: rotting wood chips, fresh-cut grass, compost heaps, potting soil, old hay and fallen leaves. The spores are 3 μm in diameter and dispersed by wind with peak spore counts seen in the autumn and winter. A seasonal trend in exacerbations of ABPA corresponds to these seasons.[3,4] *Aspergillus* is thermotolerant and grows well at 37 °C. It is capable of growing at temperatures between 15 and 53 °C.[2] Its hyphae measure 7–10 mm in diameter and branch at 45° angles.

More than 150 species of *Aspergillus* have been described.[5] The commonest to affect humans is the species *Aspergillus fumigatus* but *Aspergillus niger, Aspergillus flavus* and *Aspergillus terreus* have all been described linked with a syndrome like ABPA.[6,7] In Britain only the species *A. fumigatus* and *A. niger* are commonly found.

The features of ABPA have been described in association with other genera of fungi including *Absidia*,[8] *Candida*,[9–12] *Curvularia*,[13] *Dreschleria*,[14] *Helminthosporium*,[15,16] *Mucor*[17] and *Stemphylia*.[18]

EPIDEMIOLOGY

Following the initial report[1] of ABPA from England in 1952 cases of ABPA have been reported from all major continents. The true prevalence of ABPA remains unknown. In 1968 Henderson *et al.* noted that 20% of asthmatic patients admitted to hospital with chronic pulmonary disease in England may have ABPA.[19] Contemporary estimates suggest a prevalence of ABPA of between 1 and 6% of all asthmatic subjects[20,21] and 10% of all corticosteroid-dependent asthmatic subjects.[22]

PATHOLOGICAL FINDINGS

Pathological changes seen in lung biopsy specimens from patients with ABPA include dilated bronchi containing tenacious mucus and fibrin, as well as features of asthma such as Curschmann's spirals, Charcot–Leyden crystals within the lumen and airways inflammation with eosinophils and mononuclear cells.[23] Fungal hyphae may be seen in the bronchial lumen but do not invade the bronchial wall or parenchyma. Bronchocentric granulomatosis is a relatively common finding and is considered to arise on account of the proximal airway occlusion and sustained inflammatory insult associated with the *Aspergillus* colonization. Consistent with this there is no vasculitis, or deposition of complement or immunoglobulins in the vessel walls. However, there are increased numbers of lymphocytes, monocytes and eosinophils within the airway wall, with evidence of eosinophil activation, indicative of an inflammatory reaction rather than an immune complex-mediated mechanism, at the sites of bronchial wall destruction.[24]

PATHOGENESIS

In ABPA the pathological process remains largely unknown. It is thought that the viscid sputum present in asthmatic subjects (and cystic fibrosis patients) traps *A. fumigatus* spores permitting the thermotolerant fungus to colonize the airways. Once present in a susceptible individual *A. fumigatus* stimulates a vigorous polyclonal antibody response leading to elevated total IgE and specific IgE, IgG and IgA.[25,26] There is evidence from animal models that both IgE and IgG are essential to the pathological process as only animals challenged with both IgE-Af and IgG-Af develop pulmonary infiltrates.[27] The cellular infiltrate in ABPA is rich in eosinophils and mononuclear cells with evidence of T-cell activation. Populations of *A. fumigatus* antigen-specific T cells proliferate *in vitro* on exposure to *A. fumigatus* and are able to stimulate B-cell IgE production *in vitro*[28,29] while T-cell clones to *A. fumigatus* have been shown to recognize *A. fumigatus* antigen.[30] It is thus probable that T-cell activation orchestrates the airway inflammatory events in ABPA, as T lymphocytes have been shown to have increased gene expression for interleukin (IL)-4 and IL-5 in asthma[31] and these cells are also capable of synthesizing IL-3 and granulocyte macrophage colony stimulating factor (GM-CSF). IL-4 promotes IgE synthesis from B cells while IL-3, IL-5 and GM-CSF in concert promote the development of eosinophils from bone marrow progenitors, prime cells for activation and chemotaxis, are chemotactic themselves for eosinophils and prolong eosinophil tissue survival. Airway mast cells have been shown to generate IL-4 and IL-5 in asthmatic subjects[32] but there is no specific evidence for their increased activation in ABPA.[26]

The development of fibrosis in untreated or potentially under-treated disease is a consequence of the intensity of the local airway inflammation secondary to the persistently high IgE levels and presence of antigen. Both the eosinophils and mononuclear cells present at these sites are capable of synthesizing and releasing fibrogenic factors such as transforming growth factor β (TGF-β), platelet-derived growth factor (PDGF) and basic fibroblast growth factor (bFGF).

CLINICAL CHARACTERISTICS AND NATURAL HISTORY

The features of ABPA are the result of a chronic immune-mediated response to the colonizing fungus. Although ABPA classically occurs in asthmatic subjects it may be the first presentation of asthma, can occasionally arise in atopic individuals without asthma and is well described in patients with cystic fibrosis. It may occur at any age and has been described in children as young as 14 months[33] but is rare at the extremes of age. The syndrome is characterized by exacerbations and remissions culminating, if untreated, in widespread pulmonary fibrosis, respiratory failure and death. Five stages are described: (I) acute, (II) remission, (III) exacerbation, (IV) corticosteroid dependent and (V) end-stage lung disease with pulmonary fibrosis.

Patients with stage I disease present with symptoms of fever, malaise, deteriorating or poorly controlled asthma and cough, classically productive of golden brown plugs of sputum. On examination there may be signs of consolidation in the chest. With treatment most patients will progress to remission (stage II). During remission the patient's asthma is easily managed with bronchodilators and regular inhaled steroids. Exacerbations (stage III) can be recognized by a change in asthma severity and the recurrence of symptoms and signs as in stage I. However, in up to 33% of exacerbations of ABPA the patient may be asymptomatic,[34] the exacerbation only becoming apparent through a rise in serum IgE.[35] A doubling of the serum IgE is significant. A prolonged remission does not imply cure as exacerbations have been reported after remission of 7.5 years.[36] Patients are said to have stage IV disease when in the presence of ABPA oral corticosteroids are required to control their symptoms of asthma and it is no longer possible to wean them from their oral therapy once disease control is achieved. In stage V disease all patients have bronchiectasis and pulmonary fibrosis.

The natural history of the disease is very varied. In a review of 17 patients with stage V disease the interval between diagnosis and progression to stage V varied from 5 months to 35 years.[37] The prognosis for patients with a forced expiratory volume in 1 s (FEV_1) of less than 0.8 l at the time of diagnosis is poor with death occurring within 7 years.[37]

DIAGNOSIS AND LABORATORY FINDINGS

The diagnosis of ABPA is made based on the presence of a number of criteria. An initial seven criteria were suggested by Rosenberg et al.[34] in 1977 and one more was added by Wang and Patterson[38] in 1978 (Table 33.1).

Essential to the diagnosis of ABPA is the presence of elevated serum IgE and IgG specific for A. fumigatus. The other criteria are usual associations with ABPA but are not all essential to the diagnosis. The more of these criteria that are satisfied the more specific the diagnosis becomes.

(1) *Asthma.* ABPA is nearly universally associated with a diagnosis of asthma or cystic fibrosis but there are case reports of ABPA occurring without either.[39]

(2) *Chest X-ray infiltrates.* Fleeting chest X-ray infiltrates are inevitably found at some time in the disease history but need not be present at diagnosis.

(3) *Immediate cutaneous reactivity to A. fumigatus.* Skin testing by prick (1 : 20 weight by volume) or intradermal injection (1 : 1000 weight by volume) of A. fumigatus is invariably positive in ABPA but is also positive in 13–38% of asthmatic subjects without ABPA.[19,40–42]

(4) *Elevated total serum IgE.* Total IgE levels are generally greater than 1000 iu ml^{-1} and may be as high as 20 000 iu ml^{-1} in acute cases.[21] The greater proportion of the total serum IgE is nonspecific. The total serum IgE level acts as a useful guide to treatment response with a fall in total serum IgE of 35–50%

TABLE 33.1: *Diagnostic criteria for ABPA together with an indication of the prevalence of each criterion seen in ABPA, atopic asthma and cystic fibrosis.*

Diagnostic criteria	Comments	ABPA	Atopic asthma	Cystic fibrosis
1. Asthma	Wide range of severity			
2. Chest X-ray infiltrates	Will be present at some stage in disease	100%	0	100%
3. Skin-prick test positive to *Aspergillus*	Essential for diagnosis, not specific	100%	13–38%	30%
4. Raised serum IgE	Marker of disease activity	80–100%	50%	20%
5. Precipitating antibodies to *Aspergillus*	Not specific to ABPA	69–90%	25%	35%
6. Eosinophilia	Absent if treated with corticosteroids	100%	40%	20%
7. Raised serum IgE-Af and IgG-Af	Essential and specific to the diagnosis	100%	<5%	<5%
8. Central bronchiectasis	Absent in early disease, specific for ABPA in absence of distal bronchiectasis	60%[a]	0	100%

[a] The prevalence of central bronchiectasis in ABPA will vary depending on the stage of the disease and will be absent in ABPAs (see text).

expected with treatment. After subsequent exacerbations the IgE should return to this plateau level and failure to do so suggests that the exacerbation is ongoing. Attempts to achieve IgE levels in the normal range for the age of the patient can result in over-treatment.

(5) *Precipitating antibodies to A. fumigatus.* Serum precipitating antibodies to *A. fumigatus* are present in 69–90% of cases of ABPA[3,43,44] but are also present in 3% of non-atopic asthmatic and 25% of atopic asthmatic subjects.[42]

(6) *Eosinophilia.* A peripheral blood eosinophilia greater than 1000 cells mm^{-3} is usually found unless the patient is already treated with corticosteroids.[1,3,34,45–47]

(7) *Elevated serum IgE-Af and IgG-Af.* The presence of elevated serum IgG-Af and IgE-Af relative to control sera is specific for ABPA[38,48,49] and possibly essential for the diagnosis of ABPA.[21] Markedly elevated serum IgG-Af levels are seen in the presence of aspergillomas[44] but not elevated serum IgE-Af.[49] The differential diagnosis of an aspergilloma from ABPA can be made readily on history and chest X-ray. It is essential to use age-appropriate control serum when performing serological tests for ABPA in children, as adults with asthma can have increased serum IgE-Af concentrations when compared with children with asthma, despite having three- to ten-fold lower concentrations of total serum IgE.[50] Recently a number of *A. fumigatus*-derived antigens recognized by human IgE- and IgG- and mouse-derived monoclonal antibodies have been identified.[51] It is to be hoped that these monoclonal antibodies may lead to the development of more sensitive and specific serological tests for ABPA.[52]

(8) *Central bronchiectasis.* The presence of central bronchiectasis in the absence of cystic fibrosis and other congenital ciliary disorders is virtually pathognomonic for ABPA or other allergic bronchopulmonary fungosis.[53,54] However it has become recognized that there are a group of asthmatic subjects who satisfy all the criteria for ABPA but do not have central bronchiectasis.[55,56] It appears that this group of seropositive ABPA (ABPAs) as opposed to ABPA with central bronchiectasis (ABPAcb) have a milder form of the disease or are presenting at an earlier stage in the disease's natural history. Patients with ABPAs have significantly lower serum-specific IgG for *A. fumigatus* (IgG-Af) than ABPAcb.[55] In a small series of 11 patients with ABPAs followed for a total of 63 patient years while receiving appropriate treatment no patient progressed to end-stage lung disease.[55]

The recovery or culture of *Aspergillus* from sputum is not sensitive or specific for ABPA and is not part of the diagnostic criteria. It may be suggestive of ABPA in the appropriate clinical setting particularly if hyphae, as opposed to spores, are identified in the sputum.[21]

RADIOGRAPHIC FINDINGS

The radiological changes seen in ABPA may be fixed or transient.[54] Transient changes that resolve with corticosteroid treatment appear to be the result of parenchymal infiltrates, mucoid impaction or secretions in damaged bronchi. The radiological appearances of these pathological processes include pulmonary infiltrates, perihilar infiltrates resembling lymphadenopathy, homogeneous consolidation that may be unilateral or bilateral, "toothpaste" shadows from mucoid impactions in damaged bronchi, or "gloved finger" shadows from distally occluded bronchi filled with secretions. These radiological appearances are typically confined to one or two segments during an exacerbation, with the shadowing occurring in either the same area or elsewhere within the lung with recurrent episodes. When central bronchiectasis is present then ring shadows, 1–2 cm diameter circular markings on the chest X-ray produced by dilated bronchi viewed *en face*, or parallel hair-line shadows extending from the hilum may be seen. Previously bronchography was regarded as the gold standard for demonstrating bronchiectasis but this has now largely been replaced by high-resolution computerized tomography or hilar linear tomography.[53,57]

Late radiological findings in ABPA include cavitation, local emphysema, contracted upper lobes and honeycomb fibrosis.[58] Spontaneous pneumothorax may be a complication in very advanced ABPA especially when bullous changes are present.[59]

PULMONARY FUNCTION TESTS

Pulmonary function testing in ABPA is relatively insensitive and does not help to define the extent of disease or exclude it.[60] During an acute episode of ABPA, pulmonary function testing may demonstrate a reduction in total lung capacity, vital capacity, FEV_1 and D_{co}. These changes may be quite marked but return to baseline after treatment with corticosteroids.[60,61] Patients with stage V disease typically have reduced lung volumes, a low diffusing capacity and irreversible airflow obstruction.[37,62]

TREATMENT

INDUCTION

The cornerstone of treatment of ABPA is corticosteroids with dose modifications based on serial serum total IgE levels. The original guidelines for treatment were suggested by Wang *et al.* in 1979 and remain a good model for therapeutic regimens.[63] After diagnosis oral prednisolone 0.5 mg kg^{-1} as a single daily dose should be given for the first 2 weeks and then continued as an alternate daily dose for 3 months. After this the dose can be gradually tapered over a further 3 months. The speed at which the corticosteroids can be reduced is dictated by the clinical and objective response to treatment (see below).

Recognition of ABPA early in the disease process and effective treatment with corticosteroids and prolonged follow-up appears to prevent progression to lung damage and stage V disease.[21,55] It is not clear whether all patients with ABPA are at risk of progressing to chronic lung damage or whether exacerbations could be managed with shorter courses of steroids tailed over a period of 1 month.[26]

FOLLOW-UP

During the initial treatment period an improvement in symptoms accompanied by resolution of pulmonary infiltrates and a fall in IgE should be seen. It is important to perform regular chest X-rays to confirm the resolution of changes and then at 4-monthly intervals for the first 2 years of follow-up, extending eventually to an annual chest X-ray. Serum total IgE levels should be determined at presentation and then monthly for the following year. After this the interval between IgE measurements can be gradually extended. A fall in total serum IgE of approximately 35% is expected after 4–6 weeks of treatment[21] and a plateau level should be seen by 6 months of treatment. Failure to achieve these criteria suggests undertreatment and a more prolonged initial course of corticosteroid prior to reduction is required. Prolonged follow-up of ABPA patients is essential as exacerbations have been described as long as 7.5 years after remission.[36]

ORAL CORTICOSTEROID-SPARING AGENTS AND ANTI-FUNGALS

Attempts have been made to identify oral corticosteroid-sparing agents. Inhaled steroids are useful to control the symptoms of asthma during remissions but have not been helpful during exacerbations of ABPA.[63,64] Anti-fungal agents are very attractive in theory to reduce the antigenic load in the patient with ABPA but have not been clearly established as routine therapy by clinical trials. Older anti-fungal agents such as clotrimazole, iodoquinol and ketoconazole were abandoned because of adverse effects or failure to demonstrate useful effects in clinical trials.[65–68] A recent randomized, placebo-controlled trial of nebulized natamycin in ABPA showed no benefit of treatment over placebo in terms of steroid sparing or markers of disease activity after 1 year of treatment.[69] Trials of new oral anti-fungal agents such as itraconazole are interesting and suggest beneficial effects. The open introduction of itraconazole in the treatment of ABPA led to a reduction in oral corticosteroid dose, a fall in total serum IgE and an improvement in spirometric values when treatment was continued for up to 6 months.[70,71] These were non-controlled, non-randomized studies with small patient numbers and indicate the need for carefully conducted controlled clinical trials of this anti-fungal agent in ABPA to identify whether it should be introduced as standard adjunctive therapy.

REFERENCES

1 Hinson KFW, Moon AJ, Plummer NS. Bronchopulmonary aspergillosis: a review and a report of eight new cases. *Thorax* 1952; 7: 317–33.

2 Raper KR, Fennell DI. *The Genus Aspergillus.* Huntington, NY: Robert E. Krieger Publishing Co., 1973.

3 McCarthy DS, Pepys J. Allergic bronchopulmonary aspergillosis. Clinical immunology: (1) clinical features. *Clin Allergy* 1971; 1: 261–86.

4 Safirstein BH, D'Souza MF, Simon G, Tai EHC, Pepys J. Five year follow up of bronchopulmonary aspergillosis. *Am Rev Respir Dis* 1973; 108: 450–9.

5 Richeson RBI, Stander PE. Allergic bronchopulmonary aspergillosis. *Postgrad Med* 1990; 88: 217–22.

6 Crompton GK. Bronchopulmonary aspergillosis. In: Brewis RAL, Gibson GJ, Geddes DM (eds) *Respiratory Medicine.* London: Baillière Tindall, 1990: 1035–50.

7 Lake F, Tribe AE, McAleer R, Froudist J, Thompson PJ. Mixed allergic bronchopulmonary fungal disease due to *Pseudallescheria boydii* and *Aspergillus.* *Thorax* 1990; 45: 489–92.

8 Muscat I, Oxborrow S, Siddorn J. Allergic bronchopulmonary mycosis. *Lancet* 1988; i: 1341.

9 Akiyama K, Mathison DA, Riker JB, Greenberger PA, Patterson R. Allergic bronchopulmonary candidiasis. *Chest* 1984; 85: 699–701.

10 Lee TM, Greenberger PA, Oh S, Patterson R, Roberts M, Liotta JL. Allergic bronchopulmonary candidiasis: case report and suggested diagnostic criteria. *J Allergy Clin Immunol* 1987; 80: 816–20.

11 Sandhu RS, Mehta SK, Khan U, Singh MM. Role of *Aspergillus* and *Candida* species in allergic bronchopulmonary mycosis: a comparative study. *Scand J Respir Dis* 1979; 60: 235–42.

12 Pinson P, Stralten MVD. Fibrotic stage of allergic bronchopulmonary candidiasis. *Chest* 1991; 100: 565–7.

13 Halwig JM, Brueske DA, Dreisen RB, Greenberger PA, Sommers HM. Allergic bronchopulmonary curvulariosis. *Am Rev Respir Dis* 1985; 132: 186–8.

14 McAleer R, Kroenert DB, Elder JL, Froudist JH. Allergic bronchopulmonary disease caused by *Curvularia lunata* and *Drechslera hawaiiensis*. *Thorax* 1981; 36: 338–44.

15 Dolan CT, Weed LA, Dines DE. Bronchopulmonary helminthosporiosis. *Am J Clin Pathol* 1970; 53: 235–42.

16 Hendrich DJ, Ellithrope DB, Lyon F, Hattier P, Salvagio JE. Allergic bronchopulmonary helminthosporiosis. *Am Rev Respir Dis* 1982; 126: 935–8.

17 Kino T, Yamada Y, Honda K *et al.* Diagnosis and treatment of a case of allergic bronchopulmonary mycosis caused by *Mucor*-like fungus. *Nippon Kyobu Shikkan Gakkai Zasshi* 1983; 9: 896–903.

18 Benatar SR, Allan B, Hewitson RP. Allergic bronchopulmonary stemphyliosis. *Thorax* 1980; 35: 515–8.

19 Henderson AH, English MP, Vecht RJ. Pulmonary aspergillosis: A survey of its occurrence in patients with chronic lung disease and discussion of the significance of diagnostic tests. *Thorax* 1968; 23: 513–23.

20 Greenberger PA, Patterson R. Allergic bronchopulmonary aspergillosis and the evaluation of the patient with asthma. *J Allergy Clin Immunol* 1988; 81: 646–50.

21 Ganz MA, Greenberger PA, Patterson R. Hypersensitivity pneumonitis and allergic bronchopulmonary aspergillosis. In: Weiss EB, Stein M (eds) *Asthma: Mechanisms and Therapeutics*, 3rd edn. Boston: Little, Brown and Co., 1993: 635–43.

22 Basich JE, Graves TS, Baz MN *et al.* Allergic bronchopulmonary aspergillosis in corticosteroid-dependent asthmatics. *J Allergy Clin Immunol* 1981; 68: 98–102.

23 Bosken CH, Myers JL, Greenberger PA, Kalzenstein AL. Pathological features of allergic bronchopulmonary aspergillosis. *Am J Surg Pathol* 1988; 12: 216–22.

24 Slavin RG, Bedrossian CW, Hutcheson PS *et al.* A pathological study of allergic bronchopulmonary aspergillosis. *J Allergy Clin Immunol* 1988; 81: 718–25.

25 Patterson R, Rosenberg M, Roberts M. Evidence that *Aspergillus fumigatus* growing in the airways of man can be a potent stimulus of specific and nonspecific IgE formation. *Am J Med* 1977; 63: 257–62.

26 Wardlaw A, Geddes DM. Allergic bronchopulmonary aspergillosis: A review. *J R Soc Med* 1992; 85: 747–51.

27 Slavin RG, Fisher VW, Levine EA, Tsai CC, Winzenberger P. A primate model of allergic bronchopulmonary aspergillosis. *Int Arch Allergy Appl Immunol* 1978; 56: 325–33.

28 Knutsen AP, Mueller AP, Hutcheson PS, Slavin RG. T and B cell dysregulation of IgE synthesis in cystic fibrosis patients with allergic bronchopulmonary aspergillosis. *Clin Immunol Immunopathol* 1990; 55: 129–38.

29 Knutsen AP, Slavin RG. *In vitro* T-cell responses in patients with cystic fibrosis and allergic bronchopulmonary aspergillosis. *J Lab Clin Med* 1989; 133: 428–35.

30 Walker CA, Fitzharris P, Longbottom JL. Lymphocyte sensitization to *Aspergillus fumigatus* in allergic bronchopulmonary aspergillosis. *Clin Exp Immunol* 1989; 76: 34–40.

31 Robinson DS, Hamid Q, Ying S *et al.* Predominant TH2 like bronchoalveolar T-lymphocyte population in atopic asthma. *N Engl J Med* 1992; 326: 298–304.

32 Bradding P, Roberts JA, Britten KM *et al.* Interleukins-4, -5, -6 and TNF-α in normal and asthmatic airways. Evidence for the human mast cell as an important source of these cytokines. *Am J Respir Cell Mol Biol* 1994; 10: 471–80.

33 Turner ES, Greenberger PA, Sider L. Complexities of establishing an early diagnosis of allergic bronchopulmonary aspergillosis in children. *Allergy Proc* 1989; 10: 63.

34 Rosenberg M, Patterson R, Mintzer R, Cooper BJ, Roberts M, Harris KE. Clinical and immunological criteria for the diagnosis of allergic bronchopulmonary aspergillosis. *Ann Intern Med* 1977; 86: 405–14.

35 Rosenberg N, Patterson R, Roberts M. Immunologic responses to therapy in allergic bronchopulmonary aspergillosis: serum IgE values as an indicator and predictor of disease activity. *J Pediatr* 1977; 91: 914–7.

36 Halwing M, Greenberger PA, Patterson R, Levine M. Recurrence of allergic bronchopulmonary aspergillosis after seven years of remission. *J Allergy Clin Immunol* 1984; 74: 319–23.

37 Lee TM, Greenberger PA, Patterson R, Roberts M, Liotta JL. Stage V (fibrotic) allergic bronchopulmonary aspergillosis. A review of 17 cases followed from diagnosis. *Arch Intern Med* 1987; 147: 319–23.

38 Wang LJR, Patterson R, Rosenberg M, Roberts M, Cooper BJ. Serum IgE and IgG antibody activity against *Aspergillus fumigatus* as a diagnostic aid in allergic bronchopulmonary aspergillosis. *Am Rev Respir Dis* 1978; 117: 917–27.

39 Glancy JJ, Elder JL, McAleer R. Allergic bronchopulmonary fungal disease without clinical asthma. *Thorax* 1981; 36: 345–9.

40 Bardana EJ, Gerber JD, Craig S, Cianciulli FD. The general and specific humoral immune response to pulmonary aspergillosis. *Am Rev Respir Dis* 1975; 112: 799–805.

41 Hendrick DJ, Davis RJ, D'Souza MF, Pepys J. An analysis of skin prick test reaction in 656 asthmatic patients. *Thorax* 1975; 30(suppl): 2.

42 Longbottom JL, Pepys J. Pulmonary aspergillosis: Diagnostic and immunological significance of antigens and C-substance in *Aspergillus fumigatus*. *J Pathol Bacteriol* 1964; 88: 141–51.

43 Campbell MJ, Clayton YM. Bronchopulmonary aspergillosis. *Am Rev Respir Dis* 1964; 89: 186–96.

44 Faux JA, Shale DJ, Lane DJ. Precipitans and specific IgG antibody to *Aspergillus fumigatus* in a chest unit population. *Thorax* 1992; 47: 48–52.

45 Patterson R, Golbert F. Hypersensitivity disease of the lung. *Univ Mich Med Cent J* 1968; 34: 8–11.

46 McCarthy DS, Pepys J. Allergic bronchopulmonary aspergillosis: Clinical immunology: (2) Skin, nasal and bronchial tests. *Clin Allergy* 1971; 1: 415–32.

47 Henderson AH. Allergic aspergillosis: review of 32 cases. *Thorax* 1968; 23: 501–12.

48 Greenberger PA, Patterson R. Application of enzyme linked immunosorbent assay (ELISA) in diagnosis of allergic bronchopulmonary aspergillosis. *J Lab Clin Med* 1982; 99: 288–93.

49 Kurup VP, Resnick A, Kalbfleish J, Fink JN. Antibody isotype responses in *Aspergillus*-induced disease. *J Lab Clin Med* 1990; 115: 298–303.

50 Greenberger PA, Liotta JL, Roberts M. The effects of age on isotypic antibody responses to *Aspergillus fumigatus*: implications regarding *in vitro* measurements. *J Lab Clin Med* 1989; 114: 278–84.

51 Arruda KL, Platts-Mills TAE, Longbottom JL, El-Dahr JM, Chapman MD. *Aspergillus fumigatus*: Identification of 16, 18, and 45 kd antigens recognized by human IgG and IgE antibodies and murine monoclonal antibodies. *J Allergy Clin Immunol* 1992; 89: 1166–76.

52 Slavin RG, Knutsen AP. Purified *Aspergillus* proteins: Going where no one has gone before. *J Lab Clin Med* 1993; 121: 380–1.

53 Fisher MR, Mendelson EB, Mintzer RA, Ricketti AJ, Greenberger PA. Use of linear tomography to confirm the diagnosis of allergic bronchopulmonary aspergillosis. *Chest* 1985; 87: 499–502.

54 Mintzer R, Rogers L, Kriglik G. The spectrum of radiological findings in allergic bronchopulmonary aspergillosis. *Radiology* 1978; 127: 301–7.

55 Greenberger PA, Miller TP, Roberts M, Smith LL. Allergic bronchopulmonary aspergillosis in patients with and without evidence of bronchiectasis. *Ann Allergy* 1993; 70: 333–8.

56 Patterson R, Greenberger PA, Halwig M, Liotta JL, Roberts M. Allergic bronchopulmonary aspergillosis: natural history and classification of early disease by serological and roentgenographic studies. *Arch Intern Med* 1986; 146: 916–8.

57 Neeld DA, Goodman LR, Gurney JW, Greenberger PA, Fink JN. Computerised tomography in the evaluation of allergic bronchopulmonary aspergillosis. *Am Rev Respir Dis* 1990; 142: 1200–5.

58. McCarthy DS, Simon G, Hargreave FE. The radiological appearances in allergic bronchopulmonary aspergillosis. *Clin Radiol* 1970; 21: 366–75.

59 Ricketti AJ, Greenberger PA, Glassroth J. Spontaneous pneumothorax in allergic bronchopulmonary aspergillosis. *Arch Intern Med* 1984; 144: 181–2.

60. Nichols D, DoPico GA, Braun S, Imbeau S, Peters ME, Rankin J. Acute and chronic pulmonary function changes in allergic bronchopulmonary aspergillosis. Am J Med 1979; 67: 631–7.

61. Ricketti AJ, Greenberger PA, Mintzer RA, Patterson R. Allergic bronchopulmonary aspergillosis. Chest 1984; 86: 773–8.

62. Greenberger PA, Patterson R, Ghory A et al. Late sequelae of allergic bronchopulmonary aspergillosis. J Allergy Clin Immunol 1980; 66: 327–35.

63. Wang JLF, Patterson R, Roberts M. Management of allergic bronchopulmonary aspergillosis. Am Rev Respir Dis 1979; 120: 87–92.

64. Vaughan LM. Therapy Review: Allergic bronchopulmonary aspergillosis. Clin Pharm 1993; 12: 24–33.

65. Shale DJ, Faux JA, Lane DJ. Trial of ketoconazole in noninvasive pulmonary aspergillosis. Thorax 1987; 42: 26–31.

66. Horsefield K, Nicholls A, Cumming G, Hume M, Prowse K. Treatment of pulmonary aspergillosis with di-iodohydroxyquinoline. Thorax 1977; 32: 250–3.

67. Fournier EC, Tonnel AB, Wallaert B, Voisen C. Ketoconazole trial in prevention of acute phase of allergic bronchopulmonary aspergillosis. Am Rev Respir Dis 1984; 129: A32.

68. Crompton GK, Milne LJR. Treatment of bronchopulmonary aspergillosis with clotrimazole. Br J Dis Chest 1973; 67: 301–7.

69. Currie DC, Lueck H, Milburn HJ et al. Controlled trial of natamycin in the treatment of allergic bronchopulmonary aspergillosis. Thorax 1990; 45: 447–50.

70. Denning DW, Van Wye JE, Lewiston NJ, Stevens DA. Adjunctive therapy of allergic bronchopulmonary aspergillosis with itraconazole. Chest 1991; 100: 813–9.

71. Germaud P, Tuchais E, Canfrere I, DeLajartre M, Chailleux E, Delobel M. Therapy of allergic bronchopulmonary aspergillosis with itraconazole. Am Rev Respir Dis 1992; 145: A736.

KEY POINTS

1 *Diagnosis*
Maintain a high index of suspicion in susceptible patients (i.e. with asthma, cystic fibrosis). Look for:
(a) Skin-prick positive *Aspergillus fumigatus*
(b) Elevated total serum IgE
(c) *Aspergillus fumigatus* precipitins
(d) Fleeting shadows on chest X-ray
(e) Central bronchiectasis
(f) Specific IgE-Af and IgG-Af
(g) Eosinophilia

2   *Treatment*
Oral corticosteroids tailed according to clinical response and total serum IgE. Treatment is unlikely to reduce IgE to the normal range; the aim is to achieve a plateau response.

34

SPECIFIC PROBLEMS: EXERCISE-INDUCED ASTHMA

Sandra D. Anderson

HISTORICAL INTRODUCTION AND BACKGROUND

"Exercise-induced asthma (EIA) is the name used to describe the transitory increase in airways resistance which follows vigorous exercise in most patients with asthma."[1] The association between exercise and asthma has been recognized since the first century AD when Arateus of Cappodocia stated that "If from running, gymnastic exercises, or any other work, the breathing become difficult, it is called asthma".[2] Since Jones[3] gave the first modern clinical description of EIA in 1962, there has been considerable research interest in the topic.[4,5] Initially, this research focused on finding drugs to prevent EIA[6] and on factors that determined the severity of EIA.[7] β₂-Adrenoceptor agonists and sodium cromoglycate, when given by aerosol immediately before exercise, were found to be very effective agents for preventing EIA.[6,8] The intensity, duration and type of exercise were identified as important factors determining severity of EIA.[7,9,10] Later, however, it was shown that the ventilation rate reached and sustained during exercise[11] and the water content of the air inspired during exercise were the primary determinants of severity.[12] It was found that exercise *per se* was not necessary to provoke airway narrowing and isocapnic hyperventilation with dry air at high flow rates was developed as a laboratory challenge to substitute for exercise.[13]

By 1979 it was recognized that the stimulus to EIA was the loss of water from the airways in bringing large volumes of inspired air to alveolar conditions in a short time.[12,14,15] In the last 15 years there has been much debate as to the precise mechanism whereby water lost by evaporation leads to airway narrowing. There are currently two major hypotheses, but direct experimental evidence has not been forthcoming to support either theory.[16,17] One hypothesis suggests that it is the thermal effects of water loss acting to increase blood flow and permeability of the bronchial microcirculation, with consequent vascular engorgement and airway oedema causing the airways to narrow independently of contraction of bronchial smooth muscle.[17] This hypothesis has recently been questioned.[18] The other hypothesis suggests that EIA is a result of the dehydrating effects of water loss causing a transient increase in osmolarity of the airway surface liquid.[16,19] An increase in osmolarity is known to induce mediator release from human mast cells[20] and stimulate sensory nerves in animals.[21] Mast cell mediators and sensory neuropeptides are thought to cause the airways to narrow by contraction of bronchial smooth muscle with, or without, airway oedema.[22]

DIAGNOSIS OF EIA BY HISTORY

A diagnosis of EIA can frequently be made on history and the response to inhaled drug therapy. A patient who complains of shortness of breath that is worse after, rather than during exercise, and who reports that the symptoms are relieved by inhaling a β_2-adrenoceptor agonist has a history consistent with EIA. If the shortness of breath after exercise is prevented by taking a β_2-adrenoceptor agonist or sodium cromoglycate before exercise, this confirms the diagnosis of EIA. Obtaining a clear history of EIA suggests that the forced expiratory volume in 1 s (FEV_1) and peak expiratory flow rate (PEFR) have fallen at least 20%, as symptoms are rare with mild EIA. However, it is difficult to assess the severity of EIA by history alone or by resting lung function. Severe EIA can occur in patients with good lung function and lung function cannot be used to predict the amount of therapy required to control EIA.

It should be noted that the diagnosis of EIA cannot be simply made on a history of post-exercise cough. While it is important to recognize cough as a symptom consistent with EIA, not all those with post-exercise cough have EIA.[23,24] When there is doubt about the diagnosis, severity or the amount of medication required to control EIA, the patient should be referred to a laboratory for a standardized exercise test. Such patients should be carefully screened before referral to exclude cardiovascular disease. Although many physicians may use a "run up the stairs" to confirm a diagnosis of EIA, it should be kept in mind that a standard stimulus is required to document severity and to evaluate the effect of therapy.

Patients referred to a laboratory for testing should be told to withhold medications that could influence their response to exercise. Before visiting the laboratory the following withholding periods apply: for the shorter-acting antihistamines, 48 hours; for the long-acting antihistamines, 1 week; for the sustained-release oral bronchodilators, 24 hours; with 12 hours for ordinary release preparations. The short-acting β_2-adrenoceptor agonists (isoprenaline, salbutamol, terbutaline, ephedrine, rimiterol) and sodium cromoglycate or nedocromil sodium should not be taken for at least 6 hours. The longer-acting β_2-adrenoceptor agonists, salmeterol and formoterol, should not be taken for 24 hours. Corticosteroids, either aerosol or oral, should be withheld the morning of the study. Caffeine-containing drinks should be avoided on the day of the study. Patients should not be referred for testing unless their FEV_1 is 75% or more of the predicted value and their spirometry can be reproduced with repeated blows.

Most laboratories will use FEV_1 or PEFR to quantify EIA. As many patients own peak flow meters, they can interpret changes in PEFR and may prefer this measurement. However we recommend the documentation of FEV_1 as the most appropriate for assessing EIA as it encompasses more of the flow–volume curve (Fig. 34.1). In athletes we also document changes in the

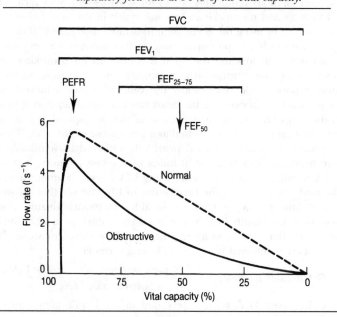

FIGURE 34.1: *The expiratory flow rate in relation to expired volume before and after exercise that has provoked airways obstruction: the portion of the flow–volume curve encompassed by the other measurements of lung function. FVC, forced vital capacity; FEV_1, forced expiratory volume in 1 s; PEFR, peak expiratory flow rate; FEF_{25-75}, forced expiratory flow rate through the middle portion of the vital capacity. FEF_{50} is the forced expiratory flow rate at 50% of the vital capacity.*

forced expiratory flow rate through the middle portion of the vital capacity (FEF_{25-75}) as a reduction in these flow rates can reduce maximal exercise performance. A specific request for these flow measurements may need to be made to the laboratory. It is also important to confirm that the protocol used in the laboratory will be sufficient to provoke EIA in a trained athlete. We choose isocapnic hyperventilation with dry air[13] as the test for athletes as the flow rates during hyperventilation are usually higher than those that can be obtained during maximal exercise of any type. In a laboratory, the type of exercise offered is often confined to running or cycling, which is appropriate for most people. However at high speeds, treadmill exercise can be dangerous and exercising on a bicycle ergometer may be inappropriate for highly trained persons or those who are trained to row or ski. Most laboratories will ensure that the air inhaled during the exercise is dry by using compressed air. In some laboratories the temperature of the inspired air is reduced to subzero values to ensure dryness of the inspired air. Sophisticated techniques for cooling the air[25] are not necessary and inhaling compressed air at room temperature is usually an adequate stimulus, providing the appropriate ventilation rate is reached and sustained.[26] In order to facilitate the laboratory in their choice of inspired air condition, the circumstances under which the patient gets EIA should be given in the referral.

Published studies demonstrate[7,27-29] that it is important for the duration of exercise to be between 6 and 8 min, and that its intensity should be sufficient to raise the ventilation to between 40 and 60% of the predicted maximum voluntary ventilation (MVV) for at least 4 min. MVV is calculated as $FEV_1 \times 35$ and the workload that will result in this ventilation can be approximated by using the nomogram illustrated in Fig. 34.2. If the test is negative for EIA it is important to confirm that pre-exercise lung function was not unusually low and the optimal conditions for provoking asthma by exercise or hyperventilation were provided in the laboratory. The laboratory report should state clearly the ventilation rate achieved during exercise, the time of exercise, the heart rate and workload during exercise and the temperature and water content of the air inspired. It is usual for the ventilation rate to be expressed as a percentage of the MVV. Unfortunately some laboratories record heart rate rather than ventilation rate. While heart rate can be a useful index of exercise intensity, it is not as good as ventilation rate for documenting EIA. Specific requests may need to be made for recording the time-course of EIA and whether recovery of the lung function was spontaneous or aided by bronchodilator. The traditional way to quantify EIA[3] is to express the reduction in PEFR or FEV_1 that occurs after exercise as a percentage of the pre-exercise value (% fall index). This is obtained using the following formula:

$$\% \text{ fall index for } FEV_1 = \frac{100 \times \text{pre-exercise } FEV_1 - \text{lowest } FEV_1}{\text{pre-exercise } FEV_1}$$

where the lowest FEV_1 value is recorded in the 15 min after exercise. A

FIGURE 34.2: *Four quadrant diagram relating FEV$_1$ (l) to the ventilation rate (V$_E$, l min^{-1}) required to be reached and sustained for 4–6 min. The ventilation rate is related to the oxygen consumption (Vo$_2$, l) it is likely to be generated by and the bicycle workload (W) producing this oxygen consumption is also given. In short the workload can be indirectly predicted from the FEV$_1$.*

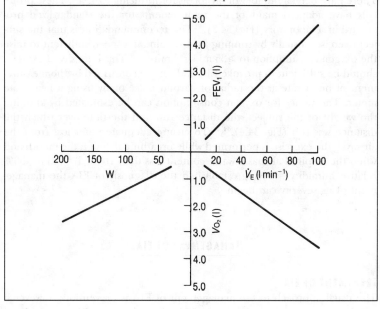

value greater than 10%, or 15% for some laboratories, is regarded as diagnostic of EIA.[4,31,32] If the % fall in FEV$_1$ is 10–25% EIA is considered to be mild. It is moderate when the fall is 26–50% and severe if the fall is >50% of the pre-challenge value. The value of 10% as the cut-off point for diagnosis of EIA is based on the responses measured in healthy subjects exercising in both temperate and cold environments.[4,31,33] The reproducibility of EIA as measured by the % fall index is good. If the tests are performed within 1 month, the % fall index will usually vary less than 20%, providing the two exercise tests are performed under standardized conditions.[8]

In addition to the % fall index, it is useful for a physician to have the pre-exercise level of FEV$_1$ and the lowest value for FEV$_1$ measured after exercise reported as a percentage of the predicted normal value. These values may reveal the benefit of treatment with aerosol steroids on pre- and post-exercise lung function and symptoms, even though the % fall index may remain the same.[34] The reason for this is that FEV$_1$ improves within days of starting steroids, whereas the severity of EIA may not be reduced for weeks or even months.[35,36] When assessing the acute effect of a drug it is useful to know what the response is after a placebo medication. The protection afforded by a drug is taken as the difference in the % fall after the placebo and the active drug expressed as a percentage of the % fall on the placebo. A value for protection greater than 50% is regarded as a significant drug effect as it takes into account the reproducibility of the test.[8]

There have been a number of protocols for inducing EIA.[37-39] These protocols have adapted many of the requirements for the standardized procedure in a laboratory (Fig. 34.3).[39] The recommendation is that the subject exercises, usually by running for 6–8 min, at a speed sufficient to raise the oxygen consumption to >35 ml kg^{-1} min^{-1}.[40] This intensity of exercise should be sufficient to provoke EIA and can be confirmed by the measurement of heart rate at the radial or carotid pulse or by using a heart rate meter. The values for oxygen consumption can be estimated by knowing the weight of the subject, the distance run and the time over which the distance was run (Fig. 34.4).[41,42] To ensure adequate water loss from the airways[43] the exercise is performed while breathing through the mouth and when the inspired air has a water content less than 10 mg l^{-1} (23 °C, 50% relative humidity). Having established the diagnosis of EIA the management of its severity can begin.

MANAGEMENT OF EIA

TREATMENT OF EIA

The usual approach to the management of EIA is prevention; however it is important to know how to treat EIA when it occurs. EIA is associated with arterial hypoxaemia and hyperinflation of the lungs.[44,45] It is the hypoxaemia associated with exercise that makes it dangerous for a person to continue or resume exercise at a time when the FEV_1 or PEFR is falling. If subjects feel an attack of asthma coming on during exercise, they should be advised to stop immediately. It can be predicted that the attack will worsen on the cessation of exercise, usually within the first 5 min but often as late as 10 min. For most asthmatic subjects, the attack of asthma can be reversed quickly by inhaling a β_2-adrenoceptor agonist. For mild to moderate EIA, two or three inhalations of a bronchodilator with 1–2 min separating each inhalation is usually all that is required. In severe cases of EIA up to 10 inhalations of a β_2-adrenoceptor agonist can be given.[46] There have been deaths after exercise, both in children and adults. As the severity of the attack is usually at its greatest 10 min after ceasing exercise, it is advisable to monitor lung function and closely watch individuals with EIA within this time. For example, they should not be allowed to leave the playing ground until their EIA has been relieved. As the flow rates return

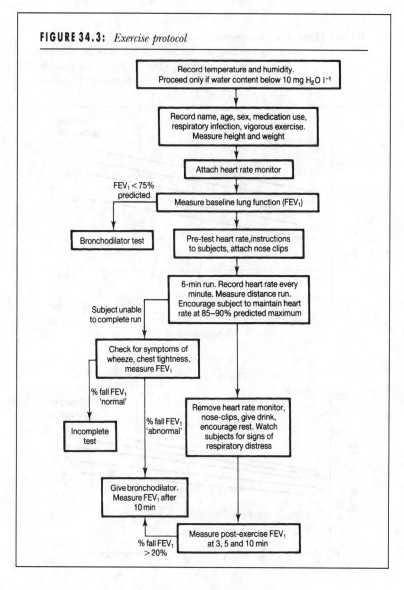

FIGURE 34.3: *Exercise protocol*

toward normal values, the arterial oxygen and lung volume also return to normal.

About 50% of people with EIA become refractory to exercise if it is repeated within 30–90 min.[47,48] In order to identify refractoriness, a person needs to recover spontaneously from an attack of EIA with lung function returning to within 5% of the pre-challenge value.[49] If an identical exercise

FIGURE 34.4: *Predicted oxygen consumption (V_{O_2}, $ml\,min^{-1}\,kg^{-1}$) during running in children and adults in relation to treadmill speed and slope. (The illustration for children is from Ref. 41 and for adults is constructed from the data given in Ref. 42.)*

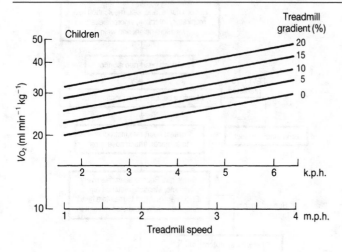

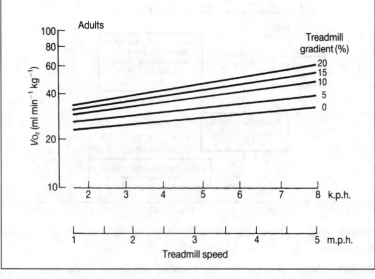

test is performed and results in less than 50% of the fall observed on the first test, the person is said to be refractory.[49] It should be noted that some people are refractory at some times but not at others.[50] The reason for this is not clear but it is known that the ingestion of non-steroidal anti-inflammatory drugs, such as indomethacin, can prevent refractoriness.[51] As these drugs are often used by athletes for injuries, a question relating to their use should be included in a work-up and the person advised as to their potential to eliminate refractoriness.

PREVENTION OF EIA

Patients taking inhaled corticosteroids

The recognition that asthma is an inflammatory disease of the airways,[52] and that EIA is a manifestation of this, has led to early introduction of inhaled corticosteroids in its treatment. Although acute administration of inhaled steroids does not affect EIA,[34] chronic treatment usually reduces the severity of EIA.[35,53–55] Further, the type and amount of medication to control EIA can be altered by chronic steroid use.[35] The decrease in severity of EIA may be due to the reduction in airway oedema by steroids. In addition, the number of mast cells are reduced by steroids[52] and they also increase the production of the enzyme responsible for removing sensory neuropeptides.[56]

It is important to know that EIA can still occur when the daily use of aerosol steroid is sufficient to achieve normal lung function, eliminate symptoms and reduce diurnal airflow variability.[55] In a study of 55 asthmatic children, 800 μg daily of budesonide halved the severity of EIA, but EIA still occurred in 55% of the children.[55] It is those patients who will still need prophylactic treatment to prevent EIA.

When aerosol steroids control symptoms of asthma and keep lung function within normal limits, EIA may be prevented by inhaling 10–20 mg of sodium cromoglycate[57–59] or 4–8 mg of nedocromil sodium.[59,60] There is recent evidence to suggest that these drugs are very effective in children taking, or within a week of completing, a course of aerosol steroids (Fig. 34.5).[32] Further, sodium cromoglycate and nedocromil sodium are free of side-effects and may be used many times throughout the day.[61] These findings in EIA are supported by the documentation of a plateau in the airway response to a known hyperosmolar stimulus.[62,63]

There is current debate about the chronic use of β_2-adrenoceptor agonists affecting airway responsiveness[64–66] and the possibility that they may reduce the beneficial effects of steroids.[67] Given that most β_2-adrenoceptor agonists in use have a protective effect less than 2 hours[26,68] it would seem advisable that β_2-adrenoceptor agonists be used with more caution than in the past. For example, β_2-adrenoceptor agonists may be added to treatment with sodium cromoglycate or nedocromil sodium rather than used initially. However a β_2-adrenoceptor agonist must be available for those who

FIGURE 34.5: *Values for % fall in FEV$_1$ in 12 asthmatic children who ran for 6 min on a treadmill set at a 10% slope and a speed adjusted to give a heart rate of 180 beats min^{-1}. The temperature of the inspired air was 22–25 °C and the relative humidity was 35–45%. Exercise was performed on 4 days: with no medication; 30 min after a placebo; 30 min after 4 mg of nedocromil sodium; and 30 min after 10 mg of sodium cromoglycate (SCG). The patients had been on inhaled steroids regularly up to 1 week before the exercise test.*

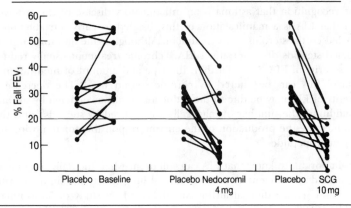

develop EIA unexpectedly, and they remain the most effective drug to be used for rescue medication.

In order to overcome the short protective effect and multiple use of β$_2$-adrenoceptor agonists, the newer longer-acting salmeterol[26,69] and formoterol[70] can be used. The only disadvantage is that the onset of action takes longer than salbutamol, terbutaline or fenoterol. In a study of 17 asthmatic subjects with moderate to severe EIA[26] we found the optimal effect of salmeterol (50 μg) at 2.5 hours after dosing rather than 0.5 hours as was the case with salbutamol (200 μg) (Fig. 34.6). Also, salmeterol did not have a prolonged effect in all subjects. In a study of patients with less severe EIA,[69] protection was afforded in some subjects for up to 12 hours. Similar findings have been made with formoterol.[70]

Patients taking these longer-acting β$_2$-adrenoceptor agonists but who still experience EIA may be advised to add sodium cromoglycate or nedocromil rather than increasing the dose or frequency of intake of the β$_2$-adrenoceptor agonist. The addition of these drugs may be particularly useful in the 2 hours before the salmeterol has its optimal effect.

FIGURE 34.6: *Values for % fall in FEV₁ in 17 asthmatic subjects who exercised by cycling for 8 min while breathing compressed dry air between 22 and 26 °C. The workload was set to give a ventilation of approximately 60% of maximum voluntary ventilation calculated at the FEV₁ predicted × 35 (see Fig. 34.2). During the first 3 min of exercise the workload was increased from 60% to 75% to 90% and, in the fourth minute to 100% of the workload calculated to produce the target ventilation. Exercise tests were performed at 0.5, 2.5, 4.5 and 6.5 hours after 200 μg of salbutamol (salb) and 50 μg of salmeterol (salm) on two separate days.*

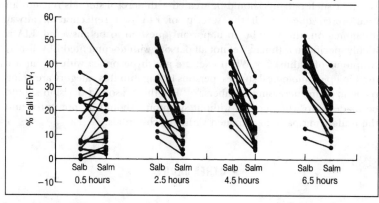

Patients not taking inhaled corticosteroids

For most patients not taking inhaled corticosteroids, who have normal lung funtion, EIA will be prevented by the standard dose of short-acting β_2-adrenoceptor agonist or sodium cromoglycate or nedocromil sodium, or the combination of the two immediately before exercise.[68,71]

For patients with airflow limitation before exercise, the use of a β_2-adrenoceptor agonist is mandatory if maximal exercise performance is to be achieved. If the patient has less than 75% of the normal predicted lung function after medication, they should be advised not to exercise and consideration should be given to the introduction of aerosol steroids.

We have previously advised patients with severe EIA to double the dose of β_2-adrenoceptor agonists.[22] In view of recent problems with multiple uses of this class of drug,[65,66] we suggest the combination with sodium cromoglycate or the introduction of inhaled corticosteroids. We have found a small number of patients who are not controlled with β_2-adrenoceptor agonists, sodium cromoglycate or nedocromil sodium or their combination, and for those we add ipratropium bromide in a dose of 80 μg.

Ipratropium bromide, an anti-cholinergic agent, when given alone is ineffective in inhibiting EIA in all but a few patients.[72]

Oral bronchodilators are not useful in the prevention of EIA. A recent, well-designed study[73] demonstrated that a sustained-release preparation of terbutaline sulphate, producing acceptably high plasma levels, and good baseline lung function, did not prevent EIA. Thus bronchodilators given orally are not recommended. Patients may feel better on their oral bronchodilator, compared with no drugs, because their flow rates before and after exercise will be higher. However the % fall in FEV_1 after exercise is usually unaffected. Similarly theophylline has a variable effect on EIA.[74,75]

For some asthmatic subjects, exercise is the only factor provoking an attack. Whether such patients should be treated with aerosol steroids remains an unanswered question. If the severity of EIA is a reflection of airway inflammation, this may be an important question to be answered. EIA is highly specific to asthma,[76] yet not all persons with documented EIA display symptoms of asthma.[39,77] When exercise and hyperpnoea with dry air are used in epidemiological studies, persons falling into this category are being recognized in increasing numbers.[39,77] For this reason, a decision should be made as to whether EIA without symptoms should be prevented and the underlying pathology treated with corticosteroids.

OTHER DRUGS

There are other drugs that are not used regularly in the treatment of asthma that have been reported to reduce the severity, and in some cases inhibit, EIA. These include the calcium antagonists, particularly nifedipine, α-receptor antagonists and the isosorbide nitrates.[1] These drugs probably act by inducing vasodilatation of the bronchial vessels and increasing the delivery of water from the circulation to the airways and thus allaying the hyperosmolar effects of evaporative water loss.[18] In addition vasodilatation may enhance the clearance of mediators from the airways. However these drugs are not recommended for treatment of EIA.

The antihistamine, terfenadine, given in a dose of 120–180 mg has been shown by several investigators to be effective in controlling EIA.[78,79] If required, this oral therapy could be added to aerosol therapy for those patients with severe EIA. It is not recommended as first-line therapy because of the large doses required, the inconvenience of having to take an oral medication 2–4 hours before exercise and the inconsistent responses between individuals studied in the same laboratory.[79,80]

Recent studies on leukotriene antagonists have shown that this class of drugs is effective in reducing EIA.[81–83] However, leukotriene antagonists still are mainly used for research purposes and are not yet available for prescription.

NON-PHARMACOLOGICAL METHODS TO PREVENT EIA

CHANGING INSPIRED AIR CONDITIONS

When it was realized that EIA could be prevented, or markedly reduced, by having the patient inhale air of alveolar conditions, i.e. 34–37 °C and 100% humidity,[12,14,15] attention was given to techniques and devices that could reduce respiratory water loss and thus the severity of EIA. A number of masks and re-breathing devices were designed and shown to reduce the severity of EIA.[84–87] These devices simply allow some of the heat and water lost during expiration to be re-breathed during inspiration. However we have found that patients are unwilling to use them regularly or in public. A similar beneficial effect on EIA can be had by nose-breathing during exercise rather than breathing through the mouth.[88,89] Because of the increase in resistance it is not natural to breathe via the nose during exercise, and normally there is a switch from nose to mouth breathing at a ventilation rate of $35 \, l \, min^{-1}$. Further, the nasal mucosa also responds to evaporative water loss and histamine and other mediators are released as a result.[90] These mediators increase nasal resistance making breathing by the nose impossible during exercise.

PHYSICAL TRAINING

Because exercise is a potent stimulus for provoking an attack of asthma it is often avoided by asthmatic subjects.[91] However there are many physical and social benefits in exercising regularly and asthmatic subjects should be encouraged to be physically active. This can easily be achieved by using the appropriate medication before exercise. Asthmatic subjects should also be encouraged to improve their fitness in order to reduce the ventilation rate required for a particular exercise intensity.

Programmes have been designed to evaluate the effects of physical training on EIA. The investigators have all concluded that there are definite social benefits to be had from physical training but the results in terms of effect on EIA have been inconsistent. Some programmes[92–95] found exercise tolerance improved after training when exercise intensity was increased after training, but there was no reduction in severity of EIA. By contrast other investigators[96–98] found both an improvement in exercise tolerance and a reduction in EIA. No change in baseline lung function was found[96] and medication was used to prevent EIA during training.

Physical training has the potential to benefit those who are unfit by raising the intensity of exercise at which EIA occurs. However, training in those who are already fit is likely to have little or no effect. If these persons have moderate to severe EIA they should be encouraged to have a trial of inhaled corticosteroids.

It should also be kept in mind that ventilating large volumes of dry and cool air may have a detrimental effect on airway calibre[98–100] as a result of dehydration. This may be the reason that there is a high prevalence of bronchial responsiveness to exercise in trained athletes.[101]

WARM-UP AND EIA

This is also an area of research that has not brought consistent results. The work of Morton and colleagues[102,103] demonstrated that warm-up of various duration was without effect in preventing EIA. However, Schnall and Landau[104] reported that multiple sprints of 30-s duration, 30 min before exercise, did reduce the severity of EIA. This has been confirmed for suboptimal exercise performed for 20 min, 30 min before exercise challenge.[105] It may be that findings on the effect of warm-up were variable because of differences in its intensity and duration used by different investigators. It would appear that there are definite benefits to be had from warming-up and, when the protocol of either Schnall and Landau[104] or Reiff *et al.*[105] is used. The mechanism whereby warm-up can lead to a reduction in EIA is not clear. It may relate to changes in the bronchial circulation as a result of warm-up. An increase in blood flow could deliver water more rapidly to the airways or clear mediators from the airways.

AIR POLLUTION AND EIA

It has been reported that the severity of EIA is enhanced when the inspired air contains sulphur dioxide or other air pollutants.[106] The reason for this may relate to the interactive effects between airway drying and sulphur dioxide, particularly on sensory nerves. It does not appear to relate to the higher doses of sulphur dioxide given as a result of the hyperpnoea of exercise.[106] It would seem sensible to advise asthmatic subjects not to exercise heavily during high pollution days.

SUMMARY

EIA is a common clinical problem and occurs in 70–80% of patients with clinically recognized asthma. Sometimes it can be diagnosed by history. A laboratory-based test is useful in assessing the severity and effects of treatment of EIA because standardized conditions for exercise are used and can be reproduced. For those patients with good lung function, EIA may be prevented by taking one to two times the clinically recommended dose of sodium cromoglycate or nedocromil sodium. For those patients who have reduced lung function before exercise, a β_2-adrenoceptor agonist is required to improve lung function and to prevent EIA. For those with moderately severe EIA, the combination of sodium cromoglycate or nedo-cromil sodium and a β_2-adrenoceptor agonist is recommended. In patients required to take this combination, a course of inhaled corticosteroids may also be tried to assess the benefits on EIA and the reduction of therapy required to control it. It should be noted that neither the severity of EIA, nor the amount of therapy required to control it, can be predicted from resting lung function. For this reason, we advise measurements of the airway response in patients who are having a change of therapy. For patients who exercise many times in a day it is useful to find out if they are refractory to the effects of repeated exercise as this will reduce the amount of drugs required to control EIA. For patients taking inhaled corticosteroids regularly EIA may be their only symptom of asthma. Many of these patients will be unwilling to accept chronic treatment with high doses of steroids in order to control their EIA. For these patients, the severity of EIA may vary and needs to be documented. β_2-Adrenoceptor agonists are the only drugs that will effect recovery from EIA and for this reason they are recommended as rescue medications. For those with severe EIA uncontrolled by a combination of sodium cromoglycate or nedocromil sodium and a β_2-adrenoceptor agonist, an anti-cholinergic such as ipratropium bromide or the antihistamine terfenadine, can be added.

There has been some controversy over warm-up and physical training and EIA but there are studies to support benefits. While fitness is something that everybody should aim for, asthmatic subjects should not be encouraged to expect that fitness alone will prevent their EIA. It will merely allow them to perform a greater amount of exercise before the response occurs. Further, while training, they should be advised always to take their medications to prevent EIA as they are unlikely to be able to perform adequate exercise without it.

REFERENCES

1 Anderson SD. Exercise-induced asthma. In: Middleton E, Reed C, Ellis E, Adkinson NF, Yuninger JW (eds) *Allergy: Principles and Practice*, 4th edn, vol 2. St Louis: C.V. Mosby Co., 1993: 1343–67.

2 Adams F. *The extant works of Arateus, The Cappadocian*. Edited and translated by Francis Adams, Sydenham Society, London, 1856.

3   Jones RS, Buston MH, Wharton MJ. The effect of exercise on ventilatory function in the child with asthma. Br J Dis Chest 1962; 56: 78–86.

4   Anderson SD, Silverman M, Godfrey S, Konig P. Exercise-induced asthma: A review. Br J Dis Chest 1975; 69: 1–39.

5   Godfrey S, Bar-Yishay E. Exercise-induced asthma revisited. Respir Med 1993; 87: 331–44.

6   Godfrey S, Konig P. Suppression of exercise-induced asthma by salbutamol, theophylline, atropine, cromolyn, and placebo in a group of asthmatic children. Pediatrics 1975; 56: 930–4.

7   Silverman M, Anderson SD. Standardization of exercise tests in asthmatic children. Arch Dis Child 1972; 47: 882–9.

8   Anderson SD, Seale JP, Ferris L, Schoeffel RE, Lindsay DA. An evaluation of pharmacotherapy for exercise-induced asthma. J Allergy Clin Immunol 1979; 64: 612–24.

9   Fitch KD, Morton AR. Specificity of exercise in exercise-induced asthma. BMJ 1971; 4: 577–81.

10   Anderson SD, Connolly N, Godfrey S. Comparison of bronchoconstriction induced by cycling and running. Thorax 1971; 26: 396–401.

11   Deal EC, McFadden ER, Ingram RH, Jaeger JJ. Hyperpnoea and heat flux: initial reaction sequence in exercise-induced asthma. J Appl Physiol: Respirat Environ Exercise Physiol 1979; 46: 476–83.

12   Strauss RH, McFadden ER, Ingram RH, Chandler E. Influence of heat and humidity on the airway obstruction induced by exercise in asthma. J Clin Invest 1978; 61: 433–40.

13   Phillips YY, Jaeger JJ, Laube BL, Rosenthal RR. Eucapnic voluntary hyperventilation of compressed gas mixture. A simple system for bronchial challenge by respiratory heat loss. Am Rev Respir Dis 1985; 131: 31–5.

14   Chen WY, Horton DJ. Heat and water loss from the airways and exercise-induced asthma. Respiration 1977; 34: 305–13.

15   Bar-Or O, Neuman I, Dotan R. Effects of dry and humid climates on exercise-induced asthma in children and preadolescents. J Allergy Clin Immunol 1977; 60: 163–8.

16.   Anderson SD. Is there a unifying hypothesis for exercise-induced asthma? J Allergy Clin Immunol 1984; 73: 660–5.

17   McFadden ER, Lenner KA, Strohl KP. Postexertional airway rewarming and thermally induced asthma. J Clin Invest 1986; 78: 18–25.

18   Anderson SD, Daviskas E. The airway microvasculature and exercise induced asthma. Thorax 1992; 47: 748–52.

19   Anderson SD, Schoeffel RE, Follet R, Perry CP, Daviskas E, Kendall M. Sensitivity to heat and water loss at rest and during exercise in asthmatic patients. Eur J Respir Dis 1982; 63: 459–71.

20 Eggleston PA, Kagey-Sobotka A, Lichtenstein LM. A comparison of the osmotic activation of basophils and human lung mast cells. Am Rev Respir Dis 1987; 135: 1043–8.

21 Umeno E, McDonald DM, Nadel JA. Hypertonic saline increases vascular permeability in the rat trachea by producing neurogenic inflammation. J Clin Invest 1990; 85: 1905–8.

22 Anderson SD. Asthma provoked by exercise, hyperventilation, and the inhalation of non-isotonic aerosols. In: Barnes PJ, Rodger IW, Thomson NC (eds) Asthma: Basic Mechanisms and Clinical Management, 2nd edn. London: Academic Press, 1992: 473–90.

23 Banner AS, Green J, O'Connor M. Relation of respiratory water loss to coughing after exercise. N Engl J Med 1984; 311: 883–6.

24 Katz RM, Siegel SC, Rachelefsky GS. Chronic cough in athletes. Clin Rev Allergy 1986; 6: 431–41.

25 Assoufi BK, Dally MB, Newman-Taylor AJ, Denison DM. Cold air test: a simplified standard method for airway reactivity. Bull Eur Physiopathol Respir 1986; 22: 349–57.

26 Anderson SD, Rodwell LT, Du Toit J, Young IH. Duration of protection of inhaled salmeterol in exercise-induced asthma. Chest 1991; 100: 1254–60.

27 Eggleston PA, Rosenthal RR, Anderson SD et al. Guidelines for the methodology of exercise challenge testing of asthmatics. J Allergy Clin Immunol 1979; 64: 642–5.

28 Cropp GJA. The exercise bronchoprovocation test: Standardization of procedures and evaluation of response. J Allergy Clin Immunol 1979; 64: 627–33.

29 Sterk PJ, Fabbri LM, Quanjer PhH et al. Airway responsiveness: Standardized challenge testing with pharmacological, physical and sensitizing stimuli in adults. Eur Respir J 1993; 6(suppl 16): 53–83.

30 Jones RS, Wharton MJ, Buston MH. The place of physical exercise and bronchodilator drugs in the assessment of the asthmatic child. Arch Dis Child 1963; 38: 539–45.

31 Burr ML, Eldridge BA, Borysiewicz LK. Peak expiratory flow rates before and after exercise in schoolchildren. Arch Dis Child 1974; 49: 923–6.

32 Comis A, Valletta EA, Sette L, Andreoli A, Boner AL. Comparison of nedocromil sodium and sodium cromoglycate administered by pressurized aerosol, with and without a spacer device in exercise-induced asthma in children. Eur Respir J 1993; 6: 523–6.

33 O'Cain CF, Dowling NB, Slutsky AS et al. Airway effects of respiratory heat loss in normal subjects. J Appl Physiol: Respirat Environ Exercise Physiol 1980; 49: 875–80.

34 Konig P, Jaffe P, Godfrey S. Effect of corticosteroids on exercise-induced asthma. J Allergy Clin Immunol 1974; 54: 14–9.

35 Henriksen JM, Dahl R. Effects of inhaled budesonide alone and in combination with low-dose terbutaline in children with exercise-induced asthma. *Am Rev Respir Dis* 1983; 128: 993–7.

36 Waalkens H, Van Essen-Zandvliet EEM, Gerritsen J *et al.* The effect of an inhaled corticosteroid (budesonide) on exercise-induced asthma in children. *Eur Respir J* 1993; 6: 652–6.

37 Mechelin W van, Hlobil H, Kemper HCG. Validation of two running tests as estimates of maximal aerobic power in children. *Eur J Appl Physiol* 1986; 55: 503–6.

38 Freeman W, Weir DC, Sapiano SB, Whitehead JE, Burge PS, Cayton RM. The twenty-metre shuttle-running test: a combined test for maximal oxygen uptake and exercise-induced asthma? *Respir Med* 1990; 84: 31–5.

39 Haby MM, Anderson SD, Peat JK, Mellis CM, Toelle BG, Woolcock AJ. An exercise challenge protocol for epidemiological studies of asthma in children: comparison with histamine challenge. *Eur Respir J* 1994; 7: 43–9.

40 Godfrey S. *Exercise Testing in Children*. London: W.B. Saunders, 1974: 168.

41 Silverman M, Anderson SD. Metabolic cost of treadmill exercise in children. *J Appl Physiol* 1972; 33: 696–8.

42 Givoni B, Goldman RF. Predicting metabolic energy cost. *J Appl Physiol* 1971; 30: 429–33.

43 Hahn A, Anderson SD, Morton AR, Black JL, Fitch KD. A re-interpretation of the effect of temperature and water content of the inspired air in exercise-induced asthma. *Am Rev Respir Dis* 1984; 130: 575–9.

44 Anderson SD, Silverman M, Walker SR. Metabolic and ventilatory changes in asthmatic patients during and after exercise. *Thorax* 1972; 27: 718–25.

45 Anderson SD, McEvoy JDS, Bianco S. Changes in lung volumes and airway resistance after exercise in asthmatic subjects. *Am Rev Respir Dis* 1972; 106: 30–7.

46 Freelander M, Van Asperen PP. Nebuhaler versus nebuliser in children with acute asthma. *BMJ* 1984; 288: 873–4.

47 Edmunds A, Tooley M, Godfrey S. The refractory period after exercise-induced asthma: its duration and relation to the severity of exercise. *Am Rev Respir Dis* 1978; 117: 247–54.

48 Schoeffel RE, Anderson SD, Gillam I, Lindsay DA. Multiple exercise and histamine challenge in asthmatic patients. *Thorax* 1980; 35: 164–70.

49 Anderson SD. Exercise-induced asthma. The state of the art. *Chest* 1985; 87(suppl): 191S–195S.

50 Gillam I, Landau LI, Phelan PD, Chennells HD. The variability of bronchoconstriction after repeated and prolonged exercise tests in asthmatics. In: Oseid S, Edwards A (eds) *The Asthmatic Child in Play and Sport*. London: Pitman Medical, 1983: 92–106.

51 O'Byrne PM, Jones GL. The effect of indomethacin on exercise-induced bronchoconstriction and refractoriness after exercise. *Am Rev Respir Dis* 1986; 134: 69–72.

52 Laitinen LA, Laitinen A, Haahtela T. A comparative study of the effects of an inhaled corticosteroid, budesonide, and a β_2-agonist, terbutaline, on airway inflammation in newly diagnosed asthma: A randomized, double-blind, parallel-group controlled trial. *J Allergy Clin Immunol* 1992; 90: 32–42.

53 Henriksen JM. Effect of inhalation of corticosteroids on exercise induced asthma: randomised double blind crossover study of budesonide in asthmatic children. *BMJ* 1985; 291: 248–9.

54 Molema J, van Herwaarden CLA, Folgering HThM. Effects of long-term treatment with inhaled cromoglycate and budesonide on bronchial hyper-responsiveness in patients with allergic asthma. *Eur Respir J* 1989; 2: 308–16.

55 Vathenen AS, Knox AJ, Wisniewski A, Tattersfield AE. Effect of inhaled budesonide on bronchial reactivity to histamine, exercise, and eucapnic dry air hyperventilation in patients with asthma. *Thorax* 1991; 46: 811–6.

56 Borson D, Gruenart DC. Glucocorticoids induce neutral endopeptidase in transformed human tracheal epithelial cells. *Am J Physiol* 1991; 260: L83–L89.

57 Tullett WM, Tan KM, Wall RT, Patel KR. Dose–response effect of sodium cromoglycate pressurised aerosol in exercise induced asthma. *Thorax* 1985; 40: 41–4.

58 Patel KR, Wall RT. Dose–duration effect of sodium cromoglycate aerosol in exercise-induced asthma. *Eur J Respir Dis* 1986; 69: 256–60.

59 Konig P, Hordvik NL, Kreutz C. The preventative effect and duration of action of nedocromil sodium and cromolyn sodium on exercise-induced asthma (EIA) in adults. *J Allergy Clin Immunol* 1987; 79: 64–8.

60 Albazzaz MK, Neale MG, Patel KR. Dose–response study of nebulised nedocromil sodium in exercise induced asthma. *Thorax* 1989; 44: 816–9.

61 Kuzemko JA. Twenty years of sodium cromoglycate treatment: a short review. *Respir Med* 1989; 83(suppl): 11–6.

62 Rodwell LT, Anderson SD, du Toit J, Seale JP. Nedocromil sodium inhibits the airway response to hyperosmolar challenge in patients with asthma. *Am Rev Respir Dis* 1993; 146: 1149–55.

63 Anderson SD, du Toit JI, Rodwell LT, Jenkins CR. The acute effect of sodium cromoglycate on airway narrowing induced by 4.5% saline in asthmatic patients, before and during treatment with aerosol corticosteroids. *Chest* 1994; 105: 673–80.

64 Crane J, Pearce N, Flatt A *et al*. Prescribed fenoterol and death from asthma in New Zealand, 1981–83: case control study. *Lancet* 1989; i: 917–22.

65 Sears MR, Taylor DR, Print CG *et al*. Regular inhaled beta-agonist treatment in bronchial asthma. *Lancet* 1990; 336: 1391–6.

66 Spitzer WO, Suissa S, Ernst P *et al.* The use of β-agonists and the risk of death and near-death from asthma. *N Engl J Med* 1992; 326: 501-6.

67 Peters MJ, Adcock IM, Brown CR, Barnes PJ. β-Agonist inhibition of steroid-receptor DNA binding activity in human lung. *Am Rev Respir Dis* 1993; 147: A772.

68 Woolley M, Anderson SD, Quigley BM. Duration of protective effect of terbutaline sulfate and cromolyn sodium alone and in combination on exercise-induced asthma. *Chest* 1990; 97: 39-45.

69 Dhillon DP. Studies in exercise-induced asthma. *Eur Respir Rev* 1991; 1: 265-7.

70 Patessio A, Podda A, Carone M, Trombetta N, Donner CF. Protective effect and duration of action of formoterol aerosol on exercise-induced asthma. *Eur Respir J* 1991; 4: 296-300.

71 Latimer KM, O'Byrne PM, Morris MM, Roberts R, Hargreave FE. Bronchoconstriction stimulated by airway cooling. Better protection with combined inhalation of terbutaline sulphate and cromolyn sodium than with either alone. *Am Rev Respir Dis* 1983; 128: 440-3.

72 Poppius H, Sovijarvi ARA, Tammilehto L. Lack of protective effect of high-dose ipratropium on bronchoconstriction following exercise with cold air breathing in patients with mild asthma. *Eur J Respir Dis* 1986; 68: 319-25.

73 Fuglsang G, Hertz B, Holm E-B. No protection by oral terbutaline against exercise-induced asthma in children: a dose–response study. *Eur Respir J* 1993; 6: 527-30.

74 Ellis EF. Inhibition of exercise-induced asthma by theophylline. *J Allergy Clin Immunol* 1984; 73: 690-3.

75 Laursen LC, Johanesson N, Weeke B. Effects of enprofylline and theophylline on exercise-induced asthma. *Allergy* 1985; 40: 506-9.

76 Godfrey S, Springer C, Noviski N, Maayan Ch, Avital A. Exercise but not methacholine differentiates asthma from chronic lung disease in children. *Thorax* 1991; 46: 488-92.

77 Weiss ST, Tager IB, Weiss JW, Munoz A, Speizer FE, Ingram RH. Airway responsiveness in a population sample of adults and children. *Am Rev Respir Dis* 1984; 129: 898-902.

78 Patel KR. Terfenadine in exercise-induced asthma. *BMJ* 1984; 285: 1496-7.

79 Finnerty JP, Holgate ST. Evidence for the roles of histamine and prostaglandins as mediators in exercise-induced asthma: the inhibitory effect of terfenadine and flurbiprofen alone and in combination. *Eur Respir J* 1990; 3: 540-7.

80 Finnerty JP, Holgate ST. The contribution of histamine release and vagal reflexes alone and in combination to exercise-induced asthma. *Eur Respir J* 1993; 6: 1132-7.

81 Manning PJ, Watson RM, Margolskee DJ *et al.* Inhibition of exercise-induced bronchoconstriction by MK-571, a potent leukotriene D_4-receptor antagonist. *N Engl J Med* 1990; 323: 1736-9.

82 Finnerty JP, Wood-Baker R, Thomson J, Holgate ST. Role of leukotrienes in exercise-induced asthma. *Am Rev Respir Dis* 1992; 145: 746-9.

83 Robuschi M, Riva E, Fuccella LM *et al.* Prevention of exercise-induced bronchoconstriction by a new leukotriene antagonist (SK&F 104353): a double-blind study versus disodium cromoglycate and placebo. *Am Rev Respir Dis* 1992; 145: 1285-8.

84 Brenner AM, Weiser PC, Krogh LA, Loren ML. Effectiveness of a portable face mask in attenuating exercise-induced asthma. *JAMA* 1980; 264: 2196-8.

85 Schachter EN, Lach E, Lee M. The protective effect of a cold weather mask on exercise-induced asthma. *Ann Allergy* 1981; 46: 12-6.

86 Gravelyn TR, Capper M, Eschenbacher WL. Effectiveness of a heat and moisture exchanger in preventing hyperpnoea induced bronchoconstriction in subjects with asthma. *Thorax* 1987; 42: 877-80.

87 Eiken O, Kaiser P, Holmer I, Baer R. Physiological effects of a mouth-borne heat exchanger during heavy exercise in a cold environment. *Ergonomics* 1989; 32: 645-53.

88 Mangla PK, Menon MPS. Effect of nasal and oral breathing on exercise-induced asthma. *Clin Allergy* 1981; 11: 433-9.

89 Shturman-Ellstein R, Zeballos RJ, Buckley JM, Souhrada JF. The beneficial effect of nasal breathing on exercise-induced bronchoconstriction. *Am Rev Respir Dis* 1978; 118: 65-73.

90 Togias AG, Proud D, Lichenstein LM *et al.* The osmolality of nasal secretions increases when inflammatory mediators are released in response to inhalation of cold, dry air. *Am Rev Respir Dis* 1988; 137: 625-9.

91 Carlson K-H, Boe J. Exercise-induced asthma in children. *Eur Respir J* 1993; 6: 614-6.

92 Fitch KD, Morton AR, Blanksby BA. Effects of swimming training on children with asthma. *Arch Dis Child* 1976; 51: 190-4.

93 Fitch KD, Blitvich JD, Morton AR. The effect of running training on exercise-induced asthma. *Ann Allergy* 1986; 57: 90-4.

94 Bundgaard A, Ingemann-Hansen T, Schmidt A, Halkjaer-Kristensen J. Effect of physical training on peak oxygen consumption rate and exercise-induced asthma in adult asthmatics. *Scand J Clin Lab Invest* 1982; 42: 9-13.

95 Nickerson BG, Bautista DB, Naney MA, Richards W, Keens TG. Distance running improves fitness in asthmatic children without pulmonary complications or changes in exercise-induced bronchospasm. *Pediatrics* 1983; 71: 147-52.

96 Henriksen JM, Nielsen TT. Effect of physical training on exercise-induced bronchoconstriction. *Acta Paediatr Scand* 1983; 72: 31-6.

97 Svenonius E, Kautto R, Arborelius M. Improvement after training of children with exercise-induced asthma. *Acta Paediatr Scand* 1983; 72: 23–30.

98 Haas F, Pasierski S, Levine N *et al.* Effect of aerobic training on forced expiratory airflow in exercising asthmatic humans. *J Appl Physiol* 1987; 63: 1230–5.

99 Schaefer O, Eaton RDP, Timmermans FJW, Hildes JA. Respiratory function impairment and cardiopulmonary consequences in long-time residents of Canadian Arctic. *Can Med Assoc J* 1980; 123: 997–1004.

100 Mahler DA, Loke J. Lung function after marathon runners at warm and cold ambient temperatures. *Am Rev Respir Dis* 1981; 124: 154–7.

101 Weiler JM, Metzger J, Donnelly AL, Crowley ET, Sharath MD. Prevalence of bronchial hyperresponsiveness in highly trained athletes. *Chest* 1986; 90: 23–8.

102 Morton AR, Fitch KD, Davis T. The effect of "warm-up" on exercise-induced asthma. *Ann Allergy* 1979; 42: 257–60.

103 Morton AR, Hahn AG, Fitch KD. Continuous and intermittent running in the provocation of asthma. *Ann Allergy* 1982; 48: 123–9.

104 Schnall RP, Landau LI. Protective effects of repeated short sprints in exercise-induced asthma. *Thorax* 1980; 35: 828–32.

105 Reiff DB, Choudry NB, Pride NB, Ind PW. The effect of prolonged submaximal warm-up exercise on exercise-induced asthma. *Am Rev Respir Dis* 1989; 139: 479–84.

106 Lin WS, Shamoo DA, Anderson KR, Whynot JD, Avol EL, Hackney JD. Effects of heat and humidity on the responses of exercising asthmatics to sulphur dioxide exposure. *Am Rev Respir Dis* 1985; 131: 221–5.

KEY POINTS

1 Severe EIA can occur in patients with good lung function and lung function cannot be used to predict the amount of therapy required to control EIA.

It should be noted that the diagnosis of EIA cannot be simply made on a history of post-exercise cough. While it is important to recognize cough as a symptom consistent with EIA, not all those with post-exercise cough have EIA.

The reason EIA should not be ignored is that it is associated with arterial hypoxaemia and hyperinflation of the lungs.

If subjects feel an attack of asthma coming on during exercise, they should be advised to stop immediately.

2   In severe cases of EIA up to 10 inhalations of a β_2-adrenoceptor agonist can be given. FEV_1 improves within days of starting steroids, whereas the severity of EIA may not be reduced for weeks or even months.

It is important to know that EIA can still occur when the daily use of aerosol steroid is sufficient to achieve normal lung function, eliminate symptoms and reduce diurnal airflow variability.

When aerosol steroids control symptoms of asthma and keep lung function within normal limits, EIA may be prevented by inhaling 10–20 mg of sodium cromoglycate or 4–8 mg of nedocromil sodium.

However β_2-adrenoceptor agonists must be available for those who develop EIA unexpectedly, and they remain the major drug to be used for rescue medication.

In order to overcome the short protective effect and multiple use of β_2-adrenoceptor agonists, the newer longer-acting salmeterol and formoterol can be used.

Oral bronchodilators are not useful in the prevention of EIA.

3   About 50% of people with EIA become refractory to exercise if it is repeated within 30–90 min.

However, training in those who are already fit is likely to have little or no effect. If these persons have moderate to severe EIA they should be encouraged to have a trial of inhaled corticosteroids.

35

SPECIFIC PROBLEMS: NOCTURNAL ASTHMA

Richard J. Martin

INTRODUCTION

To fully understand asthma, it is important for the clinician to know about alterations that occur on a circadian (24-hour cycle) basis. There are several important reasons for this concept. Symptoms of obstructive lung disease, independent of medication, occur more commonly during the sleep-related time interval with the peak at approximately 4 a.m.[1] Additionally, Turner-Warwick has shown in a large population study that "stable" asthmatic outpatients, when specifically asked, have frequent problems with their asthma at night:[2] 39% of these patients are symptomatic every night of the week, 64% three nights per week and 74% have difficulty at least one night a week.

Does this high frequency of nocturnal problems translate into anything more than a simple nuisance? Fitzpatrick and colleagues have shown that these patients have poorer daytime cognitive function than a matched control population.[3] Thus, asthmatic children with nocturnal worsening of their disease would tend to perform at a lower level in school and, similarly, adults may not function to their capacity at work. Furthermore, asthma morbidity (respiratory arrests) and mortality have the greatest occurrence during the sleeping hours.[4,5] Recent statistics show a worldwide trend for increased asthma mortality and those studies that analyse time of death have shown the majority of cases to occur at night.[6,7] This figure is probably low as the death may occur during the day, but the process begins or accelerates during the night.

ASSESSMENT

Assessment of an asthmatic patient for nocturnal asthma is, fortunately, relatively easy. However, one must always keep in mind other diseases that can mimic asthma. As an example, with the increasing prevalence of asthma in the geriatric population, cardiac problems must be differentiated in this specific asthmatic population. In fact, cardiac function normally decreases at night, which in a patient with compromised cardiac function can lead to nocturnal heart failure. This cardiac decompensation can present as nocturnal "wheezing", which can be confused with asthma. Additionally, intermittent recurrent small pulmonary emboli can present with nocturnal problems in the older population. Other types of obstructive lung diseases, e.g. chronic obstructive pulmonary disease (COPD), all have the potential to worsen during the night and give symptoms similar to asthma. One must keep in mind that most if not all disease processes have the potential for circadian alterations with symptoms and signs worse at night. This would be true for all age groups. If that particular disease process affects the upper (such as allergic rhinitis) or lower airways, symptoms may mistakenly be confused with nocturnal asthma.

Objectively measuring lung function is important in determining the severity of nocturnal asthma. The peak flow meter is relatively inexpensive and gives the patient and physician an accurate objective assessment of alterations in lung function that may occur overnight. This objectivity has an added benefit in that it allows patients to become more "aware" of changes in lung function and thus more "in tune" with their asthma. This subject awareness of asthma, particularly at night, is important. Turner-Warwick's study[2] showed that less than 50% of asthmatic patients with problems every night of the week considered their asthma to be severe. The majority considered their asthma to be mild or moderate. Many patients become "used to" the bronchoconstriction and incorporate this into their "normal" routine. Another group of asthmatic patients have a blunted perception of the degree of bronchoconstriction. Thus, objectivity (using peak flow measurements) is extremely helpful in evaluating nocturnal asthma. This has also been stressed in the recent International Asthma Consensus Report.[8]

In a very small segment of the asthma population (exact percentage unknown), the patient only has asthma during sleep. Thus, daytime spirometry, response to inhaled bronchodilators and even airway responsiveness (response to agents that produce bronchoconstriction) may be relatively normal and cast the diagnosis of asthma into doubt. Here the use of a peak flow meter at home will show the overnight changes in lung function if they are present. If further information about asthma in this situation is needed, methacholine challenge testing can be set up (with difficulty in most institutions) to be performed at 4 a.m. Airway responsiveness is much greater in nearly all asthmatic subjects during the night[9] even if nocturnal worsening of expiratory flow rates are absent.

Thus, it is important for the physician to evaluate the asthmatic patient not only during the day but also during the night. In doing so the physician truly understands the patient's asthma anad does not erroneously make assumptions of the clinical status on daytime measurements in the office. The effectiveness of any medical intervention can then also be determined in the home setting. In addition, the patient has an objective parameter to follow. This not only educates the patient to his/her disease, but also gradual impending problems can be noted and more easily dealt with compared to the time when the patient is seen in the emergency room.

MANAGEMENT (Fig. 35.1)

To understand the management of nocturnal asthma, the clinician must realize that nocturnal asthma is a multifaceted process. Figure 35.2 shows the multiple factors that can interact in producing nocturnal asthma. The nocturnal decrement in cortisol, adrenaline, body temperature and increase in vagal tone are actually normally occurring circadian rhythms. The increase in inflammation is specifically related to worsening of asthma at night. This may occur due to the decrement in cortisol and adrenaline allowing the "brakes" to be released and nocturnal inflammation to develop in those individuals primed for this event.

REVERSIBLE FACTORS

Although most patients will not have easily identifiable extrinsic factors, these still should be considered. Even if the patient is asymptomatic during the daytime, causative agents at work or home may produce delayed effects and nocturnal asthma. Examples of workplace factors are western red

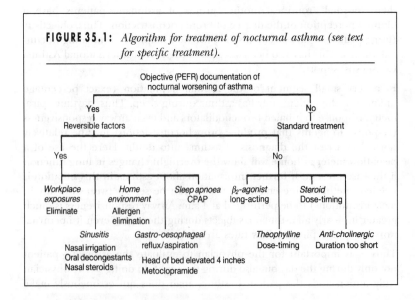

FIGURE 35.1: *Algorithm for treatment of nocturnal asthma (see text for specific treatment).*

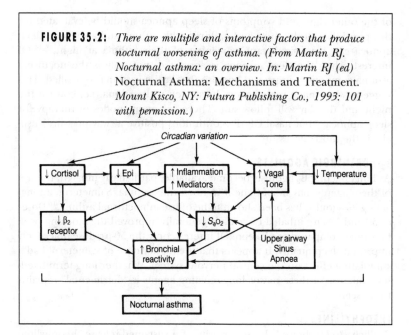

FIGURE 35.2: *There are multiple and interactive factors that produce nocturnal worsening of asthma. (From Martin RJ. Nocturnal asthma: an overview. In: Martin RJ (ed)* Nocturnal Asthma: Mechanisms and Treatment. *Mount Kisco, NY: Futura Publishing Co., 1993: 101 with permission.)*

cedar[10] and grain dust exposure.[11] At home be certain the patient is not sleeping with the family dog or cat, a not uncommon occurrence in those households with pets.

Asthma is a disease of both intra- and extra-thoracic airways and sinusitis occurs in about 40–60% of all asthmatic subjects. If aspiration of the sinus secretions occurs, this can worsen asthma. Correcting the sinusitis with nasal saline irrigation, oral decongestants and nasal steroids can improve nocturnal asthma in this subset of patients. Oral steroids and 3–4 weeks of antibiotics may be needed in severe cases of sinusitis. A sinus surgical procedure is rarely needed for control of sinusitis.

Gastro-oesophageal reflux *per se* has not been proven to be an aetiological factor in nocturnal asthma.[12] However, aspiration of reflux material may play an important and potentially correctable role in nocturnal asthma. The patient who complains of a bitter or sour taste upon arising may belong to that subset of reflux patients who aspirate during sleep. In this situation a trial of 4-inch wood or brick blocks under the head of the bed (raising the head with pillows will not work) and medication to increase gastric emptying (metoclopramide) would be indicated. Surgery to solidify the gastro-oesophageal junction is rarely indicated but should be considered if aspiration is documented and the above therapy is not of benefit.

Those asthmatic patients who have daytime hypersomnolence, loud snoring, increased irritability, restless sleep, hypertension, erythrocytosis or any of the other signs and symptoms of sleep apnoea should be evaluated for this possibility. Both adults and children with asthma and associated sleep apnoea can have significant worsening of their asthma at night.[13,14] Of interest, when the sleep apnoea is corrected, not only is the nocturnal asthma component improved but also the daytime asthma controlled. This suggests what many investigators have seen with asthma, i.e. control the night and the day will follow suit. There are many modes of therapy for sleep apnoea,[15] but nasal CPAP (continuous positive airway pressure) usually is the most successful.

β_2-ADRENERGIC AGONISTS

As longer-acting β_2 agonists become available, particularly inhaled, the use of these agents may be of benefit in nocturnal asthma. Salmeterol, a long-acting β_2 agonist, has been shown to be of use in nocturnal asthma.[16] Doses of 50 and 100 µg inhaled twice daily generally improved the morning peak flow rates compared to placebo. Of interest, only the 50-µg dose objectively improved sleep quality. It appears that the higher dose of salmeterol had a stimulating effect on the central nervous system. Whether long-term fixed-schedule use of these newer longer-acting agents is "detrimental" remains to be seen.

THEOPHYLLINES

Zwillich et al.[17] showed the superiority of a sustained-release theophylline preparation (Theo-Dur) in treating asthmatic patients with mild-to-moderate nocturnal asthma compared with a short-acting inhaled β_2 agonist (bitolterol, Tornalate). Not only was the forced expiratory volume in 1 s (FEV_1) improved in the morning, but there was also less nocturnal oxygen desaturation while on theophylline. Of importance, sleep quality and architecture were unchanged between the different preparations, demonstrating that the presence of theophylline did not alter sleep compared with the β_2 agonist.

In subjects with more significant nocturnal asthma, a chronotherapeutic approach is indicated, i.e. obtaining a higher serum theophylline concentration (STC) during the night when the disease is the worst and a lower STC during the daytime when it is easier to control the bronchoconstriction. Comparing two theophylline preparations with different pharmacokinetics, Martin et al.[18] showed that higher STCs (about 16–18 µg ml^{-1}) from 3.00 to 5.00 a.m. produced a marked improvement in the overnight worsening of lung function vs. lower therapeutic levels (about 11.5 µg ml^{-1}). During the daytime the agent that gave a higher nocturnal STC (Uniphyl, given once daily at 7.00 p.m.) exhibited a progressive decrease in STC with a nadir of about 8 µg ml^{-1} before the next dose. The other agent (Theo-Dur) given twice a day had higher daytime STCs compared with night-time. The FEV_1 levels measured every 2 hours during the daytime were not significantly different between the agents even though the STCs were different. This reinforces the importance of delivering higher concentrations of medication when most needed, i.e. at night. Furthermore, sleep quality and architecture were not altered between the higher and lower therapeutic STCs, but there was less nocturnal oxygen desaturation with the higher levels. Many other studies using theophylline in a chronotherapeutic method have shown similar beneficial results.

CORTICOSTEROIDS

Another example of chronotherapy is in the use of oral corticosteroids. If an asthma patient needs steroids, then every effort should be made to use inhaled steroids. However, inhaled steroids improve nocturnal asthma in only about 50% of patients if individual data and not group means are analysed. There are many oral steroid-dependent asthmatic patients with nocturnal asthma. Commonly, increasing the morning steroid dosing in these individuals usually leads to more steroid complications without improvement in night-time asthma control. Reinberg et al.[19,20] have suggested that the time of corticosteroid administration during the day may be relevant in attenuating the nocturnal worsening of asthma.

Beam et al.[21] have begun to clarify the contribution of timing of corticosteroids to their ability to block the circadian recruitment of inflammatory cells into the lung. Their results highlight the relevance of prednisone dose timing in attenuating the nocturnal worsening of asthmatic lung function and decrement in airways inflammation. A 3.00 p.m. dose produced significant improvement in overnight FEV_1 (placebo control, $-28\% \pm 7\%$; steroid, $-10\% \pm 4\%$). Additionally, the 3.00 p.m. dose of prednisone produced a pancellular reduction in the 4.00 a.m. bronchoalveolar lavage cytology. Neither an 8.00 a.m. nor 8.00 p.m. dose phase produced an improvement in overnight spirometry or reduction in any bronchoalveolar lavage cellular profile. It is noteworthy that Martin et al.[22] demonstrated elevations in total white cell number, neutrophil, eosinophil and lymphocyte counts in bronchoalveolar lavage fluid at 4.00 a.m. in nocturnal asthma subjects compared to 4.00 p.m. These observations support a collaborative cellular mechanism of inflammation at night that is corticosteroid sensitive, but dependent on timing in addition to dosage.

The use of inhaled steroids is of interest in patients with nocturnal asthma. One would think that these agents would be ideal for this problem. However, studies have given mixed results. Horn et al.[23] showed that in 14 asthmatic patients with nocturnal symptoms and decreased peak expiratory flow rates in the morning, only eight patients resolved the nocturnal component using inhaled beclomethasone (also taking inhaled salbutamol). The dose of beclomethasone was higher than standard, being 400 μg four times daily. Although the other six patients had improved daytime lung function, the overnight decrements in lung function did not improve. The question arises if there is also a dose time for inhaled steroids that would work better in the treatment of nocturnal asthma.

ANTI-CHOLINERGICS

Vagal tone is increased at night in everyone. This would suggest that a vagolytic would be of benefit in treating nocturnal asthma. Morrison *et al.*[24] have shown that atropine produces marked bronchodilation at 4.00 a.m. compared to 4.00 p.m. Presently, an anti-cholinergic of long enough duration is not available for this form of therapy to work. Higher bedtime dosing compared with the usual daytime dosing is needed to lengthen the duration of effective action of the drug, but side-effects are then increased. If the patient wakes during the night, then inhalation of atropine or ipratropium bromide can be of benefit.

CONCLUSION

As Eugene Robin stated 35 years ago, "the sleeping patient is still a patient. His disease not only goes on while he sleeps, but indeed may progress in an entirely different fashion from its progression during the waking state".[25] Today we can see how accurate that thought was, because any disease process of any organ system has the potential to worsen during sleep. To neglect this area of medicine hinders the care of the patient and accelerates the disease process. The future will bring tremendous advances to our understanding and ability to treat the nocturnal aspect of asthma and thus the disease itself.

REFERENCES

1. Dethlefsen U, Repgas R. Ein neues Therapieprinzip bei nachtlichen Asthma. *Klin Med* 1985; 80: 44–7.

2. Turner-Warwick M. Epidemiology of nocturnal asthma. *Am J Med* 1988; 85: 6–8.

3. Fitzpatrick MF, Engleman H, Whyte KF *et al.* Morbidity in nocturnal asthma: Sleep quality and daytime cognitive performance. *Thorax* 1991; 46: 569–73.

4. Cochrane GM, Clark TJH. A survey of asthma mortality in patients between ages 35 and 65 in the Greater London hospitals in 1971. *Thorax* 1975; 30: 300–15.

5. Hetzel MR, Clark TJH, Branthwaite MA. Asthma: Analysis of sudden deaths and ventilatory arrests in hospital. *BMJ* 1977; 1: 808–11.

6. Jackson RT, Sears MR, Beaglehole R *et al.* International trends in asthma mortality; 1970–1985. *Chest* 1988; 94: 914–8.

7   Robertson CF, Rubinfeld AR, Bowes G. Deaths from asthma in Victoria; a 12-month survey. Med J Aust 1990; 152: 511-7.

8   International Consensus Report on Diagnosis and Treatment of Asthma. National Heart, Lung and Blood Institute. National Institutes of Health, Publication No. 91-3091, June 1992.

9   Martin RJ, Cicutto LC, Ballard RD. Factors related to the nocturnal worsening of asthma. Am Rev Respir Dis 1990; 141: 33-8.

10   Gandevia B, Milne J. Occupational asthma and rhinitis due to western red cedar (*Thuja plicata*), with special reference to bronchial reactivity. Br J Ind Med 1970; 27: 235-44.

11   Davies RJ, Green M, Schofield N. Recurrent nocturnal asthma after exposure to grain dust. Am Rev Respir Dis 1976; 114: 1011-9.

12   Tan WC, Martin RJ, Pandey R et al. Effects of spontaneous and simulate gastroesophageal reflux on sleeping asthmatics. Am Rev Respir Dis 1990; 141: 1394-9.

13   Chan CS, Woolcock AJ, Sullivan CE. Nocturnal asthma. Role of snoring and obstructive sleep apnea. Am Rev Respir Dis 1988; 137: 1502-4.

14   Guilleminault C, Quera-Salva MA, Powell N et al. Nocturnal asthma: Snoring, small pharynx and nasal CPAP. Eur Respir J 1988; 1: 902-7.

15   Sanders MH. The management of sleep-disordered breathing. In: Martin RJ (ed) *Cardiorespiratory Disorders During Sleep*. Mount Kisco, NY: Futura Publishing Co., 1990: 141-88.

16   Fitzpatrick MF, Mackay T, Driver H et al. Salmeterol in nocturnal asthma: a doube blind, placebo controlled trial of a long acting inhaled β_2 agonist. BMJ 1990; 301: 1365-8.

17   Zwillich CW, Neagley SR, Cicutto L et al. Nocturnal asthma therapy: Inhaled bitolterol versus sustained release theophylline. Am Rev Respir Dis 1989; 139: 470-4.

18   Martin RJ, Cicutto LC, Ballard RD. Circadian variations in theophylline concentrations and the treatment of nocturnal asthma. Am Rev Respir Dis 1989; 139: 475-8.

19   Reinberg A, Gervas P, Choussade M et al. Circadian changes in effectiveness of corticosteroids in eight patients with allergic asthma. J Allergy Clin Immunol 1983; 71: 425-33.

20   Reinberg A, Halberg F, Falliers CJ. Circadian timing of methylprednisolone effects in asthmatic boys. Chronobiologia 1974; 1: 333-47.

21   Beam WR, Weiner DE, Martin RJ. Timing of prednisone and alterations of airways inflammation in nocturnal asthma. Am Rev Respir Dis 1992; 146: 1524-30.

22   Martin RJ, Cicutto LC, Smith HR et al. Airway inflammation in nocturnal asthma. Am Rev Respir Dis 1991; 143: 351-7.

23 Horn CR, Clark TJH, Cochrane GM. Inhaled therapy reduces morning dips in asthma. *Lancet* 1984; i: 1143–5.

24 Morrison JFJ, Pearson SB, Dean HG. Parasympathetic nervous system in nocturnal asthma. *BMJ* 1988; 296: 1427–9.

25 Robin ED. Some interrelations between sleep and disease. *Arch Intern Med* 1958; 102: 669–75.

KEY POINTS

1 *Nocturnal Asthma*
   - Occurs in the majority of stable patients at least three times a week.
   - Is a multifaceted process.
   - Treatment is based on a chronotherapeutic basis as patients are *not* homeostatic beings but have active circadian (24 hour) rhythms that respond to time-related therapy.

36

SPECIFIC PROBLEMS: ASTHMA IN PREGNANCY AND PRE-MENSES

Debora Ortega-Carr and William W. Busse

INTRODUCTION

Asthma prevalence in various age groups in the USA has been increasing and most physicians who care for asthma patients will repeatedly face the clinical problem of the asthmatic patient during pregnancy. Asthma complicates approximately 1% of all pregnancies.[1] To better understand the effect of asthma on the pregnant patient, it is necessary to understand the changes in respiratory physiology that occur during pregnancy and how these changes may produce symptoms in normal gravidas as well as in asthma. The following discussion will focus on the effects of pregnancy on asthma, the perinatal outcome in the asthmatic patient, and options for effective and appropriate medical management with emphasis on medications frequently used in pregnancy and, finally, a brief discussion on asthma and the menstrual cycle, with attention on pre-menstrual exacerbations of asthma.

PHYSIOLOGICAL CHANGES IN PREGNANCY

UPPER RESPIRATORY TRACT
Symptoms of nasal obstruction, sneezing and snoring are common complaints during pregnancy. Nasal obstruction results from hyperaemia, hypersecretion and mucosal oedema and is most noticeable in the third trimester. Oestrogen plays a major role in the mucosal changes by increasing the hyaluronic acid component of ground substance, thereby increasing tissue hydration and oedema. Oestrogen also causes capillary congestion and hyperplastic and hypersecretory mucous glands.[2] These changes may also make the mucous membranes friable and prone to epistaxis.[3]

RESPIRATORY MUSCULATURE AND THORACIC CAGE

As the uterus enlarges during pregnancy, the diaphragm is elevated by up to 4 cm. Despite this upward displacement, diaphragmatic function is not impaired.[4] This occurs because there is a 2-cm increase in the anteroposterior and transverse diameter of the thoracic cage.[5] The subcostal angle progressively broadens and there is a 5–7-cm increase in chest circumference. Respiratory muscle function does not appear to be greatly affected by pregnancy. Moreover, Contreras *et al.*,[4] by measuring transdiaphragmatic pressures with oesophageal and gastric balloons, demonstrated no significant change in maximum transdiaphragmatic pressures generated at week 37 of gestation compared with post-partum values.

PULMONARY FUNCTION

Lung Volumes

Cugell and associates found that there is a progressive decrease in both expiratory reserve volume (8–40%) and residual volume (7–22%) throughout pregnancy (Fig. 36.1). As a result, a 10–25% decrease occurs in functional residual capacity after the fifth or sixth month of pregnancy.[6–8] These changes are due to the cephalad displacement of the diaphragm and may be accentuated during recumbency.

Inspiratory capacity increases secondary to flaring of the ribs and widening of the rib cage as well as a reduced tone of the abdominal wall musculature. Consequently, vital capacity and total lung capacity are not substantially changed in most healthy gravidas.

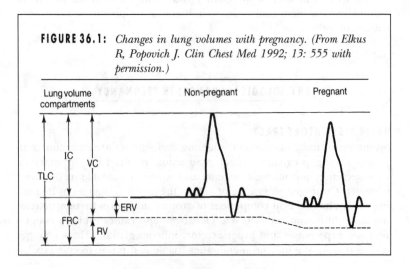

FIGURE 36.1: *Changes in lung volumes with pregnancy. (From Elkus R, Popovich J. Clin Chest Med 1992; 13: 555 with permission.)*

Ventilation and Pulmonary Mechanics

In addition to these alterations in lung volumes, hormonal changes arise (i.e. increased progesterone), which affect ventilation by direct stimulation of the respiratory centre. This leads to an increase in the respiratory rate and subsequently minute ventilation. The increased respiratory drive and rib cage volume displacement causes tidal volume to become greater. These changes may contribute to the perception of dyspnoea, but do not usually produce pulmonary compromise.

HORMONAL CHANGES

Cortisol

Cortisol increases during pregnancy. This several fold increase is noted in both total cortisol levels as well as cortisol bound to cortisol-binding globulin. Although the free cortisol level remains at 2% of the total cortisol level, the resultant cortisol is two times higher than that of the non-pregnant female. The reasons that this increase in active cortisol does not always improve asthma control are multiple. First, the rise in free cortisol is modest. Second, tissue hyporesponsiveness to cortisol decreases the biological activity of the circulating hormone.[9] Third, the cortisol increase is quite variable among individuals. Finally, as will be discussed later in the chapter, there are multiple other factors that may negatively influence pregnancy, thus offsetting the benefit from increases in cortisol.

Progesterone

Progesterone increases both resting minute ventilation and the slope of the curve of the ventilatory response to changes in alveolar P_{CO_2} or normal non-pregnant subjects. The increases in progesterone in pregnancy enhance the sensitivity of the respiratory centre to P_aCO_2 or act as a primary respiratory stimulant to promote ventilation. The effect of progesterone on airway resistance is less clear. In patients with alveolar hypoventilation and obesity, treatment with progesterone may decrease airway resistance and increase maximum expiratory flow rates. When Juniper et al. prospectively evaluated methacholine sensitivity in 16 pregnant women, they found a significant improvement in airway responsiveness; however there was no correlation of these changes with the progesterone level.[11]

Oestrogens

Whether oestrogens act to increase respiratory drive through an increased irritability of the respiratory centre has not been established.[12]

Other Hormones

The respiratory effects associated with changes in prostaglandin (PG) concentrations during pregnancy are unclear. $PGF_{2\alpha}$ a uterine smooth muscle stimulant, constricts bronchial mucosa; in contrast, PGE_1 and PGE_2 are bronchodilators. Several studies have shown reversible bronchoconstriction during intravenous or intra-amniotic administration of $PGF_{2\alpha}$ to induce abortion; therefore $PGF_{2\alpha}$ may precipitate asthma attacks in women with underlying airway disease.[13] Serum cyclic AMP concentration shows a cyclical peak during pregnancy. The first peak occurs at 14 weeks and the second at 34 weeks. Cyclic GMP excretion increases rapidly during the first trimester and then stabilizes at this level throughout the duration of pregnancy. It is not known how changes in nucleotide concentrations affect bronchomotor tone in normal pregnant women or those with obstructive lung disease.[12] The stimulus associated with these changes in cyclic nucleotides has not been established.

EFFECTS OF PREGNANCY ON ASTHMA

Asthma may improve, stabilize or worsen during pregnancy: the classical rule of thirds. Many studies have found the course of asthma to be quite variable during pregnancy. Nonetheless, Gluck and Gluck reviewed a combined series of 1087 patients and found that the course of asthma improved in 36%, worsened in 23% and was unchanged in 41% of subjects.[13] Schatz et al. identified similar ratios; asthma worsened in 35% of the patients, improved in 28% and was unchanged in 33% (by symptom diary assessment). Schatz et al. also found that asthma tended to improve during the last 4 weeks of pregnancy, and asthma attacks during labour and delivery were uncommon.[14]

Studies to evaluate pulmonary function parameters during pregnancy have shown variable responses. When spirometry was compared in 27 asthma vs. 11 non-asthma subjects, no significant effects of pregnancy on airflow obstruction were found.[15] However, Juniper et al. evaluated methacholine sensitivity in 16 pregnant women and found a two-fold improvement in airway responsiveness during pregnancy.[11] They were also able to find that the improvement in responsiveness during pregnancy was associated with a reduction in asthma severity.

Although studies differ widely on the overall effect of asthma on pregnancy, several reviews[14,16–19] find the following similar trends. First, women with severe asthma are more likely to deteriorate, while women with mild asthma are more likely to improve. Second, each individual patient has a similar clinical course with subsequent pregnancies. Third, asthma exacerbations are most likely to appear during weeks 24–36 of gestation, with few patients (10% or less) becoming symptomatic during labour or delivery. Finally, the changes in asthma noted during pregnancy usually revert toward the pre-pregnancy status within 3 months of delivery. These changes in asthma control have not necessarily been associated with fluctuations in hormonal levels. Assessment of the true course of asthma during pregnancy will require prospective, longitudinal studies with controls for additional confounding factors and repeated measures of pulmonary function.

EFFECTS OF ASTHMA ON MOTHER AND FETUS

Several studies have evaluated pregnancy outcome in asthma compared to non-asthmatic controls. The results are highly variable. Bahna and Bjerkedal found a significant increase in pre-term birth and low birthweight infants but no rise in congenital malformations in 381 asthma subjects when compared to a control population of 112530 pregnant healthy women.[20] When Gordon et al. compared pregnancy outcome in 277 asthmatic women with 30861 women controls, they found a statistically significant increase in perinatal mortality in asthmatic versus control women.[1] The majority of the perinatal morbidity appears to have arisen from poorly controlled asthma in a subset of these patients. More recently, Perlow et al. showed significant differences in Apgar score and birthweight in the offspring of steroid-dependent patients as compared to non-steroid-dependent asthma.[21] These data suggest that the severity of disease influences the likelihood of perinatal morbidity. Finally, Apter et al. examined the outcome in 28 pregnancies of adolescents with severe asthma.[22] In comparing factors such as intrauterine growth retardation, prematurity and congenital malformations, the incidence of perinatal morbidity was actually less than that typically found in non-asthmatic adolescents. Because these asthmatic patients were carefully followed, with exacerbations quickly controlled, these data reinforce the suggestion that optimally managed asthma, even severe asthma, may have few adverse effects on the fetus.

Maternal complications associated with asthma include pregnancy-induced hypertension, diabetes mellitus and gestational diabetes; these changes are seen predominantly in the steroid-dependent group. Lehrer et al. have found a significant association between pregnancy-induced hypertension and asthma symptoms during pregnancy, especially in patients with more severe hypertension.[23] Pregnant asthma patients may be more likely to receive epidural analgesia and have a Caesarean section than are non-asthmatic controls.[24]

Multiple factors may influence the perinatal morbidity and mortality that has been associated with pregnancy in asthma. Maternal hypoxaemia may cause fetal hypoxia. Acute asthma can lead to hypocapnia, alkalosis and dehydration; these changes may further reduce uterine blood flow. Asthma medications must also be considered as possible contributors to perinatal morbidity and mortality. For example, adrenaline may cause reduced uteroplacental blood flow.[25,26]

There are numerous other potential factors that affect fetal well-being such as maternal height, weight, parity, nutrition, ethnicity and cigarette smoking. However, few studies have adequately controlled for these factors. Nonetheless, recent data strongly suggest that when asthma is optimally controlled, it should not be associated with increased perinatal morbidity and mortality. Severe uncontrolled disease, however, leads to a poorer outcome.

ASTHMA MANAGEMENT DURING PREGNANCY

The goals of therapy during pregnancy are to optimize chronic maternal pulmonary function as well as to prevent acute episodes of asthma, which may lead to hypoxaemia. Essential in the overall control of the pregnant patient, as in any asthmatic individual, is the identification of potentially avoidable triggering factors, i.e. allergens or irritants such as cigarette smoke. Although the identification of allergic triggers is important, routine skin testing for allergens during pregnancy is not recommended, since a small risk of anaphylaxis exists in some patients. However, if a specific allergen is identified by history, the radioallergosorbent test (RAST) may be considered to confirm this suspicion.

Metzger *et al.* reported on 121 pregnancies in 90 women receiving inhalant allergen immunotherapy.[27] Patients on maintenance immunotherapy had no increase in prematurity, toxaemia, abortion, neonatal death and congenital malformation. In addition, no adverse effects from local or systemic reactions to immunotherapy were found. Nonetheless, anaphylaxis has been reported to contribute to abortion.[28] General recommendations on immunotherapy are that it can be continued but doses of antigen should not be increased.

PHARMACOLOGICAL MANAGEMENT

When choosing any drug in pregnancy, the potential therapeutic benefits must be weighed against possible risks to both mother and fetus. Most drugs used to treat asthma and allergic rhinitis have not shown harmful effects. Some medications have been more extensively evaluated and show documented safety and efficacy; these medications are the "drugs of choice" during pregnancy (Table 36.1). In this regard, the Food and Drug Administration (FDA) in the USA has published guidelines for prescribing medications to pregnant women. Drugs are categorized into four groups (Table 36.2) depending on their adverse effects in human or animal studies. This information can be useful in establishing a therapeutic programme in asthma.

Bronchodilators

β-Adrenergic agonists are the most frequently used bronchodilators in asthma and during pregnancy (Table 36.3). The administration of subcutaneous adrenaline during the first trimester of pregnancy has been associated with an increase in congenital malformations.[29] These data may be inconclusive and relate to the severity of the disease rather than the medication. Nonetheless, it is prudent to avoid adrenaline during the early gestational period. Studies in animals have suggested that isoproterenol and albuterol may be teratogenic in mice.[30] No teratogenic effects were identified in trials of oral ephedrine in humans; however sympathomimetics, especially systemic sympathomimetics, have the potential to reduce uteroplacental blood flow. Adrenaline has been shown to reduce uteroplacental

TABLE 36.1: *Suggested medications for use in asthma during pregnancy*

Bronchodilators
  Terbutaline by inhalation
  Theophylline

Anti-inflammatory agents
  Cromolyn sodium
  Beclomethasone dipropionate
  Prednisone

Antibiotics
  Penicillins
  Cephalosporins

Allergy medication
  Tripelennamine
  Nasal beclomethasone (for allergic rhinitis)

TABLE 36.2: *Food and Drug Administration pregnancy categories. (From Federal Registrar, Index publication 44, FR 37462, 26 June 1979 with permission)*

Category	Animal studies	Human data	Benefit outweighs risk
A	Negative	Studies negative[a]	Yes
B	Negative	Studies not done	Yes
B	Positive	Studies negative	Yes
C	Positive	Studies not done	Yes
C	Not done	Studies not done	Yes
D	Positive or negative	Studies or rep pos	Yes
X	Positive	Studies or rep pos	No

[a]Adequate and well-controlled studies in pregnant women.

TABLE 36.3: *Bronchodilators used for asthma during pregnancy*

Drug	Animal studies[a]	Malformation or other effect	Class
Inhaled β agonists			
Metaproterenol	Positive	May inhibit labour	C
Albuterol/salbutamol	Positive	May inhibit labour	C
Pirbuterol	Negative		C
	Positive (m)		
Terbutaline	Negative	May inhibit labour	B
		Preserves or increases uteroplacental blood flow	
Adrenaline	Positive	Possible malformation	C
		Associated with reduced uteroplacental blood flow in animals	
Isoproterenol/isoprenaline	Positive	Reduction in uterine blood flow (animals)	C
Ephedrine	Positive	Newborn theophylline intoxification	C
Theophylline	Positive	May inhibit labour	C
		May reduce risk of pre-eclampsia	

[a]Studies evaluating teratogenicity.

blood flow in monkeys[25] but studies with terbutaline and albuterol, in other animal species, do not show these effects.[25,31] Compared to oral agents, inhaled β-adrenergic agonists produce fewer systemic effects; consequently, the likelihood of a clinically significant vasoconstrictive effect on the uteroplacental circulation should be considered slight with inhaled products.

Intravenous β-adrenergic agents have been used as tocolytic agents in premature labour. β-Agonists relax uterine smooth muscle and cause uterine atony. Terbutaline is the most frequently used agent. As a result β-adrenergic agonists may have the theoretical potential to inhibit labour. Inhaled β agonists have minimal systemic effects so the likelihood of significant prolongation of labour is small. Systemic β agonists, however, should be avoided in the late term to term interval.

Theophylline is also a commonly used bronchodilator and does not have teratogenic effects when used at therapeutic dosages[32] (Table 36.3). Maternal theophylline pharmacokinetics may change during pregnancy causing the dosing schedule to be adjusted accordingly. In a small number of patients, theophylline clearance was reduced by 25–30% in the third trimester;[33] this has not been adequately confirmed by others.[34] Because fetal theophylline levels are similar to those of the mother[35] it is advantageous to follow maternal theophylline levels closely, particularly in the third trimester.

Xanthines also have the potential to decrease uterine contractility through an inhibition of phosphodiesterase. This effect could prolong or complicate labour. Alternatively, lower rates of perinatal death and respiratory distress syndrome[36] as well as lowered rates of pre-eclampsia[37] have been reported with theophylline use.

Theophylline rapidly crosses the placenta and appears in the breast milk with a milk to plasma ratio of 0.7.[38] Breast-feeding just before drug administration limits neonatal exposure and will minimize the transient tachycardia, jitteriness and irritability observed under these conditions. There have also been reports of infant irritability when exposed to theophylline through breast milk.

Cromolyn Sodium and Nedocromil Sodium

Cromolyn sodium (Intal) has little systemic absorption and has shown no teratogenic effects in animal studies (Table 36.4). A study of 300 patients showed no increase in fetal malformation or perinatal mortality.[39] Nedocromil sodium, a similar agent, has not been rigorously studied in pregnancy.

Corticosteroids

In animals, high doses of corticosteroids cause congenital malformations such as cleft palate.[40] Neonatal adrenal insufficiency has also been a concern.[41] Early studies reported that an increase in stillbirth and fetal mortality was found in mothers who received steroids during pregnancy; however, these studies do not control for underlying disease as a factor

TABLE 36.4: *Anti-inflammatory therapy*

Drug	Animal studies	Congenital malformation/other effect	Class
Cromolyn sodium	Negative	No congenital malformation or increase in perinatal mortality	B
Nedocromil sodium	Not well studied in pregnancy		
Corticosteroids			
Beclomethasone	Negative (inhalation)	No congenital malformation Increased LBW inf	C
Triamcinolone	Positive (inhalation)	Fetal growth retardation in patients using 40 mg daily topically	D
Flunisolide	Positive		C

affecting pregnancy outcome. Moreover, recent clinical studies have not demonstrated an increased risk of congenital malformation, stillbirth or fetal mortality with the use of inhaled or systemic corticosteroids during pregnancy.[42,43]

Dexamethasone and betamethasone cross the placenta rapidly in high concentrations.[44] In contrast, methylprednisolone appears to cross the placenta poorly.[45] Prednisone also crosses the placenta poorly, as exhibited by the low incidence of adrenal suppression in infants of mothers who require prednisone.[46] Although based on limited data, prednisone and methylprednisolone are the preferred systemic corticosteroids in treatment of acute maternal asthma.

Of the many inhaled corticosteroids available, there is the most information on beclomethasone dipropionate use during pregnancy. Greenberger and Anderson showed that inhaled beclomethasone was safe during pregnancy, and caused no increase in perinatal morbidity or congenital malformation.[43] Since inhaled triamcinolone and flunisolide have been associated with teratogenicity in animals and fetal growth retardation in humans (triamcinolone),[47,48] inhaled beclomethasone has become the inhaled corticosteroid of choice during pregnancy.

Anti-cholinergics

Inhaled ipratropium bromide (Atrovent), although more useful in the treatment of chronic obstructive pulmonary disease, is sometimes used as a bronchodilator in the treatment of asthma. Ipratropium bromide is poorly absorbed systemically, and no increased risk of congenital malformation has been observed although rigorous safety studies are not available.[49]

Other Drugs

Most antibiotics are well tolerated with few adverse perinatal effects; however tetracycline is contraindicated due to toxic effects on fetal skeletal development (Table 36.5). Some expectorants contain iodides and should be avoided during pregnancy and lactation. Conflicting data are evident on some antihistamines that have been associated with congenital malformations (i.e. diphenhydramine and hydroxyzine). The use of brompheniramine, however, was associated with an increased incidence of congenital malformation in the offspring of 65 patients in the Collaborative Perinatal Project.[50] Phenylpropanolamine and phenylephrine use has also been associated with an increased fetal risk.[51] Table 36.5 shows several medications that should be avoided during pregnancy.

MANAGEMENT

The goals of asthma therapy are to maintain both maternal and fetal health by establishing optimal maternal asthma control. Patient education plays a critical role in asthma management and should actually be initiated prior to pregnancy. Education should include methods to monitor pulmonary function with peak flow meters and avoidance of specific asthma triggers.

TABLE 36.5: *Medications to avoid in pregnancy*

Drug	Fetal toxic effects
Iodine-containing compounds	Hypothyroidism, goitre
Brompheniramine	Teratogenic in animals
	Increased teratogenicity in CPP
Antibiotics	
Ciprofloxacin	Fetal arthropathy
Sulphonamides	Hyperbilirubinaemia
Tetracycline	Discoloration of teeth
Chloramphenicol	Grey baby syndrome
Trimethoprim	Possible teratogenic effects
Rifampicin	Limb reduction defects

The fetus is most susceptible to the teratogenic effects of drugs during the first trimester and especially in the first few weeks. This is a particularly important time to avoid medications that have possible teratogenic effects. In addition, physicians should request to be alerted if a patient intends to become pregnant. This will allow for more optimal asthma control and avoidance of potential teratogenic medication.

The approach to asthma control in pregnancy is similar to that for non-pregnant adults. In general, inhaled medications are preferred, with inhaled bronchodilators, i.e. terbutaline, the appropriate choice for a patient with mild intermittent symptoms. Those patients who require frequent β_2-agonist usage should begin anti-inflammatory therapy with either inhaled cromolyn sodium or beclomethasone. Theophylline may also be used as an additional bronchodilator.

For patients perennially symptomatic, or for acute exacerbations, the timely use of corticosteroids as a short burst is appropriate and necessary. Oral prednisone is generally used and has not shown teratogenic effects in humans.[52]

For acute asthma in pregnancy aggressive therapy is necessary and supplemental oxygen essential. The inhaled β agonist, terbutaline, may be administered repeatedly, every 20 min for an hour, to provide prompt relief of acute airway obstruction. If parenteral β agonists are required, terbutaline is preferred over adrenaline, as adrenaline may decrease utero-placental blood flow and cause congenital malformations (animal studies).[25,29] Intravenous corticosteroids should be added early in therapy.

LABOUR AND DELIVERY

The majority of asthma patients, especially those who are well controlled, do not require specific asthma intervention during labour. Nonetheless, specific concerns exist during labour and delivery and should be kept in mind. First, intravenous β agonists, in substantial doses, could cause uterine relaxation, inhibit labour and alter uteroplacental blood flow. Theophylline also has the potential to inhibit myometrial contractility; intravenous aminophylline should probably be avoided during labour and delivery. Narcotic analgesia and local or regional anaesthesia has been used successfully in pregnant asthma patients;[53] this approach may reduce hyperventilation and anxiety, and thus lessen respiratory alkalosis and fetal hypoxia. Judicious use of analgesia and anaesthesia for pain relief may be beneficial.

Intravenous prostaglandins, used to induce labour, have also been reported to cause airway obstruction.[54] In the treatment of post-partum haemorrhage, oxytocin may be a preferable alternative to ergonovine or methylergonovine in stimulation of myometrial contractility, as the latter has been reported to precipitate asthma.

Patients with recent or regular use of systemic corticosteroids require stress dosages of hydrocortisone (e.g. hydrocortisone 100 mg intravenously every 8 hours for 24 hours) with the initial dose given upon administration to the labour room. This corticosteroid dose may be tapered quickly following delivery.

THE POST-PARTUM PERIOD

The changes observed in asthma with pregnancy usually revert back to their pre-pregnancy state within 3 months after delivery. Breast-feeding should be encouraged and medications that are considered safe during pregnancy can be administered during lactation. Although it has been reported to cause irritability and jitteriness, theophylline is generally well tolerated. Prednisone crosses poorly into breast milk and thus low to moderate dosages are unlikely to cause adverse effects in the infant.[55] As a rule, inhaled medications have a low systemic absorption and are well tolerated.

MENSES

The association between asthma exacerbations and the pre-menstrual period has long been of interest. In 1931, Frank described increased asthma symptoms in one patient prior to her onset of menses.[56] Repeated reports[57] have documented the variation of asthma symptoms with the onset and cessation of menses. Several studies have attempted to quantitate the prevalence of exacerbations of asthma with menses. Rees found approximately a 30% prevalence of pre-menstrual asthma.[58] Similar ratios have been determined in additional studies.[59,60] Most of these studies have been retrospective and are based on symptom scores; i.e. two studies have correlated these symptom scores with decreases in peak flow rates.[60,61] Pauli *et al.* examined the relationship between pulmonary function and the menstrual cycle and found that asthmatic subjects developed both increased asthma symptoms and decreased morning peak flows as compared to non-asthmatic controls.[62] No changes were noted in the forced expiratory volume in 1 s (FEV_1).

Mechanisms proposed to explain pre-menstrual exacerbations of asthma have included hormonal, immunological and psychological processes. There is a cyclic elevation of both oestrogen and progesterone, and a fall of progesterone immediately prior to menses. Progesterone induces uterine smooth muscle relaxation and may have a similar effect on bronchial smooth muscle. However, recent studies have failed to associate changes in pulmonary function or airway hyperresponsiveness with progesterone.[63] Oestrogen and progesterone, similar to other steroid hormones, may act to potentiate the effects of catecholamines;[64] whether or not this has clinical relevance has yet to be established.

Other hormonal influences in the menstrual cycle include the effects of prostaglandins and catecholamines. As noted previously, $PGF_{2\alpha}$ is a potent bronchoconstrictor and its level varies with different phases of the menstrual cycle. In addition, investigators have found an association between asthma and pre-menstrual symptoms. It has been proposed that pre-menstrual peaks of $PGF_{2\alpha}$ are responsible for these symptoms. However, Eliasson *et al.* were unable to confirm a pre-menstrual rise in prostaglandin metabolites.[65] Also, meclofenamate, a prostaglandin synthesis inhibitor, had no effect on pre-menstrual asthma although it did have some effect on other menstrual symptoms.

There are many additional factors that may influence pre-menstrual asthma, including increased autonomic tone and autonomic lability, higher emotional lability and increased hydration of the bronchial wall.[58] Many other aetiological agents may be involved, as the hormonal changes involved in menstruation are very complex.

Management of pre-menstrual asthma, primarily exacerbations, should be treated like other acute asthma episode. Other treatments that have been considered include diuretics, pills and non-steroidal anti-inflammatory agents. Benyon *et al.* used intramuscular injections of progesterone to prevent severe pre-menstrual attacks in three patients.[66] These therapies, however, must still be considered experimental.

SUMMARY

Asthma may be influenced by pregnancy and menses. Much has been learned about the pathophysiology of these conditions and associated asthma. Recent studies have shown that optimal control of asthma during pregnancy has little detrimental effect on the fetus. Therefore, the physician who manages asthma during pregnancy must keep in mind that the goals of therapy during pregnancy are the general overall goals of asthma therapy: minimize symptoms, normalize pulmonary function and prevent acute exacerbations. With noted exceptions, the available medication should allow the physician to achieve this goal.

REFERENCES

1   Gordon M, Niswander KR, Berendes H, Kantor AG. Fetal morbidity following potentially anoxiogenic obstetric conditions. VII. Bronchial asthma. Am J Obstet Gynecol 1970; 106: 421.

2   Paparella MM, Shumrick BA, Gluckman JL et al. Otolaryngology. Philadelphia: WB Saunders, 1991: 1892–3.

3   Fishburne JI. Physiology and disease of the respiratory system in pregnancy. J Reprod Med 1979; 22: 177–89.

4   Contreras G, Guttierrez M, Beroiza T et al. Ventilatory drive and respiratory muscle function in pregnancy. Am Rev Respir Dis 1991; 144: 837–41.

5   Bonica JJ. Maternal respiratory changes during pregnancy and partuition. In: Marx GF (ed) Partuition and Perinatology. Philadelphia: F.A. Davis, 1973: 2–19.

6   Alaily AB, Carrol KBL. Pulmonary ventilation in pregnancy. Br J Obstet Gynaecol 85: 518–24.

7   Baldwin GR, Moorthi DS, Whelton JA et al. New lung functions and pregnancy. Am J Obstet Gynecol 1977; 127: 235–9.

8   Cugell DW, Frank NR, Gaensler EA et al. Pulmonary function in pregnancy. I. Serial observations in normal women. Am Rev Tuberc 1953; 67: 568–97.

9   Nolten WE, Ruekert PA. Elevated free cortisol index in pregnancy: possible regulatory mechanisms. Am J Obstet Gynecol 1981; 139: 492.

10 Lyons HA, Huang CT. Therapeutic use of progesterone in alveolar hypoventilation associated with obesity. Am J Med 1968; 44: 881.

11 Juniper EF et al. Improvement in airway responsiveness and asthma severity during pregnancy. Am Rev Respir Dis 1989; 140: 924–31.

12 Weinberger ST, Weiss ST, Cohen WR et al. Pregnancy and the lung. Am Rev Respir Dis 1980; 121: 559–81.

13 Gluck JC, Gluck PA. The effects of pregnancy on asthma: a prospective study. Ann Allergy 1976; 37: 164.

14. Schatz M *et al.* The course of asthma during pregnancy, post partum, and with successive pregnancies: A prospective analysis. *J Allergy Clin Immunol* 1988; 81: 509–17.

15. Sims CD, Chamberlain CVP, deSwiet M. Lung function tests in bronchial asthma during and after pregnancy. *Br J Obstet Gynaecol* 1976; 83: 434.

16. Turner ES, Greenberger PA, Patterson R. Management of the pregnant asthmatic patient. *Ann Intern Med* 1980; 93: 905.

f17. Williams DA. Asthma and pregnancy. *Acta Allergol* 1967; 22: 311.

18. White RJ, Coutts II, Gibbs CJ *et al.* A prospective study of asthma during pregnancy and puerperium. *Prep Med* 1989; 83: 103.

19. Report of the Working Group on Asthma and Pregnancy, Executive Summary: Management of Asthma during Pregnancy, National Asthma Education Program, National Heart Lung and Blood Institute, NIH Publication No. 93-3279A March 1993.

20. Bahna SL, Bjerkedal T. The course and outcome of pregnancy in women with bronchial asthma. *Acta Allergol* 1972; 27: 397.

21. Perlow JH, Montgomery D, Morgan M, Towers C, Porto M. Severity of asthma and perinatal outcome. *Am J Obstet Gynecol* 1992; 167: 963–7.

22. Apter A, Greenberger PA, Patterson R. Outcome of pregnancy in adolescents with severe asthma. *Arch Intern Med* 1989; 2571–5.

23. Lehrer S *et al.* Association between pregnancy induced hypertension and asthma during pregnancy. *Am J Obstet Gynecol* 1993; 168: 1463–6.

24. Lao TT, Huensburg M. Labour and delivery in mothers with asthma. *Eur J Obstet Gynecol Reprod Biol* 1990; 35: 183.

25. Misenheimer HR, Margolies SI, Panigel M *et al.* Effects of vasoconstrictive drugs on the placental circulation of the rhesus monkey. *Invest Radiol* 1972; 7: 496.

26. Rosenfeld CR, Barton MD, Meschia G. Effects of epinephrine on distribution of blood flow in the pregnant ewe. *Am J Obstet Gynecol* 1976; 124: 156.

27. Metzger WJ, Turner E, Patterson R. The safety of immunotherapy during pregnancy. *J Allergy Clin Immunol* 1978; 61: 268–72.

28. Entman SS, Moise KJ. Anaphylaxis in pregnancy. *South Med J* 1984; 77: 402.

29. Schardein JL. *Drugs as Teratogens.* Cleveland: CRC Press, 1976.

30. *Med Lett* 1981; 23: 81.

31. Brennan SC, McLaughlin MK, Chez RA. Effects of prolonged infusion of beta-adrenergic agonist on uterine umbilical blood flow in pregnant sheep. *Am J Obstet Gynecol* 1977; 128: 709.

32. Greenberger P, Patterson R. Safety of therapy for allergic symptoms during pregnancy. *Ann Intern Med* 1978; 89: 234–7.

33 Carter BL, Driscoll CF, Smith GD. Theophylline clearance during pregnancy. *Obstet Gynecol* 1986; 68: 555–9.

34 Gardner MJ, Schatz M, Cousins L *et al.* Longitudinal effects of pregnancy on the pharmacokinetics of theophylline. *Eur J Clin Pharmacol* 1987; 31: 289–95.

35 Labovitz E, Spector S. Parental theophylline transfer in pregnant asthmatics. *JAMA* 1982; 247: 786.

36 Hadjigeorgiou E *et al.* Antepartum aminophylline treatment for prevention of respiratory distress syndrome in premature infants. *Am J Obstet Gynecol* 1979; 135: 257.

37 Dombrowski MP, Bottoms SF, Boike GM, Wald J. Incidence of preeclampsia among asthmatic patients lower with theophylline. *Am J Obstet Gynecol* 1986; 155: 265–7.

38 Wood M, Wood ATJ. Changes in plasma drug binding and α_1-acid glycoprotein in mother and newborn infant. *Clin Pharmacol Ther* 1981; 29: 522.

39 Wilson J. Utilisation du cromoglycate de sodium au cours se la grosesse. *Acta Therapeutica* 1982; 8(suppl): 45.

40 Fainstat T. Cortisol induced congenital cleft palate in rabbits. *Endocrinology* 1964; 55: 502.

41 Walsh SD, Clark FR. Pregnancy in patients on long term corticosteroid therapy. *Scott Med J* 1967; 12: 302.

42 Fitsimmons R, Greenberger PA, Patterson R. Outcomes of pregnancy in women requiring corticosteroids for severe asthma. *J Allergy Clin Immunol* 1986; 8: 349.

43 Greenberger PA, Anderson R. Beclomethasone dipropionate for severe asthma during pregnancy. *Ann Intern Med* 1983; 98: 478.

44 Ballard PL, Granberg P, Ballard RA. Glucocorticoid levels in maternal and cord serum after prenatal betamethasone therapy to prevent respiratory distress syndrome. *J Clin Invest* 1975; 56: 1548.

45 Taeusch HW, Frigoletto R, Kitzmiller J. Risk of respiratory distress syndrome after prenatal dexamethasone treatment. *Pediatrics* 1979; 63: 64.

46 Block MF, Kling OR, Corsby WM. Antenatal glucocorticoid therapy for prevention of respiratory distress syndrome in the premature infant. *Am J Obstet Gynecol* 1978; 131: 358.

47 Murphy BE *et al.* Conversion of maternal cortisol to cortisone during placental transfer to the human fetus. *Am J Obstet Gynecol* 1974; 118: 538.

48 Romero R, Lockwood C. The use of anti-asthmatic drugs in pregnancy. In: Neibyl JR (ed) *Drug Use in Pregnancy*, 2nd edn. Philadelphia: Lea & Febiger, 1988: 67–82.

49 Katz VL, Thorp JM, Bowes WA. Severe symmetric intrautereine growth retardation associated the topical use of triamcinalone. *Am J Obstet Gynecol* 1990; 162: 396–7.

50 Mawhinney H, Spector SL. Optimum management of asthma in pregnancy. Pract Ther 1986; 32: 178.

51 Heinonen OP, Slone D, Shapiro S. *Birth Defects and Pregnancy*. Littleton, MA: PSG Publishing, 1977.

52 Stablein JJ, Lockey RF. Managing asthma during pregnancy. Compr Ther 1984; 10: 45.

53 Schatz M *et al.* Corticosteroid therapy for the pregnant asthmatic. JAMA 1975; 233: 804.

54 Gottschalk W. General anesthesia in obstetrics. In: Wynn RM (ed) *Obstetrics and Gynecology Annual*. New York: Appleton-Century-Crofts, 1973.

55 Smith AP. The effects of intravenous infusion of graded doses of prostaglandin F_2 and E_2 on lung resistance in patients undergoing termination of pregnancy. Clin Sci 1973; 44: 17.

56 Frank RT. The hormonal cause of premenstrual tension. Arch Neurol Psychiatry 1931; 26: 1053.

57 Green R, Dalton K. The premenstrual syndrome. BMJ 1957; 1: 1007.

58 Rees L. An aetiological study of premenstrual asthma. J Psychosom Res 1963; 7: 191.

59 Gibbs CJ *et al.* Premenstrual exacerbation of asthma. Thorax 1984; 39: 833.

60 Hanley SP. Asthma variation with menstruation. Br J Dis Chest 1981; 75: 306.

61 Enright T *et al.* Cyclic exacerbation of bronchial asthma. Ann Allergy 1987; 58: 405.

62 Pauli BD *et al.* Influence of the menstrual cycle on airway function in asthmatic and normal subjects. Am Rev Respir Dis 1989; 140: 358.

63 Juniper EF, Kline PA, Roberts S, Hargreave FE, Daniel EE. Airway responsiveness to methacholine during the natural menstrual cycle and the effect of oral contraceptives. Am Rev Respir Dis 1987; 135: 1039-42.

64 Foster PS, Goldie RG, Paterson JW. Effect of steroids on beta-adrenoreceptor mediated relaxation of pig bronchus. Br J Pharmacol 1983; 78: 441-5.

65 Eliasson O, Densmore MJ, Scherzer HH, DeGraff AC. The effect of sodium meclofenamate in premenstrual asthma: A controlled clinical trial. J Allergy Clin Immunol 1987; 79: 909-18.

66 Benyon HLC, Garbett ND, Barnes PJ. Severe premenstrual exacerbations of asthma: Effects of intramuscular progesterone. Lancet 1988; ii: 370.

KEY POINTS

1   The influences of pregnancy on asthma can include:
● alteration in lung physiology;
● exacerbations of asthma;
● need to modify medication in use because of potential adverse
effects on the fetus.

37

SPECIFIC PROBLEMS: CORTICOSTEROID-RESISTANT ASTHMA

S. J. Lane, G. M. C. Cochrane and T. H. Lee

INTRODUCTION

Glucocorticoids are a potent and effective treatment for bronchial asthma and inhaled steroids have a major role in the preventative treatment of this disease. However, there is a small population of asthmatic individuals in whom systemic or inhaled treatment with glucocorticoids, even when given in very high doses, does not lead to an increase in forced expiratory volume in 1 s (FEV_1).[1] Corticosteroid responsiveness in asthma (corticosteroid-sensitive asthma) has been defined in most studies as an increase in FEV_1 of greater than 30% during a 14-day course of 40 mg prednisolone. Corticosteroid resistance in asthmatic subjects is defined as an improvement in the FEV_1 of less than 15% after a similar course of prednisolone despite a $\geq 20\%$ increase in FEV_1 spontaneously or in response to bronchodilator therapy.[2,3] In a large study of corticosteroid-resistant asthmatics Carmichael et al. found that these patients had similar baseline FEV_1 and bronchodilator response, however, suffered from asthma for a longer period of time.[1] Furthermore, there was a significantly greater frequency of family history of asthma in the corticosteroid-resistant as opposed to the corticosteroid-sensitive group. There was no difference between the two groups in terms of atopic status or cigarette exposure. These patients are not "Addisonian" clinically or biochemically, implying that the defect appears to be selective for the anti-inflammatory action of glucocorticosteroids. Subsequent studies suggested reduced glucocorticosteroid responsiveness in peripheral blood mononuclear cells (PBMC) in corticosteroid-resistant patients.[4] Complement receptor expression on PBMC was reduced after 1 week's treatment with oral prednisolone in corticosteroid-sensitive but not in corticosteroid-resistant asthmatic subjects.[5] Mitogen-stimulated PBMC proliferation was inhibited by dexamethasone in the sensitive but not the resistant group.[3] Furthermore, methylprednisolone substantially inhibited the growth of colonies from mitogen-stimulated PBMC cells of corticosteroid-sensitive asthmatic subjects but had little effect on colony growth from the mixed mononuclear cells of corticosteroid-resistant asthmatic individuals.[6] The origin of this *in vitro* resistance was found to be monocyte rather than lymphocyte derived.[7] We have demonstrated that the enhanced expression of the activation antigens, complement receptors 1 and 2, and Class II molecules on cultured blood monocytes seen in asthma is suppressed by hydrocortisone in corticosteroid-sensitive but not corticosteroid-resistant asthmatic subjects, suggesting ongoing monocyte activation in the presence of glucocorticoids in corticosteroid-resistant asthma.[8] There is evidence for T-lymphocyte dysfunction in steroid-resistant asthma. Corrigan *et al.* have shown enhanced interleukin-2 (IL-2) and HLA-DR receptor expression on peripheral T lymphocytes in the resistant as opposed to the sensitive individuals.[9] In addition the elaboration of interferon-γ (IFN-γ) and IL-2 from mitogen-stimulated T lymphocytes was inhibited by 10^{-7} M dexamethasone in corticosteroid-sensitive but not in corticosteroid-resistant subjects. Interestingly, cyclosporin A was seen to partially reverse this *in vitro* resistance, suggesting a potentially therapeutic role for this treatment in corticosteroid-resistant asthma.[9] Furthermore, glucocorticoid resistance in asthma is associated with an *in vivo* defect in PBMC function and appears not to be organ specific.[10,11] In a large hospital-based asthma clinic we estimate the incidence of true corticosteroid-resistant asthma to be less than 1%.

MECHANISM OF GLUCOCORTICOID ACTION (Fig. 37.1)

Glucocorticoids act through a cytoplasmic 300-kDa glucocorticoid receptor phosphoprotein complex[12] (see also Chapter 15). Upon binding the glucocorticoid, the glucocorticoid receptor undergoes dephosphorylation, dissociates two 90-kDa associated heat-shock proteins (HSP), forms dimers and translocates to the nucleus in a temperature-dependent fashion.[13] Here the glucocorticoid receptor binds to sequences of DNA known as glucocorticoid response elements (GRE), which lie in the promoter region of glucocorticoid-responsive genes and so induce or repress gene transcription.[14] The glucocorticoid receptor belongs to a highly conserved superfamily of hormone receptor proteins with impressive functional diversity that includes the receptors for the sex steroids, thyroid hormone, vitamin D_3 and the retinoids.[15] These hormone receptors are structurally organized into five homologous domains, each responsible for different functions. These are glucocorticoid and HSP90 binding, dimerization of the glucocorticoid receptor, nuclear localization of glucocorticoid receptor, DNA binding of the receptor to GRE and an N-terminal domain responsible for transactivation of gene expression.[13]

FIGURE 37.1: *Schematic representation of the mechanism of glucocorticoid action. GCS, glucocorticoid; GR, glucocorticoid receptor; HSP, heat-shock protein; P, phosphate group; GRE, glucocorticoid response element.*

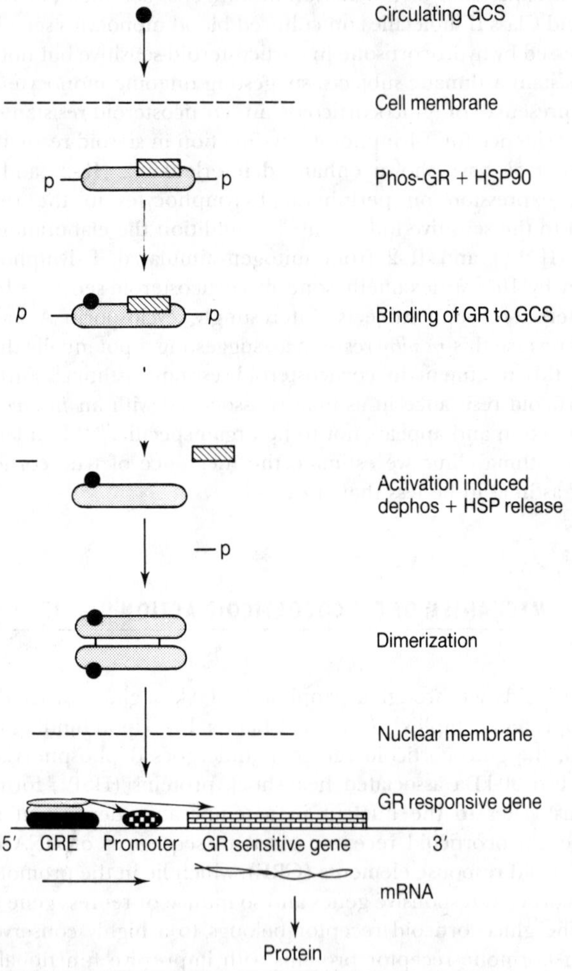

Circulating GCS

Cell membrane

Phos-GR + HSP90

Binding of GR to GCS

Activation induced
dephos + HSP release

Dimerization

Nuclear membrane

GR responsive gene

5'   GRE   Promoter   GR sensitive gene   3'

mRNA

Protein

MECHANISM OF CORTICOSTEROID-RESISTANT
BRONCHIAL ASTHMA (see also Chapter 15) (Table 37.1)

Corticosteroid-resistant asthma is not due to altered pharmacokinetics in steroid-resistant subjects.[2,3] There is no difference in peak serum levels or

TABLE 37.1: *Characteristics of corticosteroid-resistant asthma*

Chronic disease

Family history of asthma

In vitro and *in vivo* defect in mononuclear cell function

Defective regulation of specific gene(s)

Normal pharmacokinetics, ligand binding and nuclear translocation

Defective glucocorticoid receptor–glucocorticoid response element interaction

Associated extra-pulmonary glucocorticoid resistance

estimated clearances of prednisolone between sensitive and resistant patients or between either group and non-asthmatic control subjects.

In addition this defect is not caused by defective ligand binding to the glucocorticoid receptor or to subsequent nuclear translocation of the activated receptor complex.[3,16] Competitive binding studies on monocyte nuclear extracts using dexamethasone have demonstrated similar K_d (dissociation constant) and R_o (receptor density) in the sensitive and resistant groups. In collaboration with Peter Barnes we have demonstrated defective glucocorticoid receptor–GRE binding in resistant asthma using gel retardation assay.[17] These data suggest that defective receptor–GRE or receptor–transcription factor interaction may underlie the molecular basis of resistance to the anti-inflammatory effects of corticosteroids. Corticosteroid-resistant asthma may be associated with defective regulation of specific genes.[18] Cultured monocytes from asthmatic subjects generate a neutrophil priming activity (NPA) that is inhibited by glucocorticoids *in vitro* in the sensitive but not the resistant asthmatic subjects. The effect of glucocorticoids on NPA is selective as there is no difference in the steroid responsiveness on the expression and generation of other well-characterized monocyte-derived cytokines, namely tumour necrosis factor α (TNF-α) IL-1β and granulocyte macrophage colony stimulating factor (GM-CSF), between the sensitive and resistant groups.[19]

ASSESSMENT/MANAGEMENT (Figs 37.2 and 37.3)

Patients with true glucocorticoid-resistant asthma provide a difficult management problem. All patients should have a thorough clinical evaluation,

FIGURE 37.2: *Diagnostic algorithm for corticosteroid-resistant asthma. ABPA, allergic bronchopulmonary aspergillosis; CR, corticosteroid-resistant asthma; CS corticosteroid-sensitive asthma; ESR, erythrocyte sedimentation rate; FEV_1 forced expiratory volume in 1 s; PEFR, peak expiratory flow rate. For patients who demonstrate 15–30% improvement in FEV_1 or PEFR after 14 days of 40 mg prednisolone investigate as for CR asthmatic subjects.*

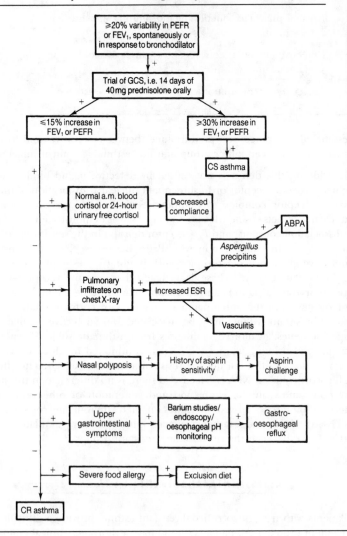

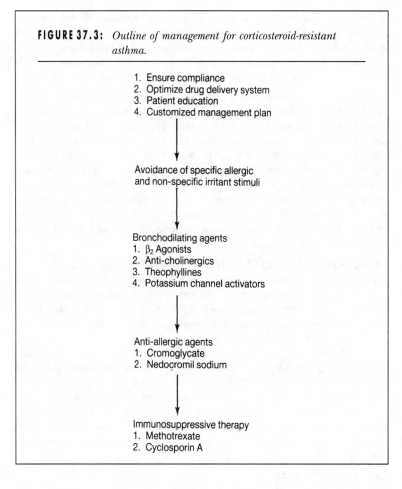

FIGURE 37.3: *Outline of management for corticosteroid-resistant asthma.*

1. Ensure compliance
2. Optimize drug delivery system
3. Patient education
4. Customized management plan

Avoidance of specific allergic and non-specific irritant stimuli

Bronchodilating agents
1. β_2 Agonists
2. Anti-cholinergics
3. Theophyllines
4. Potassium channel activators

Anti-allergic agents
1. Cromoglycate
2. Nedocromil sodium

Immunosuppressive therapy
1. Methotrexate
2. Cyclosporin A

chest X-ray, skin-prick allergy tests and full biochemical and haematological screen. Before a diagnosis of corticosteroid-resistant asthma can be entertained it is essential to rule out chronic latent occupational exposure (Chapter 31), silent gastro-oesophageal reflux (Chapter 38), aspirin sensitivity (Chapter 32), allergic bronchopulmonary aspergillosis (Chapter 33), unrecognized true food allergy (Chapter 40) and underlying systemic vasculitis. A $\geq 20\%$ improvement in FEV_1 or peak expiratory flow rate (PEFR) must be demonstrated either spontaneously or in response to a bronchodilating agent. Patients with suspected corticosteroid-resistant asthma should be given 40 mg prednisolone orally (corrected for body surface area) for 14 days and FEV_1 measured at the beginning and at the end of the trial. This trial should be repeated on at least two separate occasions. It is also important to monitor PEFR continuously throughout the trial period on at least a twice-daily basis. The vast majority of patients will demonstrate a $\geq 30\%$ improvement in spirometric values in response to this dose of prednisolone. Corticosteroid-resistant asthmatic subjects will show a $\leq 15\%$ spirometric improvement in response to a similar course of steroids although in our experience this improvement is generally only about 5%.

General management measures applicable to all asthmatic subjects should be applied rigorously in patients with corticosteroid-resistant asthma. It is essential to detect and improve upon poor compliance and to optimize a delivery system for inhaled medication that the patient finds effective and easy to use (Chapters 20 and 25). The patient should be educated concerning the nature of the underlying condition and given an easily understood customized self-management plan (Chapters 23 and 24). Specific allergic triggers and non-specific irritant exposure should be minimized wherever possible (Chapter 14). Specific pharmacotherapy in corticosteroid-resistant asthma, as in corticosteroid-sensitive asthma, is incremental depending upon severity and includes the following.

BRONCHODILATOR THERAPY IS FIRST-LINE TREATMENT (Chapter 19)

This treatment includes β_2 agonists via the inhaled, oral, subcutaneous or intravenous routes as indicated. The newer longer-acting salmeterol and bambuterol are very potent bronchodilating agents but they should be used with caution and, if possible, in combination with other non-steroidal anti-allergic drugs. Inhaled anti-cholinergics have an additional bronchodilating role and are very effective in a minority of corticosteroid-resistant asthmatic subjects. Oral and intravenous theophyllines afford additional bronchodilation in this difficult group of patients but it is important to bear in mind their narrow toxic/therapeutic ratio and their many drug interactions. Finally, it will be interesting to evaluate new agents in this group when they become more widely available, e.g. the potassium channel activators, the selective phosphodiesterase inhibitors, and the leukotriene antagonists.

ANTI-ALLERGIC DRUGS

These include the antihistamines, e.g. ketotifen, sodium cromoglycate and nedocromil sodium (Chapter 16). Our experience of the use of these drugs in corticosteroid-resistant asthma is disappointing, particularly with the antihistamines. However, they may be of use in some individuals and theoretically they can offer a degree of non-steroidal anti-inflammatory protection in patients who are often heavily β_2 stimulated.

IMMUNOSUPPRESSIVE AGENTS (Chapter 17)

The efficacy of most of these drugs has been investigated as steroid-sparing agents in glucocorticoid-dependent asthma. The most striking results have been with methotrexate and cyclosporin A. Mullarkey et al. have demonstrated a mean daily reduction from 26.9 to 6.3 mg prednisolone, which was sustained over an 18-month period in 25 patients with very little associated toxicity.[20] This implies an anti-inflammatory mechanism independent of glucocorticoids and thus a 6–18-month trial is justified in corticosteroid-resistant asthma. Alexander *et al.* have shown that in a group of 33 steroid-dependent asthmatic subjects a 12-week course of cyclosporin reduced the frequency of disease exacerbations by 48%, improved the baseline FEV_1 by 17% and reduced the diurnal variation of PEFR by 27%.[21] In view of its additional role in suppressing glucocorticoid-resistant IFN-γ and IL-2 generation from mitogen-stimulated T lymphocytes *in vitro*, a trial of cyclosporin is therefore indicated in any severe corticosteroid-resistant asthmatic subject.

ROLE OF GLUCOCORTICOIDS (Chapter 15)

Corticosteroid-resistant asthmatic subjects show a disappointing response even to large and prolonged doses of oral or intravenous glucocorticoids and they therefore have a very limited role to play; 14 days of 40 mg prednisolone effectively selects for the majority of corticosteroid-sensitive asthmatic subjects. However, there may be the very rare patient who will respond at much higher doses and thus a more aggressive therapeutic trial is indicated in any severely ill non-responsive corticosteroid-resistant patient.

SUMMARY

Corticosteroid-resistant asthma is associated with disease chronicity, positive family history for asthma and an *in vitro* and *in vivo* defect in mononuclear cell function. Glucocorticoid resistance is not organ specific and may represent a more generalized phenomenon. There is evidence of reduced binding of the glucocorticoid receptor to its GRE and of a selective resistance to glucocorticoids of certain genes. Management includes ruling out any secondary specific diseases, general asthma management and incremental pharmacotherapy. Bronchodilation is the mainstay of therapy. Anti-allergic and immunomodulatory agents may have a significant role to play in therapy. Newer agents, e.g. mediator antagonists, anti-cytokines, neuropeptide antagonists, 5-lipoxygenase inhibitors may in the future be potentially useful in this difficult condition. The results of future trials are eagerly awaited.

REFERENCES

1 Carmichael J, Paterson IC, Diaz P, Crompton GK, Kay AB, Grant IWB. Corticosteroid resistance in chronic asthma. *BMJ* 1981; 282: 1419–22.

2   Lane SJ, Palmer JBD, Skidmore IF, Lee TH. Corticosteroid pharmacokinetics in asthma. *Lancet* 1990; 336: 1265.

3   Corrigan CJ, Brown PH, Barnes NC *et al.* Glucocorticoid pharmacokinetics, glucocorticoid receptor characteristics, and inhibition of peripheral blood T cell proliferation by glucocorticoids *in vitro*. *Am Rev Respir Dis* 1991; 144: 1016–25.

4   Lee TH, Lane SJ. The role of macrophages in the mechanisms of airway inflammation in asthma. *Am Rev Respir Dis* 1992; 145: S27–S30.

5   Kay AB, Diaz P, Carmichael J, Grant IWB. Corticosteroid-resistant chronic asthma and monocyte complement receptors. *Clin Exp Immunol* 1981; 44: 576–80.

6   Poznansky MC, Gordon ACH, Dolas JG, Krajewski AS, Wyllie AH, Grant IWB. Resistance to methylprednisolone in cultures of blood mononuclear cells from glucocorticoid-resistant asthmatic patients. *Clin Sci* 1984; 67: 639–45.

7   Wyllie AH, Poznansky MC, Gordon ACH. Glucocorticoid resistant asthma: evidence for a defect in mononuclear cells. In: Kay AB (ed) *Asthma: Clinical Pharmacology and Therapeutic Progress*. Oxford: Blackwell Scientific Publications, 1986: 306–14.

8   Wilkinson JRW, Lane SJ, Lee TH. The effects of corticosteroids on cytokine generation and expression of activation antigens by monocytes in bronchial asthma. *Int Arch Allergy Appl Immunol* 1991; 94: 220–1.

9   Corrigan CJ, Brown PH, Barnes NC, Tsai J-J, Frew AJ, Kay AB. Peripheral blood T lymphocyte activation and comparison of the T lymphocyte inhibitory effects of glucocorticoids and cyclosporin A. *Am Rev Respir Dis* 1991; 144: 1026–32.

10   Brown PJ, Teelucksingh S, Matusiewicz SP, Greening AP, Crompton GK, Edwards CRW. Cutaneous vasoconstrictor response to glucocorticoids in asthma. *Lancet* 1991; 337: 576–80.

11   Lane SJ, Sousa AR, Poston RN, Lee TH. *In vivo* cutaneous tuberculin response to prednisolone in corticosteroid resistant bronchial asthma. *J Allergy Clin Immunol* 1993; 91: A221.

12   Munck A, Mendel DB, Smith LI, Orti E. Glucocorticoid receptors and actions. *Am Rev Respir Dis* 1990; 141(suppl): S2–S10.

13   Miesfeld RL. The structure and function of steroid receptor proteins. *Crit Rev Biochem Mol Biol* 1989; 24: 101–17.

14   Beato M. Gene regulation by steroid hormones. *Cell* 1989; 56: 335–44.

15   Evans RE. The steroid and thyroid hormone receptor super-family. *Science* 1988; 240: 889–95.

16   Lane SJ, Lee TH. Glucocorticoid receptor characteristics in monocytes of patients with corticosteroid-resistant bronchial asthma. *Am Rev Respir Dis* 1991; 143: 1020–4.

17   Adcock IM, Brown CR, Peters MJ *et al.* DNA binding of glucocorticoid receptor from peripheral blood monocytes of steroid sensitive and resistant patients. *Am Rev Respir Dis* 1993; 147: A244.

18 Wilkinson JRW, Crea AEG, Clark TJH, Lee TH. Identification and characterization of a monocyte-derived neutrophil-activating factor in corticosteroid-resistant bronchial asthma. *J Clin Invest* 1989; 84: 1930–41.

19 Lane SJ, Wilkinson JRW, Cochrane GM, Lee TH, Arm JP. Differential *in vitro* regulation by glucocorticoids of monocyte-derived cytokine generation in glucocorticoid-resistant bronchial asthma. *Am Rev Respir Dis* 1993; 147: 690–6.

20 Mullarkey MF, Lammert JK, Blumenstein BA. Long term methotrexate treatment in corticosteroid dependent asthma. *Ann Intern Med* 1990; 112: 577–81.

21 Alexander AG, Barnes NC, Kay AB. Trial of cyclosporin in corticosteroid dependent chronic severe asthma. *Lancet* 1992; 339: 324–8.

KEY POINTS

1   Glucocorticoid resistance is defined as failure of FEV_1 to improve by $\geq 15\%$ after 2 weeks of 40 mg oral prednisolone on two separate occasions having ruled out secondary pathology.

2   Glucocorticoid resistance is not organ specific and is associated with an *in vitro* and *in vivo* defect in mononuclear cell function.

3   Glucocorticoid resistance is associated with defective binding of the glucocorticoid receptor to its DNA binding site, the glucocorticoid response element (GRE).

4   The mainstay of current treatment is bronchodilation and "steroid-sparing" agents.

38

SPECIFIC PROBLEMS: GASTRO-OESOPHAGEAL REFLUX AND ASTHMA

Christopher J. Allen and Michael T. Newhouse

BACKGROUND

Gastro-oesophageal reflux (GOR) is very common and typically presents with heartburn and acid regurgitation. Associated symptoms may include dysphagia and choking, chest pain due to oesophageal spasm and flatulent dyspepsia due to inappropriate relaxation of the lower oesophageal sphincter. Severely affected patients may have episodes of acid or food regurgitation in the recumbent position. Population surveys suggest that 20–36% of the population have regular symptoms of heartburn and acid regurgitation. Of patients with objectively diagnosed asthma 50% complain of symptoms of heartburn and acid regurgitation, 39% show oesophagitis[1] and 82% have an abnormal degree of GOR on 24-hour pH monitoring.[2] Thus, if objective studies are carried out in patients with asthma the majority of them will have GOR. This association between asthma and reflux cannot be attributed to bronchodilator medication.[2,3]

It is not known why GOR is so common in patients with asthma. Both the oesophagus and the proximal airways develop from the foregut, resulting in cross-innervation through the vagus between the oesophagus and the airway. In patients presenting with irritable bowel syndrome who have no clinical evidence of any respiratory disease, there is a significantly higher responsiveness to methacholine inhalation when compared to asymptomatic control subjects.[4] Patients with GOR and no clinical evidence of asthma had a greater increase in airway resistance when inhaling methacholine compared to disease-free control subjects.[5] Thus, if there is a disorder in smooth muscle in the airway it may be associated with disorder of smooth muscle in the gastrointestinal tract. The mechanism of this association is unknown.

There is evidence that GOR may amplify or exacerbate naturally occurring bronchospasm. In asthmatic patients with heartburn that is reproduced by acid perfusion into the mid oesophagus (positive Bernstein test), instillation of acid into the mid oesophagus may induce >10% drop in airflow measured by either peak flow or forced expiratory volume in 1 s (FEV_1). Even more striking is that if provocative testing with hyperventilation of dry air under eucapnic conditions is undertaken and acid is then trickled down the oesophagus, the induced bronchoconstriction to dry air is more than doubled.[6] Thus, a mild asthma attack occurring under natural conditions will be amplified if acid is refluxing into the oesophagus at the same time. Aspiration of gastric contents may be suspected but is hard to prove. The patient may give a history of choking episodes, laryngitis and cough in association with acid reflux. The available evidence, however, suggests that aspiration is more likely to be associated with chronic airflow limitation or non-obstructive disease including pulmonary scars, recurrent pneumonia or interstitial fibrosis.

While it is evident that GOR is very common in patients with bronchial asthma and reflux may amplify the respiratory symptoms resulting from natural broncoconstrictor stimuli, the evidence from randomized controlled trials that control of reflux improves asthma is still controversial. Where perhaps reflux is most important is in the difficult to control asthmatic patient.[7] For example, the "asthmatic" who is unresponsive to high-dose corticosteroid therapy may not have asthma and may in reality have GOR masquerading as asthma. When reviewing patients with asthma that is not responding reflux should be considered, even if there are no typical symptoms of GOR. We do not recommend routine use of anti-reflux measures in patients presenting with asthma that is controlled and responding to standard therapy.

RECOMMENDATIONS

Enquiry for GOR should be part of any respiratory history. Pay particular attention to reflux-associated respiratory symptoms, i.e. patients who develop cough or wheeze or chest pain at the same time as they experience dyspepsia, heartburn or acid regurgitation. A symptom of choking often localizing to the upper oesophagus or crico-pharyngeal area may be obtained in 30% of asthmatic subjects and may be significant. Nocturnal symptoms, particularly cough or respiratory symptoms after meals, likewise may be suggestive. An asthmatic patient with a prominent cough or who has recurrent pulmonary infiltrates without obvious cause should also be assessed for reflux.

In general, the management of GOR in patients with asthma should proceed in three stages.

STAGE 1

In a person aged under 40 with a history of typical reflux symptoms it may be enough to give a trial of diet and life-style measures supplemented by antacid, alginate–antacid combination or perhaps an H_2 antagonist. In patients aged over 40, particularly if there are persistent or unexplained symptoms such as weight loss or anaemia, careful clinical examination and appropriate additional investigation is mandatory. Too often the focus of anti-reflux therapy in patients with asthma is on drugs and antacid. Diet and life-style measures are essential and elevation of the head of the bed may be the single most effective measure.

STAGE 2

If first-line measures do not control the reflux, or if asthma continues to deteriorate, specific investigations are necessary. An endoscopy would be considered the first line by most physicians. Oesophageal pH monitoring can be very helpful because it will document GOR in the ambulatory setting and permit correlation of symptoms with oesophageal acid reflux. If GOR is confirmed, most gastroenterologists at this point would place the patient on 3 months' treatment with omeprazole.

STAGE 3

If symptoms persist after a 3-month trial with omeprazole, the patient will need to be re-evaluated, and if reflux is refractory to medical therapy anti-reflux surgery could be considered. In carefully selected respiratory patients operated on by an experienced oesophageal surgeon, one should expect about a 90% success in controlling heartburn and acid regurgitation and about a 75% success in controlling or eliminating the respiratory complaints, particularly cough, after anti-reflux surgery.

REFERENCES

1 Sontag SJ, Schnell TG, Miller TQ *et al.* Prevalence of oesophagitis in asthmatics. *Gut* 1992; 33: 872–6.

2 Sontag SJ, O'Connell S, Khandelwal S *et al.* Most asthmatics have gastroesophageal reflux with or without bronchodilator therapy. *Gastroenterology* 1990; 99: 613–20.

3 Schindbeck NE, Muller LS. Asthmatics' gastroesophageal reflux with or without bronchodilator therapy. *Gastroenterology* 1991; 101: 876–7.

4 White AM, Stevens WH, Upton AR, O'Byrne PM, Collins SM. Airway responsiveness to inhaled methacholine in patients with irritable bowel syndrome. *Gastroenterology* 1991; 100: 68–74.

5　Surpas P, Badier M, Dupin B, Charpin D, Vervloet D. Gastroesophageal reflux and non-specific bronchial reactivity. *Am Rev Respir Dis* 1989; 139: 588A.

6　Herve P, Denjean A, Jian R, Simonneau G, Duroux P. Intraesophageal perfusion of acid increases the bronchomotor response to methacholine and to isocapnic hyperventilation in asthmatic subjects. *Am Rev Respir Dis* 1986; 134: 986–9.

7　Irwin RS, Curley FJ, French CL. Difficult-to-control asthma. Contributing factors and outcome of a systematic management protocol. *Chest* 1993; 103: 1662–9.

KEY POINTS

1　Gastro-oesophageal reflux is very common in patients with bronchial asthma – in some patients reflux may exacerbate respiratory symptoms, and enhance the bronchoconstriction resulting from natural stimuli.

2　Half the asthmatic subjects with proven gastro-oesophageal reflux do not have the typical reflux symptoms of heartburn and acid regurgitation.

3　It is particularly important to consider reflux in the "asthmatic" who appears not to respond to standard treatment for asthma.

4　A carefully monitored trial of anti-reflux therapy in addition to optimal asthma therapy may be the best way to assess the contribution of reflux.

5　Patients in whom reflux is suspected but who do not respond to anti-reflux therapy should be referred for further investigations such as endoscopy and 24-hour oesophageal pH monitoring.

39

SPECIFIC PROBLEMS: CHRONIC RHINOSINUSITIS AND ASTHMA

Robert Naclerio and Fuad M. Baroody

INTRODUCTION

Sinusitis, a common disorder, has manifestations varying from an acute illness following an upper respiratory tract viral infection to an unremitting illness associated with a genetic abnormality in the epithelium of patients with cystic fibrosis. Over 31 million Americans describe chronic sinusitis as a health problem, and it affects all age groups, including 17% of people over the age of 65. In 1989, 16 million office visits were made for sinusitis. Billions of dollars are spent on medical and surgical treatments for this enigmatic illness.[1]

Although most cases of sinusitis are acute and self-limited, a significant number of individuals develop chronic sinusitis. In the mid-1980s, a renewed interest in chronic sinusitis emerged in the USA because of the development of the techniques of functional endoscopic sinus surgery and coronal CT scans. These advances led to a renewed appreciation of the role of anatomical problems in precipitating sinus disease and resulted in a tremendous increase in the number of surgical interventions performed for this entity. With time, however, it became clear that anatomy was not the entire problem.

It is generally not known why some individuals develop chronic sinusitis. A small number have cystic fibrosis, in which there is a genetically determined abnormality of epithelial ion transport. Some individuals have atopic disease and others have abnormalities of host defence, including antibody deficiencies and ciliary dysmotility.

It is hypothesized that certain individuals have a predisposition to develop chronic sinusitis. In these persons, environmental factors, such as allergens, viruses and air pollutants, trigger epithelial alterations that induce inflammation and subsequently decrease mucociliary transport, causing sinus ostial obstruction. Stasis of mucus in the sinuses then leads to bacterial infections that may further adversely influence the epithelium. If this cycle is not interrupted, the epithelium develops metaplastic changes and the underlying mucosa proliferates, developing a self-perpetuating cycle. This cycle manifests clinically as chronic sinusitis and is no longer dependent upon either the bacteria or the anatomy that initiated the process. Despite the high prevalence of chronic sinusitis and the fact that millions of dollars are spent on treatment, there have been essentially no definitive studies of the aetiology, pathogenesis and therapy of this condition.

DEFINITION

Sinusitis implies an inflammation of the paranasal sinuses. This definition has limited intellectual, pathological and clinical significance. Sinusitis is usually divided into acute, subacute and chronic conditions based on the symptomatic duration of the illness. While there is no known pathological correlate to this classification, it is assumed that organisms and the underlying pathological mechanisms differ. Acute sinusitis implies an illness of less than 2 weeks'duration, and subacute an illness lasting 2–6 weeks. Chronic sinusitis usually implies the presence of upper respiratory tract symptoms for more than 6 weeks, with radiographic evidence of mucosal thickening within the sinuses. Major symptoms include purulent anterior nasal discharge, nasal congestion, cough and posterior nasal discharge. Minor symptoms include peri-orbital oedema, facial/dental pain, sore throat, foul breath, fever, increased wheezing, olfactory loss, headache, ear pain and tooth pain. The signs and symptoms of chronic sinusitis are non-specific in that they can be associated with other disorders that are difficult to diagnose, such as non-allergic rhinitis of unknown aetiology (vasomotor rhinitis). Many other conditions should also be considered in the differential diagnosis of rhinosinusitis, and these are shown in Fig. 39.1.

RISK FACTORS

In any large group of patients with chronic sinusitis, there appears to be a number of important parameters that affect the patient's clinical course (Table 39.1) Patients with coexisting pulmonary disease, in particular asthma and cystic fibrosis, appear to have the greatest problems with chronic sinusitis. The prevalence of sinus disease in children with cystic fibrosis approaches 100%, while 78% of extrinsic asthmatic subjects report nasal symptoms. The latter estimate may be higher, depending upon how nasal symptoms are assessed. Zimmerman *et al.* found that plain sinus films of 138 asthmatic patients showed abnormalities in 31%, compared to none of 50 patients presenting with dental complaints ($P < 0.001$), but they found no relationship to the severity of asthma.[2] De Cleyn *et al.* found that

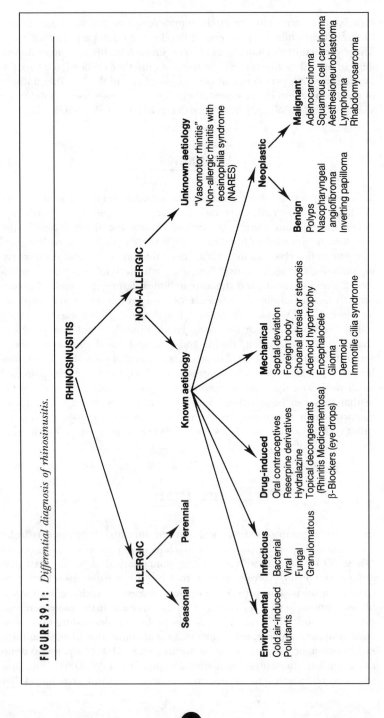

FIGURE 39.1: *Differential diagnosis of rhinosinusitis.*

TABLE 39.1: *Risk factors for sinusitis*

Lower respiratory disease
  Asthma
  Cystic fibrosis

Allergic inflammation
  Allergic rhinitis

Immune deficiencies
  Panhypogammaglobulinaemia
  Deficiencies of selective antibody responses

Anatomical abnormalities
  Septal deviation
  Concha bullosa
  Paradoxical middle turbinate
  Haller cell
  Prominent ethmoid bulla
  Atelectatic maxillary sinus

Miscellaneous
  Cigarette smoke
  Pollution
  Immotile cilia syndrome
  Foreign bodies (transnasal tubes)
  Aspirin intolerance

54% of 270 asthmatic patients had abnormal X-rays and that children had more opacifications than adults.[3] Schwartz *et al.* found that 47% of asthmatic flare-ups were associated with abnormal sinus X-rays, which was a significantly greater percentage than rhinitic patients who presented with flare-ups (29%).[4] Though these studies have several methodological flaws, they support the clinical impression of a high prevalence of simultaneously occurring sinusitis and lower respiratory tract disease.

Allergic inflammation appears to be another important factor in chronic sinusitis. Radiographic abnormalities of the sinuses are commonly found in patients with perennial allergic disease, often reaching a prevalence of over 50%.[5] How allergic rhinitis leads to chronic sinusitis is not clear. It is conceivable, particularly in subjects with underlying anatomical defects, that overwhelming allergen-induced nasal congestion could obstruct sinus drainage and lead to secondary bacterial infection. This scenario, while likely for acute sinusitis, seems unlikely to be a major factor in chronic disease, since current medications adequately control nasal congestion in the vast majority of patients with allergic rhinitis, and sinusitis can persist in allergic subjects even after they have undergone surgery to correct anatomical anomalies. Likewise, the normal anatomy and physiology of the nose and paranasal sinuses prevent pollen from directly entering the sinus cavities in patients who have not undergone surgical intervention (Fig. 39.2). Theoretical possibilities exist, but there are few, if any, data to support a mechanism by which allergic rhinitis induces chronic sinusitis.

While there is evidence that patients with panhypogammaglobulinaemia have increased susceptibility to developing infections of the paranasal sinuses, there is little information on the frequency of more limited immunodeficiencies, such as impaired antibody responses to bacterial polysaccharide antigens. In a preliminary study of 25 patients with refractory sinusitis, Sethi *et al.* found that approximately 30% had an identifiable abnormality in immune function or abnormalities limited to mucosal immune response.[6] Shapiro *et al.*, studying a group of children, found similar problems.[7] The results of an immunological survey in a larger, better defined population will determine whether the prevalence of immunological defects justifies this evaluation in all cases of refractory sinusitis and whether specific clinical presentations are associated with immunodeficiency. Other risk factors for the development of chronic sinusitis include

FIGURE 39.2: *Mucociliary clearance in the maxillary sinus. A coronal section of the nasal cavity, the osteo-meatal complex and the adjacent maxillary sinus is shown. The arrows represent the direction of mucociliary transport within the maxillary sinus. Mucus is transported superiorly to its outlet into the nasal cavity, which is bounded by the orbit and the uncinate process medially. (From Ref. 11 with permission.)*

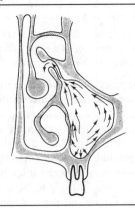

cigarette smoking, immotile cilia syndrome, foreign bodies and aspirin intolerance.

BACTERIOLOGY

The bacteriology of community-acquired acute sinusitis has been studied by antral punctures in adults and children (Table 39.2). In both adults and children, *Streptococcus pneumoniae* and *Haemophilus influenzae* are the predominant organisms.[8] In children, *Moraxella catarrhalis* is another important organism.[9] In nosocomial sinusitis (particularly in patients with tubes transversing the nasal cavity) and sinusitis in impaired hosts, a greater spectrum of organisms have been cultured, including fungi, Gram-negative organisms and methicillin-resistant *Staphylococcus aureus*. In these settings, the lack of a prompt response necessitates a culture.

In chronic sinusitis, the role of bacteria is less well established. Organisms have been cultured, but extended antibiotic usage rarely cures the problem. Thus, it is not clear whether the cultures reflect causative organisms or colonization of functionally impaired sinus cavities.

TABLE 39.2: *Microbiology of sinusitis*

Acute sinusitis
  Streptococcus pneumoniae
  Moraxella catarrhalis
  Haemophilus influenzae
  Eikenella corrodens
  Group A *Streptococcus*
  Group C *Streptococcus*
  α-*Streptococcus*

Chronic sinusitis
  α-Haemolytic *Streptococcus*
  Staphylococcus aureus
  Streptococcus pneumoniae
  Haemophilus influenzae
  Moraxella catarrhalis
  Anaerobes

Nosocomial sinusitis
  Fungi
  Gram-negative organisms
  Methicillin-resistant *Staphylococcus aureus*

EVALUATION

HISTORY

The evaluation of chronic sinusitis begins with a history of symptoms, with particular emphasis on potential risk factors. Begin by defining the onset of illness and its temporal relationship to life events (e.g. change in school or locale, acquiring a pet, trauma). Are other atopic symptoms, such as wheezing or urticaria, present? Define current symptoms with regard to the characteristics of secretions (clear vs. purulent), the presence or absence of pain, itching/sneezing (very characteristic of atopic disease), degree of air-flow obstruction, duration of symptoms, exacerbating factors (irritants and cold air) and seasonal patterns. Inquiry into the sense of smell aids in determining the degree of airflow obstruction. Severe nasal obstruction decreases the sense of smell, which is usually perceived as a loss of taste. Ocular symptoms include conjunctival itching, tearing, injection and peri-orbital oedema. Questions should be directed at disturbances of sleep. Snoring is frequently seen with nasal obstruction, but apnoeic episodes may be a sign of sleep apnoea and its sequelae. Children may also be noted to have paroxysmal nocturnal coughing spells and to awaken in the morn-ing complaining of sore throat and fatigue. Halitosis, as noted by the parent, may indicate infection. The history should detail previous treat-ments. Patients readily discuss prescription medications used but infrequently mention over-the-counter preparations, such as aspirin or top-ical medications. A family history of allergic diathesis, as well as details of the environmental history (type of home heating, presence of humidifi-cation, chemical exposures, employment), are also important.

PHYSICAL EXAMINATION

A complete ear, nose and throat examination is essential for all patients complaining of nasal symptoms. Examination of the ears may show unilat-eral or bilateral otitis media with effusion, suggesting pathology in the nasopharynx. Tenderness over the sinuses may reflect an underlying infec-tion, whereas numbness raises suspicion of a tumour. Nasal obstruction may present with discoloration beneath the lower eyelids. Chronic nasal obstruction is thought to cause under-development of the zygoma, nasal processes and maxillary sinuses, resulting in the flattened "adenoid facies". The classically described "allergic salute", in which a child attempts to relieve nasal itching and obstruction by pushing the nasal tip upward with the palm of the hand, may result in a transverse groove at the proximal nasal tip. Structural deviations or asymmetry should raise suspicion of trauma or congenital deformities.

After examining the external nares, a nasal speculum is used to examine the anterior third of the nasal cavity. This examination rules out other potential causes of similar nasal symptoms. Unilateral signs, particularly purulent drainage, should raise suspicion about foreign bodies. Pooling of secretions under the inferior turbinate hints at immotile cilia syndrome or total nasal obstruction.

Applying a topical decongestant permits better visualization of the nasal cavity. The openings to the frontal, maxillary and anterior ethmoidal sinuses are located lateral to the anterior portion of the middle turbinates in the middle meatus, and nasal polyps usually originate in this area. Septal deviations can interfere with airflow or predispose to sinusitis if they impinge and narrow the middle meatal area. Less common causes of "polyps" include dermoid cysts, encephaloceles and gliomas. A slow or absent response to a decongestant indicates a hyperplastic nasal mucosa. Rarely, a unilateral choanal atresia may be noted. Examination of the oral cavity may show a high arched palate with poor dental occlusion related to chronic mouth breathing. Posterior cervical lymphadenopathy may signal adenoiditis.

ENDOSCOPY

Following routine examination, endoscopic evaluation is considered. The introduction of a rigid or flexible fibreoptic scope provides excellent visualization of the entire nasal cavity. Subtle areas of mucosal contact can be appreciated, and pus draining from the sinuses can be cultured (Fig. 39.3).

FIGURE 39.3: *Endoscopic view of the left middle turbinate in a subject with acute sinusitis. Note the area of mucosal contact between the middle turbinate and the lateral nasal wall (to the right). The erythematous mucosa of the middle turbinate and the lateral nasal wall is suggestive of an acute inflammatory process.*

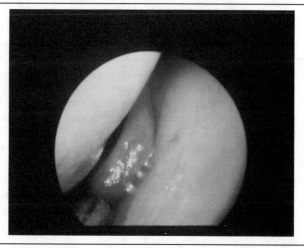

Cultures of the ostio-meatal complex have been shown to correlate with cultures obtained from within the sinuses in children undergoing sinus surgery.[10] While correlations between cultures of purulent material from the ostio-meatal area and antral punctures in patients with acute sinusitis have not been made, most clinicians suspect that there would be a strong correlation. However, random nasal cultures have a poor correlation with cultures from within the sinuses. Endoscopic examinations need not be performed in every patient with nasal complaints. However, any patient who does not respond to treatment should be referred for endoscopic evaluation.

OTHER DIAGNOSTIC TESTS

Skin testing or *in vitro* IgE measurements confirm the diagnosis of allergic rhinitis and, based on their results, the physician can provide recommendations for allergen avoidance. Nasal smears can identify eosinophils, pointing to an allergic problem or non-allergic rhinitis with eosinophilia syndrome (NARES). The presence of bacteria and neutrophils suggests infectious disease. CBC (complete blood count) with differential, CH50 levels, quantitative immunoglobulins and the response to protein and carbohydrate antigens may indicate confounding immunological defects.

Plain sinus radiographs in children are not useful, as they can be over- or under-interpreted (Fig. 39.4). In adults, they provide limited information. CT scans, though more definitive, are more expensive. Besides determining the degree of mucosal involvement, the CT scan defines anatomical abnormalities that interfere with sinus drainage (Fig. 39.5).[11] These defects are known risk factors, and their correction is the object of surgical intervention. To afford optimal demonstration of the anterior ethmoid sinuses and ostio-meatal structures, CT imaging is performed in the coronal planes (Fig. 39.6). Sectional imaging of the maxillo-facial area shows accurate soft tissue definition in the nasal cavity, paranasal sinuses, orbit and intra-cranial compartment. Highly contrasting densities identify air within the bony sinuses, fat within the orbit and soft tissue outlined by air in the nasal cavity. The CT examination is performed with the patient prone on the scanner bed with the chin in hyperextension. The parameters for CT scan can be adjusted so as to limit the radiation dose to 1 rad (0.01 Gy), which is less than the 3.5 rad (0.035 Gy) provided by the prior scanning parameters. In young children, coronal scans cannot always be obtained. In these individuals axial scans with coronal reconstructions should be obtained. Scans should be performed after the patient has had extensive medical treatment and are targeted at identifying residual disease and anatomical defects.

Magnetic resonance imaging (MRI) is excellent for demonstrating the presence of inflammatory disease in the paranasal sinuses, as the sensitivity of this modality is higher than that of CT. Its use in patients with chronic sinusitis is limited because MRI does not differentiate air from bone and therefore does not distinguish bony anatomy.

FIGURE 39.4: *Plain sinus X-ray of a child with suspected sinusitis (a) and the corresponding axial CT scan of the same patient (b) obtained within a short time interval. Whereas the plain radiograph was interpreted as opacification of both maxillary sinuses suggestive of sinusitis, the CT scan clearly shows normal maxillary sinuses. Note the prominent anterior bony wall of the maxillary sinuses on CT scan secondary to incomplete pneumatization, which probably resulted in the apparent opacification of these sinuses on the plain radiograph.*

(a)

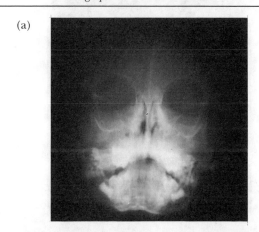

(b)

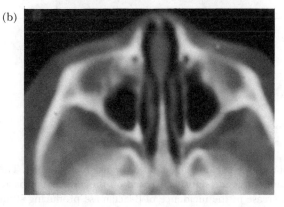

FIGURE 39.5: *Anatomical abnormalities. Coronal CT scan of the sinuses showing bilateral paradoxical middle turbinates (a) leading to narrowing of the osteo-meatal areas and the outlets to the maxillary sinuses. (b) A coronal CT scan of a patient with an atelectatic right uncinate process and maxillary sinus that is secondarily opacified and hypoplastic due to chronic infection.*

(a)

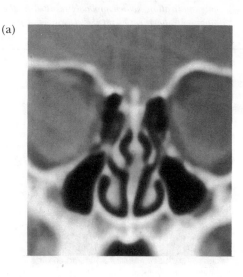

TREATMENT

MEDICAL

Antibiotics

The mainstay of medical management is the use of antibiotics. The choice of an antibiotic in acute sinusitis is based on the anticipated bacteriology. With the increase in the incidence of β-lactamase producing strains of *H. influenzae* and *M. catarrhalis*, the use of second-generation cephalosphorins, amoxycillin/clavulanate and modified derivatives of erythromycin and tri-methroprim–sulphamethoxazole has increased. Clinical cure rates are not significantly better with these medications compared to amoxycillin, but

FIGURE 39.5: *Continued.*

(b)

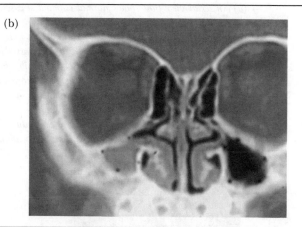

there is some evidence that bacteriological cures, based on antral puncture, are better.[8] It is important to realize that inadequate doses of antibiotics are often given and that the penetration of some antibiotics into the sinus mucosa may be inadequate. The optimal duration of antibiotic treatment is not well established. Cultures obtained after 10 days of treatment suggest sterilization of the sinuses from the offending organism. Many clinicians, however, extend the course of antibiotics beyond 10 days, although there is little scientific support for this practice. In chronic sinus disease, surgeons often treat for 6 weeks before obtaining CT scans. The rationale for the duration of pre-medication is obscure but probably relates to studies that show that mucosal abnormalities after acute sinusitis can persist for weeks and that infections of bones may necessitate prolonged therapy.

Adjuvants

Besides antibiotics, multiple other therapies have been used in the treatment of sinus disease. These include steam inhalations, saline irrigations, topical and systemic decongestants, topical and systemic steroids, muco-evacuants, anti-cholinergics, antihistamines, astringents, hot dry air and spicy foods.[12] Each adjuvant has a rationale that ranges from increasing ostial patency to providing symptomatic improvement. Unfortunately, the scientific literature regarding the use of adjuvants in the treatment of chronic sinusitis provides limited, if any, help in understanding their mechanisms of action and, therefore, appropriate usage. Well-controlled clinical trials are lacking. We follow two general principles in the use of these agents: (1) avoiding harmful side-effects, and (2) the more treatments given, the less likely the patient is to comply.

FIGURE 39.6: *Axial and coronal sinus CT scans of the same patient.*
(a) An axial view that shows normal ethmoid sinuses.
(b) An axial view depicting an opacified right
maxillary sinus. Note that the two axial cuts do not
delineate the osteo-meatal complex area or any possible
abnormalities in that area that might be responsible for
secondary disease in the maxillary sinus. (c) A coronal
CT view of the osteo-meatal complex area in the same
patient. This nicely identifies paradoxical middle
turbinates, leading to narrowing of the osteo-meatal
area and secondary right maxillary sinus opacification.

(a)

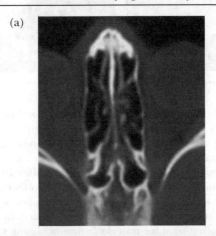

(b)

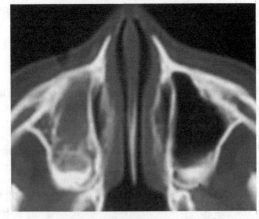

FIGURE 39.6: *Continued.*

(c)

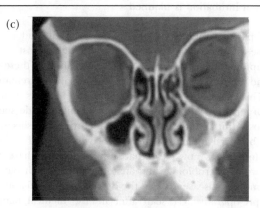

SURGERY

There are many surgical procedures for the treatment of sinus disease. Irrigation procedures, such as antral punctures and frontal sinus trephinations, are used primarily in acute disease when a culture is needed. Functional endoscopic sinus surgery, as initially described by Messerklinger and expanded upon by Kennedy and Stammberger, is a limited approach directed to the sinuses involved, as assessed by pre-operative endoscopic evaluation and CT scan.[13] This surgery has become the most commonly used technique because of its reduced morbidity in comparison with traditional procedures. It can often be performed under local anaesthesia in an outpatient setting. The major principle is that anatomical anomalies in the areas of mucociliary transport from the sinuses compromise drainage. Correction of outflow obstruction promotes drainage and leads to reversal of mucosal changes within the paranasal sinuses.

More traditional approaches remove the mucosa and create openings not necessarily within the areas of normal mucociliary transport. The classic example is the Cadwell Luc procedure, which enters the maxillary sinus anteriorly, strips out the sinus mucosa and creates an opening into the nose under the inferior turbinate (naso-antral window). Other traditional procedures employ the same principles as functional endoscopic sinus surgery but are performed via different surgical techniques. A description of all sinus surgical procedures is beyond the scope of this chapter and can be found in refs 13 and 14.

Patients with asthma need to have their asthma well controlled before surgery. Short bursts of oral steroids are often prescribed prior to surgery, particularly when intubation is planned.

In a series of patients followed by Kennedy, 45% still had evidence of mucosal disease within 18 months of surgery, although almost all reported significant symptomatic improvement.[15] The implication of these observed changes to the future clinical course of these patients remains to be determined. This observation does not negate the benefits of functional endoscopic surgery but is a reminder of the limited understanding of chronic sinusitis.[16] Initially, it was assumed that chronic sinusitis was caused by a resistant bacterial infection; later on, it was assumed to be due to abnormal anatomy. It is now clear that some individuals have problems that extend beyond microbiology and anatomy, in particular patients with coexisting pulmonary disease. In fact, the degree of mucosal abnormalities seen on the pre-operative CT scan after intense medical management seems to predict the surgical outcome, suggesting the importance of epithelial dysfunction in severe forms of chronic sinusitis. This statement does not negate evidence that sinus surgery can improve the clinical course of lower airway disease.

CONCLUSION

Chronic sinusitis is an important issue in the management of asthma. Improvement in antibiotics, endoscopy and imaging techniques has enhanced patient care and has renewed interest in this disease. Clearly, more investigation is needed to elucidate the pathophysiology of chronic sinus disease and the interrelationship between the upper and lower airways in this context.

REFERENCES

1   Loury M, Kennedy D. Chronic sinusitis and nasal polyposis. In: Getchell T, Doty R, Bartoshuk L (eds) *Smell and Taste in Health and Disease.* New York: Raven Press, 1991: 517–28.

2   Zimmerman B, Stringer D, Feanny S *et al.* Prevalence of abnormalities found by sinus X-rays in childhood asthma: Lack of relation to severity of asthma. *J Allergy Clin Immunol* 1987; 80: 268–73.

3   De Cleyn KM, Kersschot EA, De Clerck LS *et al.* Paranasal sinus pathology in allergic and non-allergic respiratory tract diseases. *Allergy* 1986; 41: 313–8.

4   Schwartz HJ, Thompson JS, Sher TH, Ross RJ. Occult sinus abnormalities in the asthmatic patient. *Arch Intern Med* 1987; 147: 2194–6.

5   Binder E, Holopainen E, Malmberg K, Salo OP. Clinical findings in patients with allergic rhinitis. *Rhinology* 1984; 22: 255–60.

6   Sethi D, Winkelstein G, Lederman H (Loury M). Immunologic defects in patients with chronic recurrent sinusitis. Diagnosis and management. *Otolaryngol Head Neck Surg* 1995; 112: 242–7.

7   Shapiro G, Virant F, Furukawa C, Pierson W, Bierman C. Immune defects in patients with refractory sinusitis. *Pediatrics* 1991; 87: 311–6.

8   Gwaltney J. Microbiology of sinusitis. In: Druce H (ed) *Sinusitis Pathophysiology and Treatment.* New York: Marcel Dekker, 1994: 41–56.

9   Wald E, Milmoe G, Bowen A, Ledosma-Modina J, Salamon N, Bluestone CD. Acute maxillary sinusitis in children. *New Engl J Med* 1981; 304: 749–54.

10 Orobello PW Jr, Park RI, Belcher LJ *et al.* Microbiology of chronic sinusitis in children. *Arch Otolaryngol Head Neck Surg* 1991; 117: 980–3.

11 Zinreich SJ, Kennedy DW, Rosenbaum AE *et al.* Paranasal sinuses: CT imaging requirements for endoscopic surgery. *Radiology* 1987; 163: 769–75.

12 Druce H. Adjuncts to medical management of sinusitis. *Otolaryngol Head Neck Surg* 1993; 103: 880–3.

13 Stammberger H. *Functional Endoscopic Sinus Surgery.* Philadelphia: BC. Decker, 1991.

14 Blitzer A, Lawson W, Friedman W. *Surgery of the Paranasal Sinuses.* Philadelphia: W.B. Saunders Co., 1985.

15 Kennedy DW. Prognostic factors, outcomes and staging in ethmoid sinus surgery. *Laryngoscope* 1992; 102: 1–18.

16 Mings R, Friedman WH, Linford PA, Slavin RG. Five-year follow-up of the effects of bilateral intranasal sphenoethmoidectomy in patients with sinusitis and asthma. *Am J Rhinol* 1988; 2: 13–6.

KEY POINTS

1   Abnormal anatomy contributes to the development of sinusitis.

2   The prevalence of chronic sinusitis in patients with asthma is high.

3   Nasal endoscopy improves ability to visualize the nasal cavity.

4   CT scan is preferred imaging modality for sinus disease.

5   Surgery plays an adjuvant role in the management of chronic sinusitis in asthmatic patients.

40

SPECIFIC PROBLEMS: FOOD ALLERGY IN ASTHMA

Jean Bousquet, Pascal Chanez and François-B. Michel

Adverse reactions to foods can be classified on the basis of the mechanisms of the reaction. Allergic reactions are immunologically mediated. The best known example of such a reaction is IgE-mediated food anaphylaxis but other types of hypersensitivity reactions have been associated with food allergy. Although IgG or IgG_4 might be involved there is no definite proof that these immunoglobulin isotypes are important in food allergy. Other reactions involve immune-complex reactions and lymphocyte activation. All other non-immunological adverse reactions such as sulphite- or aspirin-induced asthma should be classified as food intolerance.[1-3] Besides allergen-specific mechanisms, there are many non-specific mechanisms that may aggravate respiratory symptoms due to food allergy such as exercise, cold drinks, aspirin or concomitant intake of alcohol.

Food allergy has always been a difficult problem to assess, especially in asthma, where some investigators deny its existence whilst others tend to overestimate its importance. Moreover, the diagnosis of food allergy is always difficult and double-blind food challenges should often be performed to confirm the diagnosis of food-induced asthma.

CLINICAL PRESENTATION

There are several cases which demonstrate that asthma can be triggered by foods, and that this reaction can be controlled by an alteration in diet. However, many reports are only speculative and, when the delay between the ingestion and symptoms exceeds 24 hours, it is extremely difficult to ascribe an asthma attack to food allergy owing to the great variability of the airways obstruction in chronic asthmatic subjects. The best demonstration is given by double-blind food challenges but in some highly allergic individuals or in occupational allergy (e.g. bakers) inhalation challenges with foods can lead to an immediate bronchial response.[4] Elimination diets

FIGURE 40.1: *Evolution of peak flow rates in a patient allergic to eggs after an egg-free diet. (From Ref. 2 with permission.)*

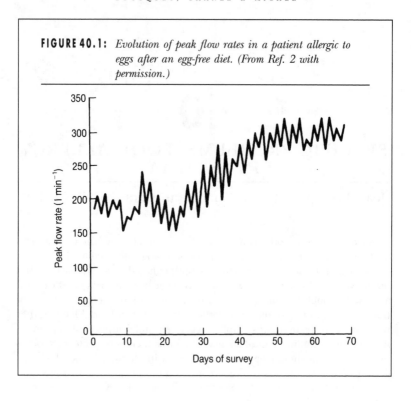

can also be demonstrative but their interpretation may be difficult when patients are allergic to both foods and inhaled allergens (Fig. 40.1).

Respiratory symptoms due to an IgE-mediated food allergic reaction can suddenly occur if the food is not routinely ingested and may be associated with other symptoms of generalized anaphylaxis. These acute outbreaks of asthma may be extremely severe and fatalities have been reported.[5,6] However, if the food is ingested routinely, the patient may present with chronic asthma that is often associated with atopic dermatitis. Often, such patients present with severe asthma that is difficult to control. The severity of chronic asthma varies widely and may in mild cases only present as a persistent cough or as exercise-induced asthma.[7] It has also been observed that foods only increase airway hyperresponsiveness without causing frank wheezing.[8]

In infants, symptoms may take the form of classical asthma but there may also be intermittent attacks of dyspnoea, tachypnoea and occasionally fever. Other symptoms of food allergy often present concomitantly.[9]

DIAGNOSIS OF FOOD ALLERGY-INDUCED ASTHMA

SUSPICION OF FOOD ALLERGY IN ASTHMA

Food allergy may be suspected (1) when asthma started early in life, especially if the patient has had or currently presents atopic dermatitis,[10] (2) in patients having suffered from anaphylactic symptoms or acute urticaria due to food allergy, and (3) in any patient, even in adults, with poorly controlled asthma and elevated total serum IgE levels. However, it must be pointed out that suspicion of food allergy alone cannot be used as the basis for diagnosis.

DIAGNOSIS OF FOOD ALLERGY IN ASTHMA

The diagnosis of food allergy in asthma is difficult because of the quality of the tests available but also because it should be demonstrated that the suspected food causes asthma. Such diagnoses are based on a suggestive clinical history, the demonstration of an IgE-mediated allergic reaction to food allergens and, at best, a food challenge.

SKIN TESTS AND ALLERGEN-SPECIFIC IgE ANTIBODIES

The value of skin tests and serum-specific IgE is dependent upon a number of variables amongst which the quality of the allergen extract used is of major importance. Allergen extracts currently available are not standardized, and their stability often remains poorly established.[11] For allergen extracts that are rapidly degraded, like those from fruit and vegetables, skin tests may be falsely negative in food-allergic individuals. Allergen extracts from egg, milk, fish, shellfish, nuts, peanuts and cereals are usually of better quality.

The diagnosis should be started using skin-prick tests with foods. For fruits and vegetables, skin-prick tests with raw fresh foods are required (prick-prick test).[12] Intradermal skin tests are more sensitive than prick tests but they are less specific. They may be used when prick tests are negative. The titration of serum food-specific IgE is available for many foods but, in contrast with better characterized inhalant allergens, the sensitivity of the test is not yet fully known for most unpurified food allergens.[13] Moreover, even more than in inhalant allergy, the presence of food-specific IgE in serum or positive skin tests to foods do not necessarily correlate with food allergy since many patients outgrow their allergy with age[14] and not all patients with food-specific IgE have a clinical sensitivity. The presence of positive skin-prick test and/or serum-specific IgE does not preclude a positive result for food challenge since only one-third of patients presenting with positive skin-prick tests and/or serum-specific IgE have asthma during food challenge,[11] so that a diet should not be started before food challenges have been performed.[15]

Patients who have developed acute urticaria or anaphylaxis often make the diagnosis of "food intolerance" by themselves, and the presence of positive skin tests and/or serum-specific IgE correlating with the claims of the patient makes it possible to establish a diagnosis without performing a food challenge. This test may cause severe untoward reactions in patients with anaphylaxis and should be performed with extreme care. However, in asthma, patients rarely identify a food as a cause of wheezing so it is necessary to confirm the diagnosis by double-blind food challenges.[15]

FOOD CHALLENGE

Food challenges should be performed in a manner similar to that reported by Bock[16] or Sampson and Albergo.[17] The food suspected of causing symptoms should be eliminated from the diet for a minimum of 2 weeks before testing. The selection of foods for administration is based upon positive skin tests and/or specific IgE or on a clear anecdotal history despite negative skin-prick tests and/or radioallergosorbent test (RAST). Patients should stop anti-asthma medications that might modify the performance of the test for an appropriate delay. However, medication withdrawal may induce a deterioration of lung function making evaluation difficult. Moreover, in patients with severe asthma it is not possible to discontinue all medications and occasionally the challenge has to be done in a patient receiving β agonists and/or theophylline and/or inhaled corticosteroids. In this case, the medications should be identical on placebo and test days. When possible, lyophilized foods should be placed in size 0 dye-free opaque capsules, or if administered as a liquid, they should be mixed in a broth or in a juice to disguise the taste. Although patients who have presented with anaphylactic symptoms should not be tested, it is advisable to increase the dose slowly from 100 mg to 10 g. Challenges should ideally be conducted in a double-blind manner, but if several foods are implicated a screening with single-blind challenges may be done first. In case of food-induced asthma, serial pulmonary function tests should be carried out for up to 8 hours since late reactions can occur.[10] During all challenges, a physician should follow up the patient since some untoward systemic reaction might occur. The challenge is only considered to be positive if the PD_{20} of forced expiratory volume in 1 s (FEV_1) is reached on a test day without any such drop in FEV_1 during a placebo day (Fig. 40.2). For asthma, the test with placebo is critical owing to the great variability of pulmonary function that is a characteristic of the disease.

In young children, pulmonary function tests are not easy to do and to interpret without sophisticated equipment, which is rarely available, and so the diagnosis of asthma may be based on clinical examination alone. Some patients develop gastrointestinal symptoms, acute urticaria or atopic dermatitis without any airways response. If the challenge is inconclusive, it has been proposed to ask the patient to eat the amount of food ingested during a usual meal and to measure the pulmonary function serially.

Food challenge data may be augmented by measuring the release of mediators in peripheral blood or the increased gut permeability.

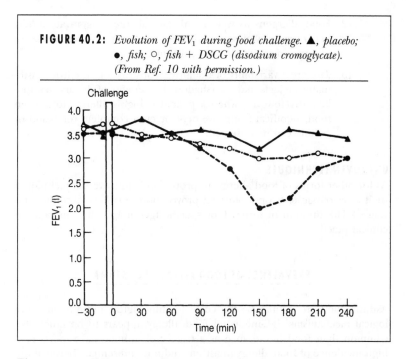

FIGURE 40.2: *Evolution of FEV_1 during food challenge.* ▲, *placebo;* ●, *fish;* ○, *fish + DSCG (disodium cromoglycate).* *(From Ref. 10 with permission.)*

The measure of airway hyperresponsiveness before and after an oral challenge was proposed by Wilson and Silverman[18] who observed that some patients only develop an increase of airway responsiveness to histamine after a food challenge without any change in basal peak flow.

A positive food challenge does not necessarily imply that the patient presents with an IgE-mediated allergy but suggests an intolerance to certain foods. If specific IgE and/or prick tests to a specific foodstuff are positive, an IgE-mediated mechanism is likely to be involved. In situations where oral cromoglycate is commercially available, a further food challenge is advisable in order to test the efficacy of this drug prior to prescribing such a treatment. The results of double-blind food challenge in asthma are similar to those observed with other food-induced symptoms and only one-quarter to one-third of patients with positive skin tests and/or specific IgE have a positive oral challenge.[10,16–19]

ELIMINATION DIETS

Elimination diets are used primarily for the diagnosis of diseases such as eczema and rhinitis. In the case of asthma, it is often difficult to make the diagnosis of food allergy by elimination diets for many reasons.[10,19]

(1) Food allergy is almost constantly associated with inhalant allergy and possibly with other triggers, and variations in the airways obstruction may be due to factors unrelated to foods.

(2) Food allergens as well as inhalant allergens aggravate airway hyperresponsiveness and it may take days or even weeks to observe an improvement of asthma.

(3) The great variability of the airways obstruction in chronic asthmatic subjects may overshadow the benefits of dietary manipulations. However, when a patient is highly allergic to a given food, significant improvement or even complete remission of asthma can be observed.

UNPROVEN TECHNIQUES

As for other forms of food allergy, unproven and controversial techniques such as cytotoxic tests or sublingual provocation tests have absolutely no value.[20] The titration of serum food-specific IgG or IgG_4 has no value in clinical practice.

PREVALENCE OF FOOD ALLERGY IN ASTHMA

Asthma due to foods may be caused by immunological and non-immunological mechanisms. IgE-mediated food allergy appears to be much less common than food intolerance as a trigger of asthma and reports of a high incidence of food allergy in asthma did not differentiate between the mechanisms of food-induced asthma (for review see ref. 21). Methodological problems limit the evaluation of the prevalence of food allergy in asthma. Only double-blind food challenges combined with skin tests or IgE can screen asthmatic subjects for allergies to foods but this method cannot be used in epidemiological studies. Thus either epidemiological studies are performed in a random population with inappropriate methods or they are performed in selected populations with appropriate techniques.

Most cases of food-induced asthma are observed in early infancy and are then often related to cow's milk hypersensitivity in which asthma has been noted in 7–29%[9,21–24] but there appear to be increasing numbers of infants allergic to egg, flour and peanuts. The incidence of food allergy decreases with age, and although some investigators have proposed that many intrinsic adult asthmatic subjects may in fact be allergic to foods, the few controlled studies performed by food challenges[9,25,26] or skin tests[21] do not substantiate this assertion. In areas where mugwort and birch pollens are rare, food allergy only represents a minor cause of perennial asthma, being present in 4–6% of asthmatic children[27] and in 1–4% of asthmatic adults.[10,28] However, when these pollen species are prevalent, allergy due to cross-reactive food epitopes, such as celery, nuts or fruits,[12] may be more important but anaphylactic or gastrointestinal and dermatological symptoms are likely to be more frequent than asthma. In non-Caucasian populations the incidence of food allergy may be greater and these figures may be increased. Finally, differences may be observed depending on the usual diet of a given country, such as the dye allergy that was reported to be relatively frequent in the UK.

TREATMENT OF ASTHMA INDUCED BY FOOD ALLERGY

The presence of a positive skin-prick test or serum IgE test to a given food should not lead to an elimination diet, because only 30–40% of patients have asthma when they are challenged orally with the offending food.[10,16,18] A positive food challenge favours dietary avoidance[29] but nutritional balance must always be maintained especially in infants and young children, since many infants are now being placed on dangerously inadequate diets.[30] Also, the reintroduction of a food, accidental or intentional, may be associated with anaphylaxis or severe respiratory obstruction, since individual patients tend to continue to react with the same symptoms as they had before.

The efficacy of oral sodium cromoglycate is not completely established but this drug was found in some studies to prevent asthma due to food allergy.[10,31] It is clear that only a fraction of patients benefit from this treatment but, when available and effective, it may be used (1) to decrease the reactivity of the gastrointestinal tract to dietary allergens and (2) to allow a less restrictive diet. Ketotifen has also been used and seems to have a greater value in the treatment of skin symptoms.

There is at present no evidence to support specific immunotherapy by either the oral or the parenteral route. If such a treatment is administered it must be done for research purposes in an intensive care setting by specialized doctors, since deaths have been reported.

In all cases, asthma is a disease of the airways and patients should always have treatment of the airway inflammation and obstruction, besides the treatment of food allergy if it is documented. The prevention of food allergy may be attempted in the newborn at high risk for allergy but at present there is no clear demonstration that breast-feeding, even prolonged, prevents the onset of allergy.[32]

REFERENCES

1   Anderson J, Sogn D. Adverse reactions to foods. AAAI Committee on Adverse Reactions to Foods and NIAID. NIH Publication no. 84-2442, July 1984.

2 Bousquet J, Chanez P, Michel FB. The respiratory tract and food hypersensitivity. In: Metcalfe DD, Sampson H (eds) *Food Allergy*. Oxford: Blackwell Scientific Publications, 1991: 139–49.

3 Kettelhut BV, Metcalfe DD. Adverse reactions to foods. In: Middleton E Jr, Ellis EF, Reed CE, Adkinson NF Jr, Yunginger JW (eds) *Allergy, Principles and Practice*, 3rd edn. St Louis: Mosby Co., 1988: 1481–502.

4 Bousquet J, Dhivert H, Clauzel AM, Hewitt B, Michel FB. Occupational allergy to sunflower pollen. *J Allergy Clin Immunol* 1985; 75: 70–4.

5 Yunginger JW, Sweeney KG, Sturner WQ *et al.* Fatal food-induced anaphylaxis. *JAMA* 1988; 260: 1450–2.

6 Sampson HA, Mendelson L, Rosen JP. Fatal and near-fatal anaphylactic reactions to food in children and adolescents. *N Engl J Med* 1992; 327: 380–4.

7 Kidd JM, Cohen SH, Sosman AJ, Fink JN. Food-dependent exercise-induced anaphylaxis. *J Allergy Clin Immunol* 1983; 71: 407–11.

8 Wilson N, Vickers H, Taylor G, Silverman M. Objective test for food sensitivity in asthmatic children: increased bronchial reactivity after cola drinks. *BMJ* 1982; 284: 1226–8.

9 Hill DJ, Firer MA, Shelton MJ, Hosking CS. Manifestations of milk allergy in infancy: clinical and immunologic findings. *J Pediatr* 1986; 109: 270–6.

10 Onorato J, Merland N, Terral C, Michel FB, Bousquet J. Placebo-controlled double-blind food challenge in asthma. *J Allergy Clin Immunol* 1986; 78: 1139–46.

11 Metcalfe DD. Food allergens. *Clin Rev Allergy* 1985; 3: 331–49.

12 Dreborg S, Foucard T. Allergy to apple, carrot and potato in children with birch pollen allergy. *Allergy* 1983; 38: 167–72.

13 Metcalfe D. Food hypersensitivity. *J Allergy Clin Immunol* 1984; 73: 749–60.

14 Dannaeus A, Inganas M. A follow-up study of children with food allergy. Clinical course in relation to serum IgE and IgG antibody level to milk, egg and fish. *Clin Allergy* 1981; 11: 533–9.

15 Yunginger JW. Proper application of available laboratory tests for adverse reactions to foods and food additives. *J Allergy Clin Immunol* 1986; 78: 220–3.

16 Bock SA. A critical evaluation of clinical trials in adverse reactions to foods in children. *J Allergy Clin Immunol* 1986; 78: 165–73.

17 Sampson HA, Albergo R. Comparison of results of skin tests, RAST and double-blind, placebo-controlled food challenges in children with atopic dermatitis. *J Allergy Clin Immunol* 1984; 75: 348–55.

18 Wilson N, Silverman M. Diagnosis of food sensitivity in childhood asthma. *J R Soc Med* 1985; 5(suppl): 11–6.

19 Atkins FM, Steinberg SS, Metcalfe DD. Evaluation of immediate adverse reactions to foods in adults. 1. Correlation of demographic, laboratory,

and skin prick test data with response to controlled oral food challenge. J Allergy Clin Immunol 1985; 75: 348–55.

20 Van Metre TE Jr. Critique of controversial and unproven procedures for diagnosis and therapy of allergic disorders. Pediatr Clin North Am 1983; 30: 807–13.

21 Bousquet J, Neukirch F, Noyola A, Michel FB. Prevalence of food allergy in asthma. Pediatr Allergy Immunol 1992; 3: 206–14.

22 Nichaman MZ, McPherson RS. Estimating prevalence of adverse reactions to foods: principles and constraints. J Allergy Clin Immunol 1986; 78: 148–54.

23 Savilahti E. Cow's milk allergy. Allergy 1981; 36: 73–8.

24 Bishop JM, Hill DJ, Hosking CS. Natural history of cow milk allergy: clinical outcome. J Pediatr 1990; 116: 862–7.

25 Oehling A, Cagnani CE. Food allergy and child asthma. Allergol Immunopathol 1980; 8: 7–14.

26 Ganderton MA. Diet and asthma. BMJ 1978; i: 1624.

27 Novembre E, Veneruso G, Sabatini C et al. Incidence of asthma caused by food allergy in childhood. Pediatr Med Chir 1987; 9: 399–404.

28 Burr ML, Fehily AM, Stott NC, Merrett TG. Food-allergic asthma in general practice. Hum Nutr Appl Nutr 1985; 39: 349–55.

29 Höj L, Osterballe O, Bundsgaard A, Weeke B, Weiss M. A double-blind controlled trial of elemental diet in severe, perennial asthma. Allergy 1981; 36: 257–62.

30 Tripp JH, Francis DEM, Knight JA, Harries JT. Infant feeding practices; a cause for concern. BMJ 1979; 2: 707–8.

31 Dannaeus A, Foucard T, Johansson SGO. The effect of orally administered sodium cromoglycate on symptoms of food allergy. Clin Allergy 1977; 7: 109–15.

32 Michel FB, Bousquet J, Dannaeus A et al. Prevention measures in early childhood allergy. J Allergy Clin Immunol 1986; 78: 1022–7.

KEY POINTS

1 Food allergy is a rare event in asthma. Its prevalence ranges from 4 to 6% in children but is less than 1% in adult asthmatic subjects.

2 In areas where birch and mugwort pollen are common sensitizers food allergy is more common due to cross-reactive allergens.

3   Except in infancy, most patients with food allergy are also sensitized to inhalant allergens.

4   Current or previous atopic dermatitis is frequently associated with asthma in patients with food allergy.

5   Although food allergy is infrequent, it should be recognized since patients often present severe symptoms that are improved by a diet.

6   An elimination diet should be based on food challenge.

41

SPECIFIC PROBLEMS: STEROID-INDUCED SIDE-EFFECTS

N. C. Barnes

Systemic corticosteroids were first used in the management of asthma in the 1930s when crude extracts of adrenocorticotrophic hormone (ACTH) were administered. The first properly conducted trials of oral corticosteroids were performed in the 1950s in two MRC-sponsored studies.[1,2] The trial in chronic asthma[1] used a low and variable dose of cortisone and showed a benefit over part of the treatment period in the steroid-treated group. The second study[2] in acute severe asthma showed compelling evidence of benefit. In the absence of other effective anti-inflammatory agents, oral corticosteroids became widely used in asthma and in other inflammatory diseases such as rheumatoid arthritis. Within a few years the serious long-term side-effects of treatment with oral corticosteroids became apparent. Since then the goal in treating asthma has been to effectively control the disease without the long-term use of oral corticosteroids. This goal has been clearly set out in various guidelines:[3,4] the objective is control of the disease with best possible lung function, minimizing the chance of a severe attack and with the least possible side-effects from drugs.

Effective anti-asthma therapy has decreased the percentage of patients who require long-term oral steroids. There remain three broad patterns of use of systemic steroids in the treatment of asthma. The first and most common is the use of short courses of oral steroids for the treatment of acute exacerbations of asthma. The second is the long-term maintenance treatment and the third pattern is repeated short courses of steroids with only short gaps between them. Although side effects are potentially the same, the principal concern differs. For instance, with a short course of oral steroids the principal concerns may be over dyspepsia, bleeding ulcers, electrolyte disturbances and impairment of glucose tolerance, whereas with long-term oral steroids the principal concerns will be over disturbances of protein metabolism, osteoporosis, skin thinning, easy bruising and cataract formation. The frequent use of short courses of oral steroids may lead to concern over both patterns of side-effects. The side-effects of oral steroids (Table 41.1) are dependent upon the dose of steroids and the duration of treatment. However, there is evidence particularly for effects on bone[5] that the

TABLE 41.1: *Complications of using systemic corticosteroids.*

	Problems occurring with both acute and chronic usage	Problems mainly related to chronic usage
Metabolic	Hypokalaemia Diabetes mellitus Hypothalamic–pituitary–adrenal axis suppression	Hyperlipidaemia Cushingoid appearance Secondary amenorrhoea Impotence
Cardiovascular	Hypertension Exacerbation of congestive cardiac failure Oedema	
Gastrointestinal tract	Peptic ulceration Oesophagitis Pancreatitis Intestinal perforation	
Infective complications	Increased susceptibility to infection Reactivation of infection Dissemination of vaccination	
Skin		Skin thinning and fragility Easy bruising Hirsuitism
CNS	Psychological changes Convulsions	
Musculoskeletal	Myopathy Aseptic necrosis of head of femur	Osteoporosis Loss of muscle mass
Ocular	Glaucoma	Cataracts

most rapid bone loss is seen early in treatment with the rate of bone loss becoming less rapid as treatment progresses. When attempting to minimize the side-effects of oral steroids two considerations are necessary: first, how can the dose or duration of treatment be minimized and, second, how can other measures be taken to counteract the side-effects?

MINIMIZING THE USE OF ORAL STEROIDS

ALLERGEN AVOIDANCE (see Chapters 14 and 31)

While the routine use of allergen avoidance in the proven control of asthma is controversial, it seems clear that in occupational asthma removal from offending allergen or improved work practices can lead to a very significant improvement in asthma. Therefore, treatment of any occupational component that can be identified is of importance.

SMOKING

Advising patients to stop smoking is a routine part of the management of asthma. There is no specific proof that this can prevent or decrease the use of oral steroids. However smoking is known to increase the risk of osteoporosis, peptic ulceration, the cardiovascular complications of hypertension and to worsen the complications of diabetes and therefore it is important that patients are strongly advised to stop smoking.

IMMUNOTHERAPY (see Chapter 21)

Immunotherapy is a treatment that remains controversial and there is no proof that it decreases the requirements for oral steroids.

β_2 AGONISTS

The possible benefits and side-effects of regular treatment with β_2 agonists for asthma remain controversial. However, there is no proof that regular β_2 agonists decrease requirement for oral steroids.

THEOPHYLLINES

Some authorities consider oral theophyllines to have an anti-inflammatory role in asthma, although this role is not clearly defined. There are a number of studies suggesting that theophyllines may decrease requirement for oral steroids.[6-8] A trial of oral controlled-release theophyllines is worth while in patients with steroid-dependent asthma.

ANTI-CHOLINERGICS

There is no well documented proof that anti-cholinergic drugs decrease requirement for oral corticosteroids.

DISODIUM CROMOGLYCATE (DSCG) AND NEDOCROMIL SODIUM

There are conflicting results of studies of DSCG and nedocromil sodium for their ability to decrease requirement for oral corticosteroids. In an early study DSCG led to an improvement in patients on oral steroids but steroid reduction was not attempted.[9] Other studies have investigated the ability to control asthma without steroids but not steroid reduction directly.[10] With nedocromil sodium both positive[11] and negative[12] trials have been reported. In practice, any oral steroid-sparing effect they have is small or non-existent in the presence of adequate doses of inhaled corticosteroids. Furthermore, as compliance with inhaled therapy is a significant problem, it is likely that any small beneficial effect obtained may well be outweighed by the fact that these drugs have to be taken three or four times a day and may decrease compliance with the more important inhaled corticosteroids.

INHALED CORTICOSTEROIDS

These are undoubtedly the most effective way of decreasing the requirement for long-term oral steroids. Early trials with beclomethasone dipropionate (BDP) were performed in patients who were dependent on oral steroids and demonstrated the ability of these drugs to decrease requirement for oral steroids.[13] Open studies have suggested that high-dose inhaled steroids can further reduce the number of patients dependent on long-term oral steroids.[14] However, these studies are open to criticism and controversy remains about the beneficial effects of increasing doses of inhaled steroids above 800–1000 µg daily.[15,16] The recent introduction of the new, more potent, inhaled steroid fluticasone propionate has allowed further research into the role of inhaled steroids in decreasing requirement for oral steroids. In a study comparing 1.5 and 2 mg daily of inhaled fluticasone with placebo for the ability to decrease the requirement for oral steroids, 88% of patients on the highest dose of inhaled steroids managed to stop their oral steroids with an increase in pulmonary function compared with only 3% of patients stopping oral steroids on placebo.[17] There was also evidence in this study of a dose-related effect. Open uncontrolled[18] and anecdotal evidence suggests that in some patients increasing the dose of BDP or budesonide above 2 mg daily may further decrease requirement for oral steroids, but as these patients provide a harder and more difficult core of oral steroid-dependent asthmatic patients the return from increasing the dose becomes smaller.

Although concern has been expressed about the side-effects of inhaled steroids when used at high dose for a long time, any effects that they have are far less than those that occur with the regular use of oral steroids. However it is important that any systemic effects are minimized. This can be achieved by using the lowest effective dose of inhaled steroids, by using a large-volume spacer with a metered dose inhaler and further decreasing the gastrointestinal deposition by gargling and spitting out. Early evidence suggests that at high dose fluticasone propionate may have an improved safety-to-efficacy ratio compared with the established inhaled steroids BDP and budesonide; if further studies continue to confirm this perhaps fluticasone should be used particularly in patients requiring oral steroids.

IMMUNOSUPPRESSANTS (see Chapter 17)

A number of trials have demonstrated that immunosuppressants can decrease the requirement for oral steroids. However, their use remains controversial. Although several immunosuppressants have been shown to decrease the requirement for oral corticosteroids in trials of several months' duration, all of these drugs have serious side-effects and it is not yet clear whether the benefit from reduction in oral steroid requirement outweighs the side-effects of these immunosuppressant drugs. At present the use of these drugs should be in clinical trials or on an individual patient basis with the clinician attempting to weigh-up the benefits and risks of the treatment for the particular patient. They should only be used once other avenues of treatment, particularly the use of high-dose inhaled corticosteroids, has been found to be inadequate.

Methotrexate

The most widely used immunosuppressant in asthma is methotrexate. This acts on all dividing cells and has an established role as a steroid-sparing agent and anti-inflammatory drug in rheumatoid arthritis. The initial observation by Mullarkey that methotrexate decreased oral steroid requirement in a patient with asthma was followed by a clinical trial demonstrating an impressive decrease in oral steroid requirement.[19] However, the group of patients studied had a very high requirement for oral steroids and the use of other anti-asthma drugs in this group was ill-defined. A well-performed study by Shiner et al.[20] investigated the steroid-sparing effect of methotrexate at a dose of 15 mg orally per week over a 24-week period in a randomized, placebo-controlled, parallel group study. The study demonstrated that methotrexate caused a 50% decrease in oral steroid requirement compared with a 14% decrease on placebo; however the effect had not maximized by the end of the study. There was also a decrease in exacerbations of asthma without any change in pulmonary function. Other studies have not shown such a marked beneficial effect of methotrexate[21,22] and there have been reports of side-effects, notably *Pneumocystis carinii* pneumonia[23] and methotrexate-induced pneumonitis.[24] Apart from an increase in opportunistic infections, the other specific side-effect of methotrexate is liver fibrosis and it is recommended by some that a liver biopsy should be performed every 2 years in patients on long-term methotrexate.[25] At present if methotrexate is to be used it should probably only be in patients on long-term oral steroids, despite high-dose inhaled steroids a trial of treatment of at least 3 months is needed to see if there is any beneficial effect. If no decrease in steroid requirement is seen at this time then it is probably best to stop. If a beneficial effect is seen it may be worth continuing until the lowest possible dose of oral steroids is reached. Regular monitoring of liver function tests and full blood count are necessary and prompt treatment of any intercurrent infection will be needed.

Azathioprine

Azathioprine was the subject of two small-scale, short-term studies.[26,27] These were most certainly of inadequate length to determine if azathioprine had a steroid-sparing role. Although it is likely that azathioprine would have a steroid-sparing role in asthma its use cannot be advocated in the absence of any controlled trials.

Cyclosporin A

With the increased understanding of the role of T lymphocytes in asthma[28] and evidence that cyclosporin A (CsA) is active in other steroid-responsive diseases, such as psoriasis and atopic dermatitis,[29,30] an investigation into the role of CsA in steroid-dependent asthma became attractive.

Three controlled trials have now been performed and there has been a report of the use of CsA on an open basis. Alexander et al.[31] showed an increase in pulmonary function with a decrease in exacerbations of asthma that required rescue courses of prednisolone in a group of steroid-dependent asthmatic subjects on high-dose inhaled steroids. Two further controlled trials have been performed specifically searching for a steroid-sparing effect. Lock et al.[32] have shown a significant steroid-sparing effect of CsA over a 36-week period with a small rise in pulmonary function. Nizankowska et al.[33] have shown a decrease in oral steroid requirement without an increase in pulmonary function in a group of steroid-dependent asthmatic subjects. In these studies and in experience with the open use of CsA[34] it seems that only 50% or so of patients respond at the dose used (5 mg kg^{-1} daily). CsA should only be used in patients dependent on oral steroids or high-dose inhaled steroids. There should be no contraindications to use, particularly previous malignancy or significant renal disease, and regular monitoring of renal function is necessary during treatment. Treatment should be given for 3 months to see if there is any beneficial effect. Anecdotal experience suggests that in patients who respond doses lower than 5 mg kg^{-1} daily can be used, and if a response is achieved then it is worth trying to wean down the dose of CsA. On stopping treatment there seems to be no long-term beneficial effect, although there is no evidence of any rebound worsening of asthma.[31-33]

Oral gold

Oral gold is well established as a steroid-sparing agent in rheumatoid arthritis and has been used for a number of years in Japan in the treatment of asthma. An open, uncontrolled study in asthma suggested benefit.[35] Recently, a well-conducted placebo-controlled study has been performed in patients with difficult asthma most of whom were on oral steroids.[36] This study suggested a small but statistically significant oral steroid-sparing effect with a slight improvement in lung function. Side-effects were mild and included rashes and slight proteinuria. In common with other steroid-sparing treatments the effect was slow in onset and a 3- or 4-month trial of therapy would be necessary to determine if oral gold was effective in an individual patient.

Intravenous Immunoglobulins

There have been anecdotal reports and small, uncontrolled studies of the use of intravenous immunoglobulins, particularly in adolescents with difficult asthma.[37] Although the effects reported have been impressive, in the absence of any controlled clinical trials it is difficult to advocate the use of this treatment.

Hydroxychloroquine

Hydroxychloroquine is established as a steroid-sparing agent in rheumatoid arthritis. There has been an uncontrolled study in steroid-dependent asthmatic subjects that indicated benefit.[38] In the absence of controlled studies it is difficult to advocate the use of this treatment.

Troleandomycin

Troleandomycin (TAO) is a macrolide antibiotic that has the odd property of slowing the metabolism of methylprednisolone.[39] Thus if methylprednisolone is the oral steroid being used in a patient, the use of TAO can decrease the number of milligrams of treatment taken while the therapeutic effect remains unaltered.[40] In addition it has been claimed that TAO has other vaguely specified immunosuppressant activity. The theoretical benefit from decreasing the number of milligrams of methylprednisolone used while steroid side-effects remain unchanged is difficult to justify. TAO also interferes with theophylline metabolism and has hepatic side-effects. A well-performed study of TAO in steroid-dependent asthma has shown no benefit and considerable side-effects.[41] Its use cannot be recommended.

Alternative Therapies (see Chapter 22)

A number of alternative therapies[42] such as homoeopathy and acupuncture[43] have been suggested. In the absence of any properly conducted, controlled trials showing benefit it is difficult to justify the use of these treatments in steroid-dependent asthma.

NEW THERAPIES

A large number of novel therapies are currently being investigated in asthma. These have mostly been studied in mild asthma. The first to be introduced will probably be the leukotriene antagonists and 5-lipoxygenase inhibitors. The leukotriene receptor antagonist Accolate (ICI204,219) has been shown to be effective in patients taking inhaled corticosteroids[44] but no trials of oral steroid reduction have been reported.

PREVENTING AND MINIMIZING SIDE-EFFECTS OF ORAL STEROIDS

The side-effects during both the acute and chronic administration of oral steroids are listed in Table 41.1. Some side-effects such as osteoporosis are mainly a problem during chronic usage, whereas others such as stomach ulceration can occur during both acute and chronic administration.

For many of the side-effects no specific preventive treatment is available. As there is a relationship between the dose of steroid and the incidence and severity of adverse events, keeping the dose of steroid to a minimum is essential. It is also important to be aware that steroids can cause this range of problems so that prompt treatment is given and needless tests for other causes are avoided. This section will concentrate on these steroid-induced problems for which specific measures need to be taken.

METABOLIC

Electrolyte imbalance, particularly hypokalaemia, can be a problem as patients may be receiving high-dose inhaled β_2 agonists and theophyllines that lower plasma potassium. Plasma potassium should be monitored and appropriate replacement therapy given as necessary.

Diabetes mellitus may be unmasked or exacerbated in patients receiving high-dose oral steroids. Plasma glucose should be monitored with either blood tests or Dextrastix and treatment with oral hypoglycaemic agents or insulin administered as required. Usually when the steroid is stopped the diabetes will resolve.

The Cushingoid appearance and weight gain is a side-effect that causes patients considerable concern. Steroids cause weight gain mainly by an increase in appetite with a minor contribution from fluid retention. Furthermore there is redistribution of body mass from the peripheries to the centre. As it is always easier to prevent weight gain rather than to treat established obesity, it is important that patients are warned of this so that dietary advice can be given.

CARDIOVASCULAR

Exacerbations of existing hypertension or mild to moderate hypertension are relatively common complications of the long-term use of oral steroids. As other cardiovascular risk factors, particularly glucose intolerance, obesity and lack of exercise, may also be present it is important to detect and control any hypertension. β-Blockers are obviously completely contraindicated in asthma, so other alternative treatment anti-hypertensive agents must be used. Thiazide diuretics are best avoided unless there is coexisting fluid retention, as they will tend to exacerbate any hypokalaemia and may theoretically increase plasma viscosity thus worsening cardiovascular risk profile. Calcium antagonists such as nifedipine or amlodipine are a good choice in hypertensive patients with asthma. Angiotensin-converting enzyme (ACE) inhibitors may be used but can precipitate cough in some patients; they may be of particular use in patients with coexisting diabetes.

Fluid retention and peripheral oedema are a particular problem in older patients who may have coexisting heart disease. A small dose of diuretic is usually sufficient to control this; however a potassium-sparing diuretic is preferable in view of the problems with hypokalaemia detailed above.

GASTROINTESTINAL TRACT

Many patients suffer from dyspepsia when taking oral steroids and these effects can be minimized by the use of enteric-coated prednisolone. The association of oral steroids with peptic ulceration and gastrointestinal haemorrhage is controversial, with conflicting results from meta-analysis of studies.[45–46] With doubt over the role of steroids in peptic ulceration the benefit of anti-ulcer drugs is also the subject of some debate. However, H_2 agonists are often given to cover courses of high-dose oral steroids; if these are going to be used ranitidine is often a good choice as it does not interact with other drugs, in particular theophyllines. The use of the new proton pump inhibitors such as omeprazole may prove more valuable as they more completely block gastric acid production.

INFECTIVE COMPLICATIONS

Oral steroids may suppress the overt signs of infection so that a patient with for instance pneumonia may present with an insidious illness rather than obvious fever, dyspnoea and malaise. The clinician needs to be alert to the masking of signs by steroids.

Controversy exists over the risk of reactivation of tuberculosis in patients on oral steroids.[47] Patients with evidence of previous tuberculosis, who have not received adequate anti-tuberculosis therapy, should be considered for isoniazid prophylaxis, particularly if doses of prednisolone above 10 mg per day are used.

The danger of the dissemination of live viral vaccinations means that they are contraindicated.

MUSCULOSKELETAL

Osteoporosis, particularly in post-menopausal women, is one of the most serious and worrying side-effects for both patients and doctors and is undoubtedly a common side-effect in patients on long-term oral steroids. Minimizing the risk of osteoporosis can be divided into non-pharmacological and pharmacological means. Many of these therapies have been developed for treating the osteoporosis of ageing and have not been directly tested in osteoporosis induced by steroids. There is evidence that the bone architecture in steroid-induced osteoporosis is different to age-related osteoporosis and that it is at least potentially reversible.[48]

Non-pharmacological Treatments

There are a number of factors that have been clearly identified as increasing the risk of osteoporosis. Smoking increases the risk of osteoporosis and patients should be strongly advised to give up smoking[49] and be given any help with smoking cessation clinics and nicotine replacement therapy. Excess alcohol consumption is associated with an increased risk of osteoporosis and a patient should be advised about sensible alcohol consumption. Physical exercise helps to maintain bone mass and, within the limits of their asthma, patients should be advised to take regular exercise.

Pharmacological Treatments

There is little evidence that calcium supplementation in patients on a normal diet is of benefit in preventing osteoporosis; however, if there are any concerns about dietary insufficiency then calcium and vitamin D supplementation should be provided.[48] In peri-menopausal women hormone replacement therapy has been shown to help to maintain bone mass;[50] however greater benefit is seen when treatment is started within 5 years of the menopause. With the risks of long-term hormone replacement therapy, particularly with regard to endometrial carcinoma, careful follow-up is necessary. In men, hypogonadism may also be present and can accelerate osteoporosis; if there is evidence of testosterone insufficiency this should be investigated and treated. There is now evidence that bisphosphonates such as etidronate may be helpful in maintaining bone mass in patients with osteoporosis.[51] A trial of intranasal calcitonin has shown benefit in maintaining bone mass in patients on long-term oral steroids, but this cannot yet be considered part of routine treatment.[52] As yet, none of these studies have demonstrated a decrease in fracture rate; however, as fracture rate has been related to a low bone density in a number of studies it seems reasonable at present to suppose that these agents will cause a decrease in osteoporotic fractures.

Sodium fluoride can increase bone mass, but may not alter fracture rate. It has significant side-effects and is difficult to use. At present treatment or prevention of osteoporosis is not routine in patients on oral steroids.

TABLE 41.2: *Prevention of osteoporosis in patients on long-term oral steroids*

1. Stop smoking
   Reduce alcohol intake
   Correct dietary calcium or vitamin D deficiency

2. Measure bone density if low
   Hormone replacement therapy in peri- or post-menopausal women
   Detect and treat hypogonadism in men
   Cyclical etidronate (2 weeks every 13 weeks)

3. If still unsatisfactory consider:
   Nasal calcitonin
   Sodium fluoride

With new treatments available more attention should now be paid to prevention and treatment (Table 41.2).

Muscle wasting and a degree of myopathy occurs in many patients on long-term steroids. A particular problem occurs in patients ventilated for acute severe asthma and treated with intravenous hydrocortisone. Whether the problem occurs to a greater extent with hydrocortisone than other steroids is not known. It has been suggested that other factors such as virally induced myopathy may also play a part.

TABLE 41.3: *A checklist to consider when treating a patient with asthma on long-term oral steroids*

Minimize allergen exposure
Stop smoking
Optimize inhaled corticosteroid therapy using doses of BDP or
    budesonide up to 2 mg per day
Trial of theophyllines
Gradually wean down oral steroids

If this fails
Consider higher doses of inhaled steroids or fluticasone
    propionate 2 mg per day

If this fails
Consider immunosuppressant trial of 3-months duration if:
    Sufficient concern over steroid dose
    No contraindications after screening

Options:
    Low-dose methotrexate 15 mg per week initial dose
        Cyclosporin A 5 mg kg^{-1} daily initial dose
        Oral gold
Patients will need to be fully informed of risks and benefits and
    closely monitored

If still on oral steroids
Regular measurement of blood pressure
Regular testing of glucose
Minimize the risk of osteoporosis (see Table 41.2)
Remember the immunosuppressant effect of steroids if
    intercurrent illness occurs
Remember infections may be masked and present insidiously

OCULAR

Glaucoma is common in the elderly and preventable. Old people on long-term steroids, particularly with a family history, should have intra-ocular pressure measured.

CONCLUSION

Although only a minority of patients now need treatment with long-term oral corticosteroids they are a group who suffer significant problems both from their disease and its treatment. Effective strategies exist to minimize or eliminate the need for oral steroids and to minimize the risk of systemic side-effects (Table 41.3).

REFERENCES

1   Medical Research Council. Controlled trial of effects of cortisone acetate in chronic asthma. *Lancet* 1956; ii: 798–803.

2   Medical Research Council. Controlled trial of cortisone acetate in status asthmatics. *Lancet* 1956; ii: 803–6.

3   British Thoracic Society, Research Unit of The Royal College of Physicians, Kings Fund Centre, National Asthma Campaign. Guidelines for management of asthma in adults. I: Chronic persistent asthma. *BMJ* 1990; 301: 651–3.

4   International Consensus Report on the Diagnosis and Management of Asthma. *Clin Exp Allergy* 1992; 22(suppl 1).

5   Smith R. Corticosteroids and osteoporosis. *Thorax* 1990; 45: 573–8.

6   Scherr MS *et al. Ann Allergy* 1980; 44: 82–8.

7   Nassif EG, Weinberger M, Thompson R, Huntley W. The value of maintenance theophyllines in steroid dependent asthma. *N Engl J Med* 1981; 304: 71–5.

8   Brenner M, Berkowitz R, Marshall N, Strunk RC. Need for theophylline in severe steroid requiring asthmatics. *Clin Allergy* 1988; 18: 143–50.

9   Howell JBL, Altounyon REC. A double-blind trial of disodium cromoglycate in the treatment of allergic bronchial asthma. *Lancet* 1967; ii: 539–42.

10 Brompton Hospital/Medical Research Council Collaborative Trial. Long-term study of disodium cromoglycate in treatment of severe extrinsic or intrinsic bronchial asthma in adults. *BMJ* 1972; 4: 383–8.

11 Boulet L-P, Cartier A, Cockroft DW *et al.* Tolerance to reduction of oral steroid dosage in severely asthmatic patients receiving nedocromil sodium. *Respir Med* 1990; 84: 317–23.

12 Goldin JG, Bateman EA. Does nedocromil sodium have a steroid sparing effect in adult asthmatic patients requiring maintenance oral corticosteroids. *Thorax* 1988; 43: 982–6.

13 Morrow-Brown H, Storey G, George WMS. Beclomethasone dipropionate: a new steroid aerosol for the treatment of allergic asthma. *BMJ* 1971; 1: 585–90.

14 Smith MJ, Hodson ME. High dose beclomethasone inhaler in the treatment of asthma. *Lancet* 1983; i: 265–9.

15 Hummel S, Lehtonen L. Comparison of oral steroid sparing by high and low dose inhaled steroid in maintenance treatment of severe asthma. *Lancet* 1992; 340: 1483–7.

16 Geddes DM. Inhaled corticosteroids: benefits and risks. *Thorax* 1992; 47: 404–7.

17 Noonan MJ, Chervinsky P, Weisberg SC *et al.* Fluticasone propionate aerosol therapy permits reductions of prednisolone while improving pulmonary function and asthma symptoms (abstract). *Am J Respir Crit Care Med* 1994; 149(suppl): A214.

18 Otulana BA, Varna N, Bullock A, Higenbotham T. High dose nebulised steroid in the treatment of chronic steroid-dependent asthma. *Respir Med* 1992; 86: 105–8.

19 Mullarkey MF, Blumenstein BA, Andrade WP, Bailey GA, Ulason I, Wetzel CE. Methotrexate in the treatment of corticosteroid-dependent asthma. *N Engl J Med* 1988; 318: 603–7.

20 Shiner RJ, Nunn AJ, Chung KF, Geddes DM. Randomized, double-blind, placebo-controlled trial of methotrexate in steroid-dependent asthma. *Lancet* 1990; 336: 137–40.

21 Erzurum SC, Leff JA, Cochran JE *et al.* Lack of benefit of methotrexate in severe steroid-dependent asthma: a double-blind, placebo-controlled study. *Ann Intern Med* 1991; 114: 353–60.

22 Trigg CJ, Davies RJ. Comparison of methotrexate 30 mg per week with placebo in chronic steroid-dependent asthma: a 12-week double-blind, cross-over study. *Respir Med* 1993; 87: 211–6.

23 Kuitert LM, Harrison AC. *Pneumocystis carinii* pneumonia as a complication of methotrexate treatment of asthma. *Thorax* 1991; 46: 936–7.

24 White DA, Rankin JA, Storer PE, Gellene RA, Gupta S. Methotrexate pneumonitis. Bronchoalveolar lavage findings suggest an immunologic disorder. *Am Rev Respir Dis* 1989; 139: 19–21.

25 Health and Public Policy Committee, American College of Physicians. Methotrexate in rheumatoid arthritis. *Ann Intern Med* 1987; 107: 418–9.

26 Hodges NG, Brewis RAL, Howell JBL. An evaluation of azathioprine in severe chronic asthma. *Thorax* 1971; 26: 734.

27 Asmundsson T, Kilburn KH, Lazzlo J, Krock CJ. Immunosuppressive therapy of asthma. *J Allergy* 1971; 47: 136–47.

28 Corrigan CJ, Kay AB. T-Lymphocytes. In: Barnes PJ, Rodger IW, Thomson NC (eds) *Asthma Basic Mechanisms and Clinical Management*, 2nd edn. London: Academic Press, 1992: 125–41.

29 Ellis CN, Fradin MS, Messona JM *et al.* Cyclosporine for plaque-type psoriasis. Results of a multidose, double-blind trial. *N Engl J Med* 1991; 324: 277–84.

30 Sourden JM, Berth-Jones J, Ross JS *et al.* Double-blind controlled crossover study of cyclosporin in adults with severe refractory atopic dermatitis. *Lancet* 1991; 338: 137–40.

31 Alexander AG, Barnes NC, Kay AB. Trial of cyclosporin A in corticosteroid-dependent chronic severe asthma. *Lancet* 1992; 339: 324–8.

32 Lock SH, Barnes NC, Kay AB. Cyclosporin A (CsA) as a corticosteroid sparing agent in corticosteroid dependent asthma. *Thorax* 1994; 49: 1051P (Abstract).

33 Nizankowska E, Soja J, Pinis G. Treatment of steroid-dependent asthma with cyclosporin (abstract). *Am Rev Respir Dis* 1993; 147(suppl): A294.

34 Szczeklik A, Nizakowska E, Dworski R, Danagalen B, Pinis G. Cyclosporin for steroid-dependent asthma. *Allergy* 1992; 47: 349–54.

35 Bernstein DI, Bernstein L, Bodenheimer SS, Pietrusko RG. An open study of Auranolin in the treatment of steroid-dependent asthma. *J Clin Immunol* 1988; 81: 6–16.

36 Nierop G, Gijzel WP, Bel EM, Zwinderman AM, Dijkman JM. Auranofin in the treatment of steroid-dependent asthma: a double-blind study. *Thorax* 1992; 47: 349–54.

37 Mazer BD, Gelford EW. An open-label study of high dose intravenous immunoglobulin in severe childhood asthma. *J Allergy Clin Immunol* 1991; 87: 976–83.

38 Charous BL. Open study of hydroxychloroquine in the treatment of severe symptomatic or corticosteroid-dependent asthma. *Ann Allergy* 1990; 65: 53–8.

39 Szeler SJ, Rose JQ, Ellis EF, Spector SL, Green AW, Jusko WJ. The effect of troleandomycin on methylprednisolone elimination. *J Allergy Clin Immunol* 1980; 66: 447–51.

40 Zeiger RS, Schatz M, Sperling W, Simon RA, Stevenson DD. Efficacy of troleandomycin in out-patients with severe corticosteroid-dependent asthma. *J Allergy Clin Immunol* 1980; 66: 438–66.

41 Nelson HS, Hamilos DL, Corsello PR, Levesque NV, Buchmeier AD, Bucher BL. A double-blind study of troleandomycin and methylprednisolone in asthmatic subjects who require daily corticosteroids. *Am Rev Respir Dis* 1993; 147: 398–404.

42 Alternative and complementary medicine for asthma. *Thorax* 1991; 46: 787–97.

43 Kleijnen J, ter Reit G, Knipschild P. Acupuncture and asthma: a review of controlled trials. *Thorax* 1991; 46: 799–802.

44 Hui KP, Barnes NC. Lung function improvement in asthma with a cysteinyl-leukotriene receptor antagonist. *Lancet* 1991; 337: 1062–3.

45 Conn HU, Blitzer BL. Non association of adrenocorticosteroid therapy and peptic ulcer. *N Engl J Med* 1976; 294: 473–9.

46 Messer J, Reitman D, Sacks HS, Smith H, Chalmers TC. Association of adrenocorticosteroid therapy and peptic ulcer disease. *N Engl J Med* 1983; 309: 21–4.

47 Bateman ED. Is tuberculosis chemoprophylaxis necessary for patients receiving corticosteroids for respiratory disease? *Respir Med* 1983; 87: 485–7.

48 Hosking DJ. Effects of corticosteroids on bone turnover. *Respir Med* 1993; 87(suppl A): 15–21.

49 Hopper JL, Seeman E. The bone density of female twins discordant for tobacco use. *N Engl J Med* 1994; 330: 387–92.

50 Lindsay R, Aitken JM, Anderson JB, Hart DM, MacDonald EB, Clarke AC. Long-term prevention of osteoporosis by oestrogen. *Lancet* 1976; i: 1038–41.

51 Storm T, Thamsburg G, Stenicke T, Genart HK, Sorensen OM. Effect of intermittent cyclical etidronate therapy on bone mass in women with post-menopausal osteoporosis. *N Engl J Med* 1990; 322: 1265–71.

52 Luengo M, Pons F, de Osaba MJM, Picado C. Prevention of further bone mass loss by nasal calcitonin in patients on long-term gluco-corticoid therapy for asthma a two year follow-up. *Thorax* 1994; 49: 1099–102 .

KEY POINTS

1 The most important method of preventing steroid side-effects is to minimize the dose of oral steroids and the most effective way of doing this is with inhaled steroids.

2 Poor compliance with inhaled steroids or poor inhaler technique is a common cause of treatment failure.

3   It is important to minimize side-effects and the following need to be considered.
      (a)   Monitor and treat hypertension.
      (b)   Check for hypokalaemia.
      (c)   Check for diabetes mellitus.
      (d)   Warn about weight gain.
      (e)   Avoid live vaccines.

4   Osteoporosis is a serious side-effect. It can be minimized by:
      (a)   hormone replacement therapy;
      (b)   cyclical etidronate;
      (c)   correcting calcium or vitamin D deficiency.

5   A trial of immunosuppressants may be justified in some patients. Proven agents are:
      (a)   methotrexate;
      (b)   oral gold;
      (c)   cyclosporin A.

6   Avoiding smoking is very important as it worsens asthma and increases the risk of cardiovascular, gastrointestinal and bone side-effects.

42

ACUTE COMPLICATIONS OF ASTHMA

Bernadette Hickey and E. Hayden Walters

Despite better understanding of the pathophysiology of acute asthma attacks, asthma remains a life-threatening disease. Little attention has been paid to the morbidity of acute exacerbations: one might infer from the current literature that acute asthma is a condition in which the patient either dies or makes a predictable recovery. However, this is not the case. There are a number of complications related either to the asthma disease process or its treatment.

COMPLICATIONS OF THE DISEASE

CONSEQUENCES OF AIRFLOW OBSTRUCTION

Airflow obstruction, the hallmark of acute asthma, generates major changes in respiratory mechanics. The inspiratory muscles must generate an increased negative thoracic pressure to overcome the rise in airway resistance. Expiratory flow is limited by the increased airway resistance and inspiratory muscle activity continuing through expiration. Airway closure occurs before expiration is complete and "gas trapping" results. These changes produce increases in both functional residual capacity (FRC) and residual volume (RV) as an acute attack progresses. This is called dynamic hyperinflation, and the resulting positive alveolar pressure at the completion of expiration has been described as auto PEEP (positive end-expiratory pressure) or intrinsic PEEP.[1] This positive pressure may have a protective role, opposing early airway closure and atelectasis during acute asthma. However, as the attack continues increased negative pressure must be generated during inspiration to "overcome" this intrinsic PEEP, thus increasing the work of breathing.[2,3]

Work of breathing is a term used to describe the energy cost of breathing. It is a function of the pressure the respiratory muscles are required to generate and the volume of gas displaced per unit time. This energy is used to overcome the pulmonary resistance, which is a combination of

TABLE 42.1: *Markers of fatigue*

Subjective difficulty: "the asthmatic knows best"!

Falling oxygenation despite increasing peak expiratory flow rate

No longer able to speak

Floppy, lethargic, unable to cough

airflow obstruction, intrinsic PEEP and elastic resistance. During acute asthma all these components of lung resistance are increased and in addition the expiratory muscles are recruited, further increasing energy requirement and oxygen consumption. At the same time inspiratory muscle power is compromised because the inspiratory muscles are stretched beyond their optimal length. If asthma remains unresponsive to therapy these factors may lead to respiratory muscle fatigue and contribute to ventilatory failure. Fatigue is identified by a combination of patient characteristics (Table 42.1) and changes in the arterial blood gases.

The expanding lungs may compress the heart, increase the pericardial pressure, limit venous return and diastolic filling and essentially tamponade right and left ventricular stroke volume. As the acute asthmatic atttack develops the thoracic and adjacent structures are subjected to substantial swings in pressure. Elevated intra-thoracic pressure may have adverse effects on visceral and muscle function (Table 42.2).

Coughing is a consequence of airway inflammation. It produces transient massive rises in intra-thoracic pressure. These increases are superimposed

TABLE 42.2: *Extra-thoracic effects of increased intra-thoracic pressure*

Gastro-oesophageal reflux[4]

Rectal or urethral incontinence or prolapse

Diaphragmatic, inguinal and abdominal hernias

Vaginal prolapse

Ruptured viscus, e.g. hydrocele, stomach, spleen[5,6]

on the already increased intra-thoracic pressure and may cause further tissue damage (Table 42.3).

Air leaks from alveolar rupture may occur. These are caused by a rise in intra-alveolar pressure and radial wall tension, especially distal to airways that are "slow" to empty during expiration. When gas escapes from the pulmonary tree it will follow the pathway of least resistance finding its way to pleural space (pneumothorax), mediastinum, peritoneum, subcutaneous tissue and even the epidural space. Airflow obstruction ensures high airways pressures are maintained during expiration, which assists gas leakage out of a ruptured alveolus. The gas itself is of little consequence but it may exert considerable pressure if localized in a confined space, causing compression of surrounding structures. The most serious situation is "tension" in the pleura or mediastinum causing impairment of myocardial function. This requires emergency drainage.

In the setting of acute asthma most pneumothoraces should be drained to protect against large volumes of gas escaping under the elevated airway pressure. Accumulation of gas in the pleural space will decrease ventilation to the affected side and contribute to hyperventilation of the opposite lung, so predisposing to the disastrous situation of bilateral pneumothoraces. Very small uncomplicated air leaks may be managed conservatively, without drainage, except in mechanically ventilated patients when all air leaks should be drained to minimize the morbidity from rapidly evolving tamponade.

CONSEQUENCES OF ALTERED GAS EXCHANGE: HYPOXIA, HYPERCAPNIA, ACIDOSIS

Hypoxaemia is the initial manifestation of the gas exchange defect that occurs during an acute asthma attack. Obstructed lung units participate in gas transfer roughly proportional to the degree of obstruction. This varies between different lung units, from complete obstruction with mucous

TABLE 42.3: *Cough complications*

Musculoskeletal chest pain

Rib fractures

Subconjunctival haemorrhage

Syncope

Ruptured viscus

Nausea and vomiting

plugs to minimal obstruction. Ventilation varies across the lung as different lung units develop different time constants. Hypoxia is initially associated with hypocapnia due to an increase in total minute ventilation. As the asthma attack continues hypoxia may worsen, with increases in ventilation–perfusion mismatch and oxygen consumption as well as falling alveolar ventilation.

Severe, prolonged or inadequately treated attacks may progress to ventilatory failure. As the minute ventilation falls, hypoxia worsens and is accompanied by hypercapnia and acidosis. Compromised tissue oxygen delivery contributes a metabolic component to the evolving acidosis. These changes affect most organ systems producing severe physiological impairment as hypercapnia and acidosis progress (Table 42.4).

Normal circulatory responses to hypoxia, hypercapnia and acidosis are impaired in the severe asthmatic patient. Right and left ventricular filling may be limited by the rise in intra-thoracic pressure. Cardiac output is maintained by increasing heart rate but this may be at the expense of decreasing myocardial oxygen delivery. This is of most concern for the right ventricle where the raised intra-pulmonary pressure increases the right ventricular afterload and therefore the stroke work and oxygen consumption. Although ECG abnormalities consistent with right ventricular strain have been reported[7] there is limited published data describing the haemodynamic changes during acute asthma using direct measurements. This may be due to difficulties in inserting, and interpreting the data from, pulmonary artery catheters in patients with severe airflow obstruction. The

---

TABLE 42.4: *Complications of hypercapnia and effects of acidosis*

Complications of hypercapnia
Circulatory: hypotension, vasodilatation, decreased myocardial contractility

Respiratory: dyspnoea, impaired respiratory muscle function, increased $\dot{V}/Q$ mismatch

CNS: cerebral vasodilatation and oedema, confusion, coma, seizures

Effects of acidosis
Decreased intracellular enzyme activity
Altered drug absorption
Decreased plasma protein binding, e.g. muscle relaxants
Decreased drug–receptor binding, e.g. β agonists
Impaired pathways for drug elimination

trace may be "damped" by the raised intra-thoracic pressures, and there is no uniform practice for referencing the transducers, either to atmospheric or to intra-thoracic pressure.

There is a real risk of myocardial ischaemia in the setting of acute asthma, although it is probably only of clinical significance in patients who have underlying heart disease. Both right and left ventricular failure have been described during acute asthma, but this remains uncommon. It is worth remembering that "capillary leak" is a component of airway inflammation that, when combined with pulmonary venous congestion, produces a predisposition to oedema formation.[8] Volume replacement therapy should be administered with these conditions in mind.

Cerebral hypoxaemia is an important sequela of this combination of hypoxaemia and hypotension during an acute asthmatic attack. A proportion of patients who die from acute asthma despite arriving at hospital have irreversible cerebral hypoxia.

MUCUS, SECRETIONS, INFECTION

Increased mucus production, alteration in its viscosity and impaired mucociliary clearance are typical of the inflammation of asthma.[9] They combine to exacerbate airway narrowing and cause plugging and atelectasis. Although this most commonly occurs in subsegmental bronchi, lobar obstruction with resultant collapse is well described. This usually resolves with appropriate bronchodilator and physical therapy but fibreoptic bronchoscopy may be required if airway obstruction persists, or collapse is associated with major physiological impairment. Prolonged collapse of lung tissue should be avoided as it predisposes to superimposed infection and possibly permanent airway damage and bronchiectasis. Patients who require intubation and assisted ventilation have an increased risk of developing nosocomial lower respiratory tract infection.

COMPLICATIONS OF TREATMENT

PHARMACOLOGICAL

Much has been written about the relationship between use of pharmacological agents and morbidity in asthma (Table 42.5). These issues are considered in other chapters of this book.

MECHANICAL

Mechanical ventilation is necessary in a small number of asthmatic patients with respiratory failure. The mortality of ventilated asthmatic patients during the 1980s was reported as between 10 and 38%.[10] Recently, methods of controlled hypoventilation designed to limit pulmonary hyperinflation have been implemented with significant decrease in mortality.[11,12]

TABLE 42.5: *Complications of pharmacological treatment*

Class of drug	Complication
β Agonist	Tremor, restlessness, anxiety, dreams, tachycardia rarely, arrhythmias, myocardial ischaemia, dilated cardiomyopathy, lactic acidosis, hypokalaemia, hyperglycaemia
Theophylline	Gastrointestinal disturbances, seizures, arrhythmias
Corticosteroid	Psychosis, metabolic alkalosis, hypokalaemia, glucose intolerance, myopathy
Sedative	Decreased cough, impaired mucociliary clearance, ventilatory failure
Muscle relaxant	Skeletal muscle dysfunction, rhabdomyolysis, anaphylaxis, malignant hyperpyrexia

As the majority of hospital morbidity in acute asthma occurs in mechanically ventilated patients it is preferable to avoid assisted ventilation if possible.[11] However, a number of patients become unable to maintain adequate gas transfer and require intubation despite optimal treatment.

Intubation and initiation of assisted ventilation pose special problems in asthmatic patients. These patients are more liable to laryngospasm and to allergic reactions to induction agents or muscle relaxants. They may be hypovolaemic from prolonged hyperventilation and systemic venous return may be further impaired by rising intra-thoracic pressure as well as hypoxia and hypercapnia causing peripheral vasodilatation. The combination of hypovolaemia, hypoxia and sympathetic activation during severe asthma when followed by the use of sedatives and relaxants for intubation, and the application of positive pressure to the thorax, can precipitate circulatory collapse and cardiac arrest.[10]

Because of the difficulty of evaluating over-inflation during "hand" ventilation, asthmatic patients should be promptly connected to a volume-cycled preferably pressure-limited ventilator with, initially, slow breath rates, high inspiratory flow rates and low inspiration to expiration ratios.

Pulmonary Hyperinflation

Pulmonary hyperinflation, which can occur in spontaneously breathing acute asthma, is exacerbated during positive pressure ventilation because the tidal volume is no longer limited by the patient's ability to generate a high inspiratory pressure gradient. Large increases in intra-thoracic volume may occur during artificial ventilation as modern ventilators are able to generate high "working pressures" and deliver large tidal volumes despite elevated airway resistance. The sequelae of hyperinflation are limited in the spontaneously breathing asthmatic patient by the increased work of breathing, failing inspiratory muscles and fatigue. In the mechanically ventilated patient this protection is lost and hyperinflation and circulatory compromise occur more rapidly. It has been suggested that dynamic hyperinflation is the variable that best correlates with significant asthma morbidity.[12]

A range of strategies have been described over the last 10 years to avoid the morbidity of over-ventilating acute asthmatic patients but the optimal method is still debated.[13,14] The aim is to ensure oxygenation, relieve the mechanical load and clear secretions using a ventilatory pattern that permits hypercapnia so as to prevent the complications of over-inflation. The normalization of ventilation is achieved when the airway obstruction resolves; if necessary acidosis may be controlled with intravenous sodium bicarbonate.

One difficulty in designing this type of controlled hypoventilation has been the absence of an accepted objective measurement of "over-inflation". Tuxen and Lane have described a method for grading pulmonary hyperinflation by measuring the volume at end inspiration (V_{EI}) and report that it predicts the incidence of complications.[15] They use this measurement to control the mechanical ventilation of all asthmatic patients and report a resulting fall in the incidence of hypotension.

To tolerate these methods of permissive hypercapnia patients require sedation and often paralysis. These pharmacological agents may be additive to hypoxia, acidosis and hypercapnia as insults to intracellular metabolism. This concern is highlighted by the growing evidence for acute myopathy occurring in ventilated patients.[16,17]

Barotrauma

Barotrauma is a poorly defined term that is used to describe physical damage to the lung from the application of positive pressure. There are three currently recognized variants.

(1) Extra-alveolar gas is due to rupture of the alveolar membrane as discussed above for spontaneously breathing patients. There are increased risks when this occurs in a patient receiving positive pressure ventilation. The intra-thoracic pressure may rise rapidly producing tamponade of the circulation. One must

have a high level of suspicion to detect air leaks in the intensive care unit setting. A lateral decubitus X-ray of the chest may be more sensitive at confirming a pneumothorax than the traditional supine AP views.

(2) Systemic gas embolism occurs when alveolar gas enters the systemic circulation. This is uncommon but recorded in ventilated patients with very high airway pressures, as seen in severe acute asthma.

(3) Diffuse lung injury with plasma extravasation and hyaline membrane formation is proposed in patients ventilated for pulmonary oedema or acute respiratory distress syndrome, where high pressures and oxygen concentrations are applied to the lung for extended periods. It is unusual for these conditions to be required for prolonged periods in acute asthma and therefore the risk and incidence of this type of diffuse lung injury in ventilated asthmatic patients is uncertain.

Myopathy

Myopathy is a well-described complication in asthmatic patients who require mechanical ventilation.[16,17] It is associated with increased duration of assisted ventilation and difficulty with weaning. Initial reports implicated high-dose glucocorticoids as the cause, referring to the myopathy in Cushing's original description of hypercortisolaemia. However, as more cases are reported the aetiology of this condition becomes less clear. In view of the increasing use of paralysis in the management of asthma the most worrisome association is with the "steroidal" muscle relaxants such as pancuronium and vecuronium.[17] Animal studies have shown an increase in glucocorticoid receptors in denervated muscle.[18] If this effect can be extrapolated to humans then muscles subject to pharmacological denervation may become hypersensitive to steroid effects, such as atrophy. To date there have not been reports of "non-steroidal" muscle relaxants such as atracurium being associated with muscle dysfunction. For the present time the benefits of paralysis and controlled hyperventilation would seem to outweigh these concerns over muscle damage in patients with severe obstruction and pulmonary hyperinflation. However, the routine use of muscle relaxants in less severe asthmatic patients should be discouraged.

REFERENCES

1 Pepe PE, Marini JJ. Occult positive end expiratory pressure in mechanically ventilated patients with airflow obstruction. *Am Rev Respir Dis* 1982; 126: 166–70.

2 Smith TC, Marini JJ. Impact of PEEP on lung mechanics and work of breathing in severe airflow obstruction. *J Appl Physiol* 1988; 65: 1488–99.

3 Fleury D, Murciano C, Talmo C, Aubier M, Pariente R, Milic-Emili J. Work of breathing in patients with chronic obstructive lung disease in acute respiratory failure. *Am Rev Respir Dis* 1985; 131: 822–7.

4 Sontag JS, Schnell TG, Miller TQ *et al.* Prevalence of oesophagitis in asthmatics. *Gut* 1992; 33: 872–6.

5 McQueen M, Gollock RJ. Spontaneous gastric rupture complicating acute asthma. *BMJ* 1982; 285: 692–3.

6 Quint HJ, Miller JI, Drach GW. Rupture of a hydrocele: an unusual event. *J Urol* 1992; 147: 1375–7.

7 Rebuck AS, Read J. Assessment and management of severe asthma. *Am Med J* 1971; 51: 788–98.

8 Stalcup SA, Mellins RB. Mechanical forces producing pulmonary odema in severe asthma. *N Engl J Med* 1977; 297: 592–6.

9 O'Riordan TG, Zwang J, Smaldone GC. Mucocilary clearance in adult asthma. *Am Rev Respir Dis* 1992; 146: 598–603.

10 Webb AK, Bilton AH, Hanson GC. Severe bronchial asthma requiring ventilation. *Postgrad Med J* 1979; 55: 161–70.

11 Mansel KJ, Stonger SW, Petrini MF, Norman RJ. Mechanical ventilation in acute severe asthma. *Am J Med* 1990; 89: 42–8.

12 Williams T, Tuxen DV, Scheinkestel CD, Czarny D, Bowes G. Risk factors for morbidity in mechanically ventilated patients with acute severe asthma. *Am Rev Respir Dis* 1992; 146: 607–15.

13 Tuxen DV, Williams T, Scheinkestel CD, Czarny D, Bowes G. Use of a measurement of pulmonary hyperinflation to control the level of mechanical ventilation in patients with acute severe asthma. *Am Rev Respir Dis* 1992; 146: 1136–42.

14 Darioli R, Perret C. Mechanically controlled hypoventilation in status asthmaticus. *Am Rev Respir Dis* 1984; 129: 385–7.

15 Tuxen DV, Lane S. The effects of ventilatory pattern on hyperinflation, airway pressures and circulation in mechanical ventilation of patients with severe airflow obstruction. *Am Rev Respir Dis* 1987; 136: 872–9.

Douglas SJA, Tuxen DV, Horne M *et al.* Myopathy in severe asthma. *Am Rev Respir Dis* 1992; 146: 517-9.

17 Griffin D, Fairman N, Coursin D, Rawsthorn L, Grossman JE. Acute myopathy during treatment of status asthmaticus with corticosteroids and steroidal muscle relaxants. *Chest* 1992; 102: 510-4.

18 Hansen-Flaschen J, Cowen J, Raps EC. Neuromuscular blockade in the intensive care unit. *Am Rev Respir Dis* 1993; 147: 234-6.

KEY POINTS

1   Acute asthma is a potentially lethal condition.

2   Beware not only airflow obstruction but also gas trapping and over-inflation.

3   The side-effects of therapy are a major cause of asthma complications.

4   Prevention remains the best approach to acute asthma complications.

43
CHRONIC COMPLICATIONS OF ASTHMA

D. S. Postma, C. I. M. Panhuysen and H. A. M. Kerstjens

INTRODUCTION

Despite many recent advances in understanding of asthma, the causes of the chronic sequelae of asthma are as yet unsolved and methods for the prevention or resolution are unknown. Chronic complications may show in severe symptomatology as well as in work disability.[1] However, unlike many conditions that affect primarily older persons, asthma disproportionally affects those of working ages, indeed those in the prime of their careers. It is thus worth while to investigate whether the chronic consequences of the disease can be prevented. Chronic complications are most likely the result of the inflammatory process that underlies the clinical presentation of asthma. The nature of the inflammatory reaction has been discerned by advanced immunohistochemical and molecular biological techniques of bronchial biopsy and lavage specimens. Inflammation has thus been found even in newly diagnosed asthmatic subjects with clinically mild disease,[2] and not only in those with far advanced disease[3] or dying from intractable asthma.[4-7] As a result of activation of inflammatory cells an array of mediators and cytokines are produced and/or released, causing bronchoconstriction, plasma exudation, vasodilatation, mucus hypersecretion and activation of sensory nerves, all contributing to the clinical presentation of asthma. Although acute inflammation has been the main focus of research on the pathophysiology of asthma, it is evident that asthma is a chronic inflammatory condition. As a result structural changes may occur, i.e. subepithelial fibrosis, hyperplasia of airway smooth muscle and angiogenesis. Therefore, it is likely that in some asthmatic subjects irreversible damage to the lungs may occur. This has indeed been found after long-term follow-up of asthmatic subjects, resulting in irreversible airflow limitation.[8-10] In this chapter, the little knowledge available from cross-sectional and prospective studies on the long-term outcome of asthma will be discussed. The possible influence of treatment on acute (i.e. death) and long-term outcome of disease will be discussed as well.

LONG-TERM OUTCOME MEASURES OF ASTHMA

What defines a positive outcome of disease? One has no difficulty to argue that for a patient this will be absence of symptoms and a good quality of life, much more than a near normal value of laboratory parameters like lung function or airway hyperresponsiveness (AH). However, symptoms may remain unchanged while lung function deteriorates[11] and it has been shown that the annual decline in forced expiratory volume in 1 second (FEV_1) is the most important measure for the progression of asthma or chronic obstructive pulmonary disease (COPD).[12–14] It therefore can be postulated that meaningful outcome measures will be both symptoms and lung function.

SYMPTOMS

There are a few studies looking at the relationship between development of respiratory symptoms and either the diagnosis of asthma or the rate of change in ventilatory function in asthma. Fortunately they cover the whole age range cross-sectionally, although virtually no longitudinal study is available. Wheeze is the most common symptom reported in asthma. It occurs in up to 40% of children in an epidemiological setting[15] and 11% of the non-asthmatic elderly population[16] and is thus not a specific parameter for asthma diagnosis. However, almost all asthmatic subjects do wheeze. In many studies wheezing is related to AH, even after taking into account smoking and pre-challenge lung function.[17–19]

In childhood it has become clear that wheeze and cough, next to the presence of atopy are independently associated with respiratory morbidity as quantified by both objective and subjective parameters.[20,21] Thus, wheeze was, even more than cough, associated with a lower level of AH and FEV_1, greater within-day and between-day variability of peak expiratory flow rate (PEFR) and greater chronicity of symptoms.[20] Wheezing and other symptoms disappear in a substantial proportion of asthmatic subjects during teenage years (Fig. 43.1).[22–24] To outgrow symptoms of asthma a better FEV_1 and level of AH in childhood are important factors.[23,24] Symptoms and AH improve during childhood asthma irrespective of improvement in FEV_1.[22,24] Many children in Kondo's study did not completely normalize their PC_{20} values, and it was therefore suggested that this incomplete improvement was related to irreversible damage of the bronchial wall produced by long-standing inflammation.[21] However, symptoms improved dramatically, showing that an asymptomatic state does not imply normalization of airflow limitation or AH, which has also been found in another study.[25] Wheeze in childhood is a poor predictor of remission of asthma by the

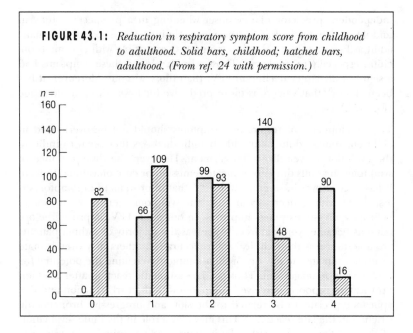

FIGURE 43.1: *Reduction in respiratory symptom score from childhood to adulthood. Solid bars, childhood; hatched bars, adulthood. (From ref. 24 with permission.)*

time of maturity.[26] There appears to be a gender difference effect in this respect in that active wheeze was necessary for female asthmatic children to experience a reduction in lung function over 8 years of follow-up.[27] Wheeze should thus direct the doctor at stronger caution for deterioration of lung function at follow-up, especially in female children with asthma.

The presence of symptoms in young adults with asthma is associated with lower levels of lung function.[22,23,28,29] Jaakkola *et al.*[30] studied 391 young adults (15–40 years) during a study period of 8 years. Subjects who developed wheeze and dyspnoea and in whom a doctor diagnosed asthma had a significantly greater average decline in FEV_1 than asthmatic subjects without respiratory symptoms. The association was even stronger in atopic individuals, showing that atopy is a significant modifier of disease outcome. The association was also stronger in ex-smokers, suggesting that they are the susceptible individuals who develop respiratory symptoms and lung function impairment concurrently, which leads them to quit smoking. This confirms cross-sectional studies[31] showing that adverse effects of smoking on lung function were restricted to those who were wheezing.

Asthma in the elderly is not a rare disease and is also accompanied by wheeze, although chronic cough is also frequent. A large proportion of patients have had their disease for many years[32] and most individuals claiming late onset appear to have had subclinical symptoms years prior to the age they state that their disease started. Current smoking is the strongest independent predictor of new-onset wheezing in a prospective study in middle-aged individuals.[33] Furthermore Almind *et al.* showed that many adult asthmatic subjects develop symptoms compatible with chronic bronchitis, especially in smokers.[34] Those who developed these symptoms had a significantly larger decline in FEV_1 than those without. Moreover, it has been shown[35] that wheeze is more predictive for lower FEV_1 at older age (Fig. 43.2).

The development of respiratory symptoms should not be overlooked in children, young adults or in elderly individuals, as they seem to indicate the evolution of ventilatory impairment. However, the disappearance of symptoms in adults does not indicate remission or cure of asthma. Indeed, it has been shown in several studies[36–39] that improvement in symptoms is associated with a decrease in AH, but symptoms generally ameliorate before hyperresponsiveness improves. In one study FEV_1 improved before patients became symptom-free.[39] Whereas the majority of asthma patients are able to assess their clinical status accurately, others may overestimate or underestimate the severity of their symptoms, creating the potential for problems in management. Thus the late asthmatic reaction after allergen provocation is poorly perceived compared with the early reaction and this appears especially to be related to the slow and progressive bronchoconstriction in the late reaction.[40] This may play a role in the under-evaluation of the severity of asthma. Finally in long-standing asthma symptoms are

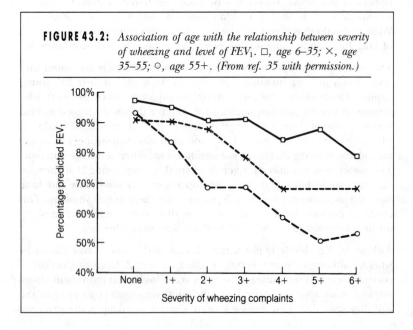

FIGURE 43.2: *Association of age with the relationship between severity of wheezing and level of FEV_1. □, age 6–35; ×, age 35–55; ○, age 55+. (From ref. 35 with permission.)*

less perceived,[41] making it more dangerous to assess the outcome of asthma by symptoms only.

LUNG FUNCTION

Achievement of a maximal level of FEV_1 is of potential importance, as it is an indicator of future risk of chronic obstructive lung disease. Thus it is important to investigate both the rate of lung growth in children as well as the rate of decline in adults with asthma. Epidemiological studies on growth of lung function from childhood to adulthood show that, even in asthma with initial normal lung function, the growth patterns lie outside the 95% confidence limits of non-asthmatic children.[25,28,42] However, it is unknown whether these observed differences result from under-treatment, airway abnormalities or are linked to hormonal, nutritional or other influences, as yet unknown, on lung growth. In adults, some epidemiological studies show a less rapid decline of FEV_1 in adult asthmatic as compared to normal subjects.[43,44] Burrows et al. selected non-smoking or atopic individuals with a doctor's diagnosis of asthma (group I) and showed them to have less loss of lung function over long-term follow-up than individuals who had never had an asthma diagnosis and were non-atopic smokers (group III) (Table 43.1). Though decline was very low, it cannot be ruled out that selection of the population migrated to Tucson for reasons of their symptoms of asthma, or long-standing therapy has affected the results. Nevertheless it suggests a more beneficial course of FEV_1 in individuals with asthma than with COPD. In another report[45] Burrows et al. showed that in newly diagnosed asthma in individuals over 60 years, decline in lung function was more rapid (-42 ml per year) than in normal subjects (-23 ml per year) and even higher than in individuals who were excluded in their analyses because of the presence of an asthma diagnosis at the

TABLE 43.1: *Characteristics of three groups enrolled in follow-up. (From ref. 43 with permission)*

	Group I	Group II	Group III
Number	27	45	45
Male (%)	30	58	64
Age (years)	62	63	65
FEV_1 (% predicted)	51	47	47
Allergy (%)	68	38	0
Never smokers (%)	56	13	0
Asthma diagnosis	100	56	0
FEV_1 decline (ml year^{-1})	4	24	42

start of the follow-up (-15.4 ml per year). Thus, results may be variable in one and the same population. Finally, parental smoking had progressive, more serious and clinically significant effects on the FEV_1/Forced Vital Capacity (FVC) ratio among adolescents with wheeze and asthma.[46]

The few prospective studies in asthmatic adults[13,34,47–51] almost invariably show an overall increased decline in FEV_1 over time, and declines in the range of those with emphysema are even reported.[34,47] Though this may possibly be due to bias in selection of more severely ill cases in a clinical setting, it may also give a warning that not all asthmatic subjects have a benign course of disease. It remains to be determined what is the natural course of FEV_1 in adult asthma and, most likely, results will have to come from epidemiological studies, as clinical studies are always and persistently influenced by the doctor's institution or change of therapy. Nevertheless it appears that asthmatic subjects with long-standing disease have lower lung function than those with recent development of asthma in adulthood.[52] In this respect it is important to follow up both pre- and postbronchodilator FEV_1, the latter being indicative of changes in non-muscular (inflammatory) components of airway narrowing.[36]

In recent years, CT scans have shown that emphysema can occur not only in asthmatic subjects who smoke but also in non-smokers.[53] Parenchymal destruction has also been mentioned in a pathological examination of a 37-year-old non-smoker with fatal asthma.[54] Thus, the damage caused by chronic inflammation in the lung, whether aggravated by smoking or not, may also lead to emphysema. Whether this is related to more progressive decline in lung function is, however, not certain.

ASTHMA DEATHS

Although only 1% died of asthma during an 8-year follow-up of 2547 individuals, there was a tremendous excessive risk of asthma compared to non-asthmatic individuals (relative risk 8–∞).[55] Mortality of asthma has increased over recent years in many countries. The cause of this is unclear: it cannot be completely explained by increased prevalence of the disease and it is very worrisome that despite improved access to medical care and better treatments for asthma this rise in mortality can occur. Fatal asthma mostly occurs in severe forms of asthma and it has been proposed that patients who over-rely on symptomatic bronchodilator and arrive late for medical care are especially at risk.[56–59] Other factors, such as increased levels of allergen exposure, more peripheral deposition of allergens after bronchodilation and air pollution have also been mentioned. Recently, seemingly unavoidable deaths due to sudden, extremely rapid onset of bronchoconstriction have been reported,[60] which may also occur in milder forms of asthma and are associated with a more neutrophilic, rather than eosinophilic, inflammation in the airways.[61] It is uncertain why this occurs; one possibility may be a toxic phenomenon or viral disease.

It has been shown that individuals with very severe AH are at risk for a fatal asthma attack,[57] even when peak flow values are stable.[62] Thus, in all individuals who have had a near fatal attack of asthma, intensive coordination between the patient, the family (passive smoking) and the health care team is essential for optimal reduction in AH to prevent further risk. General rules, like allergen avoidance, are of course of utmost importance in these individuals.

Pathological investigations in fatal and non-fatal asthma have shown that membranous airways show more airway wall thickening in fatal asthma than in non-fatal asthma.[63,64] Moreover, an increase in submucosal vascular volume may contribute to reduction in airway calibre in fatal asthma. Structural changes that may increase AH occur both in large and small airways in fatal asthma, but they occur predominantly in small airways in non-fatal cases.[65] Whether these changes, when widespread, predispose to death from asthma or are attributable to the long-term effects of severe asthma is not yet clear. However, the observations have great implications for the following reasons.

(1) Small airways disease appears to be an important factor in asthma and it is debatable whether current forms of anti-inflammatory therapy alter inflammation in this part of the airways.

(2) It is well known that exaggerated airways constriction may occur upon airway challenge in asthmatic individuals. The elegant investigations of Wiggs et al.[66] have shown that this is largely attributable to increase in peripheral airway resistance, while a plateau in airflow obstruction is associated with increased central airway narrowing (Fig. 43.3). These data suggest that pathology of peripheral airways is the key to asthma and that the fall in FEV_1 associated with the challenge could be the result of continuous closure of unstable airways.[5]

The consequences of the above findings are that future research should include investigations of small airways either by old or new lung function techniques or pathology studies, and also assessment of whether this affliction is associated with increased risk of death, with increased risk for decline in lung function or AH, and whether therapy can also improve small airways disease. It may well be that there are individuals who show hardly any change in FEV_1 over time but who have small airways disease that is either decreasing or progressing unnoticed by routine lung function testing.

FIGURE 43.3: *Effects of central (a) and peripheral (b) airway narrowing in asthma. (From ref. 66 with permission.)*

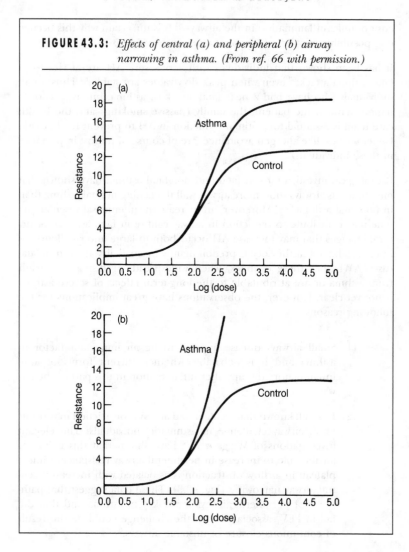

FACTORS INFLUENCING THE OUTCOME OF ASTHMA

It is an attractive hypothesis to assume that those risk factors associated with the development of asthma may also be important for the progressive nature of the disease. This hypothesis makes it possible to assess whether

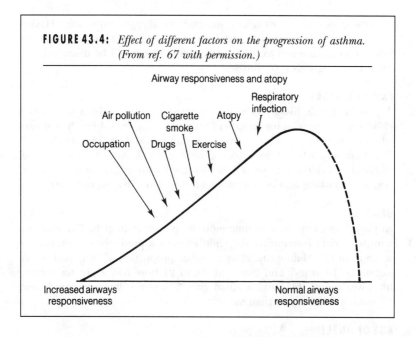

FIGURE 43.4: *Effect of different factors on the progression of asthma. (From ref. 67 with permission.)*

intervention in these factors affects the course of the disease. Epidemiological studies, the best available studies to predict the outcome of asthma, show some factors to be related consistently with the outcome of asthma (Fig. 43.4, Table 43.2). Thus, maternal smoking, presence of atopy (as

TABLE 43.2: *Factors influencing the outcome of asthma*

Family history of atopy	Unfavourable
Sex	Variable
Age of onset	Unknown
Respiratory infections	Unknown
Allergy	Unfavourable
Airway hyperresponsiveness	Unfavourable
Smoking	Unfavourable
Environmental exposure	Unfavourable
Low level of PFT	Unfavourable
Severe wheezing	Unfavourable
Treatment	Unknown

PFT, pulmonary function test.

assessed by skin testing or IgE measurements), allergen exposure, AH, viral infections, environmental factors and possibly personal smoking may be interesting parameters to investigate. These factors will be discussed with regard to progression of disease.

FAMILY HISTORY

A positive family history of atopy, elevated IgE and asthma increases a child's risk of developing persistent asthma. From several family and twin studies it has become clear that total serum IgE and positive skin tests,[68–70] asthma and AH[71–73] are under genetic control. Nevertheless from all studies it is evident that several factors modify the effects of heredity, i.e. sex, age, smoking and environmental factors like allergen exposure.

GENDER

At young ages boys have asthma more frequently than girls. There are no consistent data concerning the child's sex as a predictor of outcome of asthma. In the Melbourne study a higher proportion of boys had severe asthma at 14 years[42] and from age 14 to 21 boys had a greater relative improvement of their asthma than girls.[26] However, between age 21 and 28 women fared better than men.[27]

AGE OF ONSET

The available data are conflicting in this respect. There are studies showing an early onset to be related with a more favourable prognosis,[74] a worse prognosis[75] or with no effect on prognosis.[26,76,77]

RESPIRATORY INFECTIONS

In a prospective study to investigate risk factors for development of asthma in childhood, respiratory infections appeared to be a high-risk factor.[78] Furthermore, children are thought to be more affected by respiratory syncytial virus and parainfluenza virus and adults more by rhinovirus and influenza. However, a recent report mentioned that respiratory syncytial virus was as important as influenza in causing morbidity and excess death in older individuals.[79] Whether these viral infections affect the disease outcome in the long term remains to be established. It is of course clear that they affect asthmatic individuals severely in the acute phase.

ALLERGY

Allergy by itself is an established risk factor for the development of asthma in childhood and adulthood.[8,80–84] In children, the odds ratios for the association between increased AH and skin-test reactivity range between 1.5 and 9.2, and in adults from 0.6 to 2.6,[14] suggesting that atopy plays a more prominent role in children than in adults. The reason for this is unknown and may be related to diagnostic bias. Nevertheless a longitudinal study of blood IgE levels showed that even in males with a mean age of 64 a rise in IgE antibody against house-dust mite preceded the onset of wheeze,[83] a finding compatible with higher age-adjusted IgE levels in elderly individuals with recent diagnosis of asthma as compared to asymptomatic individuals.[16] At least two reports suggest that the age of onset of atopy may be predictive of the persistence of AH and asthma.[84,85]

The results of studies examining the relationship of allergy to the development of asthma from childhood to adulthood are conflicting; some investigations show no relationship with allergy[23,76] while others do.[20,86] The latter studies, showing lower lung function, PC_{20} and more symptoms in atopic individuals, were cross-sectional but suggest that atopy at one point in time does correlate with asthma severity. However, this does not imply that the same is true for the long-term prognosis, although a study by De Grooijer et al.[87] showed that atopy at age 8–11 was associated with a greater risk for symptoms 27 years later.

Atopy has been proposed as a risk factor for decline in lung function independent of the presence of clinical asthma[50,86] in an epidemiological setting. Other studies have not shown this effect in working or general populations.[13,49] Ulrik et al.[51] showed that decline was more rapid in intrinsic asthmatic subjects compared with extrinsic asthmatic subjects, but this difference was not observed by Almind et al.[34] However, patient selection and duration of disease may have affected the difference in outcome. Moreover, documentation of allergic status in the latter study was made at the end of follow-up and investigated with skin testing only. As the expression of allergy may change with age this may have affected the results. Also, an influence of therapy on the outcome cannot be ruled out, as 66% of non-atopic asthmatic and 47% of atopic individuals were treated with corticosteroids in the study of Ulrik et al. Van Schayck et al.[47] showed in a prospective study in corticosteroid-naive asthmatic subjects that more severe AH in atopic individuals was associated with a steeper decline in FEV_1, an association not observed in non-atopic individuals. Another study[31] showed that adults who developed respiratory symptoms and asthma had a significantly greater average decline in FEV_1 than those without. As the association was stronger in atopic individuals, this suggests that atopy is a significant modifier of disease outcome in asthma.

The above observations, together with findings that allergen avoidance reduces the development of asthma and the severity of symptoms and AH,[88–92] suggest that allergen avoidance may beneficially affect the outcome of asthma. Finally, treatment of allergic rhinitis with intranasal corticosteroids also improves AH, suggesting that appropriate treatment of this atopy is also beneficial.[93]

AIRWAY HYPERRESPONSIVENESS

Increased AH usually precedes the development of asthma,[94] which has not only been observed in children or young adults[94,95] but also in middle-aged men not selected for an allergic history.[18] More severe AH is associated with more symptoms[50,96–98] and steeper fall in FEV_1.[50,97] The combination of wheeze and AH discriminates the asthmatic group with ongoing significant respiratory impairment.[97] AH is persistent in children with persisting symptoms[99] but it generally improves in young asthmatic subjects in their teens,[21,87] although one study did not show improvement despite a better clinical course of disease.[100] However, this may be due to the fact that anti-inflammatory therapy was only withheld for 72 hours, while many were instituted on this therapy. The possible reasons for the improvement in AH may be related to growing airway diameter. However, this cannot be the sole solution, as this also occurs in those with persistent AH. Finally, the importance of persistent AH in predicting ongoing respiratory symptoms has been demonstrated in two long-term epidemiological studies.[21,101]

Severity of AH defines individuals with a better response on inhaled corticosteroids.[36] Long-term treatment with corticosteroids may diminish the number of inflammatory cells in the airways dramatically, but nevertheless does not normalize AH.[36–38]

SMOKING

Parental smoking affects the development of atopy and asthma. This is true for *in utero* cigarette smoke exposure and exposure in the first few months of life.[102–105] However, smoking itself almost never shows up as a risk factor for progressive airflow limitation, when asthma is present. This may be the result of the so-called "healthy smoker effect", in that those with more susceptible airways do not take up smoking or quit at an early stage. Thus a negative effect may not become apparent. However, the observation that active smoking during adolescence is associated with shortening of the plateau phase of FEV_1 that generally occurs between 20 and 35 years[105] suggests that there is an overall negative effect of smoking in adolescence, which may also be present in asthmatic subjects. Further observations have shown that cessation of smoking during adolescence had a positive impact on lung growth.[106]

ENVIRONMENTAL EXPOSURE

Whether environmental exposure affects the outcome of asthma is largely determined by the type of exposure. Environmental air pollution may not increase the prevalence of atopic status, but may enhance the development and duration of clinical symptoms among already sensitized subjects.[92] Whether it affects long-term outcome is still uncertain. Toluene diisocyanate exposure, on the other hand, may affect the outcome negatively when exposure is continued and not resolved within 6 months.[107]

LEVEL OF PULMONARY FUNCTION

As described above, both in children and in adults, a low level of FEV_1 appears to be predictive for continuation of wheezing into adulthood and a low level of lung function in adulthood, as well as for more rapid decline of FEV_1. Moreover low lung function is even a predisposing factor for first wheezing illness in infants.[108]

TREATMENT

Although treatment has reduced the morbidity of asthma, it has not been definitely shown to alter the course of disease (see below).

THERAPEUTIC INTERVENTION IN THE COURSE OF DISEASE

There is an urgent need to know whether treatment can improve the disease outcome of asthma both in children, adults and the elderly. This is all the more important as it has been shown that the expected eventual outcome is a crucial factor in decision making about a patient's management.[109] Therapy is generally directed at improvement of symptoms. Although attractive in a clinical setting, it seems not advisable to allow treatment to be solely regulated by symptoms as (1) patients do not comply with taking more medication when PEFR variability increases, symptoms deteriorate or additional use of β agonists increases,[110] and (2) symptomatic deterioration does not relate to objective worsening of lung function or AH,[11] especially not when slow and progressive bronchoconstriction occurs.[40]

Inhaled corticosteroids (IC) are at the present time the first step in treatment of asthmatic subjects, from very young ages onwards. This is largely based on the short-term beneficial effects on both symptoms, diurnal and day-to-day variability in PEFR, level of lung function and AH.[36–38,111–122] The longest double-blind study is 2.5 years.[36,121] IC do improve lung function during regular therapy given for weeks or months, but this may not be obvious in all asthmatic subjects, as asthma may very well start off with normal lung function. Thus, greater improvements are usually obtained in individuals with more severe degrees of airway obstruction. It is important to note that both pre- and post-bronchodilator FEV_1 improve, which is indicative of effects on non-muscular (inflammatory) components of airway narrowing.[36]

There is growing concern that despite increased use of prophylactic treatments some children may have a chronically high functional residual capacity (FRC), which may put them at risk of COPD in later life.[123] However, they are as yet not discernible from those who react with normalization of FRC and spirometry.

Non-smoking, atopic and severely hyperresponsive individuals respond the best by improving their FEV_1 in the first 3 months of IC treatment, the improvement being maintained throughout 2.5 years of follow-up.[36] However, these factors do not influence the course of FEV_1 during IC therapy once the initial improvement has been gained. Such a predictive effect on the long-term course after the first few months of treatment has been demonstrated for reversibility of airflow obstruction, i.e. 80 ml FEV_1 per year improvement per 10% predicted increase with a bronchodilator for those treated with IC vs. 57 ml FEV_1 per year decline per 10% predicted improvement in FEV_1 with a bronchodilator in those who were not treated with IC. A high reversibility may thus be a sign to institute IC for prevention of decline in lung function in asthma.

Whether this treatment will prevent irreversible damage to the airways is as yet not certain. However, cessation of treatment, even after 36 months,[112,124,125] negates the beneficial effects, i.e. symptoms recur within 5 days followed by deterioration of lung function (visible in PEFR after ± 16 days and after 2–3 months by worsening of hyperresponsiveness).[124,125] Gradually tapering off the treatment has been tried as well and one study in children (Fig. 43.5) suggests that even gradual diminution of IC does not prevent final deterioration.[126] A follow-up study by Haahtela et al.[127] shows that reduction of the dose from 1200 μg for 2 years to 400 μg of inhaled budesonside for 1 year was feasible without deterioration of lung function and AH in most asthmatic subjects in this study.

There is some evidence that early institution of IC is of importance for preventing irreversible damage. Thus it has been shown that PC_{20} histamine values deteriorate after 2 years of treatment with bronchodilators only,[113] but PC_{20} values after 1 year of IC improved only to the same level as at the start of the first 2 years. Thus, it did not show the rapid and large increase that one would have expected in the treatment of asthma.[36,38]

FIGURE 43.5: *Effect of gradual reduction of inhaled corticosteroids on FEV_1 (a) and airway hyperresponsiveness (b) in asthmatic children. (From ref. 126 with permission.)*

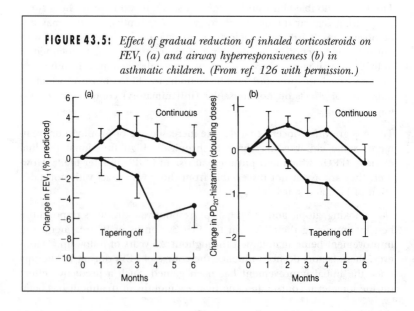

There are also some reports that later institution does not improve AH to the same extent as earlier institution regimens.[128,129]

On a pathological basis beneficial effects have been investigated in mucosal biopsies of the large airways. Diminution in numbers of inflammatory cells in the submucosa,[129,131] as well as of activated eosinophils in the epithelium and submucosa[132] and activated CD4[+] T cells and interleukin (IL)-5 levels in peripheral blood,[133] have been observed. Favourable effects have also been shown by reduction of mRNA expression for IL-4 and IL-5[134] after 2 weeks' oral prednisolone treatment and reduction of eosinophilic activity, as reflected by the amount of eosinophilic cationic protein in broncho-alveolar lavage fluid after 4 weeks of IC treatment.[135] All these studies did not show reduction of sub-basement membrane thickening, and it can be argued that this might affect AH in a negative way.

Some studies suggest that regular use of β_2 agonists may actually worsen asthma[136,137] and are a risk factor for (near) death from asthma.[138] Irrespective of the presence or absence of symptoms, regular bronchodilator use may negatively affect lung function.[11] This has been attributed to the lack of effect in reducing inflammation, masking of ongoing deterioration in lung function by relieving symptoms almost continuously, and possibly an increase in exposure to allergens and environmental toxins. Other studies show worsening of AH, which is opposite to the improvement in AH with inhaled corticosteroids.[115,116] Furthermore, cessation of long-acting inhaled β_2 agonists also worsened AH. If these studies relate to clinical practice they suggest that prolonged treatment with β_2 agonists may affect the outcome of asthma negatively. It has to be determined whether these findings can be reproduced over longer periods of follow-up. Nevertheless, it seems reasonable to accept that anti-inflammatory therapy is the first step in the treatment of asthma.

SUMMARY

Little is known about the long-term outcome of asthma. Symptoms are not the only focus for direction of asthma treatment, as severe and irreversible airflow limitation may develop without the patient noticing it. Early treatment of asthma with IC may give optimal control and preliminary results of studies in both adults and children suggest that delaying institution may result in irreversible damage. However, cessation of treatment results in rapid recurrence of symptoms, AH and airflow limitation.

There are many problems left to unravel. It is uncertain whether the use of IC in the management of asthma alters the disease in the small airways or cures the disease. It seems that once the trigger is activated, the inflammatory process takes its own course. Optimal avoidance of allergens, environmental toxins and smoke may, next to optimal anti-inflammatory therapy, alter the course of asthma. It remains to be established whether the observation that physiological plasma cortisol levels modulate the process responsible for the deterioration of ventilatory function with ageing has clinical relevance for asthma as well.[139] Future new strategies are still needed for a treatment that either prevents the occurrence of asthma, switches the disease off in childhood once present, or prevents relapse in adult life.

REFERENCES

1   Blanc PD, Jones M, Besson C, Katz P, Yelin E. Work disability among adults with asthma. Chest 1993; 104: 1371-7.

2   Laitinen LA, Laitinen A, Haahtela T. Airway mucosal inflammation even in patients with newly diagnosed asthma. Am Rev Respir Dis 1993; 147: 697–704.

3   Sobonya RE. Quantitative structural alteration in long-standing allergic asthma. Am Rev Respir Dis 1984; 130: 289–92.

4   Carroll N, Eliott J, Morton A, James A. The structure of large and small airways in nonfatal and fatal asthma. Am Rev Respir Dis 1993; 147: 405-11.

5   Hogg JC, Pathology of asthma. J Allergy Clin Immunol 1993; 92: 1-5.

6   Wiggs BR, Moreno R, Hogg JC, Hilliam C, Pare PD. A model of the mechanics of airway narrowing. J Appl Physiol 1990; 69: 849-60.

7   Wiggs BR, Bosken CH, Pare PD, James A, Hogg JC. A model of airways narrowing in asthma and in chronic obstructive pulmonary disease. Am Rev Respir Dis 1992; 145: 1251-8.

8   Dodge R, Burrows B, Lebowitz MD, Cline MG. Antecedent features of children in whom asthma develops during the second decade of life. J Allergy Clin Immunol 1993; 92: 744-9.

9   Brown PJ, Greville HW, Finucane KE. Asthma and irreversible airflow obstruction. Thorax 1984; 39: 131-6.

10 Connolly CK, Chan NS, Prescott RJ. The relationship between age and duration of asthma and the presence of persistent obstruction in asthma. Postgrad Med J 1988; 64: 422-5.

11 Van Schayck CP, Folgering H, Den Otter JJ, Tirimanna P, van Weel C. Does the continuous use of bronchodilators mask the progression of asthma of chronic bronchitis? Fam Pract 1992; 9: 397–404.

12 Burrows B, Knudson RJ, Camilli AE, Lyle SK, Lebowitz MD. The horse-racing effect and predicting decline in forced expiratory volume in one second from screening spirometry. Am Rev Respir Dis 1987; 135: 788-93.

13 Peat JK, Woolcock AJ, Cullen K. Rate of decline of lung function in subjects with asthma. *Eur J Respir Dis* 1987; 70: 171–9.

14 Weiss ST, Sparrow D, O'Connor GT. The interrelationship among allergy, airway responsiveness and asthma. *J Asthma* 1993; 30: 329–49.

15 Pearce N, Weiland S, Keil U *et al.* Self-reported prevalence of asthma symptoms in children in Australia, England, Germany and New Zealand: an international comparison using ISAAC protocol. *Eur Respir J* 1993; 6: 1455–61.

16 Burrows B, Lebowitz MD, Barbee RA, Cline MG. Findings before diagnoses of asthma among the elderly in longitudinal study of a general population sample. *J Allergy Clin Immunol* 1991; 88: 870–7.

17 Trigg CJ, Bennett JB, Tooley M, Sibbald B, D'Souza MF, Davies RJ. A general practice based survey of bronchial hyperresponsiveness and its relation to symptoms, sex, age, atopy and smoking. *Thorax* 1990; 45: 866–72.

18 Sparrow D, O'Connor G, Colton T, Barry CL, Weiss ST. The relationship of nonspecific bronchial responsiveness to the occurrence of respiratory symptoms and decreased levels of pulmonary function. *Am Rev Respir Dis* 1987; 135: 1255–60.

19 Burney PG, Chinn S, Britton JR, Tattersfield AE, Papacosta AO. What symptoms predict the bronchial response to histamine? *Int J Epidemiol* 1989; 18: 165–73.

20 Clough JB, Williams JD, Holgate ST. Effect of atopy on the natural history of symptoms, peak expiratory flow, and bronchial responsiveness in 7- and 8-year-old children with cough and wheeze. *Am Rev Respir Dis* 1991; 143: 755–60.

21 Kondo S. Spontaneous improvement in bronchial responsiveness and its limit during preadolescence and early adolescence in children with controlled asthma. *Chest* 1993; 104: 1359–63.

22 Martin AJ, McLennan LA, Landay LJ, Phelan PD. The natural history of childhood asthma to adult life. *BMJ* 1980; 280: 1397–400.

23 Gerritsen J, Koëter GH, Postma DS, Schouten JP, Knol K. Prognosis of asthma from childhood to adulthood. *Am Rev Respir Dis* 1989; 140: 1325–30.

24 Roorda RJ, Gerritsen G, Van Aalderen WMC *et al.* Risk factors for the persistence of respiratory symptoms in childhood asthma. *Am Rev Respir Dis* 1993; 148: 1490–5.

25 Borsboom GJJM, Van Pelt W, Quanjer PH. Pubertal growth curves of ventilatory function: relationship with childhood respiratory symptoms. *Am Rev Respir Dis* 1993; 147: 372–8.

26 Martin AJ, Landau LI, Phelan P. Lung function in young adults who had asthma in childhood. *Am Rev Respir Dis* 1980; 122: 609–16.

27 Kelly WJW, Hudson I, Phelan PD, Pain MCF, Olinsky A. Childhood asthma and adult lung function: a further study at 28 years of age. *BMJ* 1987; 294: 1059–62.

28　Weiss ST, Tosteson TD, Segal MR, Tager IB, Redline S, Speizer FE. Effects of asthma on pulmonary function in children. A longitudinal population-based study. *Am Rev Respir Dis* 1992; 145: 58–64.

29　Kelly WJW, Hudson I, Phelan PD, Pain MCF, Olinsky A. Childhood asthma and adult lung function. *Am Rev Respir Dis* 1988; 138: 26–30.

30　Jaakkola MS, Jaakkola JJK, Ernst P, Becklake MR. Respiratory symptoms in young adults should not be overlooked. *Am Rev Respir Dis* 1993; 147: 359–66.

31　Jaakkola MS, Ernst P, Jaakkola JJK, Nganga LW, Backlake MR. Effect of cigarette smoking on evolution of ventilatory lung function in young adults. An eight year longitudinal study. *Thorax* 1991; 128: 17–23.

32　Burrows B, Barbee RA, Cline MG, Knudson RJ, Lebowitz MD. Characteristics of asthma among elderly adults in a sample of the general population. *Chest* 1991; 100: 935–42.

33　Sparrow D, O'Connor GT, Basner RC, Rosner B, Weiss ST. Predictors of the new onset of wheezing among middle-aged and older men. *Am Rev Respir Dis* 1993; 147: 367–71.

34　Almind M, Viskum K, Evald T, Dirksen A, Kok-Jensen A. A seven-year follow-up study of 343 adults with bronchial asthma. *Danish Med Bull* 1992; 39: 561–5.

35　Traver GA, Cline MG, Burrows B. Asthma in the elderly. *J Asthma* 1993; 302: 81–91.

36　Kerstjens HAM, Brand PLP, Hughes MD *et al.* A comparison of bronchodilator therapy with or without inhaled corticosteroid therapy in obstructive airways. *N Engl J Med* 1992; 327: 1413–9.

37　Van Essen-Zandvliet EE, Hughes MD, Waalkens HJ *et al.* Effects of 22 months of treatment with inhaled corticosteroids and/or beta-2-agonists on lung function, airway responsiveness, and symptoms in children with asthma. *Am Rev Respir Dis* 1992; 146: 547–54.

38　Haahtela T, Järvinen M, Kava T, Kiviranta K, Koskinen S, Lehtonen K. Comparison of beta-agonist, terbutaline, with an inhaled corticosteroid, budesonide, in newly detected asthma. *N Engl J Med* 1991; 325: 388–92.

39　Kawasaki A, Mitzushima Y, Hoshino K, Oosaki R, Kobayashi M. Bronchial hypersensitivity in asthmatics in long-term symptom-free state. *Chest* 1993; 103: 370–5.

40　Turcotte H, Boulet L-P. Perception of breathlessness during early and late asthmatic responses. *Am Rev Respir Dis* 1993; 148: 514–8.

41　Boulet L-P, Milot J, Turcotte H. Relationship between changes in diurnal variation of expiratory flows, lung volumes and respiratory symptoms after acute asthma. *Respir Med* 1991; 85: 487–93.

42　McNicol KN, Williams HB. Spectrum of asthma in children. Clinical and physiological components. *BMJ* 1973; 4: 7–11.

43 Burrows B, Bloom JW, Traver GA, Cline MG. The course and prognosis of different forms of chronic airways obstruction in a sample from the general population. *N Engl J Med* 1987; 317: 1309–14.

44 Frew AJ, Kennedy SM, Can-Yeung M. Methacholine responsiveness, smoking and atopy as risk factors for accelerated FEV_1 decline in male working populations. *Am Rev Respir Dis* 1992; 146: 878–83.

45 Burrows B, Lebowitz MD, Barbee RA, Cline MG. Findings before diagnoses of asthma among an elderly in a longitudinal study of a general population sample. *J Allergy Clin Immunol* 1991; 88: 870–7.

46 Sherill D, Sears MR, Lebowitz MD *et al*. The effects of airway hyperresponsiveness, wheezing, and atopy on longitudinal pulmonary function in children: A 6 year follow-up study. *Pediatr Pulmonol* 1992; 13: 78–85.

47 Van Schayck CP, Dompeling E, Van Herwaarden CAL, Wever AMJ, Van Weel C. Interacting effects of atopy and bronchial hyperresponsiveness on the annual decline in lung function and the exacerbation rate in asthma. *Am Rev Respir Dis* 1991; 144: 1297–301.

48 Schachter EN, Doyle CA, Beck GJ. A prospective study of asthma in a rural community. *Chest* 1983; 85: 623–30.

49 Peat JK, Salome CM, Sedgwick CS, Kerrebijn J, Woolcock AJ. A prospective study of bronchial hyperresponsiveness and respiratory symptoms in a population of Australian schoolchildren. *Clin Exp Allergy* 1989; 19: 299–306.

50 Burrows B, Halonen M, Lebowitz MD, Knudson RJ, Barbee RA. The relationship of serum immunoglobulin E, allergy skin test and smoking to respiratory disorders. *J Allergy Clin Immunol* 1982; 70: 199–204.

51 Ulrik CS, Backer V, Dirksen A. A 10 year follow up of 180 adults with bronchial asthma: factors important for the decline in lung function. *Thorax* 1992; 47: 14–8.

52 Braman SS, Keammerlen JT, Davis SM. Asthma in the elderly. A comparison between patients with recently acquired and long-standing disease. *Am Rev Respir Dis* 1991; 143: 336–40.

53 Paganin F, Trussard V, Seneterre E *et al*. Chest radiography and high resolution computed tomography of the lungs in asthma. *Am Rev Respir Dis* 1992; 146: 1084–7.

54 Fabbri LM, Danieli D, Crescioli S *et al*. Fatal asthma in a subject sensitized to toluene diisocyanate. *Am Rev Respir Dis* 1988; 137: 1494–8.

55 Markowe HL, Bulpitt CJ, Shipley MJ, Rose G, Crombie DL, Fleming DM. Prognosis in adult asthma: a national study. *BMJ* 1987; 295: 949–52.

56 Birkhead G, Attaway NJ, Strunk RC, Townsend MC, Teutsch S. Investigation of a cluster of deaths of adolescents from asthma: evidence implicating inadequate treatment and poor patient adherence with medications. *J Allergy Clin Immunol* 1989; 84: 484–91.

57 Pouw EM, Koëter GH, Monchy JGR, Homan AJ, Sluiter HJ. Clinical assessment after a life-threatening attack of asthma; the role of bronchial hyperreactivity. *Eur Respir J* 1990; 3: 861–6.

58 Marquette CH, Saulnier F, Leroy O *et al.* Long-term prognosis of near-fatal asthma. A 6-year follow-up study of 145 asthmatic patients who underwent mechanical ventilation for a near-fatal attack of asthma. *Am Rev Respir Dis* 1992; 146: 76–81.

59 Ruffin RE, Latimer KM, Schembri DA. Longitudinal study of near fatal asthma. *Chest* 1991; 99: 77–83.

60 Strunk RC. Death due to asthma. *Am Rev Respir Dis* 1993; 148: 550–2.

61 Sur S, Grotty TB, Kephart GM *et al.* Sudden-onset fatal asthma: a distinct entity with few eosinophils and relatively more neutrophils in airway submucosa. *Am Rev Respir Dis* 1993; 148: 713–9.

62 Saetta M, Thiene G, Crescioli S, Fabbri LM. Fatal asthma in a young patient with severe bronchial hyperresponsiveness but stable peak flow record. *Eur Respir J* 1989; 2: 1008–12.

63 Dunnill MS, Massarella GR, Anderson JA. A comparison of the quantitative anatomy of the bronchi in normal subjects, in status asthmaticus, in chronic bronchitis, and in emphysema. *Thorax* 1969; 69: 39–42.

64 Kuwano K, Bosken CK, Pare P, Bai TR, Wiggs BR, Hogg JC. Small airways dimensions in asthma and in chronic obstructive pulmonary disease. *Am Rev Respir Dis* 1993; 148: 1220–5.

65 Carroll J, Elliott J, Morton A, James A. The structure of large and small airways in nonfatal and fatal asthma. *Am Rev Respir Dis* 1993; 147: 405–10.

66 Wiggs BR, Bosken C, Pare PD, James A, Hogg JC. A model of airway narrowing in asthma and in chronic obstructive pulmonary disease. *Am Rev Respir Dis* 1992; 145: 1251–8.

67 Weiss ST, O'Connor GT, Sparrow D. The role of allergy and airway responsiveness on the natural history of chronic airflow obstruction. In: West ST, Sparrow D (eds) *Airways Responsiveness and Atopy in the Development of Chronic Lung Disease.* New York: Raven Press, 1990: 218–20.

68 Hopp RJ, Bewtra AK, Watt GD, Nair NM, Townley RG. Genetic analysis of allergic disease in twins. *J Allergy Clin Immunol* 1984; 73: 265–70.

69 Meyers DA, Beaty TH, Freidhoff LR, Marsh DG. Inheritance of serum IgE (basal levels) in man. *Am J Hum Genet* 1987; 41: 51–62.

70 Cookson WOCM, Sharp PA, Faux JA, Hopkin JM. Linkage between immunoglobulin E responses underlying asthma and rhinitis and chromosome 11q. *Lancet* 1989; i: 1292–5.

71 Edfors-Lubs ML. Allergy in 7000 twin pairs. *Acta Allergol* 1971; 26: 249–85.

72   Hopp RJ, Bewtra AK, Nair NM, Townley RG. Bronchial reactivity patterns in nonasthmatic parents of asthmatics. *Ann Allergy* 1987; 61: 184–6.

73   Tager IB, Tishler PV, Rosner B, Speizer FE, Litt M. Studies of the familial aggregation of chronic bronchitis and obstructive airways disease. *Int J Epidemiol* 1978; 7: 55–62.

74   Foucard T, Sjoberg O. A prospective 12 year follow-up study of children with wheezy bronchitis. *Acta Paediatr Scand* 1984; 73: 577–83.

75   Johnsson JA, Boe J, Berlin E. The long-term prognosis of childhood asthma in a predominantly rural Swedish county. *Acta Paediatr Scand* 1987; 76: 950–4.

76   Blair H. Natural history of childhood asthma: a 20 year follow-up. *Arch Dis Child* 1977; 52: 613–9.

77   Park ES, Golding J, Carswell F, Stewart-Brown S. Preschool wheezing and prognosis at 10. *Arch Dis Child* 1986; 61: 642–6.

78   Yarnell JWG, St Leger S. Respiratory infections and their influence on lung function in children: a multiple regression analysis. *Thorax* 1981; 36: 847–51.

79   Fleming DM Cros KW. Respiratory syncytial virus or influenza? *Lancet* 1993; 342: 1507–10.

80   Burrows B, Lebowitz MD, Barbee RA, Knudson RJ, Halonen M. Interactions of smoking and immunologic factors in relation to airways obstruction. *Chest* 1983; 84: 657–61.

81   Crane J, O'Donnell TV, Prior IA, Waite DA. The relationships between atopy, bronchial hyperresponsiveness and a family history of asthma: A cross-sectional study of migrant Tokelauan children in New Zealand. *J Allergy Clin Immunol* 1989; 84: 768–72.

82   Burrows B, Martinez FD, Halonen M, Barbee RA, Cline MG. Association of asthma with serum IgE levels and skin-test reactivity to allergens. *N Engl J Med* 1989; 320: 271–7.

83   Ohman JL, Sparrow D, McDonald MR. New onset of wheezing in an older male population: evidence of allergen sensitisation in a longitudinal study. *J Allergy Clin Immunol* 1993; 91: 752–7.

84   Peat JK, Salome CM, Woolcock AJ. Longitudinal changes in atopy during a 4-year period: relation to bronchial hyperresponsiveness and respiratory symptoms in a population sample of Australian school children. *J Allergy Clin Immunol* 1990; 85: 65–74.

85   Van Asperen PP, Kemp AS, Mirkhiu A. Atopy in infancy predicts the severity of bronchial hyperresponsiveness in late childhood. *J Allergy Clin Immunol* 1990; 85: 790–5.

86   Kelly WJW, Hudson I, Phelan PD, Pain MCF, Olinsky A. Atopy in subjects with asthma followed to the age of 28. *J Allergy Clin Immunol* 1990; 85: 548–57.

87 De Gooijer A, Brand PLP, Gerritsen J, Koëter GH, Postma DS, Knol K. Changes in respiratory symptoms and airway hyperresponsiveness after 27 years in a population-based sample of school children. *Eur Respir J* 1993; 6: 648–54.

88 Sears MR, Herbison GP, Holdaway MD, Hewitt CJ, Flannery EM, Silva PA. The relative risks of sensitivity to grass pollen, house dust mite and cat dander in the development of childhood asthma. *Clin Exp Allergy* 1989; 19: 419–24.

89 Luczynska CM, Li Y, Chapman MD, Platts-Mills TAE. Airborne concentrations and particle size distribution of allergen derived from domestic cats (*Felis domesticus*). *Am Rev Respir Dis* 1990; 141: 361–7.

90 Ehnert B, Lau-Schadendorf S, Weber A, Buettner P, Schou C, Wahn U. Reducing domestic exposure to dust mite allergen reduces bronchial hyperreactivity in sensitive children with asthma. *J Allergy Clin Immunol* 1992; 90: 135–8.

91 Arshad SH, Matthews S, Gant C, Hide DW. Effects of allergen avoidance on development of allergic disorders in infancy. *Lancet* 1992; 339: 1493–7.

92 Corbo GM, Forastiere F, Dell'Orco V *et al.* Effects of environment on atopic status and respiratory disorders in children. *J Allergy Clin Immunol* 1993; 92: 616–23.

93 Watson WTA, Becker AB, Simons FER. Treatment of allergic rhinitis with intranasal corticosteroids in patients with mild asthma: effect on lower airway responsiveness. *J Allergy Clin Immunol* 1993; 91: 97–101.

94 Hopp RJ, Townley RG, Biven RE, Bewtra AK, Nair NM. The presence of airway reactivity before the development of asthma. *Am Rev Respir Dis* 1990; 141: 2–8.

95 Zhong NS, Chen RC, O-Yang M, Wu JY, Fu WX, Shi LJ. Bronchial hyperresponsiveness in young students of southern China: relation to respiratory symptoms, diagnosed asthma, and risk factors. *Thorax* 1990; 45: 860–5.

96 Peat JK, Salome CM, Woolcock AJ. Factors associated with bronchial hyperresponsiveness in Australian adults and children. *Eur Respir J* 1992; 5: 921–9.

97 Peat JK, Toelle BG, Salome CM, Woolcock AJ. Predictive nature of bronchial responsiveness and respiratory symptoms in a one year cohort study of Sydney schoolchildren. *Eur Respir J* 1993; 6: 662–9.

98 Britton JR, Burney PGJ, Chinn S, Papacosta AO, Tattersfield AE. The relation between change in airway reactivity and change in respiratory symptoms and medication in a community study. *Am Rev Respir Dis* 1988; 135: 530–4.

99 Radford P, Hopp RJ, Biven RE, Degan JA, Bewtra AK, Townley RG. Longitudinal changes in bronchial hyperresponsiveness in asthmatic and previous asthmatic children. *Chest* 1992; 101: 624–9.

100 Adachi Y, Murakami G, Matsuno M *et al.* Longitudinal study of bronchial hyperreactivity in preschool children with bronchial asthma. *Ann Allergy* 1992; 68: 261–6.

101 Redline S, Tager IB, Speizer FE, Rosner BB, Weiss ST. Longitudinal variability in airway responsiveness in a population-based sample of children

and young adults. Intrinsic and extrinsic contributing factors. *Am Rev Respir Dis* 1989; 140: 172–8.

102 Sherrill DL, Martinez FD, Lebowitz MD *et al.* Longitudinal effects of passive smoking on pulmonary function in New Zealand children. *Am Rev Respir Dis* 1992; 145: 1136–41.

103 Martinez FD, Antognoni G, Macri F *et al.* Parental smoking enhances bronchial responsiveness in nine-year old children. *Am Rev Respir Dis* 1988; 138: 518–23.

104 Murray AB, Morrison BJ. Effect of passive smoking on asthmatic children who have and who have not had atopic dermatitis. *Chest* 1992; 101: 16–8.

105 Tager IB, Segal MR, Speizer FE, Weiss ST. The natural history of expiratory volumes. Effect of cigarette smoking and respiratory symptoms. *Am Rev Respir Dis* 1988; 138: 837–49.

106 Lebowitz MD, Holberg CJ, Knudson RJ, Burrows B. Longitudinal study of pulmonary function development in childhood, adolescence and early adulthood. *Am Rev Respir Dis* 1987; 136: 69–75.

107 Fabbri LM, Danieli D, Crescioli P *et al.* Fatal asthma in a subject sensitized to toluene diisocyanate. *Am Rev Respir Dis* 1988; 137: 1494–8.

108 Martinez FD, Morgan WJ, Wright AL, Holberg CJ, Taussig LM. Diminished lung function as a predisposing factor for wheezing respiratory illness in infants. *N Engl J Med* 1988; 319: 1112–7.

109 Murray LS, Teasdale GM, Murray GD *et al.* Does prediction of outcome alter patient management? *Lancet* 1993; 341: 1487–91.

110 Mann MC, Eliasson O, Patel K, Zu Wallack RL. An evaluation of severity-modulated compliance with q.i.d. dosing of inhaled beclomethasone. *Chest* 1992; 102: 1342–6.

111 Molema J, Herwaarden CLA, Folgering HThM. Effects of long-term treatment with inhaled cromoglycate and budesonide on bronchial hyperresponsiveness in patients with allergic asthma. *Eur Respir J* 1989; 2: 308–16.

112 Bel EH, Timmers MC, Hermans J, Dijkman JH, Sterk PJ. The long-term effects of nedocromil sodium and beclomethasone dipropionate on bronchial responsiveness to methacholine in nonatopic asthmatic subjects. *Am Rev Respir Dis* 1990; 141: 21–8.

113 Dompeling E, Van Schayck CP, Molema JM, Folgering H, van Grunsven PM, van Weel C. Inhaled beclomethasone improves the course of asthma and COPD. *Eur Respir J* 1992; 5: 945–52.

114 Kraan J, Koëter GH, van der Mark ThW *et al.* Dosage and time effects of inhaled budesonide on bronchial hyperreactivity. *Am Rev Respir Dis* 1988; 137: 44–8.

115 Kraan J, Koëter GH, van der Mark ThW, Sluiter HJ, de Vries K. Changes in bronchial hyperreactivity induced by 4 weeks of treatment with anti-asthmatic drugs in patients with allergic asthma: a comparison between budesonide and terbutaline. *J Allergy Clin Immunol* 1985; 76: 628–36.

116 Kerrebijn KF, Van Essen-Zandvliet EEM, Neijens HJ. Effect of long-term treatment with inhaled corticosteroids and beta-agonists on the bronchial responsiveness in children with asthma. *J Allergy Clin Immunol* 1987; 79: 653–9.

117 Svendsen UG, Frolund L, Madsen F, Nielsen NH. A comparison of the effects of nedocromil sodium and beclomethasone dipropionate on pulmonary function, symptoms, and bronchial responsiveness in patients with asthma. *J Allergy Clin Immunol* 1989; 84: 224–31.

118 de Baets FM, Goetheyn M, Kerrebijn KF. The effect of two months of treatment with inhaled budesonide on bronchial responsiveness to histamine and house dust mite antigen in asthmatic children. *Am Rev Respir Dis* 1990; 142: 581–6.

119 Juniper EF, Kline PA, Vanzieleghem MA, Ramsdale EH, O'Bryne PM, Hargreave FE. Long-term effects of budesonide on airway responsiveness and clinical asthma severity in inhaled steroid-dependent asthmatics. *Eur Respir J* 1990; 3: 1122–7.

120 Juniper EF, Kline PA, Vanzieleghem MA, Ramsdale EH, O'Bryne PM, Hargreave FE. Effect of long-term treatment with an inhaled corticosteroid (budesonide) on airway hyperresponsiveness and clinical asthma in non-steroid-dependent asthmatics. *Am Rev Respir Dis* 1990; 142: 832–6.

121 Kerstjens HAM, Overbeek SE, Schouten JP, Brand PLP, Postma DS. Airways hyperresponsiveness, bronchodilator response, allergy and smoking predict improvement in FEV_1 during treatment with inhaled corticosteroid treatment. *Eur Respir J* 1993; 6: 868–76.

122 Kerstjens HAM, Brand PLP, Quanjer PhH, van der Bruggen-Bogaarts BAHA, Koëter GH, Postma DS. Variability of bronchodilator response and effects of inhaled corticosteroid treatment in obstructive airway disease. *Thorax* 1993; 48: 722–9.

123 Greenough A, Everett L, Pool J, Price JF. A 2-year longitudinal study of lung hyperinflation in young asthmatics. *Respir Med* 1991; 85: 379–82.

124 Gibson PG, Wong BJO, Hepperle MJE *et al.* A research method to induce and examine a mild exacerbation of asthma by withdrawal of inhaled corticosteroid. *Clin Exp Allergy* 1992; 22: 523–32.

125 Juniper EF, Kline PA, Vanzieleghem MA, Hargreave FE. Reduction of budesonide after a year of increased use: a randomized controlled trial to evaluate whether improvements in airway responsiveness and clinical asthma are maintained. *J Allergy Clin Immunol* 1991; 87: 483–9.

126 Waalkens HJ, van Essen-Zandvliet EEM, Hughes MD *et al.* Cessation of long-term treatment with inhaled corticosteroid (budesonide) in children with asthma results in deterioration. *Am Rev Respir Dis* 1993; 148: 1252–7.

127 Haahtela T, Jarvinen M, Kava T *et al.* First-line treatment of newly detected asthma: an inhaled steroid? One year's follow-up after two years' treatment. *Eur Respir J* 1992; 5(suppl): 13S.

128 Pedersen S, Agertoft L. Effect of long term budesonide treatment on growth, weight and lung function in children with asthma. Am Rev Respir Dis 1993; 147: A265.

129 Overbeek SE, Kerstjens HAM, Bogaard JM, Mulder P, Postma DS and the Dutch CNSLD study group. Is delayed institution of inhaled corticosteroids harmful? Am Rev Respir Dis 1993; 147: A291.

130 Laitinen LA, Laitinen A, Haahtela T. A comparative study of the effects of an inhaled corticosteroid, budesonide, and a beta2-agonist, terbutaline, on airway inflammation in newly diagnosed asthma: A randomized, double-blind, parallel-group controlled trial. J Allergy Clin Immunol 1992; 90: 32–42.

131 Lundgren R, Soderberg M, Horstedt P, Stenling R. Morphological studies of bronchial mucosal biopsies from asthmatics before and after ten years of treatment with inhaled corticosteroids. Eur Respir J 1988; 1: 883–9.

132 Djukanovic R, Wilson JW, Britten KM et al. Effect of an inhaled corticosteroid on airway wall inflammation and symptoms in asthma. Am Rev Respir Dis 1992; 145: 669–74.

133 Corrigan CJ, Jaczku A, Gemou-Engesath V et al. CD4-T lymphocyte activation in asthma is accompanied by increased serum concentrations of interleukin-5. Effect of glucocorticoid therapy. Am Rev Respir Dis 1993; 147: 540–7.

134 Robinson D, Hamid Q, Ying S et al. Prednisone treatment in asthma is associated with modulation of bronchoalveolar lavage cell interleukin-4, interleukin-5 and interferon gamma cytokine gene expression. Am Rev Respir Dis 1993; 148: 401–6.

135 Adelroth E, Rosenhall L, Johansson S-A, Linden M, Venge P. Inflammatory cells and eosinophil activity in asthmatics investigated by bronchoalveolar lavage. The effects of antiasthmatic treatment with budesonide or terbutaline. Am Rev Respir Dis 1990; 142: 91–9.

136 Van Schayck CP, Dompeling E, Van Herwaarden CLA et al. Bronchodilator treatment in moderate asthma or chronic bronchitis: continuous or on demand? A randomized controlled study. BMJ 1991; 303: 1426–31.

137 Sears MR, Taylor DR, Print CG et al. Regular inhaled beta-agonist treatment in bronchial asthma. Lancet 1990; 336: 1391–6.

138 Crane J, Flatt A, Jackson R et al. Prescribed fenoterol and death from asthma: The New Zealand experience. Lancet 1989; i: 917–22.

139 Sparrow D, O'Connor GT, Rosner B, Demolles D, Weiss ST. A longitudinal study of plasma cortisol concentration and pulmonary function decline in men. Am Rev Respir Dis 1993; 147: 1345–8

KEY POINTS

1   Little is known about the long-term outcome of asthma in adulthood.

2   A better FEV_1 and level of airway hyperresponsiveness in childhood are important factors in determining that an individual patient will outgrow asthma.

3   Persistent wheeze suggests a deterioration of lung function especially in female children with asthma.

4   Disappearance of symptoms in adults does not indicate remission or cure of asthma.

5   Asthma is generally a benign disease with a good prognosis.

6   Delay in institution of anti-inflammatory drugs may result in irreversible damage in the airways.

7   Optimal allergen, environmental and smoke avoidance may, next to optimal anti-inflammatory drugs, alter the course of asthma.

Running an Asthma Service

44

PRIMARY CARE

Mark L. Levy

Asthma care in the community is comprised of three interlinked components: (1) diagnosis, i.e. the initial recognition and application of a disease label for the patient's problem; (2) organization and delivery of ongoing supervision and care, i.e. the maintenance of good health, ideally free from symptoms and attacks; and (3) acute asthma management. The goal should be to make the transition between these areas as seamless as possible. These three facets form the focus for this chapter on primary care of patients with asthma.

DIAGNOSIS

Diagnosis of asthma is the most important task for health professionals in primary care; without the label "asthma" the patient cannot be cared for properly. Diagnosis of asthma in childhood is the main topic for this section because most of the research on asthma diagnosis in primary care has focused upon children. However, a few studies indicate that asthma is under-diagnosed in adults and, although not discussed in depth here, this area is important for future study. Although there is no evidence of long-term positive outcome for children diagnosed and treated early, there is good evidence that undiagnosed asthmatic children are inappropriately treated[1-3] and could benefit substantially from improved management. Children do not outgrow their asthma:[4,5] it goes into remission, hospital admissions are increasing, and there is some evidence that permanent lung damage may result from asthma. Therefore early diagnosis is a major goal for asthma care in the community. In 1978, Speight postulated unacceptable levels of under-diagnosis and under-treatment of childhood asthma,[6] and later confirmed the level of the problem[2] by showing that only a small minority of asthmatic children were actually given a diagnostic label of "asthma". Recent studies of general practice management of asthma continue to demonstrate that asthma is still under-diagnosed in the community.[7]

Levy and Bell identified a particular aspect of poor asthma management in children: a delay in diagnosis of up to 5 years with an average of 16 respiratory consultations before the diagnosis of childhood asthma in primary care.[8] This delay was verified by others.[9–11] In the UK, the delay could possibly be explained by the nature of general practice (National Health Service) in the early 1980s: poor continuity of care, which resulted from mobility of patients coupled with long delays in obtaining past medical records; doctors working in large group practices with patients consulting different doctors each time they attended; and a general reluctance by doctors and patients to use the term "asthma".[12] Lack of awareness of the presenting symptoms (Table 44.1) of asthma could also explain the delayed recognition and under-diagnosis in primary care.[13]

A peer-group audit of asthma diagnosis suggested that there has been a marked improvement in the speed of diagnosis of asthma in general practices in the UK. This audit[18] set out to assess the possible impact of the raised awareness of the presenting features of asthma in childhood, in the mid 1980s, on the diagnosis of childhood asthma. Two cohorts of children born in 1981 and 1986 were simultaneously audited in two self-selected

---

TABLE 44.1: *Some of the symptoms which asthmatic patients present to the general practitioner. Any patient presenting with any of these symptoms on more than three occasions a year should be considered asthmatic until proved otherwise*

Well known
Cough
   "still coughing"
   "coughing for months"
   "no better despite antibiotics"
   "worse when laughing"
   "induced by exercise"
Wheeze
Shortness of breath
Chest tightness

Less well known
Difficulty in sleeping
Spoilt holiday (spent time in hospital)
Chest pain[13]
Vomiting[13–15]
Itching[13,16,17] (children, usually preceding attacks, usually upper body)

groups of doctors responding to a postal invitation: (1) the General Practitioner's in Asthma Group (GPIAG), a UK-based special interest group of general practitioners; 70 out of the membership (at that date) of 300 practices participated (23.3%); and (2) 63 out of a total of 225 general practices in north-west London (28%).

Summary data for these 133 practices is shown in Table 44.2 where: (1) the prevalence of diagnosed asthma in these practices increased from 8.7 to 10.2% in the 1981 and 1986 cohorts respectively; and (2) the average (median) age of diagnosis reduced from 5.7 to 3.2 years from 1981 to 1986 in the two cohorts respectively ($P < 0.001$). There was no difference in the ages diagnosed between the GPIAG and the north-west London practices and therefore this improvement in care was not limited to practices with a special interest in asthma.

Similarly a retrospective study of family doctor records in Ireland of 769 children under 5 years of age found that the mean age of diagnosis is 2.59 years.[19] In addition Barritt and Staples[20] in their second audit, 3 years after introducing the use of a specially designed asthma record card for use in their practice, found that 92% of their asthmatic children were diagnosed within 1 month of their first presentation with respiratory symptoms.

TABLE 44.2: *Asthma audit results autumn 1992: GPIAG and two FHSA districts*

Total number of patients audited	
Born 1981	9 871
Born 1986	10 216
Asthmatics	
Born 1981	974
Born 1986	1 164
Prevalence: median (IQR[a])	
1981	8.7 (4.7–13)
1986	10.2 (5.3–17.6)
Age diagnosed: median (IQR[a])	
Born 1981	5.7 (4.6–7.9)
Born 1986	3.2 (2.8–3.7)
	$P < 0.001$

[a]Inter-quartile ranges.

These data provide evidence of a reduction in the time taken to diagnose asthma, signifying an improvement in asthma care by general practitioners in the UK over the last decade. In effect general practitioners are provided with a target standard for diagnosing childhood asthma, i.e. the majority of children with asthma should be diagnosed before their fourth birthday.

POSSIBLE SOLUTIONS: EARLIER DIAGNOSIS OF ASTHMA

There are many possible reasons for the demonstrated reduction in time to diagnose asthma and these deserve discussion. Increased awareness of asthma and the more unusual presenting features of this condition, following the publication of studies on under-diagnosis and under-treatment, has probably played a major role in earlier diagnosis. In the early 1980s general practitioners were not aware that childhood asthma presents very differently from the pattern taught and seen in hospitals (Table 44.1). It is known now that medical records often provide important clues to the diagnosis[8,21–23] and histories such as "still coughing" or "coughing for months" now alert doctors to the possibility of missed asthma. It is also appreciated that asthma is a chronic condition, characterized by exacerbations of ill health. Children presenting to the doctor with recurrent episodes of respiratory symptoms, often provoked by upper respiratory tract infections, otitis media, exercise or increased allergen levels are regarded as asthmatic until proven otherwise. By maintaining this high level of awareness health professionals suspect asthma in any patient presenting repeatedly with respiratory symptoms, undiagnosed chest pain, disturbed sleep or, more rarely, vomiting or itching.[13]

In childhood, coughing is the commonest symptom while wheezing is a relatively infrequent presenting feature of asthma; in adults, asthma should be suspected if the records indicate frequent consultations for nocturnal respiratory symptoms, particularly following infections and in the absence of a history of smoking. Patients whose past medical record indicates a possible diagnosis of asthma should be recalled to see the doctor or nurse, for confirmation of the diagnosis by taking a detailed history and examination, which should include reversibility tests or daily peak expiratory flow rate (PEFR) diary charts. Prospectively, the diagnosis in childhood could be hastened by numbering recorded respiratory consultations from birth onwards; and because asthmatic children consult more frequently than normal patients[24] any child consulting the doctor more than three times in any one year with respiratory symptoms has asthma until proved otherwise.[13] These principles, aimed at earlier childhood diagnosis, could also be applied to improve the recognition of late-onset or undiagnosed asthma in adults.

ORGANIZATION OF ASTHMA CARE IN THE COMMUNITY

Asthma accounts for a substantial proportion of the workload in primary care. The third (1990/1991) Australian national survey of morbidity in general practice[25] found that respiratory consultations accounted for 23% of patient encounters ($n = 145\ 799$ patient encounters with 495 doctors). Annual asthma consultations as a proportion of all encounters totalled 2.5% in all ages and 7.2% in children ($n = 42\ 131$ patient encounters). The mean weekly incidence in the UK of new episodes of asthma are shown in Fig. 44.1. From these data it is clear that significantly more general practitioners are recording new episodes of asthma, indicating an increased awareness of asthma. Flemming and Crombie[26] confirmed that there were real increases in the age-standardized consulting rates for males and females in the data between the second and third National Morbidity Surveys of primary care in the UK.[27]

Ian Gregg, one of the pioneers of primary care management of asthma asserted that, "Asthma is a disease that should be managed in the community, by primary care physicians and trained asthma nurses with access to secondary and tertiary care for emergencies and guidance on management". In support of this statement, he wrote: "i) a general practitioner can deliver as good, if not better, care than that of an outpatient department or chest clinic where patients often see a succession of junior doctors who may have had little experience in the long term management of asthma;

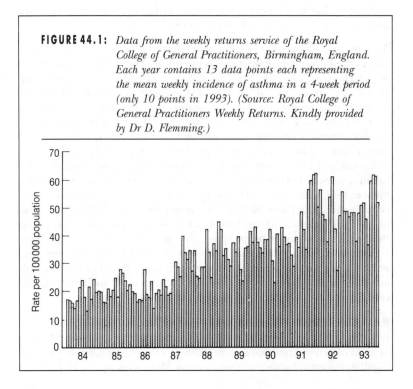

FIGURE 44.1: *Data from the weekly returns service of the Royal College of General Practitioners, Birmingham, England. Each year contains 13 data points each representing the mean weekly incidence of asthma in a 4-week period (only 10 points in 1993). (Source: Royal College of General Practitioners Weekly Returns. Kindly provided by Dr D. Flemming.)*

and ii) the principles of treating asthma are perfectly straightforward and every aspect of its management including diagnosis, assessment and education of patients, embodies those elements of clinical practice which are the most distinctive features of primary medical care".[28] In 1983, Pereira Gray found that over 95% of asthmatic patients were being cared for exclusively by general practitioners.[29] The UK national acute asthma audit estimated that 14.3 per 1000 patients consulted their general practitioner annually for acute asthma, and found that 86% (1546/1805) of these episodes were managed within the community.[30]

Guidelines exist to enable health professionals to select appropriate asthma management and to maintain high standards of care for their patients. Many of these have been prepared mainly by hospital specialists. However, a survey[31] of general practitioner members of the GPIAG found a high level of agreement with the principles of management set out in the first UK guidelines.[32–34] Having made the diagnosis of asthma the main role of the general practitioner and asthma nurse is to enable the asthmatic patient to enjoy life without symptoms or attacks. Patients should be regularly reviewed, two or three times a year in most cases, more or less frequently during the rest of the year depending upon the severity and timing of exacerbations; they should understand clearly how to recognize attacks and know what to do when these occur. In theory this is fine; however, there is evidence of poor adherence to existing guidelines.

An Australian postal survey[35] compared selected general practitioners' self-reported asthma management practices with the Asthma Management Plan of the Thoracic Society of Australia and New Zealand.[36] Their results suggested that most general practitioners in Australia know and practise appropriate asthma management. However, they concluded that there was room for improvement in the understanding of the use of preventive medications and use of crisis planning for severe asthma attacks and lung function measurement. Another study in Wellington, New Zealand,[37] which examined general practitioners' prescriptions for 228 asthmatic children, found a marked deviation from international guidelines on the management of childhood asthma: 84% of the children were prescribed β_2-adrenoceptor agonists; of these, 80% of those under 5 years, and 27% over 5 years of age, received these agents by the oral route. In almost half of the cases these drugs were prescribed on a regular basis, rather than intermittently as instructed by the guidelines. Fifty-two per cent of patients were prescribed some form of anti-inflammatory therapy (inhaled or oral steroids, ketotifen or sodium cromoglycate); only 2% received sodium cromoglycate.

WHAT CAN BE DONE ABOUT NON-ADHERENCE TO GUIDELINES?
In 1983 Colmer and Pereira Gray[38] had the foresight to recognize the value of audit of general practice care in defining current standards of care and highlighting areas for further investigation. More recently, the Department

of General Practice at the University of Leicester[39] has produced an extremely practical paper suggesting structured asthma audit. The idea is that practices select quality criteria for providing asthma care and divide these into three groups: "must do", "should do" and "could do" criteria (Table 44.3). Practices interested in adopting this approach may wish to amend or add to some of them. This methodology for structuring general practitioners' approach to the provision of care could be complemented by the use of asthma record cards[40] in the patient's medical notes.

ORGANIZATION OF CARE: ASTHMA CLINICS IN GENERAL PRACTICE

The following section contains extracts from another book,[13] with permission, and the reader is referred to this text for further information and examples of practice protocols.

Reports of nurse-run asthma clinics in the UK started appearing during the late 1980s, largely modelled upon similar care for the care of diabetic patients in the community. In 1990 general practitioners in the UK National Health Service had new contracts imposed upon them by the Government. As a result the numbers of trained asthma nurses soared, many of whom completed the Stratford-Upon-Avon distance learning course,[41] pioneered by Greta Barnes, a practice nurse, and Dr Robert Pearson, a general practitioner. Unfortunately, in April 1993, the general practitioners' remuneration for these clinics was substantially reduced with the possible result that research in this field will probably dwindle. The relatively few published studies on the efficacy of these UK-based nurse-run clinics have shown increased patient satisfaction, reduced doctor consultations in favour of nurse consultations and reduced episodes of acute asthma and home visits for these episodes, as well as reduced feelings of stigma,[42-44] which had been previously recognised.[45] Ian Charlton, who has also led the way in setting up nurse-run asthma clinics[44,46,47] found a marked drop in doctor consultations, out of hours visits and acute attacks of asthma during the 6 months after setting up a nurse-run asthma clinic in one practice.[46] It is unclear which aspect of these clinics brought about the changes and this is an area for further study; increased levels of education, organized follow-up and monitoring are possibilities. A controlled trial of the effect of asthma education did not improve morbidity or self-management of asthma.[48]

Usherwood and Barber's[49] doctor-run mini-clinic reduced their patients' school absence and the need for home visits for acute asthma; however their workload increased markedly. Barritt's 6-year audit of asthma care in general practice showed an initial improvement in care and outcome; however this was not enhanced significantly by the subsequent introduction of a nurse-run asthma clinic.[50]

Inappropriate self-management of acute asthma may be the reason for increased or prolonged morbidity due to asthma. A controlled study (23 active patients; 19 controls) that included monthly interviews of the effects

TABLE 44.3: *Three suggested levels of criteria for asthma audit. (From Ref. 39 with permission)*

"Must do" criteria

1. Diagnosed asthmatics will be recorded in the practice asthma register
2. The diagnosis has been confirmed
3. The records show that at least annually an assessment is made of the level of control of asthma by assessment of nocturnal and daytime symptoms and limitations on activities
4. The records show that at least annually the daily dose of bronchodilator has been checked and that those patients who require more than one dose daily are also receiving prophylactic medication
5. The records show that the patient's smoking habits are recorded at least annually, and for children, the smoking habits of adults in the household are recorded and advice given
6. The records show that at least annually, the inhaler technique has been checked

"Should do" criteria

7. The records show that at least annually asthmatic patients and/or their carer(s) have received education about asthma management
8. Each patient will be reviewed at regular intervals agreed with the patient, but not exceeding 12 months
9. The records show that at least annually assessment has been made about the role of precipitating factors including drugs
10. At least annually the patient's need and suitability for a peak flow meter has been assessed and a meter prescribed if required and the patient is able to use it
11. The target (ideal) peak flow should be recorded annually

"Could do" criteria

12. Information about complications of asthma including deaths, acute admissions to hospital and severe attacks is recorded on the asthma register
13. The annual assessment of the patient has been undertaken either by a hospital physician, a general practitioner or a nurse who has received additional training about asthma.

of asthma education by a trained asthma nurse found that self-treatment of episodes of asthma was significantly better in those patients attending the nurse-run clinic (89 out of 138, 65% episodes of uncontrolled asthma) compared to the control group (58 out of 113, 51% episodes) ($P < 0.05$). This study[51] utilized self-management plans that had been modified from Beasley *et al.*[52] The original plan had been modified[13] by drawing action lines on the PEFR charts, thus making it easier for patients to see when their readings were dropping and approaching the zones where action was needed (Fig. 44.2).

PRACTICALITIES OF NURSE-RUN ASTHMA CLINICS

Certain issues need to be addressed before a practice decides to include a nurse to care for the needs of asthma patients in the practice. Training

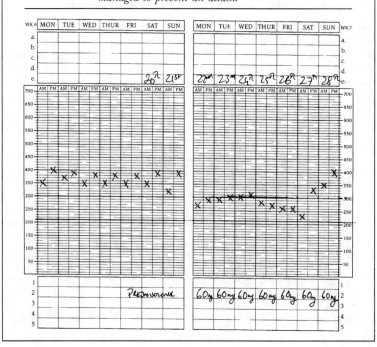

FIGURE 44.2: *This patient's PEFR was fairly constant between 350 and 400 l min⁻¹ when she became unwell with influenza on the 20th of the month. Her readings soon dropped below her 75% action line, and because her asthma is usually very bad under these circumstances, she commenced a short course of oral prednisolone and managed to prevent an attack.*

is essential but costly and the practice needs to be committed to fully support nurses by assisting them to learn quickly and effectively. They will need considerable "hands-on" experience and the doctors will need to help by allowing them to sit-in on consultations with asthmatic patients as often as possible. They will need some protected time to learn and later to run the clinic. Once they are trained, they will need to work autonomously, within the limits of their ability; however they will also need to feel reassured that an experienced doctor is available on site to assist them when they have difficulty in managing a patient. Clear guidelines need to be agreed within the practice regarding when the nurse should seek the doctor's opinion.[13] In addition, they will soon become as expert (if not more so) in the management of asthma than the doctors in the practice and they should be respected for this, rather than "shouted down" as is the experience of many nurses having attained considerable experience in this field. The level to which the nurse is involved in the four aspects of care (Table 44.4) will obviously vary according to expertise and experience. Barnes describes three levels of nurse involvement.[41] With minimum involvement, they will record PEFR, demonstrate and check inhaler technique and set up an asthma register. With medium involvement, they will carry out reversibility and exercise tests, teach home monitoring and educate patients. With maximum involvement, they will have considerable autonomy in management and will quite likely be involved in treating acute episodes, particularly if the doctor is temporarily unavailable.

In an emergency the nurse needs to know how to deal with a severe attack if patients arrive at the surgery when the doctor is out on calls. As this is an emergency, it is not being suggested that acute asthma management should be delegated to the practice nurse. The fact is that once the practice becomes known amongst its asthmatic patients as "asthma aware", they may choose to arrive at the surgery instead of emergency departments. In this event, the staff need to know what to do while contacting the doctor. It is

---

TABLE 44.4: *Tasks for the doctor or nurse running asthma clinics*

Diagnosis of patients (case finding)

Monitoring and review at regular intervals
  Inhaler technique, adherence to drug regimens

Education of patients
  Self-management plans

Management of acute attacks

recommended that the practice develops a protocol for the management of acute asthma, perhaps modelled upon those already available.[36,53-61.]

Asthma clinics in general practice do not necessarily mean that a specific slot of time is allocated to asthma care, although this is probably the preferred method ensuring protected time for the doctor or nurse running the clinic. In practice, many asthma nurses work according to appointment systems, allowing for flexible accommodation to the needs of their patients. What is important, however, is that there is a protocol for asthma care in force within the practice. In addition there needs to be a system for ensuring that comprehensive care is provided that covers all aspects of asthma care, not necessarily at each appointment. One group[62] developed a very elegant method of educating asthma patients over a period of time by using a checklist of items (e.g. inhaler technique, self-management, effect on life-style) that were each covered in time slots of about 6 min on different occasions. A specially designed record card[50] helped to ensure comprehensive coverage of the practice protocol; another group in Tayside developed a rubber stamp for use in the records (Fig. 44.3). Figure 44.4 is an example of a record card that could be used for asthma care in general practice.

FIGURE 44.3: *The Core Information Recording Stamp for use in the record when patients consult the nurse or doctor. (Source: Tayside Asthma Group, with permission.)*

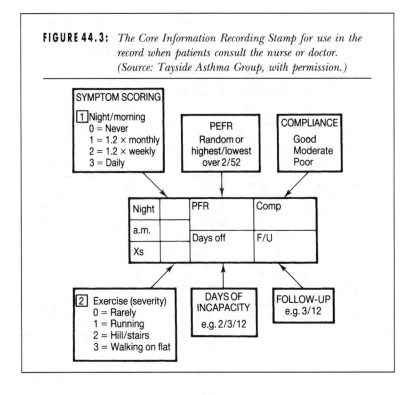

FIGURE 44.4: *The Asthma Training Centre Asthma Clinic Record card, designed to fold into the general practitioner's records. (Source: The Asthma Training Centre, Stratford-Upon-Avon, with permission.)*

ASTHMA TREATMENT *(include oral & inhaled steroid therapy)*
Previous ....
....
....
Current ....
....

Other medical conditions & drug therapy
....
....
....

INVESTIGATIONS
Height: cms   ft. ins.
Weight: Kg.   st. lbs.
Smoking (Y or N)
If Y, how many?
If ever, when stopped
  and how many?
Blood pressure (adults only) ....
Urine (if patient taking oral steroids): Glu .... Prot ......
If requested: Hb ☐☐ · ☐   Skin tests ....
CXR ....
EDUCATION
Present level of understanding: High/Med/Low
Booklet given (Y or N)   ☐

COMMENTS AND PLANS
....
....
....

FOR LUNG FUNCTION TESTS SEE INSIDE

ASTHMA CLINIC
Name ....   Sex ....
Address ....   Marital status ....
....   Dr's name ....
Date of birth ....

INITIAL ASSESSMENT
    Date ....

ASTHMATIC HISTORY
Year of onset of symptoms
Year of asthma diagnosis
Age at asthma diagnosis
Family History ....
Occupational history ....
Eczema *(please put Y or N as appropriate in all following boxes)*
Hay Fever
Urticaria
Wheezy Bronchitis
Drug allergies
Specify ....

PROVOCATION   **PRESENT SYMPTOMS**
Exercise   Respiratory infection
Cold air   Sputum
Respiratory infection   Cough
Emotion   If Y, specify Night or Day ....
Cough/sneeze   Wheezy
Laugh   If Y specify worse time ....
Work related   ....
Animals
Seasonal element   **ASTHMA STATE**
Specify season .... Persistent
....   Episodic
                               CONTINUE ON BACK OF CARD
© *Bridge House Medical Centre, Stratford-upon-Avon*

Date	Time	Specify assessment, peripeol & election exercise test, etc.	Weight PEF Meas. Pred.	Inhalation Technique	Comp	SYMPTOMS (Always check symptoms against the following list: cough, respiratory infection, bronchitis, sputum, exercise-induced asthma. Wheeziness worse at night and first thing in the morning?) HOME CHARTING RESULTS, EDUCATION, PLANS & THERAPY.	APPT.

There is opportunity for further development of a team approach to asthma care. General practitioners should not be afraid to involve nursing colleagues in the day-to-day management and follow-up of patients with asthma.

MANAGEMENT OF ACUTE ASTHMA

Studies investigating asthma deaths clearly demonstrate a failure on the part of patients, their families and their doctors to recognize the danger signs of asthma and to take early and appropriate action.[63,64] Despite this well-known danger, health professionals are extremely resistant to change their management of asthma from being reactive to a more pro-active approach. Two recent innovations are possible means to this end: self-management plans and nurse-run asthma clinics. Self-management plans are of practical help in management and education of patients and their families and, most importantly, in recognizing the danger signs preceding asthma attacks. Asthma clinics run by appropriately trained practice nurses offer an opportunity to implement the use of self-management plans.

SELF-MANAGEMENT PLANS

Basic to self-management is the availability of accurate,[65,66] cheap, robust, portable peak flow meters and an individually constructed education plan.

First, patients need to be taught to recognize the signs of uncontrolled or acute asthma (self-diagnosis). Asthmatic subjects may recognize acute asthma by increase in symptoms, decreased efficacy of their medication, or by objective measurement of their PEFR. Use of PEFR action levels or zones for recognizing uncontrolled asthma and subsequent adjustment of therapy[24,47,52,55] has become accepted by many health professionals and there is evidence of successful outcome of asthma care resulting from their use.[67]

Next, patients need to understand clearly what action needs to be taken when their asthma goes out of control. The medical records should reflect that the patient has been advised how to recognize the danger signs indicating asthma attacks, what to do under these circumstances and when to seek medical help (Table 44.5).

It is important to consider each patient's individual clinical history when advising on self-management plans, which should be tailored to their own particular circumstances. Some patients experience attacks of asthma without a corresponding drop in PEFR, and these people are best advised to adjust their medication at the onset of symptoms or during exposure to known trigger factors. For the majority of patients, however, a PEFR management plan is better because it is easier to take action based on actual figures. These plans are discussed in detail elsewhere (see Chapter 24) but

TABLE 44.5: *Essential information that should be made available to all patients and parents of asthmatic children*

Patients should know that their relief medication (e.g. inhaled β_2 bronchodilators can, and indeed must, be used in high doses in emergency situations

Patients should know that their relief medication should work immediately, and this improvement should last at least 4 hours. If neither of these apply, they should seek immediate assistance from their GP and if this is not possible they should go directly to the nearest emergency treatment facility

Patients should record their PEFR in the event of symptoms of asthma and they should know what to do at various action levels of PEFR, e.g. if the patient's usual best PEFR is $400\,l\,min^{-1}$ they should increase their inhaled steroids if the readings are tending to drop towards $320\,l\,min^{-1}$ (80%); they should initiate a short course of oral steroids if the readings are dropping towards $240\,l\,min^{-1}$ (60%); and should seek immediate attention or call an ambulance if the readings are dropping towards $120\,l\,min^{-1}$ (33%)

Relative as opposed to absolute PEFR values act as clues to uncontrolled asthma. If patients' readings are tending to go down or are increasing in variation from morning to evening or from day to day, urgent action needs to be taken according to a previously agreed plan with their health professional adviser

are mentioned here because the primary care team have a major role to play in their implementation. There are a number of practical points to note in connection with the use of PEFR management plans.

(1) Rather than rely entirely on single readings or predicted values, it is better to use a series of readings, when the patient is well, to determine the target "best" PEFR.

(2) Different meters may give different results, even if they are of the same manufacturer type. Therefore the patient's own PEFR readings (preferably using their PEFR diary card) should always be used in making management decisions.

(3) Depending upon which scales are used on PEFR meters, there is a risk of underestimating the readings in the higher ranges (e.g. in tall people or adults) and of overestimating those in patients in the lower ranges of PEFR.[65,66] It is also important to realize that PEFR action levels selected at the time of diagnosing the patient's asthma will need to be adjusted upwards as the patient improves with therapy.

Once patients become familiar with the treatment protocol, they feel in control and are in a position to decide at what stage extra medication or indeed help should be sought. Figure 44.5 shows a PEFR chart with action lines drawn at 75% and 50% of the patients best PEFR. It was easy for her to decide to initiate a short course of oral prednisolone when she developed influenza, which resulted in a drop in her PEFR.

HOW ARE WE MANAGING ACUTE ASTHMA NOW?

A UK national asthma attack audit, which aimed to determine how acute asthma is currently managed, found that the majority of asthma attacks

FIGURE 44.5: *Peak flow chart with action lines drawn on it to help the patient recognize episodes of uncontrolled asthma.*

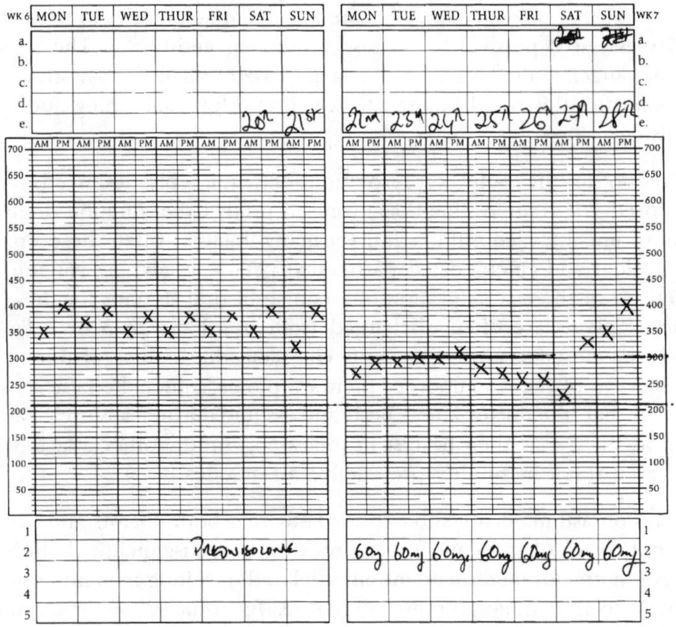

were managed by general practitioners in the community.[30] Asthma attacks were defined as "an episode of respiratory symptoms which prompts an urgent consultation with a doctor, is of sufficient severity to prevent the patient working or attending school or performing domestic duties or playing, and results in increased use of anti-asthma medication". This national study by the GPIAG provided useful data to enable comparison of actual care of acute asthma in the community with nationally accepted guidelines available at the time in the UK.[32–34] Overall the standard of clinical care provided by the 218 participating practices was judged less than acceptable. In particular, the use of systemic steroids by general practitioners in patients breathless and distressed (52% patients) and too breathless to talk (85% patients) and the use of nebulized bronchodilator therapy in those breathless and distressed (54%) and those patients who were too breathless to talk (82%) was unacceptably low according to guidelines. Poor adherence to guidelines on asthma care is not limited to primary care: a recent interface audit of the provision of care in three district general hospitals outside London found that only 35% of 85 patients deemed severe enough to require nebulized bronchodilators were prescribed systemic steroids.[68]

POSSIBLE SOLUTIONS: MANAGEMENT OF ACUTE ASTHMA

The first step is, as in the case of other chronic diseases, to reduce the possibility of patients developing acute asthma attacks. The aim is to reduce the overall levels of asthma morbidity.[69–71] The scheme suggested in Table 44.3 may help towards this end by raising the quality of care within the practice. Next, management of acute asthma attacks needs to be assessed and reassessed, possibly by means of ongoing audit.[13,30,39] The national asthma attack audit[30] has provided some baseline data for assessing acute asthma care; this could be used to set criteria for establishing audit standards.

Follow-up to the point of resolution of acute episodes needs to be improved.[13] It is impossible for anyone to predict the duration of an episode of uncontrolled asthma and yet many doctors (often those working in accident and emergency departments) persist in advising patients prospectively of the exact duration of a course of oral steroids for these episodes. Patients are often discharged from hospital with 5 or 6 days of prednisolone tablets: these patients complete the "course of treatment", irrespective of the resolution of their symptoms, under the false sense of security that "the doctor knows best" and assume the attack is over. Patients such as these may then be lost to follow-up, until another attack, which may even result in another preventable asthma death.

Studies on asthma death show consistently that both doctors and patients are not aware of the danger signs of asthma. Consequently, help is not sought in time or medical attention is delayed, resulting in many avoidable asthma deaths. Although most asthma deaths occur in the community, a significant proportion of these had been recently treated in hospital for an acute attack.[64] It seems sensible therefore to intensify follow-up of asthmatic patients in the community, during the few weeks following an acute attack. Without objective measurements, the timing of resolution of an attack is guesswork and it is logical to make more use of daily PEFR diary charts to help practitioners as well as patients decide when the danger has passed and whether or not to step down the treatment (Fig. 44.6).

Primary care physicians are in a unique position to influence outcome for patients following an acute attack, whether this has been treated in the community or hospital emergency room. An appointment with the general practitioner or nurse within 24 hours of the initial presentation with uncontrolled asthma with subsequent frequent review (daily if necessary) over the next few weeks should be included as routine in any practice protocols for acute asthma.[13] In this way patients can be monitored very closely during the vulnerable post-attack period and are given the opportunity to learn first hand how to manage their next attack. The doctor–

FIGURE 44.6: *This 47-year-old woman's first ever asthma attack took about 10 days to resolve. After she was returned to the care of the general practitioner (a few hours after the onset of the attack) daily management decisions were assisted greatly by the PEFR readings.*

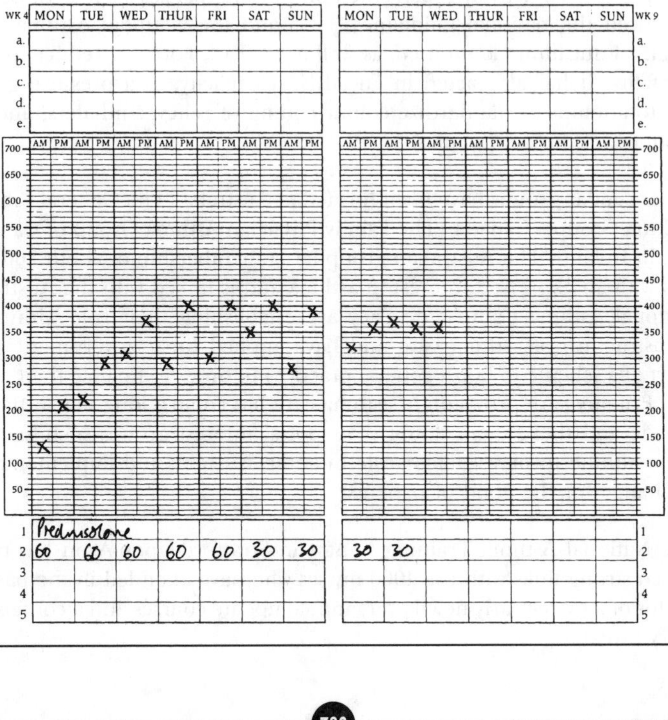

patient (or nurse–patient) relationship of trust and understanding is therefore enhanced and it is more likely that the patient will return for routine follow-up and review as requested.

SPECIAL INTEREST GROUPS

Groups of health professionals with a special interest in asthma exist to share experience, audit and research to improve the management of asthma in the community. In 1987, six general practitioners formed the GPIAG in the UK (500 members, 1993). In 1995, the Eighth Annual Scientific Meeting was held and, as in the past, the programme consisted almost entirely of peer-reviewed presentations from within the membership. The last two meetings established a tradition of inviting practice nurses and hospital specialist speakers (on the conference theme of the year) in order to facilitate better understanding and cooperation across the hospital–community interface of care. The Research Unit of the GPIAG was formed in 1991 and has been invaluable in facilitating and conducting high-quality research on behalf of the group. In addition to its academic activities, the group has been actively represented on working parties such as those that produced the national guidelines,[32–34,53] and the National Asthma Campaign's Education Committee, as well as its Task Force to reduce asthma mortality. It has also acted in an advisory capacity, as a pressure group, e.g. to attempt to standardize colour coding of reliever inhalers, and has produced reports on clinics.[30,31,72–76]

Other similar groups have been formed in Australia (The General Practice Asthma Group), Canada (The Family Physician Asthma Group of Canada) and in Ireland. The Australian group has a membership of about 200 doctors with an expressed interest in asthma and is linked with the Australian National Asthma Campaign. They are establishing their role within the infrastructure of asthma care and have applied for a government grant (part of a scheme to boost general practice) in order to finance their activities. Primary care provision of asthma care has come a long way in the last decade and there is no doubt that special interest groups such as these will continue to play a major role in audit, research and implementation of change for the good of patients.

The National Asthma Training Centre in Stratford-Upon-Avon has maintained strong links with the 4000 nurses who have attended in the past, by means of a twice-yearly newsletter, annual update courses and a conference every 2 years.

THE FUTURE

The problem of facilitating health professionals' adherence to guidelines remains a major challenge for all right across the interface of health care. Most patients with asthma are treated in the community and it seems that most acute attacks are managed exclusively by general practitioners.[30] Hospital specialists are involved with care of those asthmatic patients who are either so severe that their general practitioners have sought assistance or admitted for acute episodes of asthma. This "distorted view" from the hospital perhaps leads to the erroneous, but often quoted, conclusion that general practitioners cannot manage asthma. On the other hand, general practitioners see their patients discharged too early[77] or even denied hospital admission when this is clearly in keeping with guidelines (see Fig. 44.6). Both parties, together with the patients, want the same thing – to reduce asthma attacks and morbidity. If preventable asthma deaths are caused by problems across the interface, the way forward is to try and smooth out the transition between the hospital and community when this is required.

REFERENCES

1   Hill R, Williams J, Britton J, Tattersfield A. Can morbidity associated with untreated asthma in primary schools be reduced? A controlled intervention study. *BMJ* 1991; 303: 1169–74.

2   Speight ANP, Lee DA, Hey EN. Underdiagnosis and undertreatment of asthma in childhood. *BMJ* 1983; 286: 1256–8.

3   Anderson HR, Bailey PA, Cooper JS, Palmer JC, West S. Influence of morbidity illness label and social, family and health service factors on drug treatment of childhood asthma. *Lancet* 1981; ii: 1030–2.

4   Gerritsen J. *Prognosis of Childhood Asthma.* Assen, The Netherlands: Van Gorcum, 1989.

5   Kelly WJW, Hudson I, Phelan PD, Pain MCF, Olinsky A. Childhood asthma in adult life: a further study at 28 yrs of life. *BMJ* 1987; 294: 1059–62.

6   Speight ANP. Is childhood asthma being underdiagnosed and undertreated. *BMJ* 1978; 2: 331–2.

7   Tse M, Cooper C, Bridges-Webb C, Bauman A. Asthma in general practice. Opportunities for recognition and management. *Aust Fam Physician* 1993; 22: 736–41.

8   Levy M, Bell L. General practice audit of asthma in childhood. *BMJ* 1984; 289: 1115–6.

9   Tudor-Hart J. Wheezing in young children: problems of measurement and management. *J R Coll Gen Pract* 1986; 36: 78–81.

10   Jones A, Sykes A. The effect of symptom presentation on delay in asthma diagnosis in children. *Respir Med* 1990; 84: 139–42.

11   Charlton I, Jones K, Bain J. Delay in diagnosis of childhood asthma and its influence on respiratory consultation rates. *Arch Dis Child* 1993; 66: 633–5.

12   Levy M. Delay in diagnosing asthma – is the nature of general practice to blame? (editorial). *J R Coll Gen Pract* 1986; 36: 52–3.

13   Levy M, Hilston S. *Asthma in Practice.* London: Royal College of General Practitioners, 1993.

14   Osundwa VM, Dawod ST. Vomiting as the main presenting symptom of acute asthma. *Acta Paediatr Scand* 1993; 78: 968–70.

15   Boggs PB. Asthma and bronchitis. *J Allergy Clin Immunol* 1993; 84: 1055–8.

16   Orr AW. Prodromal itching in asthma. *J R Coll Gen Pract* 1979; 29: 287–8.

17   David TJ, Wybrew M, Hennessen U. Prodromal itching in childhood asthma. *Lancet* 1984; i: 154–5.

18   General Practitioners in Asthma Group (GPIAG), Levy ML. An audit of diagnosis of asthma in children (abstract). *Thorax* 1993; 48: 451–2.

19   Steen HJ, Stewart MC, McAuley D, Parker S. Changing trends in approach to wheezy children by family doctors. *Ir Med J* 1993; 85: 59–60.

20   Barrit PW, Staples E. Measuring success in asthma care: a repeat audit. *Br J Gen Pract* 1991; 41: 232–6.

21   Den BJH. Prevalence and management of asthma in children under 16 in one practice. *BMJ* 1986; 292: 175–6.

22   Toop LJ. Active approach to recognising asthma in general practice. *BMJ* 1985; 290: 1629–31.

23   Neville RG, Bryce FP, Robertson FM, Crombie IK, Clark RA. Diagnosis and treatment of asthma in children: usefulness of a review of medical records. *Br J Gen Pract* 1992; 42: 501–3.

24   Levy M, Parmar M, Coetzee D, Duffy SW. Respiratory consultations in asthmatic compared with non-asthmatic children in general practice. *BMJ* 1985; 291: 29–30.

25   Bridges-Webb C, Britt H, Miles D *et al.* Morbidity and treatment in general practice in Australia 1990–1991. *Med J Aust* 1992; 157: S1–S56.

26   Flemming DM, Crombie DL. Prevalence of asthma and hay fever in England and Wales. *BMJ* 1987; 294: 279–83.

27   Royal College of General Practitioners, Office of Population Censuses and Surveys and Department of Health and Social Security. *Morbidity Statistics from General Practice 1981–82. Third National Study.* London: HMSO, 1986.

28 Gregg I. The importance of asthma to the general practitioner. *Practitioner* 1987; 231: 471-7.

29 Pereira Gray D. Asthma in general practice. *Practitioner* 1983; 227: 196-201.

30 Neville RG, Clark RC, Hoskins G, Smith B. National asthma attack audit 1991–2. General Practitioners in Asthma Group. *BMJ* 1993; 306: 559-62.

31 Hilston SR, GPs in Asthma Group. General practice survey of acceptability and impact of the 1990 guidelines for management of adult asthma (abstract). *Thorax* 1991; 46: 741 p.

32 Warner JO, Gotz M, Landau LI *et al.* Management of asthma: a consensus statement. *Arch Dis Child* 1993; 64: 1065-79.

33 British Thoracic Society. Guidelines for the management of asthma in adults: 1. Chronic persistent asthma. *BMJ* 1990; 301: 651-3.

34 British Thoracic Society. Guidelines of asthma in adults: II. Acute severe asthma. *BMJ* 1990; 301: 797-800.

35 Tse M, Bauman A, Bridges-Webb C. Asthma management in general practice. *Aust Fam Physician* 1991; 20: 1085, 1088-9, 1092.

36 Woolcock A, Rubinfeld AR, Seale JP *et al.* Thoracic Society of Australia and New Zealand. Asthma management plan, 1989. *Med J Aust* 1993; 151: 650-3.

37 Thompson R, Dixon F, Watt J, Crane J, Beasley R, Burgess C. Prescribing for childhood asthma in the Wellington area: comparison with international guidelines. *N Z Med J* 1993; 106: 81-3.

38 Colmer LJ, Pereira Gray DJ. An audit of the care of asthma in a general practice. *Practitioner* 1983; 227: 271-9.

39 Eli Lilly National Clinical Audit Centre. Monitoring Asthma (working draft). Full report available from Department of General Practice, University of Leicester, Gwendolien Road, Leicester LE5 4PW.

40 Barritt P, Staples EB. Measuring success in asthma care: a repeat audit. *Br J Gen Pract* 1991; 41: 232-6.

41 Asthma Training Centre. Asthma Training Centre (ATC)/Royal College of General Practitioners (RCGP) Asthma Diploma Programme. Straford-Upon-Avon: Stratford Repro, 1993.

42 Charlton I, Charlton G, Broomfield J, Campbell M. An evaluation of a nurse-run asthma clinic in general practice using an attitudes and morbidity questionnaire. *Fam Pract* 1992; 9: 154-60.

43 Charlton I, Charlton G, Broomfield J, Mullee MA. Audit of the effect of a nurse run asthma clinic on workload and patient morbidity in a general practice. *Br J Gen Pract* 1991; 41: 227-31.

44 Charlton I. Asthma clinics: audit. *Practitioner* 1989; 233: 1522-3.

45 Sibbald B. Patient self care in acute asthma. *Thorax* 1989; 44: 97-101.

46 Charlton I. Asthma clinics: setting up. *Practitioner* 1989; 233: 1359–60.

47 Charlton I. Asthma clinics: how to run one. *Practitioner* 1989; 233: 1440–5.

48 Hilton S, Sibbald B, Anderson HR, Freeling P. Controlled evaluation of the effects of patient education on asthma morbidity in general practice. *Lancet* 1986; i: 26–9.

49 Usherwood TP, Barber JH. Audit of process and outcome in a mini-clinic for children with asthma. *Fam Pract* 1988; 5: 289–93.

50 Barritt PW. Repeated asthma audits in family practice (abstract). *Asthma Gen Pract* 1993; 2: 12.

51 Levy M, Hayward SA, Jordan M, Golden G. A nurse-run asthma clinic in general practice: guided self-management. *Am Rev Respir Dis* 1993; 147(suppl): A587.

52 Beasley R, Cushley M, Holgate ST. A self management plan in the treatment of adult asthma. *Thorax* 1989; 44: 200–4.

53 Statement by the British Thoracic Society, The British Paediatric Association, the Research Unit of the Royal College of Physicians of London, the Kings Fund Centre, the National Asthma Campaign, the Royal College of General Practitioners, the General Practitioners in Asthma Group, the British Association of Accident and Emergency Medicine and the British Paediatric Respiratory Group following a meeting at the Royal College of Physicians, London on the 4th and 5th June 1992. Guidelines for the Management of Asthma. *Thorax* 1993; 48(suppl): S1–S24.

54 Gibson PG, Talbot PI, Hancock J, Hensley MJ. A prospective audit of asthma management following emergency asthma treatment at a teaching hospital. *Med J Aust* 1993; 158: 775–8.

55 International Consensus Report on Diagnosis and Treatment of Asthma. National Heart, Lung, and Blood Institute, National Institutes of Health, Bethesda, Maryland 20892. Publication no. 92-3091, March 1992. *Eur Respir J* 1993; 5: 601–41.

56 Mitchell EA. Consensus on acute asthma management in children. Ad Hoc Paediatric Group. *N Z Med J* 1993; 105: 353–5.

57 Davies DP. Asthma: a follow up statement from an international paediatric asthma consensus group. *Arch Dis Child* 1993; 67: 1059.

58 Levison H. Canadian consensus on the treatment of asthma in children. Toronto, September, 1990. *Can Med Assoc J* 1993; 145: 1449–55.

59 van der Laag J, van Aalderen WM, Duiverman EJ, van Essen-Zandvliet EE, Nagelkerke AF, van Nierop JC. Asthma in children; consensus by pediatric pulmonologists on long-term treatment. II. Treatment (Dutch). *Ned Tijdsc Geneesk* 1993; 135: 2319–23.

60 Anonymous. Management of childhood and adolescent asthma – 1991 consensus. South African Childhood Asthma Working Group. *South Afr Med J* 1991; 81: 38–41.

61 Janson-Bjerklie S. Assessment and management of adults with asthma: guidelines for nurse practitioners. *Nurse Practitioner Forum* 1993; 4: 23–9.

62 Crosby FRG, Whyte E, Ogston S *et al.* Improving asthma control in general practice (abstract). *Thorax* 1989; 44: 344.

63 British Thoracic Association. Death from asthma in two regions of England. *BMJ* 1982; 285: 1251–5.

64 Anonymous. Proceedings of the Asthma Mortality Task Force. November 13–16, 1986, Bethesda, Maryland. *J Allergy Clin Immunol* 1987; 80: 361–514.

65 Burge PS. Peak flow measurement. *Thorax* 1992; 47: 903.

66 Miller MR, Dickinson SA, Hitchings DR. The accuracy of portable peak flow meters. *Thorax* 1992; 47: 904–9.

67 Beasley R, D'Souza W, Te Karu H *et al.* Trial of an asthma action plan in the Maori community of the Wairarapa. *N Z Med J* 1993; 106: 336–8.

68 Levy ML, Robb M, Bradley JL, Winter RJD. Presentation and self management in acute asthma: a prospective study in two districts (abstract). *Thorax* 1993; 48: 460–1.

69 Horn CR, Cochrane GM. An audit of morbidity associated with chronic asthma in general practice. *Respir Med* 1989; 83: 71–5.

70 Turner-Warwick M. Nocturnal asthma: a study in general practice. *J R Coll Gen Pract* 1989; 39: 239–43.

71 Gellert AR, Gellert SL, Iliffe SR. Prevalence and management of asthma in a London inner city general practice. *Br J Gen Pract* 1990; 40: 197–201.

72 Jones K. Impact of an interest in asthma on prescribing costs in general practice. *Quality in Health Care* 1992; 1: 110–3.

73 Hilton S. An audit of inhaler technique among asthma patients of 34 general practitioners. *Br J Gen Pract* 1990; 40: 505–6.

74 Levy M. The General Practitioners in Asthma Group. *Primary Health Care Management* 1993; 3: 10.

75 Levy M. The General Practitioners in Asthma Group: a personal report by the outgoing chairman. *Asthma in General Practice* 1993; 2: 2.

76 Levy M. A survey of FHSA practice regarding asthma clinics (letter). *BMJ* 1993; 306: 521.

77 Bucknall CE, Robertson C, Moran F, Stevenson RD. Management of asthma in hospital: a prospective audit. *BMJ* 1988; 296: 1637–9.

USEFUL ADDRESSES

General Practitioners in Asthma Group (GPIAG), Secretariat, The Medical Marketing Interface, Bath Brewery, Toll Bridge Road, Bath BA1 7DE, UK. Telephone: 01225 858880. Fax: 01225 859977.

National Asthma Training Centre, Winton House, Church Street, Stratford-Upon-Avon, Warwickshire CV37 6HB, UK. Telephone: 01789 296974. Fax: 01789 261027.

National Asthma Campaign, Providence House, Providence Place, London N1 0NT, UK. Telephone: 0171 226 2260. Fax: 0171 704 0740. Helpline: 01345 01 02 03.

The General Practice Asthma Group (GPAG), Dr Ian Charlton, 7 Tilba Street, Kincumber, NSW 2251, Australia. Telephone: 043 692444. Fax: 043 631664.

Family Physician Asthma Group Of Canada, Dr Mervyn Dean, West Coast Medical Center, 3 Church Street, Corner Brook, NF, Canada A2H 2Z4. Telephone: 709 634 2818. Fax: 709 634 5649.

Dr R. Spellman, Health Centre, Bridgtown, Wexford, Ireland. Telephone: (053) 35296.

KEY POINTS

1	The majority of children with asthma should be diagnosed before their fourth birthday.
2	Any child consulting the doctor more than three times in any one year with respiratory symptoms has asthma until proved otherwise.

45

HOSPITAL PRACTICE

Jeff Garrett

The rationale behind a coordinated team approach to the hospital-based management of asthma is principally a philosophical one, since the approach has never been validated by a well-conducted trial. Although patients who attend a specialist asthma clinic have less subsequent morbidity than those randomized to usual follow-up,[1-3] it is difficult to evaluate which aspect of care contributed most to the patients' outcome, namely education, peak flow monitoring, self-management plans, evaluation by an asthma specialist, the prescription of inhaled steroids or even that it may have been due to attendance (selection) bias.[4] On the other hand, it is probably beyond the scope of any hospital-based approach to medical management to substantially influence factors that are directly under the control of the patient (illness behaviour or health care utilization), dependent upon the organization and quality of medical care within the community[5] or to social, economic or psychological problems[5-7] (Fig. 45.1). Such factors are likely to have a greater influence on the patient's subsequent outcome than anything that can be achieved by way of a time-limited intervention from a team of hospital-based health care professionals. As such, the goals of hospital-based asthma management should be realistic, relevant and reinforced over time. The aims should be to maximize the potential of the resources available with the hope of reducing morbidity of asthma by improving patients' knowledge and self-management skills while maintaining continuity of care and good communication between all health professionals involved in the care of patients (Fig. 45.2). This chapter takes a pragmatic look at the development of a hospital-based approach to asthma management. However, once experience is gained utilizing a multidisciplinary model of hospital-based care, the model needs to evolve into the community, specifically where good-quality primary health care is deficient in order to improve standards of care for all people with asthma.

The hospital-based coordinated team approach to asthma care has usually arisen out of the needs of patients and/or their caregivers and in response to either high or escalating admission rates. Since a variety of personnel are available within hospitals, multidisciplinary models of health care are

FIGURE 45.1: *Interacting factors contributing to hospital admissions for asthma.*

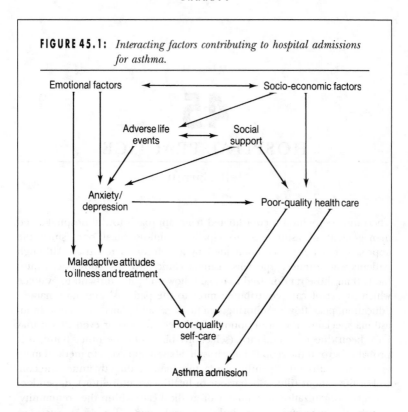

able to evolve easily. However, because of the nature of hospitals, patients admitted with asthma may be managed by a variety of services, e.g. emergency room (ER), general medical team, respiratory medical team, general medical or asthma outpatient clinic, and intensive care unit (ICU). Whether to admit people with asthma to a specialist respiratory unit or to a general medical ward will usually be determined by local policy, although the outcome is superior for patients admitted to respiratory wards.[3,8,9] As a rule, patients should be admitted to the care of the same team under whom they were previously admitted or whose care they have been under in the outpatient clinic. Where general medical wards exist, it remains logical to improve levels of care by introducing guidelines and by allowing members of the asthma management team to contribute to the management of patients admitted to a general medical ward. This approach allows medical and nursing staff working outside of specialist respiratory services to attain and then maintain expertise in asthma management. The development of an asthma management team also enables the philosophy of good asthma management to be endorsed, gives asthma an elevated status, ensures the maintenance of good practice and increases the potential for continuity of care.

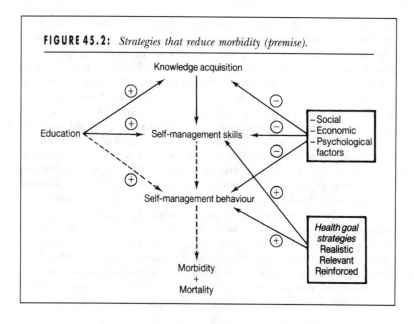

FIGURE 45.2: *Strategies that reduce morbidity (premise).*

THE ASTHMA MANAGEMENT TEAM

A variety of health professionals have skills that may be useful to an asthma management team (Table 45.1). Key people include: the physician(s), paediatrician(s) and the asthma educator. The asthma educator is more often a nurse, particularly in the hospital setting where they are closely involved with coordination of patient care and frequently function in a patient advocacy role. However, there is no reason why a physiotherapist

TABLE 45.1: *Asthma management team personnel*

Physician
Paediatrician
Asthma educator
Physiotherapist
Clinical psychologist
Dietitian
Community health worker
Pharmacist
Social worker

or pharmacist cannot perform the role of asthma educator. The final decision will often depend on the availability of skilled health care workers who not only have the appropriate background of training in asthma but also the necessary management, education, communication and inter-personal skills needed to successfully fill the position. The final make-up of the team and its size should be influenced by the size of the hospital or by the number of people with asthma requiring hospital care and thus more comprehensive management. In small hospitals, the asthma educator's role may merge with that of a traditional nursing role, or may be combined with a nurse specialist role in another condition (e.g. rehabilitation, cystic fibrosis or diabetes). Alternatively, the role may evolve into the community. In New Zealand, the asthma educator has occasionally been funded by both hospital and lay asthma society with responsibilities to both employers. Conversely, in large hospitals or hospitals serving a large population, the asthma educator's role may evolve into that of a liaison one, providing the link between hospital-based care and community services (general practitioner, social worker, asthma society, etc.). Subsequent aims may include establishing education programmes for health care workers (either within or outside of the hospital) and the coordination of activities of workers involved in asthma management.

Before the final composition of the team is established and before its goals are defined, it is important to define the socio-demographic and clinical characteristics of the population of asthmatic patients who are to be targeted. For example, if the group responsible for the majority of asthma admissions are from ethnic minority groups, are socially and economically disadvantaged or disenfranchised, then attendance at a hospital-based clinic, even if it is free, is likely to be poor.[10–12] The decision to admit a patient with asthma to hospital is subject to three factors: illness behaviour, the organization of the medical care system and medical practice.[13] Whilst a common goal is to reduce the patient's severity of asthma by appropriate use of medication and avoidance of triggers (with the hope of reducing the need for subsequent hospitalization), factors outside the control of the hospital-based asthma team may influence the final results of the intervention. Poor organization of after-hours care, poor quality or absent primary health care[15,16] or financial barriers to primary health care[17] may lead to patients becoming more dependent on ER services and which tend to be used later in the course of an attack than do community-based services.[18,19] This trend is particularly strong for patients living in disadvantaged neighbourhoods, and more so if they belong to ethnic minority groups.[5] As such, and if the hospital serves a population with a high density of ethnic minority groups, then community health workers from the same ethnic background will be essential to the asthma team. If primary health care is either of poor quality or insufficient to meet the needs of the community, then the service developed within the hospital will need to subsequently evolve into the community.[20]

A physician and a paediatrician should both be associated with the programme and should either be trained in respiratory medicine or have a subspecialty interest in the area. They should ensure that good standards of asthma care are attained and subsequently maintained. Guidelines based on a variety of consensus statements on asthma management[21–24] should be introduced to medical wards, ERs, ICUs and outpatient clinics. In association with the asthma educator, the physician/paediatrician should develop education programmes for both patients and health care workers. A large number of education programmes are in existence[25,26] and should be adapted to meet the needs of patients using the service, and which accommodate the modern approach to asthma management. In general, patients from disadvantaged communities with little formal education, in our experience, need only a basic understanding of the pathophysiology of asthma and of how asthma medicines work, and rather more time spent on basic survival skills. An individualized self-management plan explaining when and how to seek medical attention when confronted with worsening asthma, and how to access community support networks if social isolation exists, are needed. Physicians should develop links with the community through lay organizations such as the asthma society and through meetings with primary health care physicians that include postgraduate workshops. They should also develop a database to monitor in their hospital(s): ICU admissions,[27] hospital admissions and re-admissions,[28] ER attendances and re-attendances including relapse rate within 1 week,[29] outpatient clinic attendances including origin of referral[4,10] and non-attendance rates for asthma clinic to help evaluate the overall success of the team. They should, of course, manage asthmatic patients admitted to the ward under their care, consult on asthmatic patients admitted to other wards and review their patients in specialist asthma clinics.

Asthma educators should develop asthma education programmes for both patients and health care professionals. Ideally they should visit all patients who are admitted to hospital with an acute exacerbation of asthma. They should visit all patients on the ward who are to be referred to the asthma clinic for follow-up and all patients already under their care within the asthma clinic. They should ensure that all patients discharged from hospital have a basic understanding of asthma management, including how and when to monitor peak flow rates, and how to use a basic self-management plan. A basic self-management plan should include what asthma treatment to use and when, how to predict the onset of an attack and what to do if confronted with an attack. They should also ensure that the patient can satisfactorily use the inhaler device prescribed. They may advise the general medical team as to which patients should be followed up within the specialist asthma clinic, and they may share follow-up on some patients with the general medical team. They may seek to follow up some patients in their own homes or workplace. They see all patients who require asthma clinic follow-up in association with the physician or paediatrician.

The physiotherapist (physical therapist) is a health professional experienced in managing acute exacerbations of asthma, helping the patient to reduce the work of breathing by teaching relaxation techniques and breathing control and to improve the pattern of breathing. Whilst vigorous mucociliary clearance techniques such as percussion should be discouraged during the acute phase, the physiotherapist can teach the patient self-management techniques to assist in removal of mucous plugs when they occur, particularly in conjunction with nebulization.[30] The forced expiration-technique, which uses breathing control and "huffing",[31] has been noted to be beneficial in patients with bronchopulmonary suppuration[32,33] and is helpful in reducing the tendency to bronchospasm, which can accompany coughing. For the above reasons, it is beneficial to involve the physiotherapist early in the management of an acute exacerbation of asthma, whether it be on the medical ward or in the ER. Physiotherapy can play an important role in managing patients with factitious asthma, hyperventilation syndrome[34] and in those who exhibit panic at the time of acute exacerbations of asthma. The physiotherapist visiting the medical ward can also check on inhaler technique, ensure nebulizers are being properly administered, perform spirometry and reinforce the message of good management by the asthma management team.

Psychosocial factors (recent bereavement, loss of employment, marriage break-up, psychiatric illness) have consistently been associated with an increased risk of mortality, severe life-threatening attacks and morbidity.[7,35–38] Anyone involved in asthma management will be aware of the importance of psychological factors in preventing patients from gaining control over their asthma. Clinical psychologists improve the ability of the asthma management team to evaluate the psychological dimension and, where appropriate, apply psychological treatments. This is invariably a very sensitive component of care. The value of working closely with a clinical psychologist with whom the asthma team develops a trust cannot be overstated.[39] Both denial and, conversely, over-anxiety have been associated with an increased risk of morbidity and may benefit from psychological intervention.[40] The personalities of some patients are incompatible with chronic illness and its management or contribute to psychosomatic exacerbations of symptoms.[41] Some patients may not respond to education about self-management because of psychological problems, which the clinical psychologist can assess, treat or advise the asthma team with regard to future management.

Whilst the contribution food allergy and, to a lesser extent, chemical sensitivity makes to poorly controlled or severe asthma is relatively small in our experience, there is some evidence to suggest otherwise.[42,43] If patients are concerned about the possibility of a food allergy, it is important to take this seriously and to assess by way of a double-blind exclusion diet, which can be overseen by a dietitian.[44] None of our patients who underwent a double-blind exclusion diet were found to be allergic to dairy, wheat or beef products. Detailed "laboratory" assessment of possible chemical sensitivity is beyond the scope of most asthma teams,[45] but preservative-free (particularly metabisulphite-free) diets should be available to patients who have a clear history of chemical sensitivity.

Pharmacists may contribute to asthma management.[46,47] Their depth of knowledge of asthma medicines can be useful to the asthma team and the principles of good asthma management are more likely to be reinforced through retail pharmacies if a pharmacist in the region has taken an active interest in asthma management.

COMPONENTS OF SERVICE

EMERGENCY ROOM
A tendency for patients to become more dependent on the ER for the management of acute exacerbations of asthma appears to be happening worldwide, particularly amongst the poor.[48-50] As a result, there is a tendency for care to become fragmented and for the patient's primary physician, if they have one, to underestimate the severity of the asthma if they are not consulted at the time of an acute attack. Further, ER physicians tend to look at managing the acute attack rather than considering the attack in the context of the patient's overall management. Therefore, it should be the aim of the ER to maintain good communication with the patient's usual health care provider. One way of achieving this is to have a triplicated health record of the attack within the ER, one copy being kept in the ER, one handed to the patient and the other posted to their usual doctor. Patients fulfilling the criteria for asthma clinic referral (Table 45.2) should be referred. Since patients referred to outpatient clinics from the ER are traditionally poor attenders[10,51] then, if possible, a member of the asthma management team should see the patient at the time of their ER attendance, or very soon after discharge.

MEDICAL WARD
Whilst assessment and comprehensive management of the acute attack remains the principal aim of the medical ward, a hospital admission provides the opportunity to improve upon the patient's knowledge of asthma and asthma medicines and to improve upon self-management skills. Whilst the medical ward may not be an ideal environment for health education, after a significant life event most patients are keen to learn more about their asthma and how to manage it better. Therefore, they may benefit from a referral to the asthma educator, respiratory physiotherapist or ward-based physiotherapist. Prior to discharge all patients should have basic skills taught, including how to identify early symptoms of worsening asthma, and when and how to access the medical care system if confronted with another attack. They should also be discharged with a peak flow meter

TABLE 45.2: *Guidelines for specialist consultation. (Adapted from Ref. 22)*

Adults	Children
A life-threatening asthma attack	A life-threatening asthma attack
Poor self-management ability requiring intensive education	Poor parental asthma management skills requiring intensive education
Uncertain diagnosis	Uncertain diagnosis, atypical symptoms or signs
Patient not responding to therapy	Patient not responding to therapy
Unexpected side-effects from medications	Unexpected side-effects from medications
Requiring frequent courses or continuous oral corticosteroids	Requiring frequent courses or continuous oral corticosteroids
Requiring >1600 µg daily of inhaled corticosteroid	Requiring >600 µg daily in children less than 5 years and >1000 µg daily in older children or adolescents or toddler or infant needing continuous inhaled steroid
Occupational asthma	
Abnormal lung function tests despite apparently well-controlled symptoms	
Previous admission to hospital or frequent ER attendance within the previous year	Previous admission to hospital or frequent ER attendance within the previous year

and diary, a written individualized self-management plan, inhaler(s) (with good technique) and should be followed up in either the asthma clinic or outpatient clinic within 2–4 weeks of discharge, since relapses occur more often within 1 month. Patients should be referred to the asthma specialist as an inpatient if their course is complicated or their response to therapy unusual. Patients from an ethnic minority group should ideally be referred to a community health worker of the same ethnicity.

INTENSIVE CARE UNIT

Principal aims of therapy include assessment and comprehensive management of acute, severe, life-threatening attacks of asthma. Ideally, all patients admitted to ICU should see an asthma specialist during their hospital stay and all patients should be referred to the asthma clinic for follow-up within 2 weeks of discharge. Patients who have suffered an exacerbation of asthma sufficiently severe to warrant ICU admission are at greatest risk of either mortality[37,52,53] or further severe attacks of asthma.[4] Follow-up should be intensive until good control has been achieved, and knowledge regarding appropriate self-management obtained and observed to have been put into practice, without the need for hospital admission for 2 years (since subsequent ICU admissions or death are most likely to occur in this time).[4] Since these patients are more likely to have psychosocial problems[38,39] then they may benefit particularly from a multidisciplinary approach to care.

ASTHMA CLINIC

Patients should be followed within the outpatient clinic until satisfactory control of asthma has been obtained and self-management skills learnt. The exact timing of discharge is dependent on the quality of primary health care available to the patient and whether or not there is an ongoing need for ER attendance or hospital admission. Those patients who require continuous oral corticosteroids or an inhaled corticosteroid dose of >1600 μg daily in adults, >1000 μg daily in older children or adolescents and >600 μg daily in children under 5 years should continue to be followed in the clinic (Table 45.2). Patients and their primary care physician should be informed of the need to refer back to the asthma clinic should good control not be maintained. Some patients may have difficulty obtaining permission from their workplace to attend an asthma clinic.[53] If they reside in areas where unemployment is high they may be afraid to admit to a medical condition that is sufficiently severe to warrant outpatient clinic attendance. If this is the case, then evening clinics may need to be introduced. Patients from lower socio-economic group neighbourhoods or who are from an ethnic minority group have a poorer attendance rate at asthma clinic.[10,11] In this instance new strategies of health care may need to be developed. The development of a community-based asthma education centre[19] run by an asthma educator and community health workers, in association with hospital-based and ambulatory asthma clinics, within a community of 167 000 that was defined as having the highest medical and social need in New Zealand was associated with a two-fold increase in prescription of inhaled steroids and a 67% reduction in asthma admissions (and which are now 30% below the national average (Fig. 45.3)). Whilst we remain unsure as to which component contributed most to this downward trend, the services developed were established to meet those needs defined by our epidemiological studies. In the final analysis, it is not so much which component of care is most important to overall management, but rather that a low-cost multidisciplinary approach to asthma care has been shown to be successful.

SUMMARY

A hospital-based approach to asthma management must be realistic in the goals it establishes for itself. For knowledge and self-management skills to be acquired during an admission to hospital or referral to an asthma clinic, then the educational message must be realistic, relevant and consistently reinforced. Because social, economic and psychological factors have a negative impact on our ability to teach these strategies (Fig. 45.2) then a multidisciplinary team is required. This allows a more consistent approach to medical care to be introduced and leads to the establishment of continuity of care. Due to the newer patterns of health care that have developed, then the traditional doctor–patient relationship is being replaced by short-term encounters with numerous specialists and other health workers.[55] The asthma management team must aim to overcome this tendency by limiting

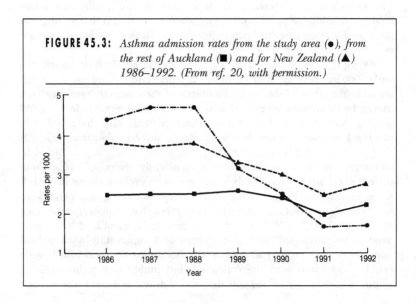

FIGURE 45.3: *Asthma admission rates from the study area (●), from the rest of Auckland (■) and for New Zealand (▲) 1986–1992. (From ref. 20, with permission.)*

the number of team members involved with an individual's care and by providing continuity of care by visiting and assisting with management when patients are admitted under other services.

Illness behaviour is more likely to be influenced over time. Since it is unrealistic of hospital-based asthma teams to manage patients over a prolonged period of time, then the strategies need to be moved out into the community and to be reinforced by primary health care physicians. Where primary health care is deficient, then improvement in access to ambulatory care and in the quality of such care can lead to fewer hospitalizations among both medically indigent and non-indigent persons with asthma.[56] Community-based education and support centres may complement the care offered by primary health care physicians in disadvantaged neighbourhoods and may be helpful in either establishing education to improve self-management skills or in reinforcing that which has been instituted whilst the patient was in hospital.[20,57]

ACKNOWLEDGEMENT

The author would like to acknowledge the contributions of Ms Kathy McGregor (Asthma Nurse Manager), Pam Young (Physiotherapist), Grant Taylor (Clinical Psychologist) and John Kolbe to this chapter.

REFERENCES

1 Mayo PH, Richman J, Harris HW. Results of a program to reduce admissions for adult asthma. *Ann Intern Med* 1990; 112: 864–71.

2 Zeiger RS, Heller S, Mellon MH, Wald J, Falkoff R, Schatz M. Facilitated referral to asthma specialist reduces relapse in asthma emergency room visits. *J Allergy Clin Immunol* 1991; 87: 1160–8.

3 Bucknall CE, Moran F, Robertson C, Stevenson RD. Differences in hospital asthma management. *Lancet* 1988; i: 748–50.

4 Kolbe J, Every S, O'Hagen A, Richards G, Garrett J, Rea HH. Outcome following a severe life threatening attack of asthma: influence of asthma clinic. *Aust N Z J Med* 1990; 20(suppl 1): 515.

5 Garrett JE, Mulder J, Wong-Toi H. Reasons for racial differences in A & E attendance rates for asthma. *N Z Med J* 1989; 102: 121–4.

6 Wissow LS, Gittelsohn AM, Szklo M, Starfield B, Mussman M. Poverty, race and hospitalisation for childhood asthma. *Am J Public Health* 1988; 78: 777–82.

7 Sibbald B, White P, Pharaoh C, Freeling P, Anderson HR. Relationship between psycho-social factors and asthma morbidity. *Fam Pract* 1988; 5: 12–7.

8 Baldwin DR, Ormerod LP, Mackay AD, Stableforth DE. Changes in hospital management of acute severe asthma by thoracic and general physicians in Birmingham and Manchester during 1978 and 1985. *Thorax* 1990; 45: 130–4.

9 Osman J, Ormerod LP, Stableforth DE. Management of acute asthma: a survey of hospital practice and comparison between thoracic and general physicians in Birmingham and Manchester. *Br J Dis Chest* 1987; 81: 232–42.

10 McClellan VE, Garrett JE. Attendance failure at Middlemore Hospital asthma clinic. *N Z Med J* 1989; 102: 211–3.

11 Oppenheim GL, Bergman MD, English EC. Failed appointments: a review. *J Fam Pract* 1979; 8: 789–91.

12 Deyo RA, Thomas SI. Dropouts and broken appointments. *Med Care* 1980; 18: 1146–57.

13 Anderson HR. The epidemiological value of hospital diagnostic data. In: Bennett AE (ed) *Recent Advances in Community Medicine.* Edinburgh: Churchill Livingstone, 1978: 175–94.

14 Karetsky MS. Asthma in the South Bronx: clinical and epidemiological characteristics. *J Allergy Clin Immunol* 1977; 60: 383–90.

15 Garrett JE, Mulder J, Veale A. Characteristics of asthmatics using an urban accident and emergency department. *N Z Med J* 1988; 101: 359–61.

16 Schneider KC, Dove HG. High uses of VA emergency room facilities: Are outpatients abusing the system or is the system abusing them? *Inquiry* 1983; XX: 57–64.

17 Weiss KB, Gerger PJ, Hodgson TA. An economic evaluation of asthma in the United States. *N Engl J Med* 1992; 326: 862–6.

18 Dalby BCS, Farrer JA, Harvey PW. Casualty activity analysis coding and computing. *Comput Program Biomed* 1974; 3: 254–66.

19 Torrens PR, Yedvab DG. Variations among emergency room populations: a comparison of four hospitals in New York City. *Med Care* 1970; 8: 60–75.

20 Garrett JE, Mercer Fenwick J, Taylor G, Mitchell E, Stewart J, Rea H. Prospective controlled evaluation of the effect of a community-based education centre in a multiracial working class neighbourhood. *Thorax* 1994; 49: 976–83.

21 National Asthma Education Program. Guidelines for the Diagnosis and Managementt of Asthma. *National Institutes of Health Publication No. 91-3042,* 1991.

22 Guidelines on the Management of Asthma. *Thorax* 1993; 48(suppl): S1–24.

23 Asthma Management Handbook. National Asthma Campaign Limited (Australia), 1993.

24 Thoracic Society of Australia and New Zealand 1990. Consensus of Asthma: Asthma Management Plan 1989. *N Z Med J* 1990; 103: 16–8.

25 Wigal JK, Creer TL, Kutses H, Lewis P. A critique of 19 self-management programs for childhood asthma I. Development and evaluation of the programs. *Paediatr Asthma Allergy Immunol* 1990; 4: 17–39.

26 Creer TL, Wigal JK, Kutses H, Lewis P. A critique of 19 self management programs for childhood asthma II. Comments regarding the scientific merit of the programs. *Paediatr Asthma Allergy Immunol* 1990; 4: 41–55.

27 Richards GN, Kolbe J, Fenwick J, Rea HH. Demographic characteristics of severe life threatening asthma: comparison with asthma deaths. *Thorax* 1993; 48: 1105–9.

28 Mitchell EA, Elliot RB. Hospital admissions for asthma in children: a prospective study. *N Z Med J* 1981; 94: 331–4.

29 Rea HH, Garrett JE, Mulder J, Chapman KR, White JG, Rebuck AS. Emergency room care of asthmatics: a comparison between Auckland and Toronto. *Ann Allergy* 1991; 66: 48–52.

30 Sutton PP, Gemmell HG, Innes N *et al.* Use of nebulised saline and nebulised terbutaline as an adjunct to chest physiotherapy. *Thorax* 1988; 43: 57–60.

31 Thompson BJ. The physiotherapists' role in rehabilitation of the asthmatic. *N Z J Physiotherapy* 1973; 4: 11–6.

32 Pryor JA, Webber BA. An evaluation of the forced expiration technique as an adjunct to postural drainage. *Physiotherapy* 1979; 65: 304–7.

33 Pryor JA, Webber BA, Hodson ME, Batten JC. Evaluation of the forced expiration technique as an adjunct to postural drainage in the treatment of cystic fibrosis. *BMJ* 1979; 2: 417–8.

34 Howell JBL. Behavioural breathlessness. *Thorax* 1990; 45: 287–92.

35 Cohen SI. Psychological factors. In: Clark TJH, Goodfrey S (eds) *Asthma.* London: Chapman & Hall, 1977: 177–89.

36 Knapp PH, Mathe AA. Psychophysiologic aspects of bronchial asthma. In: Weiss EB, Segal MS, Stein M (eds) *Bronchial Asthma: Mechanisms and Therapeutics*, 2nd edn. Boston: Little, Brown, 1976: 914–31.

37 Rea HH, Scragg R, Jackson R, Beaglehole R, Fenwick J, Sutherland PC. A case-control study of deaths from asthma. *Thorax* 1986; 41: 833–9.

38 Gordon GMF, Ayres JG. Psychiatric and social aspects of brittle asthma. *Thorax* 1993; 48: 501–5.

39 Miklich DR. Health psychology practice with asthmatics. *Professional Psychology* 1979; 10: 580–8.

40 Yellowlees PM, Ruffin RE. Psychological defenses and coping styles in patients following a life-threatening attack of asthma. *Chest* 1989; 95: 1298–303.

41 Kinsman RA, Luparello T, O'Banion K, Spector S. Multidimensional analysis of the subjective symptomotology of asthma. *Psychosom Med* 1973; 35: 250–67.

42 Taylor SL, Bush RK, Selner JC *et al.* Sensitivity to sulfited foods among sulfite-sensitive subjects with asthma. *J Allergy Clin Immunol* 1988; 81: 1159–67.

43 Stevenson DD, Simon RA, Lumry WR, Mathison DA. Adverse reactions to tartrazine. *J Allergy Clin Immunol* 1986; 78: 182–90.

44 Bernstein M, Day JH, Welsh A. Double-blind food challenge in the diagnosis of food sensitivity in the adult. *J Allergy Clin Immunol* 1980; 70: 205–10.

45 Simon RA. Sulfite challenge for the diagnosis of sensitivity. *Allergy Proc* 1989; 10: 357–62.

46 Self T. The value of demonstration and role of the pharmacist in teaching the correct use of pressurised bronchodilators. *Can Med Assoc J* 1983; 128: 129–31.

47 Smith NA. The potential for pharmacists as patient educators in asthma. *Aust J Hosp Pharm* 1988; 18: 244–8.

48 Garrett JE, Mulder J, Veale A. Trends in the use of an urban accident and emergency department by asthmatics. *N Z Med J* 1988; 101: 253–5.

49 Halfon N, Newacheek PW. Childhood asthma and poverty: differential impacts and utilization of health services. *Paediatrics* 1993; 91: 56–61.

50 Strachan DP, Anderson HR. Trends in hospital admission rates for asthma in children. *BMJ* 1992; 304: 819–20.

51 Straus JH, Tangerose S, Charney E. Referrals from an emergency room to primary care practices of an urban hospital. *Am J Public Health* 1983; 73: 57–61.

52 Sears MR, Rea HH. Patients at risk for dying of asthma: New Zealand experience. *J Allergy Clin Immunol* 1987; 80: 477–80.

53 Strunk RC. Identification of the fatality-prone subject with asthma. *J Allergy Clin Immunol* 1989; 83: 477–85.

54 McClellan VE, Garrett JE. Asthma and the employment experience. *N Z Med J* 1990; 103: 399–401.

55 Korsch BM, Gozzi EK, Francis V. Gaps in doctor–patient communication. I. Doctor–patient interaction and patient satisfaction. *Pediatrics* 1968; 42: 855–71.

56 Hughes DM, McLeod M, Garner B, Goldbloom RM. Controlled trial of a home and ambulatory program for asthmatic children. *Pediatrics* 1991; 87: 54–61.

57 Clark NM, Feldman CH, Evans D, Levison MJ, Wasilewski Y, Mellins RB. The impact of health education on frequency and cost of health care use by low income children with asthma. *J Allergy Clin Immunol* 1986; 78: 108–15.

KEY POINTS

1 There are many interacting factors that contribute to hospital admissions for asthma and which include: psychosocial, quality of health care and self-care, ethnicity and economic factors.

2 To accommodate these factors the hospital approach to management must be multidisciplinary, well coordinated and of good quality.

3 Strategies that are likely to reduce morbidity must be implemented and this includes education to improve self-management skills.

46

AUDIT IN ASTHMA

Brian D.W. Harrison

INTRODUCTION

QUALITY ASSURANCE AND MEDICAL AUDIT

High quality in medicine, like pornography, is difficult to define but easy to recognize. It includes good professional performance, efficient use of resources, minimal risk to the patient and patient satisfaction.[1] High-quality medicine meets the users' needs effectively, efficiently and expertly and conforms to the users' requirements.[1] The most important users are the patients, but other users in this context include medical colleagues, other health care professionals and funders.

Quality is assessed under the three headings of *structure, process* and *outcome.* Structure comprises the basic resources of personnel, buildings and equipment. Process describes the procedures and processes involved in the use of the structure to achieve the desired outcome. Outcome is the effect of managing the condition, hopefully the restoration of the patient to as good health as possible in terms of the disease and the actual or potential side-effects and complications of the treatment.

Quality assurance is the process of recognizing and maintaining high-quality services and identifying areas of less than optimal quality and then taking steps to improve those aspects of poor quality. *Medical audit* is quality assurance applied to medicine. Both medical audit and quality assurance have four key elements that are encapsulated in the feedback loop[1] (Fig. 46.1).

Effective medical audit will reveal high-quality practices and high-quality outcomes. High quality when recognized requires praise and preservation. Most time in medical audit involves the detection, analysis and correction of deficiencies in care, but forgetting to praise and preserve the existing high quality risks the audit process degenerating into a "witch hunt" with loss of the support and collaboration of those most required to correct the deficiencies and improve the service.

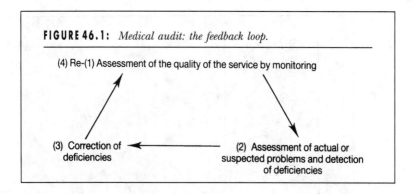

FIGURE 46.1: *Medical audit: the feedback loop.*

(4) Re-(1) Assessment of the quality of the service by monitoring

(3) Correction of deficiencies

(2) Assessment of actual or suspected problems and detection of deficiencies

ASTHMA AUDIT: THE FEEDBACK LOOP

ASSESSING THE QUALITY OF THE SERVICE BY MONITORING

There are four methods of monitoring asthma care, which are listed in Table 46.1.

Sentinel-case audit and criterion-based audit require high-quality medical record systems and medical notes, though formats designed to assist the clerking of patients admitted with asthma or to provide a summary of their admission to hospital are available.[2]

Sentinal-case Audit

Sentinel-case audit involves an in-depth analysis of particularly serious departures from the norm, such as death from asthma. Between 1975 and 1993 there have been ten studies of asthma deaths[3-12] (Table 46.2). These

TABLE 46.1: *Methods of monitoring asthma care*

Sentinel-case audit: variation from the norm in structure, process or outcome

Criterion-based audit
  Departure from specified criteria (of structure, process or outcome)
  Comparison of care by different groups of physicians

Patient satisfaction surveys

Peer review

TABLE 46.2: *Studies of asthma deaths: potentially preventable factors. (From Ref. 13 with permission).*

Year	Authors	Under-treatment with steroids	Inappropriate therapy	Under-estimation of condition by doctor	Under-estimation of condition by patient	Failure to recognize or treat months or weeks prior to acute attack	Psychosocial factors
1975	Cochrane GM, Clark TJH[3]	*	*	*	*		
1976	Macdonald JB, Seaton A, Williams DA[4]	*	*	*	*	*	
1976	Macdonald JB, Macdonald ET, Seaton A, Williams DA[5]	*	*	*	*	*	
1979	Bateman JRM, Clarke SW[6]	*			*	*	
1980	Ormerod LP, Stableforth DE[7]	*	*	*		*	

1982 British Thoracic Association[8]	*			*	*	*
1985 Sears MR, Rea HH, Beaglehole RG et al.[9]	*	*	*	*	*	*
1987 Eason J, Markowe HLJ[10]	*		*	*	*	
1993 Wareham NJ, Harrison BDW, Jenkins PF, Nicholls J, Stableforth DE[11]	*	*	*	*	*	*
1993 Somerville M, Ryland I, Williams EMI, Pearson MG[12]	*	*	*	*	*	

studies have highlighted the same potentially preventable factors that repeatedly contributed to deaths during this period of almost two decades.

The two largest studies in Britain and New Zealand revealed potentially preventable factors in over 80% of the deaths. Nine of these studies have assessed the quality of the service by monitoring and have detected deficiencies in care, but have not progressed any further around the audit loop. One study is attempting to close the audit loop by reporting the results to the local medical community and then continuing the confidential enquiry into asthma deaths on an annual basis.[11] This enquiry is analogous to the report on British Confidential Enquiry into Maternal Deaths in the UK[14] and the Confidential Enquiry into Perioperative Death.[15]

The methodology developed from the earlier British[8] and New Zealand[9] asthma death studies has several unique features[11] (Tables 46.3 and 46.4) and has been adopted by the UK Asthma Task Force of the National Asthma Campaign for ongoing confidential enquiries into asthma deaths in Scotland, Wales and four regions of England.

Criterion-based Audit

Departure from specified criteria (Table 46.5) Frustration with the findings during the 1970s and 1980s that the same preventable factors were repeatedly found in surveys of asthma deaths led to the development during 1989 and 1990 of the British Guidelines on the Management of Asthma in Adults.[16,17] These have already been revised and updated.[18] One of the original intentions of these guidelines was that they should be used for auditing care of patients with asthma. Judged by the number of papers presented at British Thoracic Society meetings in the last 3 years, this intention of using the criteria in the National Guidelines has certainly been achieved.

Lim and Harrison[2] using an earlier but similar set of local asthma management guidelines have shown that the standards recommended in such guidelines are achievable, at least on a specialist respiratory medical ward. The three pages of the history and summary proforma are reproduced in Fig. 46.2. To summarize the results: 78 patients were admitted, mainly from their general practitioner or via the accident and emergency department, with a small number admitting themselves directly to the ward. Peak expiratory flow (PEF) had been measured before admission to the ward in 76% of the patients and systemic steroids given to 74%. Full objective assessment of the severity of asthma (heart rate, systolic paradox, respiratory rate, PEF and arterial blood gases) on admission was recorded in all but one patient and all patients received systemic steroid and high-dose nebulized bronchodilator therapy. Problems with the checking of inhaler technique before discharge and of discharging patients before their PEF variability had fallen to the agreed level were identified at the first audit.

A further audit,[19] this time of care of asthma by general practitioners, has also used the criteria published in the British National Guidelines. Good

TABLE 46.3: *Unique features of the confidential enquiry into asthma deaths*

Continuing enquiry

Multidisciplinary team (Table 46.4)

Quality of care compared against recommendations in the British Thoracic Society Guidelines[15–17]

Results are fed back to the local medical community, i.e. general practitioners and hospital physicians, annually

TABLE 46.4: *Confidential enquiry into asthma deaths: personnel and their roles*

General practitioner	Reviews patient's GP notes and interviews GP
Specialist respiratory nurse	Interviews next-of-kin with agreement of GP
Public health physician	Chairs review meeting
Consultant chest physician	Coordinates enquiry, reviews hospital notes (if any)
Local chest physician	Reviews hospital notes (if any)
Research assistant	Collects names from death register, requests GP and hospital notes, administers enquiry

practical assessment of the severity of the attack was reflected by the patient's state of breathlessness or distress being recorded in 97% and PEF recorded in 82%. However, the treatment of the attack was much less satisfactory, with only 56% of those having an attack severe enough to prevent normal activities being given systemic steroids and only 31% nebulized bronchodilators. Furthermore, maintenance treatment was not increased or stepped up according to the recommendations in the guidelines in over 75% of the patients already taking anti-inflammatory medication.

TABLE 46.5: *Criterion-based audit. (From Ref. 13 with permission)*

1. Define and agree the standard (e.g. protocols of management)

2. Measure the performance against the standard

3. Agree changes to improve the performance against the standard

4. Repeat audit to ensure the changes have had the desired and intended effect

Comparison of care of patients admitted to hospital with asthma by different groups of physicians (Fig. 46.3) Since 1987 several British studies[20–23] have shown that the processes and outcomes of care of patients with asthma are significantly better for those looked after by teams including a specialist respiratory physician than by teams containing no such specialist. In Glasgow, patients looked after by teams including a specialist respiratory physician had significantly fewer symptoms during the first 2 weeks following discharge from hospital and significantly fewer re-admissions for asthma within 1 year of discharge.[21] Repeat studies in Birmingham, Manchester and Glasgow[22,24] have shown significant improvements in management of asthma following the feedback of results from the initial surveys and further education. This improvement applies to care provided by both respiratory physicians and by general physicians, though respiratory physicians continue to provide a higher-quality service.

A more recent multicentre audit of hospital inpatient asthma care in 36 British hospitals undertaken by the British Thoracic Society, Royal College of Physicians and National Asthma Campaign has confirmed that patients are significantly more likely to be managed in a way that matches up to the National Guidelines if they are admitted under the care of a respiratory physician[25] (Table 46.6). This assessment of asthma care of 766 patients was conducted in August and September 1990 immediately before publication of the British Guidelines. The audit was repeated in the same months a year later when the Guidelines had been widely disseminated and discussed.

The second audit, involving 900 patients, showed there had been no significant improvement in any of the variables relating to process and outcome of asthma management, but the marked differences between the management provided by specialist and non-specialist physicians persisted (M. G. Pearson, personal communication).

These audits have highlighted differences in the quality of care received by patients admitted with asthma under the care of specialist respiratory physicians and their teams and by general physicians. They also show that when deficiencies in care and problems are demonstrated improvements can be made, but the care provided by general physicians has in no study risen to the higher quality of care provided by respiratory physicians, even when district protocols have been formulated and locally agreed.

Patient Satisfaction Surveys

Little has been published in this area in the field of asthma management. Such surveys enquire into how satisfied patients are with their outpatient or inpatient care. They can include specific questions about, for example, the acceptability, painfulness or otherwise of arterial blood sampling, or about aspects of treatment such as waiting times or drug therapy. They can also, more importantly, question the well-being and overall function of the patient with asthma.

One survey sponsored by the National Asthma Campaign asked 1490 patients what they expected of their asthma care; 94% opted for care under a respiratory physician or asthma specialist rather than a general physician (National Asthma Campaign, personal communication).

Patient satisfaction surveys have tended to concentrate on the hotel aspects of care. Whilst these are clearly not unimportant, such relatively simplistic surveys must not be allowed to proliferate at the expense of surveys that are more difficult to conduct, relating to patients' medical and nursing care. A further problem with patient satisfaction surveys is that it remains difficult to ensure that enough patients complete the survey to allow the results to be representative of the whole population. Questionnaires need to be simple, specific and repeatable if the necessary compliance rates of more than 70–80% are to be obtained.

Peer Review

The British Thoracic Society has established a peer review scheme in which respiratory departments in one district are visited by two consultants from separate districts in different regions of the country. Consultant members of the British Thoracic Society were asked to volunteer to participate in this scheme. Volunteers agreed to be either visitors or to be visited, but could not express a preference. The pair selected to visit a particular department were provided with a demographic profile of the population served by the hospital and a statistical summary of the workload and facilities available in the department. They were also given a checklist developed specifically for the purpose of the audit or review based on published guidelines and recommendations[26–28] (R. Page, personal communication).

After a 2-day visit, during which the visitors were allowed unrestricted access to the department, the hospital and the staff, they gave a verbal report to the visited consultant or consultants. Errors of fact were corrected

(a)
WEST NORWICH HOSPITAL

DEPARTMENT OF RESPIRATORY MEDICINE

ASTHMA INPATIENT ADMISSION RECORD

Surname: Firstname: Hospital No:

Address: Birthdate:

⟨MALE⟩   ⟨FEMALE⟩

Occupation: G.P.:   Age at onset of asthma:

Smoker: ⟨YES⟩ ⟨NO⟩   Smoked in past: ⟨YES⟩ ⟨NO⟩

Average cigarettes/day: Total years smoking:

Average units of alcohol/week:

Consultant: Ward:

Date admitted: Date discharged:

No of admissions in past year: Date of last admission:

Number of days since patient last quite well (*eg no nocturnal disturbances*):

Duration of immediate attack (hours):

History of present attack:

Reason(s) for deterioration:

Trigger factors: (*Circle relevant items*) ⟨URTI⟩ ⟨COLD AIR⟩ ⟨EXERCISE⟩

⟨MENSTRUAL⟩ ⟨ORGANIC DUST⟩

Objective assessment before admission? ⟨YES⟩ ⟨NO⟩

Heart rate   [   ]   Respiratory rate   [   ]   (*If yes, circle each quantity*
Peak flow   [   ]   *measured & record the value*).

Usual medication before admission: (*Circle as appropriate*).   NIL

β-agonist β-ag. in high dose Inhaled steroid <800 μg/day Inh. ster. >800 μg.day

Oral steroid Atrovent Cromone Xanthine Other What other?

Emergency medication before admission: (*Circle as appropriate*).   NIL

β-agonist β-ag. in high dose Inhaled steroid <800 μg/day Inh. ster. >800 μg.day

Oral steroid i/v steroid Atrovent i/v β-agonist i/v xanthine Oxygen

Other What other?

FIGURE 46.2: *History/summary proforma: (a) page 1, (b) page 2, (c) page 3.*

(b)

Coexisting medical problems:

Other past diseases:

Other relevant history
(*personal, social, family, drug therapy*):

Date of last menstrual period:

EXAMINATION AND INVESTIGATION

OBJECTIVE ASSESSMENT OF SEVERITY

Heart rate: Respiratory rate: BP:

PEF: Pulse oximeter: ? SaO2 > 92%   〈YES〉   〈NO〉

Arterial blood gases (kPa)   PaO2:   PaCO2:   pH:

Chest X-ray: NORMAL   HYPERINFLATED   CONSOLIDATION

PNEUMOTHORAX

Was the patient **conscious?** 〈YES〉 〈NO〉   **...confused?** 〈YES〉 〈NO〉

...cyanosed? 〈YES〉 〈NO〉 **...able to speak in sentences?** 〈YES〉 〈NO〉

Did the patient have a silent chest?   〈YES〉   〈NO〉

Abnormalities in other systems:

Other relvant or abnormal investigations:

TREATMENT AND MONITORING

INITIAL TREATMENT (*Circle treatment. N.B. Oxygen must be recorded on Drug treatment card*)

Oxygen   oral steroid   i/v ster   Neb. β-agon.   Neb. Atrovent   i/v β-agon.

i/v xanth.   oral xanth.   antibiotic

Throughout admission: Lowest PEF: Highest PEF:

During last 24 hours: Lowest PEF: Highest PEF:

Admitted to ITU? 〈YES〉   〈NO〉   Given IPPV?   〈YES〉   〈NO〉

CIRCUMSTANCES PRECEDING ADMISSION

Was there an avoidable precipitating cause?   〈YES〉   〈NO〉

Was this a catastrophic sudden attack ...   〈YES〉   〈NO〉
(*ie no period of recognisable deterioration before the acute attack*)

Did the patient (or relatives) react appropriately   〈YES〉   〈NO〉
when the asthma deteriorated?

Was the patient complying with regular therapy?   〈YES〉   〈NO〉

Can we do anything to help?   〈YES〉   〈NO〉

If so, what?

Was medical management appropriate?   〈YES〉   〈NO〉

(c)   *Asthma inpatient admission record – Page 3*

DISCHARGE AND FOLLOW UP

If answer is YES, circle ✓   *If answer is NO, circle* ✗

Inhaler technique checked pre-discharge: ✓   ✗

– by nurse ✓ ✗   – by doctor ✓ ✗   – by other ✓ ✗

Treatment on discharge:

Oral steroids:	✓	✗	Inhaled steroids:	✓	✗
Inhaled β-agonist:	✓	✗	Nebulised β-agonist:	✓	✗
Oral β-agonist:	✓	✗	Atrovent:	✓	✗
Oral theophylline:	✓	✗	Other:	✓	✗

What other?

Please record drug names and dosage regime for treatment given on discharge.

Drug 1: _____

Drug 2: _____

Drug 3: _____

Drug 4: _____

Drug 5: _____

Drug 6: _____

Is nebuliser treatment required?   ✓   ✗

  Does patient have a home nebuliser?   ✓   ✗

Will patient conduct self monitoring?   ✓   ✗

  Does patient have a peak flow meter?   ✓   ✗

Does patient have written instructions?   ✓   ✗

  Has patient been given thresholds?   ✓   ✗

To be followed as an outpatient?   ✓   ✗

Outpatient appoint date: **With:**   ⟨Consultant⟩   ⟨Asssoc. spec.⟩   ⟨Reg.⟩

Has self admission access been agreed?   ✓   ✗

Is there a copy of the GP discharge letter in the notes?

                                                       ✓   ✗

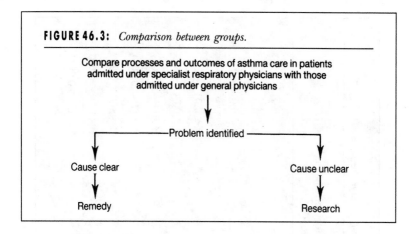

FIGURE 46.3: *Comparison between groups.*

Compare processes and outcomes of asthma care in patients admitted under specialist respiratory physicians with those admitted under general physicians

↓

Problem identified

Cause clear → Remedy

Cause unclear → Research

and the visitors were then asked to submit a written report, which they first showed to the visited consultant(s), to the coordinator of the review within 1 month.

Twenty-two reviews have now been completed. Both reviewers and reviewed have commented upon how much they learned from the visits, how they were able to exchange ideas and good practices and how problems, often recognized by the local physicians, were highlighted in a supportive way by the visitors.

It is clear that colleagues in respiratory medicine in British hospitals are generally working extremely hard and providing by and large an extremely good service. Their workload reflects the fact that respiratory diseases are responsible for 25% of acute medical admissions, 20% of new medical outpatient consultations and account for an enormous load of morbidity and mortality in society.[27]

The confidential intra-professional approach has allowed frank constructive exchanges. Inadequate staffing levels and facilities and whether or not the department uses national or local guidelines and protocols for the management of common disorders, including asthma,[16–18] can be discussed and identified. To determine whether or not the peer reviews have any impact on the provision of the service, the intention is to evaluate changes that have occurred, if any, 1 year after the visit.

ASSESSMENT AND IMPROVEMENT

Monitoring allows the identification and assessment of problems. Further analysis will suggest possible ways of improving and correcting the problems. When the cause of the problems is unclear this should stimulate questions and research (Fig. 46.3) with the aims of determining the cause and suggesting improvements.

TABLE 46.6: *Differences between respiratory and non-respiratory physicians care. (From Ref. 25 with permission)*

	General physicians ($n = 340$) (%)	Respiratory physicians ($n = 426$) (%)	χ^2 (P)
Patients admitted by general practitioner	40	60	$P < 0.01$
Measurement of PEF on admission	83	89	$P < 0.05$
Measurement of arterial blood gases on admission	58	79	$P < 0.01$
No steroid therapy in first 24 hours	12	6	$P < 0.01$
PEF monitored and recorded on the ward	63	83	$P < 0.01$
PEF variability not measured on ward	32	19	$16.6 (P < 0.001)$
Home management plan not given	94	87	$7.6 (P < 0.005)$
No steroids at all on discharge	10	6	$3.98 (P < 0.05)$
No outpatient appointment made	44	9	$124.0 (P < 0.001)$
Not seen in outpatient department within 2 months of discharge	56	27	$64.6 (P < 0.001)$

Improvements can be achieved by re-education, re-training, facilitation in small groups, or by more active persuasion. Four examples that exemplify this are discussed below.

Example 1

Compared with earlier British studies[8,10] the most recent study of asthma deaths[11] has shown improved routine treatment (appropriate in 79%), improved objective monitoring with PEF measurement (adequate in 65%), but continuing deficiencies in advice, education and written management plans given to patients. When all aspects of care are combined only 4 of 24 patients dying of asthma had received routine care that was appropriate in all respects. Most striking was the finding that 71% of patients had psychological or social factors considered to have had an important bearing on the patient's death from asthma. This ongoing confidential enquiry has recorded a halving of asthma deaths since it began in 1988. As a result of the enquiry three changes have been introduced into the process of care.

(1) A joint clinic has been established by a chest physician and a psychiatrist, specializing in adolescent and family psychiatry, to see young people with asthma. The aim is to detect and hopefully correct behaviour and attitudes that make asthma control much more difficult.

(2) When patients thought to be at risk from dying from asthma because of their psychosocial background fail to attend clinic appointments, attempts are made to contact them in their own home at a time convenient to them by a respiratory liaison health visitor.

(3) We now seek to interview the next of kin of such "at-risk" patients with the patient at the clinic review in the same way as we always see the parents of children with asthma.

Example 2

In the inpatient asthma audit[2] problems were revealed with the recording of a check on inhaler technique in patients before their discharge from hospital and in patients being discharged from hospital before their diurnal PEF variability had fallen to the recommended level.

To address the first of these, a rubber stamp was introduced for use on the patient's PEF chart. This required the signature of a trained nurse or doctor to state that they had checked the patient's inhaler technique. This, with further encouragement from senior medical and nursing staff, resulted in a significant improvement in this parameter being recorded. Adherence to the PEF variability criterion was improved by relaxing the criterion following publication of the National Guidelines,[17] by encouragement from senior medical staff, and by the requirement to specify in the notes the reason why patients were discharged before their diurnal variability had fallen to 25% or less, when this occurred.

Re-monitoring the service demonstrated marked improvement in both areas.[2] This improvement has been maintained in subsequent audits.

Example 3

The results of the multicentre audit of inpatient asthma care[24] were fed back to the coordinators in each hospital so that the results of their own hospital were identified and could be compared with the overall results. Disappointingly, the second audit 1 year later showed no significant improvement in any of the criteria audited. This led to two suggestions. The first is that all patients admitted with asthma should be admitted according to a protocol agreed by the local chest physicians, that they should be transferred to the local chest physician's care within 24 hours of admission during the week and on Mondays following the weekend, and that all patients requiring hospital outpatient follow-up should be seen by a respiratory physician or a member of the respiratory team. Furthermore, purchasers could help significantly in this area of quality by requiring explicitly that all patients with asthma seen in the hospital should be cared for in this way.

One result from the British Thoracic Society multicentre audit of inpatient asthma care has been the recognition that the detection of pulsus paradoxus as a sign indicative of severe asthma is of little or no value.[29] Paradox was recorded in 41% of patients and in only 4% of them was paradox of 10 mmHg or greater the only abnormal measurement. The recommendation to measure paradox and use levels of 10 mmHg or greater as an indicator of severe asthma in the original British Guidelines[17] has been dropped from the revised Guidelines.[18]

Example 4

The reports from the peer review teams have been sent by local physicians to their hospital management and to purchasers in an attempt to facilitate improvements.

FURTHER MONITORING AND ASSESSMENT

Clearly after the first monitoring and assessment, attempts at improvement can only be evaluated by repeated monitoring and assessment and in this way the audit loop is closed. Experience suggests that once satisfactory care is achieved further audits at regular intervals are required to maintain a high-quality service and once again recognition of high quality will be praised and rewarded.

CONCLUSIONS

Some measures of the structure, process and outcome of ambulatory and inpatient asthma care that are amenable to audit are listed in Table 46.7.

TABLE 46.7: *Measures in asthma care that are amenable to audit.*
(Modified from Ref. 1 with permission)

Structure of respiratory care[26–28]

Medical staff
  Senior
  Middle grade
  Pre-registration

Nursing staff
  Trained
  Untrained

Clinical facilities
Beds
Secretarial and administrative support
Pulmonary function laboratory facilities
Bronchoscopy facilities
Access to imaging facilities, ICU, pathology

Some measures of the process of outpatient asthma care[16,18]

Evidence of written action/management plan
Evidence of step-wise management
Recorded checks on inhaler technique
Evidence of PEF chart
Treatment
  Regular inhaled steroids   Y/N Dose
  Regular DSG/nedocromil   Y/N Dose
  Regular inhaled bronchodilator   Y/N Dose
  Regular oral bronchodilator   T/N Type Dose
  Maintenance oral steroids   Y/N Dose
  Theophylline levels monitored in patients on oral
    theophyllines
  Recorded evidence of spacer use if inhaled steroid dose
    exceeds 800 μg daily
Smoking
  Active: current/ex/never
  Passive

Some outcome measures for outpatient asthma care[16,18,30]

Symptoms
  Nocturnal wakening
  Time off school/work

TABLE 46.7: *Continued*

Pulmonary function
PEF
  Actual value
  Best in previous 2–5 years
FEV_1
  Actual value
  Best in previous 2–5 years
Home PEF >80% of best
Maximum diurnal variation in last week/month/3
  months <25%

Treatment and its appropriateness to symptoms and function
  Regular inhaled steroids   Y/N Daily dose
  Regular DSG/nedocromil   Y/N Daily dose
  Regular bronchodilator   Y/N Daily dose
  Maintenance oral steroids   Y/N Daily dose
  Boosts of oral steroid/courses of oral steroids during
    previous month/in last year
  Number of β agonist inhalers per month

Events
  Emergency visits to accident and emergency department in
    last month/year
  Urgent (unplanned) calls to, or visit to or from, GP in last
    month/year
  Admissions to hospital with asthma in last month/year
  Death

*Some measures of the process and outcome of inpatient asthma
care*[17,18]

Objective assessment of severity
  PEF
  Heart rate
  Respiratory rate
  Presence/absence of cyanosis
  Oxygen saturation/blood gases

Treatment
  Systemic steroids
  High dose β agonists inhaled/intravenous

TABLE 46.7: *Continued*

Pre-discharge
  PEFR diurnal variation <25%
  Written check on inhaler technique
  Oral steroid to take home

Post-discharge
  PEFR meter for home monitoring
  Treatment "stepped up" compared with maintenance
    therapy before admission
  Written management plan
  Follow-up appointment

Outcome
  Death
  Re-admission within 8 weeks

DSG, disodium cromoglycate; FEV_1, forced expiratory volume in 1 s; ICU, intensive care unit; PEF, peak expiratory flow.

Asthma audit, like quality assurance, can be used to maintain and improve high-quality services and to assess and improve aspects of care where there are problems. To undertake such audits and to achieve the potential benefits, resources of information technology, time and money are required. In industry between 1 and 3% of turnover is spent on quality assurance. Investment on that scale in clinical audit would transform the way our health care is delivered.

Asthma is the commonest chronic disease affecting all age groups in the developed world. Why are patients still dying unnecessarily? Why are so many patients admitted when well-established treatment strategies could have prevented those admissions? Why in survey after survey are so many patients with asthma still waking at night and still failing to lead full and unlimited lives?

High-quality excellent care is not necessarily the most expensive care. High-quality care may be expensive, but frequently low-quality care is even more expensive in terms of death, preventable morbidity and the time, hassle and litigation involved in dealing with complaints and with professional staff not performing at an acceptable level.

Asthma audit is our responsibility, the responsibility of respiratory physicians, nurses, physiotherapists, pharmacists and other health care professionals involved in the care of patients with asthma. To be most effective professionals involved in audit need support and rewards, not sanctions. It obviously requires commitment from the senior staff, who then enable high standards and high quality to permeate throughout the system that they lead. When this happens such departments and services become "magnetic" and attract high-quality staff and provide care that is both rewarding to the patient and to those delivering and purchasing that care.

Medical audit fosters and supports the altruism of physicians wishing to provide the best possible care for their patients with asthma. It also stimulates us to maintain high-quality standards. It fosters both the effectiveness and efficiency of the service that we provide to the population of patients we serve. It helps us to ensure that patients with asthma under our care receive optimal care, that we are not denying them effective care and that we are avoiding unnecessary risks when we provide that care.

Finally, audit gives us information with which to defend ourselves against criticism and to support our claims for additional resources.

REFERENCES

1 Harrison BDW. Audit in respiratory disease. *Respir Med* 1991; 85(suppl B): 47–51.

2 Lim KL, Harrison BDW. A criterion based audit of inpatient asthma care. Closing the feedback loop. *J R Coll Physicians Lond* 1992; 26: 71–5.

3 Cochrane GM, Clark TJH. A survey of asthma mortality in patients between ages 35 and 64 in the Greater London hospitals. *Thorax* 1975; 30: 300–5.

4 Macdonald JB, Seaton A, Williams DA. Asthma deaths in Cardiff 1963–74: 90 deaths outside hospital. *BMJ* 1976; 1: 1493–5.

5 Macdonald JB, Macdonald ET, Seaton A, Williams DA. Asthma deaths in Cardiff 1963–74: 53 deaths in hospital. *BMJ* 1976; 2: 721–3.

6 Bateman JRM, Clarke SW. Sudden death in asthma. *Thorax* 1979; 34: 40–4.

7 Ormerod LP, Stableforth DE. Asthma mortality in Birmingham 1975–7: 53 deaths. *BMJ* 1980; 280: 687–90.

8 British Thoracic Association. Death from asthma in two regions of England. *BMJ* 1982; 285: 1251–5.

9 Sears MR, Rea HH, Beaglehole RG *et al.* Asthma mortality in New Zealand: a two year national study. *N Z Med J* 1985; 98: 271–5.

10 Eason J, Markowe HLJ. Controlled investigation of deaths from asthma in hospital in the North East Thames region. *BMJ* 1987; 294: 1255–8.

11 Wareham NJ, Harrison BDW, Jenkins PF, Nicholls J, Stableforth DE. A district confidential enquiry into deaths due to asthma. *Thorax* 1993; 48: 1117–20.

12 Somerville M, Ryland I, Williams EMI, Pearson MG. Asthma deaths in Mersey in 1989–90. *Thorax* 1993; 48: 420P.

13 Harrison BDW, Pearson MG. Audit in acute severe asthma – who benefits? *J R Coll Physicians Lond* 1993; 27: 387–90.

14 Department of Health. Report on British Confidential Enquiries into Maternal Deaths in the UK 1985–7. London: Department of Health, 1991.

15 Campling EA, Devlin HB, Hoile RW, Lunn JN. The Report of the National Confidential Enquiry into Perioperative Deaths. London: National Confidential Enquiry into Perioperative Deaths, 1992.

16 Statement by the British Thoracic Society, Research Unit of the Royal College of Physicians of London, King's Fund Centre, National Asthma Campaign. Guidelines for management of asthma in adults: I. Chronic persistent asthma. *BMJ* 1990; 301: 651–3.

17 Statement by the British Thoracic Society, Research Unit of the Royal College of Physicians of London, King's Fund Centre, National Asthma Campaign. Guidelines for management of asthma in adults: II. Acute severe asthma. *BMJ* 1990; 301: 797–800.

18 Guidelines on the management of asthma. *BMJ* 1993; 306: 776–82 and *Thorax* 1993; 48: S1–S24.

19 Neville RG, Clark RG, Hoskins G, Smith B. National asthma attack audit 1991–2. *BMJ* 1993; 306: 559–62.

20 Osman J, Ormerod LP, Stableforth DE. Management of acute asthma: a survey of hospital practice and comparison between thoracic and general physicians in Birmingham and Manchester. *Br J Dis Chest* 1987; 81: 232–41.

21 Bucknall CE, Robertson C, Moran F, Stevenson RD. Differences in hospital asthma management. *Lancet* 1988; i: 748–50.

22 Baldwin DR, Ormerod LP, Mackay AD, Stableforth DE. Changes in hospital management of acute severe asthma by thoracic and general physicians in Birmingham and Manchester during 1978 and 1985. *Thorax* 1990; 45: 130–4.

23 Bell D, Layton AJ, Gabbay J. Use of a guideline based questionnaire to audit hospital care of acute asthma. *BMJ* 1991; 302: 1440–3.

24 Bucknall CE, Robertson C, Moran F, Stevenson RD. Improving management of asthma: closing the loop or progressing along the audit spiral? *Quality in Health Care* 1992; 1: 15–20.

25 Pearson MG, Ryland I, Harrison BDW. A national audit of acute severe asthma in adults admitted to hospital. *Quality in Health Care* 1995; 4: 24–36.

26 Muers MF, Chappell AG, Farebrother M, Farrow SC, Harrison BDW, Laszlo G. Facilities for the diagnosis of respiratory disease in the UK. *J R Coll Physicians Lond* 1988; 22: 180–4.

27 Pearson MG, Littler J, Davies PDO. Analysis of medical workload – evidence of patient to specialist mismatch. *J R Coll Physicians Lond* 1994: 28; 230–4.

28 Corris P, Page R, Rudolf M, Wolstenholme R. Requirements for Good Practice in Respiratory Medicine. London: British Thoracic Society, 1993.

29 Pearson MG, Spence DPS, Ryland I, Harrison BDW. Value of pulsus paradoxus in assessing acute severe asthma. *BMJ* 1993; 307: 659.

30 Connolly CK. Management of asthma in outpatients. *J R Coll Physicians Lond* 1983; 17: 115–20.

KEY POINTS

1   Medical audit is the process of recognizing and maintaining high-quality services and identifying areas of less than optimal quality and then taking steps to improve them.

2   Sentinal case audit is best exemplified by an ongoing confidential enquiry into asthma deaths.

3   Criterion-based audit requires agreed standards with which actual practice can be compared. National guidelines and local protocols can provide these and are also of value in sentinal-case audits.

4   Repeat audits (closing the feedback loop) have demonstrated improvements in the processes of asthma care.

5   Audits of hospital inpatient practice and of asthma care in general practice have demonstrated high-quality care and also areas such as checking and recording inhaler technique, and increasing treatment during exacerbations, where improvements were necessary.

6   Audits of inpatient management of asthma have repeatedly shown significant differences between the care provided by chest physicians and that provided by general physicians.

7   Most asthmatic patients requiring hospital management and most of their general practitioners opt, wherever possible, for care under a respiratory physician.

8   High-quality *optimal* care may be expensive, but frequently low-quality care is even more expensive.

9   Asthma audit is the responsibility of the health care professionals involved in the care of patients with asthma. It requires commitment from senior staff and will contribute to the service becoming attractive to high-quality staff.

Index